SMALL ANIMAL
DERMATOLOGY
A COLOR ATLAS AND THERAPEUTIC GUIDE

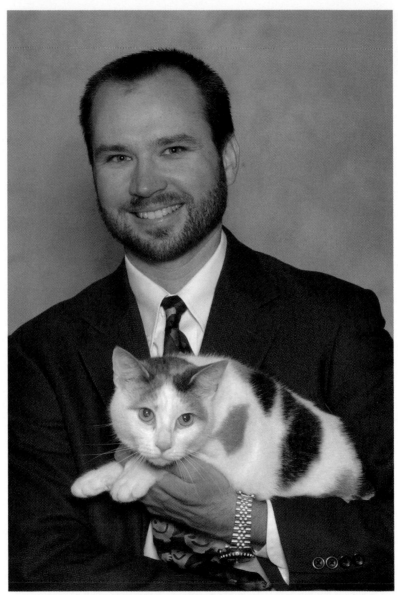

KEITH A. HNILICA

SMALL ANIMAL
DERMATOLOGY
A COLOR ATLAS AND THERAPEUTIC GUIDE

KEITH A. HNILICA, DVM, MS, DACVD, MBA
www.itchnot.com
Pet Wellness Center
Allergy and Dermatology Clinic
Knoxville, Tennessee

ELSEVIER
SAUNDERS

3251 Riverport Lane
St. Louis, Missouri 63043

SMALL ANIMAL DERMATOLOGY: A COLOR ATLAS AND THERAPEUTIC GUIDE, THIRD EDITION

ISBN: 978-1-4160-5663-8

Library of Congress Cataloging-in-Publication Data
Hnilica, Keith A.
    Small animal dermatology : a color atlas and therapeutic guide / Keith A. Hnilica.—3rd ed.
        p. ; cm.
    Rev. ed. of: Small animal dermatology / Linda Medleau, Keith A. Hnilica. 2nd ed. c2006.
    Includes bibliographical references and index.
    ISBN 978-1-4160-5663-8 (hardcover : alk. paper) 1. Dogs–Diseases. 2. Cats–
Diseases. 3. Veterinary dermatology. I. Medleau, Linda. Small animal dermatology. II. Title.
    [DNLM: 1. Dog Diseases. 2. Skin Diseases–veterinary. 3. Cat Diseases. SF 992.S55]
    SF992.S55M44 2011
    636.089′65—dc22

                                                                2010038399

Vice President and Publisher: Linda Duncan
Acquisitions Editor: Heidi Pohlman
Senior Developmental Editor: Shelly Stringer
Publishing Services Manager: Catherine A. Jackson
Senior Project Manager: Karen M. Rehwinkel

Printed in Canada

Last digit is the print number: 9 8 7 6 5 4 3 2 1

Contributors

Cheryl Greenacre, DVM, DABVP, DABVP (Exotic Companion Mammal)
Professor
Avian and Zoological Medicine
Department of Small Animal Clinical Sciences
College of Veterinary Medicine
The University of Tennessee
Knoxville, Tennessee

Amy LeBlanc, DVM, DACVIM
Director of Medical Oncology
College of Veterinary Medicine
The University of Tennessee
Knoxville, Tennessee

To Be Brilliant

To be brilliant is to look past want to what you have.
To be brilliant is to be streaming with the line of the law but always one step ahead.
To be brilliant is to be thinking without stopping, without yielding, without procrastination.
To be brilliant is to be yet graceful when inside stress and frustration.
To be brilliant is to always be brilliant.
    Sam T.

One who is with their culture, is trapped,
While the one who is of their own mind is set free.
    Sara H.

Minute variations in religion result in war and conflict.
Hope will overcome; love prevails; faith endures.
Why? Why the hell not!
    Max T.

Love is the closest thing we have to heaven on Earth.
    Keith H.

Preface

This atlas began as a companion text for Muller and Kirk's *Small Animal Dermatology*. We designed the book to be a practical color atlas that includes current treatments for each disorder. Great effort has gone into making this book an easy-to-use reference for practicing small animal veterinarians.

This third edition has been revised to eliminate useless, overly historic, or downright dangerous treatments. Additionally, the diagnostic chapter has been expanded and includes multiple methods to arrive at the diagnosis of a patient's skin disease. As many diseases can appear very similar, every attempt has been made to compare and contrast similar diseases throughout the text, differential lists, images, and figure legends. For itchy dogs, the Novartis Dermatology System has been included because it represents the most simple and elegant starting point for differentiating common allergic diseases, identifying the secondary infections, and combining primary disease treatment with symptomatic therapy. The Novartis Dermatology System, developed by multiple dermatologists over 3 years, has been implemented in numerous clinics across the United States and has a proven track record for improving clinical outcomes and ultimately reducing the use of steroid therapy for allergy.

A key feature of this text is the relevant clinical images. Numerous new images have been added to provide a useful perspective of the most common lesions and patterns caused by each disease. Dermatology relies heavily on the identification of patterns in the patient's signalment, history, and lesion type and pattern. The images in each disease section were selected not for their extreme nature but rather because each image demonstrates a common feature of the disease. By reviewing all of the images for a given disease, the practitioner should acquire a working knowledge of the most common presentations for that disease. This will hopefully result in arriving at the most likely and shortest differential diagnosis list possible for each dermatology patient.

New to this edition are Author's Notes, which were included in an attempt to provide a contemporary feeling for the most important issues surrounding select disorders. The Author's Notes are ultimately the opinion of the author; however, the information has been collected from many sources, human and otherwise, over many years and reflects an endless pursuit of practical knowledge, which truly makes a difference in the diagnosis and treatment of each disease.

Finally, a chapter on exotic animal dermatology was incorporated to provide a useful reference for the most common skin diseases affecting the most common species a general practitioner is likely to be asked to diagnose and treat.

I hope you find the special efforts taken to provide a practical approach to veterinary dermatology useful.

Keith A. Hnilica

Acknowledgments

Much thanks to the many people whose generosity made this book possible: Donna Angarano, John MacDonald, Anthony Yu, Gail Kunkle, Michaela Austel, Craig Greene, Alice Wolfe, Karen Campbell, Richard Malik, Linda Frank, Lynn Schmeitzel, Patricia White, Dunbar Gram, Jim Noxon, Linda Messinger, Elizabeth Willis, Terese DeManuelle, William Miller, Thomas Manning, Kimberly Boyanowski, Norma White-Weithers, Manon Paradis, Robert Dunstan, Kelly Credille, Pauline Rakich, Charles Martin, Clay Calvert, Sherry Sanderson, Mary Mahaffey, Sue McLaughlin, E. Roberson, Gary Norsworthy, Michael Singer, Sandy Sargent, Cheryl Greenacre, and any whom I mistakenly missed.

Keith A. Hnilica

Contents

SMALL ANIMAL
DERMATOLOGY
A COLOR ATLAS AND THERAPEUTIC GUIDE

CHAPTER 1

Differential Diagnoses

- Essential Questions
- Ten Clinical Patterns
- What Are the Infections?
- Why Are They There?
- Differentials Based on Body Region
- Diseases Primarily Limited to the Face
- Diseases of Nasal Depigmentation
- Diseases With Oral Lesions
- Ear Margin Dermatitis
- Nasodigital Hyperkeratosis
- Interdigital Pododermatitis
- Diseases of the Claw
- Diseases of the Footpads
- Differentials Based on Primary and Secondary Lesions
- Vesicular and Pustular Diseases
- Erosive and Ulcerative Diseases
- Papules
- Miliary Dermatitis
- Plaques
- Follicular Casts
- Epidermal Collarettes
- Comedones
- Lichenification
- Inflammatory/Pruritic Alopecic Diseases
- Noninflammatory/Nonpruritic Alopecic Diseases
- Cellulitis and Draining Lesions
- Nodular Diseases
- Pruritic Diseases
- Seborrheic Diseases
- Hyperpigmentation
- Hypopigmentation

Almost all dermatology patients have a primary/underlying disease that causes secondary infections. These infections must be eliminated and prevented but will recur rapidly unless the primary disease is identified and controlled.

Most skin cases seen in a veterinary practice can be successfully managed if two essential questions can be answered: (1) What are the secondary infections? (2) Why are these secondary infections there?

Essential Questions

1. What are the infections?
   - Folliculitis
     - Pyoderma
     - *Demodex*
     - Dermatophyte
   - Pododermatitis
     - Bacterial
     - Yeast
   - Otitis
     - Bacterial
     - Yeast
   - Yeast dermatitis
2. Why are they there?
   - Allergies
     - Atopy
     - Food allergy
     - Scabies
   - Endocrinopathy
     - Hypothyroidism
     - Cushing's

Once the origin of a patient's dermatosis is known, it is a simple matter of therapeutic follow-through to resolve the problem.

Recognition of basic patterns allows a practical approach to most of the common skin diseases.

Ten Clinical Patterns

What are the secondary infections? (always secondary)
1. Folliculitis
2. Pododermatitis
3. Otitis
4. Yeast dermatitis

Why are they there? (the key to preventing relapse of infections)
5. Pruritus (allergies, mites, fleas)
6. Nonpruritic alopecia (endocrine)
7. Autoimmune/Immune-mediated skin disease
8. Keratinization defects
9. Lumps, bumps, and draining tracts
10. Weirdopathies

What Are the Infections?

A vast majority of dogs with allergy or endocrine disease have or will have a secondary bacterial or yeast infection. Yeast dermatitis is the most commonly missed diagnosis in general practice dermatology. Bacterial pyoderma is often identified but is usually mistreated with too low doses of antibiotics administered for too short a time. Otitis is now recognized and treated better than it was in years past; however, treatment for otitis that is based on actual documented organism types and relative counts on follow-up evaluations is a rare occurrence.

So, what is the solution?

For **every** dermatitis case **every** time you evaluate the patient, ask yourself, "What are the infections?"

Unless you have microscopic vision, answering this question will require the use of cytology. Unfortunately, most general practices do not routinely perform skin and ear cytology for dermatitis; instead they rely on the doctor's best guess. Sometimes this can be successful (even a broken clock is correct twice a day); however, a more precise method is available. Use of diarrhea and the fecal exam as a comparison and as a model for improvement works well because both skin cytology and fecal exams involve the use of a microscope, can easily identify the type of infection, and can be performed by trained technical staff.

■ So why does your clinic perform fecal exams?
■ When is a fecal exam performed (before the doctor's exam or during)?
■ Who performs the fecal exam?
■ Does the clinic charge for the fecal exam?

The answers to these questions should be the same for skin cytology (skin scrapings, impression smears, tape preps, and otic swabs).

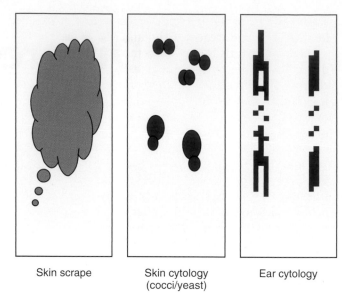

| Skin scrape | Skin cytology (cocci/yeast) | Ear cytology |

FIGURE 1-1 The 3-Slide Technique. Skin scrapes, cutaneous cytology, and otic swabs.

The practical solution for determining the best method by which to answer the question, "What are the infections?" is to implement a minimum database infection screening procedure to be performed by the technician before the veterinarian examines the patient. Every dermatology patient should undergo otic cytology, skin cytology (an impression smear or a tape prep), and a skin scrape at every examination (initially and at every recheck visit). The **3-slide technique** (Figure 1-1) can be performed easily and interpreted by a technician before the doctor completes an evaluation—which is exactly how diarrhea and fecal examinations are handled in most clinics. Moving the cytologic evaluation to the beginning of the dermatology appointment and thereby empowering the technical staff to accomplish the evaluation optimizes the dermatology appointment and provides essential information in the most efficient manner.

When an owner brings a pet into the clinic for a small hairless spot, it would be appropriate to question the necessity for an otic cytology when the hairless spot is the problem. However, the 3-slide technique is most helpful in these exact types of cases. If focal pruritus occurs in a dog and the patient has a secondary otitis (which the technician identified during the infection screen), the veterinarian should more aggressively discuss this and work up the patient for possible allergy. If the patient did not have otitis, the pruritus could be minimized in the hope that it was a short-term problem that is likely to self-resolve.

Similarly, there is no excuse for mistreating a patient who has demodicosis. Lesions caused by demodicosis can look identical to folliculitis lesions caused by bacterial pyoderma and dermatophytosis. Clinical appearance is not an acceptable criterion for ruling in or ruling out demodicosis. When the technician performs a skin scrape as part of the infection screen, demodicosis can be identified and treated easily and accurately.

Yeast dermatitis is one of the most frequently missed diagnoses in the United States as of this writing. The clinical presentation is unique; however, initial cytologic evaluation is often omitted, and follow-up cytology to determine the effectiveness of treatment rarely happens.

Why Are They There?

Infections are always secondary to a primary disease; however, all too often, the patient is not evaluated or treated for the primary disease for three main reasons: (1) only the secondary infections are treated over and over again, (2) the nature of the allergy is confusing, and (3) cheap steroids that have delayed repercussions are accessible.

Why are the infections there? This question should be asked and answered for every dermatology patient if successful outcomes are to be achieved.

Most dermatology patients suffer from allergy or endocrine disease. Through signalment, a good patient history, and recognition of unique patterns of lesions, a prioritized differential list can be formulated quickly.

By knowing the most unique and frequent symptoms associated with each allergic disease, an astute clinician can determine the most likely allergy with approximately 85% accuracy; this rate rivals many other diagnostic testing results for some of the most common assays.

For example, a dog that is foot licking is likely atopic. If the owner reports a seasonal pattern to the podopruritus, then you have a reasonably accurate diagnosis—EASY.

Atopy: Foot licking, seasonal, when pruritus first started, typically between 1 and 3 years of age

Food allergy: Perianal dermatitis (erythema, alopecia, lichenification), gastrointestinal disease; younger than 1 year old or older than 5 years of age when started; German breeds

Flea allergy: Dermatitis predominantly affecting the lumbar region (caudal to the last rib)

Scabies: Positive pinnal-pedal reflex (ear scratch test)

Hypothyroidism: Large-breed dog that is disproportionately obese for food intake and has a poor hair coat

Cushing's disease: Patient with a long history of steroid abuse, or small-breed dog with polyphagia, polyuria (PU), and polydipsia (PD).

Author's Note

Could clinical dermatology really be this easy?

Yes. Unfortunately, most of us were taught dermatology from the perspective of a NASA engineer who is determined to address and eliminate every possible scenario regardless of how rare its occurrence. Based on any standard of logic, statistics, or common sense, the most likely disease should be addressed first. It is illogical to perform diagnostic tests or therapeutic trials for rare or unlikely diseases as part of the initial dermatologic workup, yet this is exactly how most veterinarians are taught to diagnose atopy: "a diagnosis of exclusion." If a patient is seasonally foot licking, the most likely diagnosis is atopy.

Text continued on p.10

WHAT IS MAKING MY DOG SO ITCHY?

Evaluation Form

A thorough history can help us find the source of your dog's itching more quickly.
Please answer the following questions to help guide the diagnostic process.

Date _____ Pet owner name _____

Name of dog _____ Age _____ Breed _____ Weight _____

PHYSICAL EVALUATION

Please check any that describe your dog and circle problem areas on the drawing.

- ❑ Hair loss
- ❑ Foul odor
- ❑ Inflammation or redness
- ❑ Itching/Scratching
- ❑ Otitis (ear infections)
- ❑ Licking/Chewing
- ❑ Skin lesions (sores)
- ❑ Changes in skin (reddish brown stains, discolorations and/or areas that are thick and leathery)
- ❑ Other _____

CIRCLE PROBLEM AREAS
(Itching, hair loss, lesions, etc.)

- Has your dog ever had ear problems?   ❑ Yes ❑ No
- Does your dog have any chronic gastrointestinal signs like diarrhea or vomiting?   ❑ Yes ❑ No

SEVERITY EVALUATION On a scale of 0 to 10 rank the severity of your dog's symptoms.

SEVERITY OF CONDITION OVERALL

0	1	2	3	4	5	6	7	8	9	10
No symptoms										Severe

SEVERITY OF SKIN LESIONS

0	1	2	3	4	5	6	7	8	9	10
No lesions										Severe

SEVERITY OF SCRATCHING/LICKING/CHEWING

0	1	2	3	4	5	6	7	8	9	10
No signs										Severe

ONSET AND SEASONALITY EVALUATION

- Is this the first time your dog has experienced these symptoms?   ❑ Yes ❑ No
  - If no, at what age did the symptoms first occur?   ❑ <1 yr ❑ 1-3 yrs ❑ 4-7 yrs ❑ 7+ yrs
  - If no, has it occurred around the same time of year each time?   ❑ Yes ❑ No
  - If no, approximate time of year symptoms occur. _____
- How long have the current symptoms been going on? _____
- Did the itch start gradually and over time become worse?   ❑ Yes ❑ No
- Did the itch come on suddenly without warning?   ❑ Yes ❑ No
- Was there a "rash" first or itching first? Or simultaneous?   ❑ Rash first ❑ Itch first ❑ Simultaneous

PARASITE CONTROL

- Is your dog on a flea/heartworm preventative?   ❑ Yes ❑ No
  - If yes, what product(s)? _____
- What months do you administer the preventative? _____
- When was the last time you administered the parasite control? _____

ὑ NOVARTIS
ANIMAL HEALTH

FIGURE 1-2 Medical history and information forms to be filled out by the owner. *(Courtesy Novartis Animal Health US, Inc.)*

LIFE STYLE EVALUATION

- Where does your dog live? ❑Indoors ❑Outdoors ❑Both
  – If outdoors, please describe environment:_____
- Are there other pets in your household? ❑Yes ❑No
  – If yes, do these pets have the same symptoms? ❑Yes ❑No
  – If these pets are cats, do they go outside? ❑Yes ❑No
- Do you board your dog, take him or her to obedience school, training or groomers? ❑Yes ❑No
  – If yes, when was the last time you took your dog?_____
- Have you taken your dog on a trip to another location? ❑Yes ❑No
  – If yes, please indicate when and location:_____
- Have you recently moved? ❑Yes ❑No
- Have you been to a new dog park or walking trail? ❑Yes ❑No
- Have you used any new shampoo or topical skin treatments recently? ❑Yes ❑No
- Are any humans in your household exhibiting signs? ❑Yes ❑No

DIETARY EVALUATION

- What pet food are you feeding?_____
- Do you feed the same food all the time or provide a variety? ❑Always same ❑Variety
- Have you changed his or her diet recently? ❑Yes ❑No
- Do you give your dog packaged treats? ❑Yes ❑No
- Do you feed your dog "human" food? ❑Yes ❑No

RELATIONSHIP/BEHAVIORAL EVALUATION

Indicate if and how your dog's itching has affected his/her behavior and relationship with you. (CIRCLE ALL APPROPRIATE ANSWERS)

SLEEPS THROUGH THE NIGHT
Always   Usually   Occasionally   Never

ACTIVITY LEVEL
Inactive   Much less active   Somewhat less active   No change

SOCIAL BEHAVIOR
Unsocial   A lot less social   Somewhat less social   No change

RELATIONSHIP CHANGES
Fewer walks   No longer sleeps in bed/same room   Interacts less with family

PRIOR TREATMENTS

- Has your dog been treated for itching before? ❑Yes ❑No
- Indicate previous treatments administered to your dog: (CHECK ALL THAT APPLY)
  ❑ Steroids ❑ Shampoos ❑ Sprays ❑ Ointments ❑ Antibiotics ❑ Hypoallergenic food
  ❑ Essential fatty acids ❑ Antihistamines ❑ Immunotherapy
  ❑ Other (PLEASE SPECIFY) _____

Next Steps	
Physical Exam: A thorough physical evaluation of your dog will help us identify obvious problems and conditions like parasites.	**Laboratory Testing:** Ear Swab–To identify any infections in the ear including yeast and/or bacteria. Skin Scrape/Hair Pluck–To detect scabies or demodex mites. Impression Smear/Tape Prep–To detect other parasites and check for presence of yeast and/or bacteria.

FIGURE 1-2, cont'd.

SEVERITY OF ITCHING   PET'S NAME: _____

1	2	3	4	5	6	7	8	9	10
Minor									Severe

DERMATOLOGY WORK-UP

1 | WHAT ARE THE INFECTIONS?

Perform 3-Slide Technique™ during the physical exam.

Slide 1 Skin Scrape: ___ Positive for _____ /___ Negative

Slide 2 Ear Swab: ___ Positive for _____ /___ Negative

Slide 3 Tape Prep/Impression Smear: ___ Positive for _____ /___ Negative

❑ Pyoderma   ❑ Otitis (Cocci, yeast, pseudomonas)

❑ Demodex   ❑ Pododermatitis (Cocci, yeast)

❑ Dermatophytosis   ❑ Yeast Dermatitis

COMMON ALLERGIC SIGNS[1]

A. LUMBAR DERMATITIS

- Dermatitis on the lower back is usually indicative of a flea allergy
- Supports positive finding of fleas/flea dirt

B. EAR SCRATCH TEST

- Positive pinnal-pedal reflex: a reflexive rear-leg itch induced by scratching the ear tip is 80% diagnostic of scabies[2]
- Confirm with 3-Slide Technique

C. PERIANAL DERMATITIS

- Usually related to food allergy
- Should be suspected if age of onset is less than one year or older than five years
- Particularly in Labradors and German breeds

D. FOOT LICKING

- 85% of the time foot-licking dogs are atopic (pollen allergy, house dust mite allergy)[3]
- 15% will have food allergy

FIGURE 1-2, cont'd.

2

LOOK FOR THE OBVIOUS

- ❏ Flea Allergy (Lumbar dermatitis)
- ❏ Scabies (Positive pinnal-pedal reflex)
- ❏ Perianal Dermatitis (Food allergy)
- ❏ Foot Licking (Atopic dermatitis)

*Note: 15% of foot-licking dogs will have a food allergy or mixed (atopy and food allergy).

COMMENTS:_____

3

TREATMENT OPTIONS

Treat the Infections

- ❏ Antibiotics
- ❏ Antifungals
- ❏ Shampoos

Treat the Obvious Conditions

- ❏ Lumbar Dermatitis (Flea allergy/flea control)
- ❏ Perianal Dermatitis (Food allergy/diet change)
- ❏ Foot Licking (Atopy/Atopica or allergy testing)
- ❏ Ear-Scratch Response (+Scabies/scabicidal treatment)

Short-Term Control: Symptomatic Relief Only

- ❏ Steroids (Dex Na Phos)
- ❏ Antihistamines
- ❏ EFA
- ❏ Anti-Itch Conditioner
- ❏ Sleep Promoter

COMMENTS:_____

RECHECK TIME: _____

[1]Source: Keith Hnilica, DVM, MS, DACVD.
[2]Source: R.S. Mueller DipACVD, FACVSc, S.V. Bettenay BVSc, FACVSc, and M.Shipstone BVSc, DipACVD, FACVSc: Value of the pinnal-pedal reflex in the diagnosis of canine scabies, *The Veterinary Record*, Vol 148, Issue 20, 621-623.
[3]Source: The ACVD task force on canine atopic dermatitis (XIV): clinical manifestations of canine atopic dermatitis, 2001
[4]Source: Craig Griffin, DVM, DACVD

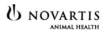

NOVARTIS
ANIMAL HEALTH

FIGURE 1-2, cont'd.

HOW ITCHY IS YOUR DOG?
DAILY ITCH REPORT CARD

Keep track of how itchy your dog is for the next 30 days. Measure the severity of itch on a scale of 1-10, 1 being mild and 10 being the most severe. Bring this report card back on your next visit.

PET'S NAME: _____

PET OWNER: _____

START DATE: _____

SEVERITY OF ITCHING

	1	2	3	4	5	6	7	8	9	10
DAY 1	1 Minor	2	3	4	5	6	7	8	9	10 Severe
DAY 2	1	2	3	4	5	6	7	8	9	10
DAY 3	1	2	3	4	5	6	7	8	9	10
DAY 4	1	2	3	4	5	6	7	8	9	10
DAY 5	1	2	3	4	5	6	7	8	9	10
DAY 6	1	2	3	4	5	6	7	8	9	10
DAY 7	1	2	3	4	5	6	7	8	9	10
DAY 8	1	2	3	4	5	6	7	8	9	10
DAY 9	1	2	3	4	5	6	7	8	9	10
DAY 10	1	2	3	4	5	6	7	8	9	10
DAY 11	1	2	3	4	5	6	7	8	9	10
DAY 12	1	2	3	4	5	6	7	8	9	10
DAY 13	1	2	3	4	5	6	7	8	9	10
DAY 14	1	2	3	4	5	6	7	8	9	10
DAY 15	1	2	3	4	5	6	7	8	9	10

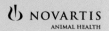
NOVARTIS
ANIMAL HEALTH

FIGURE 1-2, cont'd.

	SEVERITY OF ITCHING									
DAY 16	1 Minor	2	3	4	5	6	7	8	9	10 Severe
DAY 17	1	2	3	4	5	6	7	8	9	10
DAY 18	1	2	3	4	5	6	7	8	9	10
DAY 19	1	2	3	4	5	6	7	8	9	10
DAY 20	1	2	3	4	5	6	7	8	9	10
DAY 21	1	2	3	4	5	6	7	8	9	10
DAY 22	1	2	3	4	5	6	7	8	9	10
DAY 23	1	2	3	4	5	6	7	8	9	10
DAY 24	1	2	3	4	5	6	7	8	9	10
DAY 25	1	2	3	4	5	6	7	8	9	10
DAY 26	1	2	3	4	5	6	7	8	9	10
DAY 27	1	2	3	4	5	6	7	8	9	10
DAY 28	1	2	3	4	5	6	7	8	9	10
DAY 29	1	2	3	4	5	6	7	8	9	10
DAY 30	1	2	3	4	5	6	7	8	9	10

NOVARTIS
ANIMAL HEALTH

FIGURE 1-2, cont'd.

Differentials Based on Body Region

Diseases Primarily Limited to the Face

Dogs

Mucocutaneous pyoderma
Nasal pyoderma
Chin pyoderma
Eosinophilic furunculosis of the face
Pemphigus erythematosus
Pemphigus foliaceus
Discoid lupus erythematosus
Uveodermatologic syndrome
Juvenile cellulitis
Nasal depigmentation
(Early) Familial canine dermatomyositis

Cats

Pemphigus erythematosus
Discoid lupus erythematosus
Feline acne
Idiopathic facial dermatitis of Persian cats
Indolent ulcer
Feline solar dermatosis

Diseases of Nasal Depigmentation

Dogs

Contact dermatitis
Pemphigus erythematosus
Pemphigus foliaceus
Pemphigus vulgaris
Bullous pemphigoid
Discoid lupus erythematosus
Systemic lupus erythematosus
Vesicular cutaneous lupus erythematosus
Uveodermatologic syndrome
Vitiligo
Neoplasia

Diseases With Oral Lesions

Dogs

Candidiasis
Pemphigus vulgaris
Bullous pemphigoid
Systemic lupus erythematosus
Vesicular cutaneous lupus erythematosus
Eosinophilic granuloma
Cutaneous drug reaction

Contact dermatitis
Epitheliotropic lymphoma
Melanoma
Squamous cell carcinoma

Cats

Indolent ulcers
Eosinophilic granuloma
Pemphigus vulgaris
Bullous pemphigoid
Systemic lupus erythematosus
Cutaneous drug reaction
Contact dermatitis
Squamous cell carcinoma
Epitheliotropic lymphoma

Ear Margin Dermatitis

Dogs

Canine leproid granuloma syndrome
Scabies
Fly bite dermatitis
Ear margin dermatitis
Vasculitis
Pemphigus erythematosus
Pemphigus foliaceus
Pemphigus vulgaris
Bullous pemphigoid
Discoid lupus erythematosus
Systemic lupus erythematosus
Vesicular cutaneous lupus erythematosus
Drug reactions
Solar dermatitis
Squamous cell carcinoma

Cats

Atopy
Food allergy
Eosinophilic plaque
Feline scabies
Vasculitis
Pemphigus foliaceus
Pemphigus vulgaris
Bullous pemphigoid
Systemic lupus erythematosus
Drug reactions
Solar dermatitis
Squamous cell carcinoma

Nasodigital Hyperkeratosis

Dogs

Canine distemper
Leishmaniasis
Zinc-responsive dermatosis
Hepatocutaneous syndrome
Idiopathic nasodigital hyperkeratosis
Hereditary nasal parakeratosis of Labrador retrievers
Familial footpad hyperkeratosis
Pemphigus foliaceus
Systemic lupus erythematosus
Cutaneous horn

Interdigital Pododermatitis

Dogs

Bacterial infections
Malassezia
Dermatophytosis
Demodicosis
Trombiculiasis
Hookworm dermatitis
Pelodera dermatitis
Atopy
Food hypersensitivity
Contact dermatitis
Interdigital pyogranuloma
Neoplastic tumor

Cats

Bacterial infections
Dermatophytosis
Malassezia
Trombiculiasis
Neoplastic tumor

Diseases of the Claw

Dogs

Trauma
Bacterial infections
Dermatophytosis

Leishmaniasis
Vasculitis
Symmetrical lupoid onychodystrophy
Squamous cell carcinoma
Melanoma

Cats

Trauma
Bacterial infections
Dermatophytosis
Vasculitis
Squamous cell carcinoma

Diseases of the Footpads

Dogs

Contact dermatitis
Canine distemper
Leishmaniasis
Cutaneous neosporosis
Pemphigus foliaceus
Pemphigus vulgaris
Bullous pemphigoid
Systemic lupus erythematosus
Vesicular cutaneous lupus erythematosus
Vasculitis
Hepatocutaneous syndrome
Familial footpad hyperkeratosis
Idiopathic nasodigital hyperkeratosis
Zinc-responsive dermatosis
Cutaneous horn

Cats

Plasma cell pododermatitis
Mosquito bite hypersensitivity
Contact dermatitis
Pemphigus foliaceus
Pemphigus vulgaris
Bullous pemphigoid
Systemic lupus erythematosus
Vasculitis
Hepatocutaneous syndrome
Cutaneous horn

Differentials Based on Primary and Secondary Lesions

Vesicular and Pustular Diseases

(Uncommon but specific lesions associated with folliculitis or autoimmune skin diseases)

Dogs

Chin pyoderma
Superficial pyoderma
Impetigo
Dermatophytosis
Contact dermatitis
Pemphigus foliaceus
Pemphigus erythematosus
Pemphigus vulgaris
Bullous pemphigoid
Systemic lupus erythematosus
Vesicular cutaneous lupus erythematosus
Cutaneous drug reaction
Epidermolysis bullosa
Canine familial dermatomyositis
Subcorneal pustular dermatosis
Sterile eosinophilic pustulosis

Cats

Superficial pyoderma
Impetigo
Dermatophytosis
Contact dermatitis
Pemphigus foliaceus
Pemphigus erythematosus
Pemphigus vulgaris
Cutaneous drug reaction
Epidermolysis bullosa

Erosive and Ulcerative Diseases

(Uncommon and nonspecific lesions often subsequent to a vesicle or pustule usually caused by infection or autoimmune skin diseases)

Dogs

Mucocutaneous pyoderma
Pyotraumatic dermatitis
Deep pyoderma
Candidiasis
Protothecosis
Blastomycosis
Cryptococcosis
Fly bite dermatitis
Rocky Mountain spotted fever (RMSF)
Cutaneous leishmaniasis
Neosporosis
Pemphigus vulgaris

Bullous pemphigoid
Systemic lupus erythematosus
Vesicular cutaneous lupus erythematosus
Vasculitis
Erythema multiforme/Toxic epidermal necrolysis
Cutaneous drug reaction
Epidermolysis bullosa
Canine familial dermatomyositis
Perianal fistulae
Neoplasia

Cats

Pyotraumatic dermatitis
Candidiasis
Sporotrichosis
Blastomycosis
Feline calicivirus
Feline rhinotracheitis virus
Cutaneous leishmaniasis
Neosporosis
Pemphigus vulgaris
Vasculitis
Erythema multiforme/Toxic epidermal necrolysis
Cutaneous drug reaction
Epidermolysis bullosa
Eosinophilic plaque
Indolent ulcer
Plasma cell pyodermatitis
Idiopathic ulcerative dermatosis
Feline solar dermatosis
Neoplasia

Papules

(Nonspecific lesions caused by a cellular infiltrate)

Dogs

Chin pyoderma
Superficial pyoderma
Impetigo
Dermatophytosis
Canine scabies
Cheyletiellosis
Ear mites
Trombiculiasis
Pediculosis
Atopy
Flea allergy
Food allergy
Contact dermatitis
Pemphigus foliaceus
Pemphigus erythematosus
Pemphigus vulgaris

Bullous pemphigoid
Systemic lupus erythematosus
Vesicular cutaneous lupus erythematosus
Cutaneous drug reaction
Epidermolysis bullosa
Canine familial dermatomyositis
Subcorneal pustular dermatosis
Sterile eosinophilic pustulosis
Calcinosis cutis
Squamous cell carcinoma
Early neoplasia

Cats

Superficial pyoderma
Dermatophytosis
Demodicosis
Canine scabies
Cheyletiellosis
Ear mites
Trombiculiasis
Pediculosis
Feline immunodeficiency virus (FIV) infection
Atopy
Food hypersensitivity
Flea allergy dermatitis
Contact dermatitis
Cutaneous drug reaction
Pemphigus foliaceus
Pemphigus erythematosus
Pemphigus vulgaris
Cutaneous drug reaction
Epidermolysis bullosa
Squamous cell carcinoma
Early neoplasia

Miliary Dermatitis

Cats

Superficial pyoderma
Dermatophytosis
Demodicosis
Cheyletiellosis
Ear mites
Atopy
Food hypersensitivity
Flea allergy dermatitis
Pemphigus foliaceus
Lupus
Cutaneous drug reaction
FIV infection

Plaques

(Larger lesions that usually are formed by numerous papules that coalesce)

Dogs

Dermatophytosis
Contact dermatitis
Cutaneous drug reaction
Calcinosis cutis
Squamous cell carcinoma
Early neoplasia

Cats

Dermatophytosis
Demodicosis
Cheyletiellosis
Ear mites
Trombiculiasis
FIV infection
Contact dermatitis
Cutaneous drug reaction
Squamous cell carcinoma

Follicular Casts

(Specific lesions associated with primary keratinization defects)

Dogs

Primary seborrhea
Vitamin A–responsive dermatosis
Sebaceous adenitis

Epidermal Collarettes

(Specific lesions that develop subsequent to a pustule or vesicle; most often found in association with folliculitis)

Dogs

Superficial pyoderma
Impetigo
Demodicosis
Dermatophytosis
Pemphigus foliaceus

Differentials Based on Primary and Secondary Lesions—*cont'd*

Comedones

(Specific lesions that are caused by plugging of the hair follicles)

Dogs
Chin pyoderma
Demodicosis
Dermatophytosis
Canine hyperadrenocorticism
Schnauzer comedone syndrome
Vitamin A–responsive dermatosis
Hairless breeds
Color dilution alopecia
Follicular dysplasias

Cats
Feline acne

Lichenification

(Characteristic lesion of yeast dermatitis in dogs but can also be caused by chronic inflammatory disease)

Dogs
Malasseziasis
Chronic inflammation
    Parasitic infections
    Hypersensitivities
    Keratinization diseases

Inflammatory/Pruritic Alopecic Diseases

(Nonspecific lesions caused by any inflammatory dermatitis)

Dogs
Superficial pyoderma
Mucocutaneous pyoderma
Pyotraumatic dermatitis
Malasseziasis
Canine scabies
Cheyletiellosis
Ear mites
Trombiculiasis
Pediculosis
Hookworm dermatitis
Pelodera dermatitis
Atopy
Food hypersensitivity
Flea allergy dermatitis
Contact dermatitis
Pemphigus foliaceus

Acral lick dermatitis
Subcorneal pustular dermatosis
Sterile eosinophilic pustulosis
Superficial necrolytic migratory erythema

Cats
Superficial pyoderma
Pyotraumatic dermatitis
Malasseziasis
Feline scabies
Cheyletiellosis
Ear mites
Trombiculiasis
Pediculosis
Atopy
Food hypersensitivity
Flea allergy dermatitis
Contact dermatitis
Idiopathic facial dermatitis of Persian cats
Psychogenic alopecia
Feline lymphocytic mural folliculitis
Eosinophilic plaque
Idiopathic ulcerative dermatosis
Feline paraneoplastic alopecia
Superficial necrolytic migratory erythema

Noninflammatory/Nonpruritic Alopecic Diseases

(Relatively specific lesions associated with endocrine disease or follicular dysplasia)

Dogs
Hyperadrenocorticism
Hypothyroidism
Sex hormone imbalance
Alopecia X
Recurrent flank alopecia
Congenital hypotrichosis
Color dilution alopecia
Black hair follicular dysplasia
Canine pattern baldness
Idiopathic bald thigh syndrome of Greyhounds
Anagen and telogen defluxion
Postclipping alopecia
Traction alopecia
Injection reaction
Alopecia areata

Cats
Allergic alopecia
Hyperadrenocorticism
Congenital hypotrichosis
Feline preauricular and pinnal alopecia

Anagen and telogen defluxion
Injection reaction
Alopecia areata
Feline lymphocytic mural folliculitis

Cellulitis and Draining Lesions

(Nonspecific lesions caused by severe cellular infiltrates; usually associated with infection or neoplasia)

Dogs

Deep pyoderma
Actinomycosis
Nocardiosis
Opportunistic mycobacteriosis
Tuberculosis
Pythiosis
Lagenidiosis
Zycomycosis
Blastomycosis
Coccidiomycosis
Juvenile cellulitis
Blepharitis
Perianal fistulas

Cats

Subcutaneous abscess
Actinomycosis
L-form infection
Nocardiosis
Opportunistic mycobacteriosis
Tuberculosis
Plague
Phaeohyphomycosis
Pythiosis
Lagenidiosis
Sporotrichosis
Zycomycosis
Blastomycosis
Coccidiomycosis
Blepharitis
Anal sac disease

Nodular Diseases

(Nonspecific lesions caused by any cellular infiltrate; most often associated with neoplasia or infection)

Dogs

Botryomycosis
Actinomycosis
Nocardiosis
Opportunistic mycobacteriosis
Subcutaneous abscess
Tuberculosis
Canine leproid granuloma syndrome
Dermatophytosis

Eumycotic mycetoma
Phaeohyphomycosis
Protot022hecosis
Pythiosis
Lagenidiosis
Sporotrichosis
Zygomycosis
Blastomycosis
Coccidiomycosis
Histoplasmosis
Cuterebra
Dracunculiasis
Viral papillomatosis
Leishmaniasis
Cutaneous neosporosis
Systemic lupus erythematosus
Vesicular cutaneous lupus erythematosus
Cutaneous vesicular lupus erythematosus
Sterile nodular panniculitis
Idiopathic sterile granuloma and pyogranuloma
Tail gland hyperplasia
Acral lick dermatitis
Callus
Hygroma
Eosinophilic granuloma
Canine solar dermatosis
Neoplastic tumors
Nodular dermatofibrosis
Fibropruritic nodule
Collagenous nevus
Follicular cyst–intraepidermal inclusion cyst
Calcinosis circumscripta

Cats

Botryomycosis
Actinomycosis
Nocardiosis
Opportunistic mycobacteriosis
Subcutaneous abscess
Feline leprosy
Plague
Tuberculosis
Dermatophytosis
Eumycotic mycetoma
Phaeohyphomycosis
Protot022hecosis
Pythiosis
Lagenidiosis
Sporotrichosis
Zygomycosis
Blastomycosis
Coccidiomycosis
Cryptococcosis
Histoplasmosis
Cuterebra
Dracunculiasis

Differentials Based on Primary and Secondary Lesions—*cont'd*

Feline cowpox
Viral papillomatosis
Leishmaniasis
Cutaneous neosporosis
Sterile nodular panniculitis
Eosinophilic granuloma
Neoplastic tumors
Follicular cyst–intraepidermal inclusion cyst

Pruritic Diseases

(Nonspecific symptoms caused by any inflammatory dermatitis; some diseases have characteristic patterns that are more clinically relevant)

Dogs

Superficial pyoderma
Malasseziasis
Canine scabies
Cheyletiellosis
Ear mites
Trombiculiasis
Pediculosis
Hookworm dermatitis
Pelodera dermatitis
Atopy
Food hypersensitivity
Flea allergy dermatitis
Contact dermatitis
Pemphigus foliaceus
Acral lick dermatitis
Subcorneal pustular dermatosis
Sterile eosinophilic pustulosis
Hepatocutaneous syndrome

Cats

Superficial pyoderma
Malasseziasis
Feline scabies
Cheyletiellosis
Ear mites
Trombiculiasis
Pediculosis
Atopy
Food hypersensitivity
Flea allergy dermatitis
Contact dermatitis
Idiopathic facial dermatitis of Persian cats
Psychogenic alopecia
Feline lymphocytic mural folliculitis
Eosinophilic plaque
Idiopathic ulcerative dermatosis
Feline paraneoplastic alopecia
Hepatocutaneous syndrome

Seborrheic Diseases

(Nonspecific lesions that usually are secondary to a primary dermatologic disease but can be caused by a primary keratinization defect)

Dogs

Superficial pyoderma
Malasseziasis
Dermatophytosis
Demodicosis
Canine scabies
Cheyletiellosis
Pediculosis
Leishmaniasis
Cutaneous neosporosis
Food hypersensitivity
Pemphigus foliaceus
Pemphigus erythematosus
Systemic lupus erythematosus
Cutaneous drug reaction
Hyperadrenocorticism
Hypothyroidism
Sex hormone imbalances
Canine primary seborrhea
Vitamin A–responsive dermatosis
Ichthyosis
Epidermal dysplasia of West Highland White terriers
Sebaceous adenitis
Zinc-responsive dermatosis
Hepatocutaneous syndrome
Canine ear margin seborrhea
Neoplasia

Cats

Superficial pyoderma
Dermatophytosis
Malasseziasis
Demodicosis
Feline scabies
Cheyletiellosis
Cat fur mite
Pediculosis
Pemphigus foliaceus
Pemphigus erythematosus
Systemic lupus erythematosus
Cutaneous drug reaction
Hepatocutaneous syndrome
Tail gland hyperplasia
Idiopathic facial dermatitis of Persian cats
Neoplasia

Hyperpigmentation

(Common, usually nonspecific, change caused by inflammation of long duration)

Dogs

Lentigo
Chronic trauma
Chronic inflammation
　Allergy
　Post-infection
Cushing's

Sex hormone alopecia
Alopecia X
Recurrent flank alopecia
Melanoma

Hypopigmentation

(Uncommon lesion)
Autoimmune skin disease
Vitiligo
Uveodermatologic syndrome

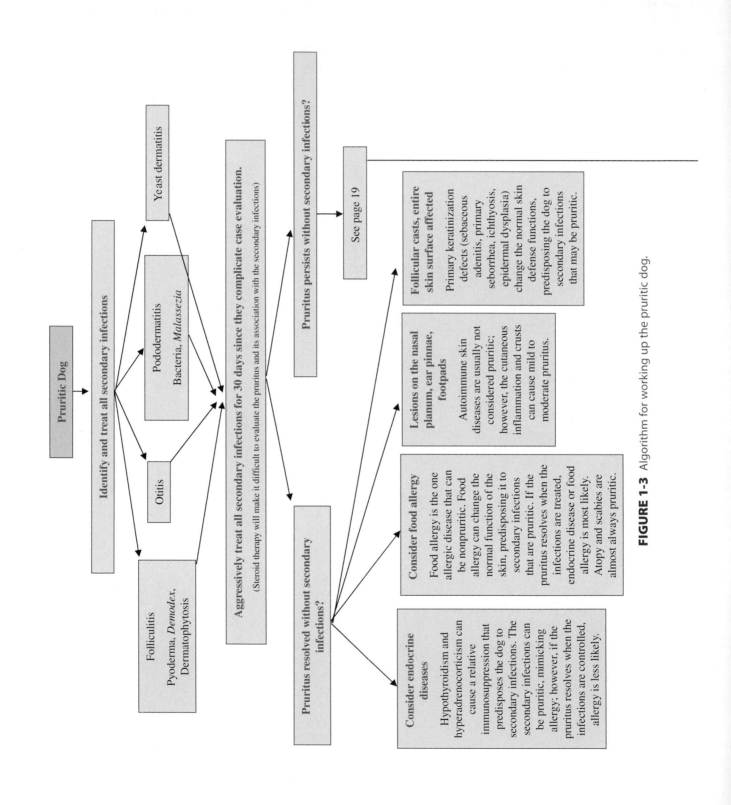

FIGURE 1-3 Algorithm for working up the pruritic dog.

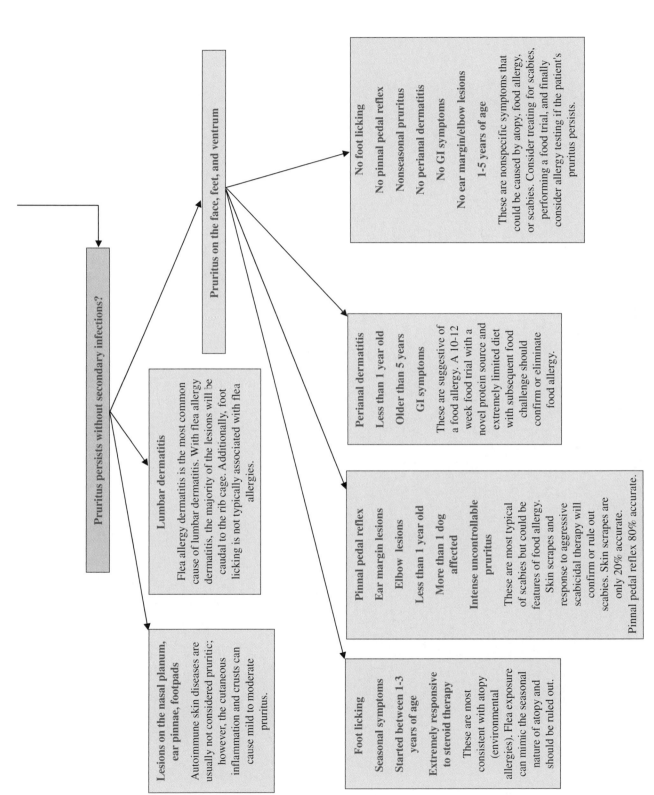

Pruritus persists without secondary infections?

Lumbar dermatitis

Flea allergy dermatitis is the most common cause of lumbar dermatitis. With flea allergy dermatitis, the majority of the lesions will be caudal to the rib cage. Additionally, foot licking is not typically associated with flea allergies.

Lesions on the nasal planum, ear pinnae, footpads

Autoimmune skin diseases are usually not considered pruritic; however, the cutaneous inflammation and crusts can cause mild to moderate pruritus.

Pruritus on the face, feet, and ventrum

No foot licking

No pinnal pedal reflex

Nonseasonal pruritus

No perianal dermatitis

No GI symptoms

No ear margin/elbow lesions

1-5 years of age

These are nonspecific symptoms that could be caused by atopy, food allergy, or scabies. Consider treating for scabies, performing a food trial, and finally consider allergy testing if the patient's pruritus persists.

Perianal dermatitis

Less than 1 year old

Older than 5 years

GI symptoms

These are suggestive of a food allergy. A 10-12 week food trial with a novel protein source and extremely limited diet with subsequent food challenge should confirm or eliminate food allergy.

Pinnal pedal reflex

Ear margin lesions

Elbow lesions

Less than 1 year old

More than 1 dog affected

Intense uncontrollable pruritus

These are most typical of scabies but could be features of food allergy. Skin scrapes and response to aggressive scabicidal therapy will confirm or rule out scabies. Skin scrapes are only 20% accurate. Pinnal pedal reflex 80% accurate.

Foot licking

Seasonal symptoms

Started between 1-3 years of age

Extremely responsive to steroid therapy

These are most consistent with atopy (environmental allergies). Flea exposure can mimic the seasonal nature of atopy and should be ruled out.

FIGURE 1-3, cont'd.

Differentials Based on Primary and Secondary Lesions—*cont'd*

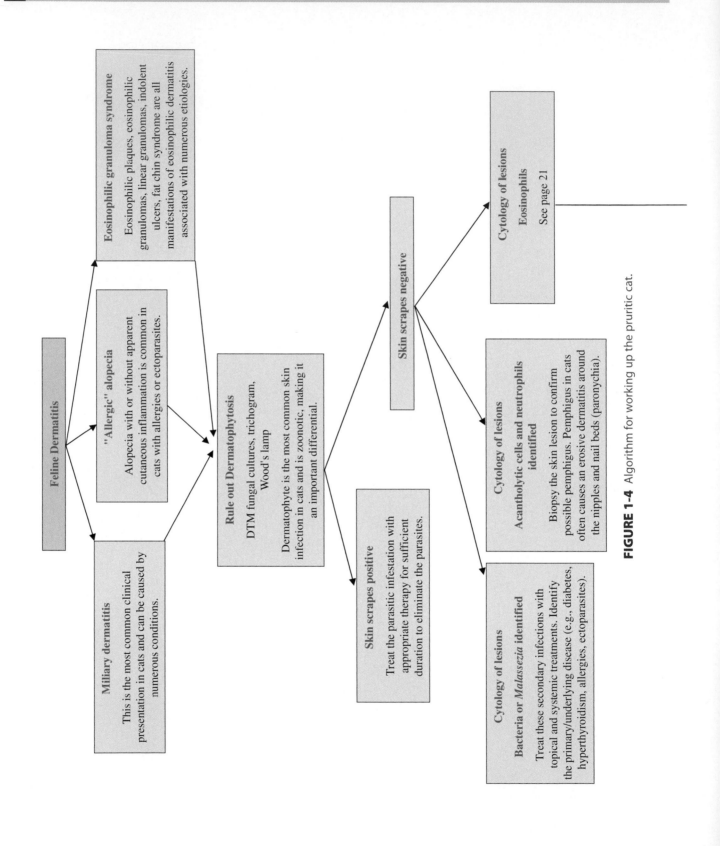

Feline Dermatitis

"Allergic" alopecia
Alopecia with or without apparent cutaneous inflammation is common in cats with allergies or ectoparasites.

Miliary dermatitis
This is the most common clinical presentation in cats and can be caused by numerous conditions.

Eosinophilic granuloma syndrome
Eosinophilic plaques, eosinophilic granulomas, linear granulomas, indolent ulcers, fat chin syndrome are all manifestations of eosinophilic dermatitis associated with numerous etiologies.

Rule out Dermatophytosis
DTM fungal cultures, trichogram, Wood's lamp

Dermatophyte is the most common skin infection in cats and is zoonotic, making it an important differential.

Skin scrapes positive
Treat the parasitic infestation with appropriate therapy for sufficient duration to eliminate the parasites.

Skin scrapes negative

Cytology of lesions
Bacteria or *Malassezia* identified

Treat these secondary infections with topical and systemic treatments. Identify the primary/underlying disease (e.g., diabetes, hyperthyroidism, allergies, ectoparasites).

Cytology of lesions
Acantholytic cells and neutrophils identified

Biopsy the skin lesion to confirm possible pemphigus. Pemphigus in cats often causes an erosive dermatitis around the nipples and nail beds (paronychia).

Cytology of lesions
Eosinophils
See page 21

FIGURE 1-4 Algorithm for working up the pruritic cat.

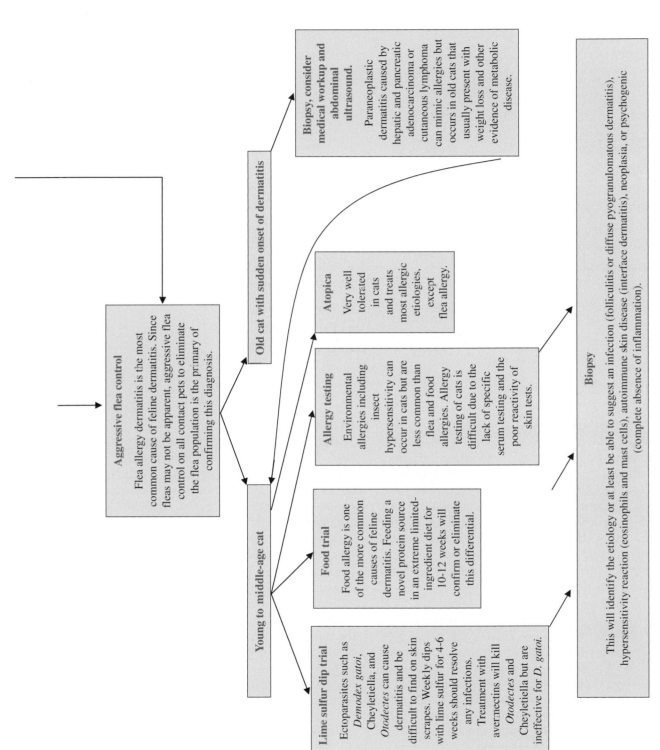

Aggressive flea control

Flea allergy dermatitis is the most common cause of feline dermatitis. Since fleas may not be apparent, aggressive flea control on all contact pets to eliminate the flea population is the primary of confirming this diagnosis.

Old cat with sudden onset of dermatitis

Biopsy, consider medical workup and abdominal ultrasound.

Paraneoplastic dermatitis caused by hepatic and pancreatic adenocarcinoma or cutaneous lymphoma can mimic allergies but occurs in old cats that usually present with weight loss and other evidence of metabolic disease.

Young to middle-age cat

Atopica

Very well tolerated in cats and treats most allergic etiologies, except flea allergy.

Allergy testing

Environmental allergies including insect hypersensitivity can occur in cats but are less common than flea and food allergies. Allergy testing of cats is difficult due to the lack of specific serum testing and the poor reactivity of skin tests.

Food trial

Food allergy is one of the more common causes of feline dermatitis. Feeding a novel protein source in an extreme limited-ingredient diet for 10-12 weeks will confirm or eliminate this differential.

Lime sulfur dip trial

Ectoparasites such as *Demodex gatoi*, *Cheyletiella*, and *Otodectes* can cause dermatitis and be difficult to find on skin scrapes. Weekly dips with lime sulfur for 4-6 weeks should resolve any infections. Treatment with avermectins will kill *Otodectes* and *Cheyletiella* but are ineffective for *D. gatoi*.

Biopsy

This will identify the etiology or at least be able to suggest an infection (folliculitis or diffuse pyogranulomatous dermatitis), hypersensitivity reaction (eosinophils and mast cells), autoimmune skin disease (interface dermatitis), neoplasia, or psychogenic (complete absence of inflammation).

FIGURE 1-4, cont'd.

CHAPTER 2

Diagnostic Techniques

- ■ Diagnostic Testing
- ■ Skin Scrapes
- ■ Cutaneous Cytology
- ■ Acetate Tape Preparations
- ■ Otic Swabs
- ■ Dermatophyte Test Medium Fungal Cultures
- ■ Trichogram
- ■ Wood's Lamp Examination
- ■ Biopsy

- ■ Cultures
- ■ Polymerase Chain Reaction Assays
- ■ Serology
- ■ Immunostaining Techniques
- ■ Diascopy
- ■ Allergy Testing
- ■ Patch Testing
- ■ Therapeutic Trials

Diagnostic Testing

The dermatologic diagnostic minimum database includes skin scrapes, otic swabs, and cutaneous cytology. The goal should be to identify all secondary infections (e.g., pyoderma, demodicosis, dermatophytosis, otitis, *Malassezia* dermatitis, infectious pododermatitis), then formulate a diagnostic plan for identifying and controlling the underlying/primary disease (i.e., allergies, endocrinopathies, keratinization defects, and autoimmune skin diseases) (Box 2-1).

Skin Scrapes

Skin scrapes are the most common dermatologic diagnostic tests (slide #1 in the 3-slide technique). These relatively simple and quick tests can be used to identify many types of parasitic infections (Table 2-1). Although they are not always diagnostic, their relative ease and low cost make them essential tests in a dermatologic diagnostic minimum database.

Many practitioners reuse scalpel blades when performing skin scrapes; however, this practice should be stopped because of increased awareness of transmittable diseases (e.g., *Bartonella*, *Rickettsia*, feline leukemia virus [FeLV], feline immunodeficiency virus [FIV], herpes, papillomavirus).

Procedure

Superficial Skin Scrapes (for Sarcoptes, Notoedres, Demodex gatoi, Cheyletiella, Otodectes, chiggers). A dulled scalpel blade is held perpendicular to the skin and is used with moderate pressure to scrape in the direction of hair growth. If the area is covered with hair, it may be necessary to clip a small window to access the skin. In an attempt to find the relatively few sarcoptic mites that may be present on a dog, large areas (1–2 inches) are scraped. Applying mineral oil directly to the skin to be scraped helps dislodge debris and makes it easier to collect the scraped material. Because these mites do not live deep within the skin, it is not necessary to visualize capillary oozing or blood. The most productive sites for sarcoptic mites include the ear margin and the lateral elbows. Anecdotal reports suggest that *Demodex gatoi* in cats may be found more easily on the lateral shoulder. Usually, several slides are needed to spread the collected material thinly enough for microscopic examination.

Deep Skin Scrapes (for Demodex spp. except D. gatoi). A dulled scalpel blade is held perpendicular to the skin and is used with moderate pressure to scrape in the direction of hair growth. If the area is covered with hair (usually, alopecic areas caused by folliculitis are selected), it may be necessary to clip a small window to access the skin. After several scrapes, the skin should appear pink, with the capillaries becoming visible and oozing blood. This ensures that the material collected comes from deep enough within the skin to allow the collection of follicular *Demodex* mites. Most people also squeeze (pinch) the skin to express mites from deep within the follicles into a more superficial area, so that they may be collected more easily. If scraping fails to provide a small amount of blood, then the mites may have been left in the follicle, resulting in a false-negative finding. In some situations (with Shar peis or deep inflammation with scarring), it may be impossible to scrape deeply enough to harvest *Demodex* mites. These cases are few in number but require biopsy for identification of mites within the hair follicles. Hair-plucks from an area of lesional skin may be used to help find

---

BOX 2-1 What Are the Infections?

For every dermatitis case, every time you evaluate the patient, ask yourself, "What are the infections?"

Using diarrhea and the microscopic fecal exam as a comparison works well because both skin cytology and fecal exams involve the use of a microscope, can easily identify the type of infection, and can be performed by trained technical staff. So why does your clinic perform fecal exams? When is a fecal exam performed (before the doctor's examination)? Who performed the fecal? Does the clinic charge for the fecal exam? The answers to these questions should be the same for skin cytology (skin scrapings, impression smears, tape preps, and otic swabs).

The practical solution for determining the best method by which to answer the question, "What are the infections?" is to implement a minimum database "infection screening" procedure to be performed by the technician before the veterinarian examines the patient. Every dermatology patient should undergo otic cytology, skin cytology (an impression smear or a tape prep), and a skin scrape at every examination (initially and at every recheck visit). This 3-Slide Technique can be performed easily and interpreted by a technician before the doctor completes an evaluation—which is exactly how diarrhea cases and fecal exams are handled in most clinics.

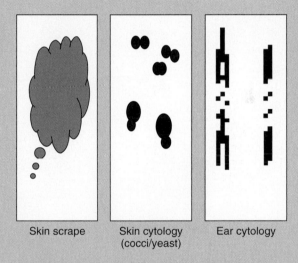

| Skin scrape | Skin cytology (cocci/yeast) | Ear cytology |

FIGURE 2-1 The 3-Slide Technique. Skin scrapes, cutaneous cytology, and otic swabs.

TABLE 2-1 Diagnosing Common Cutaneous Parasites

Mite	Diagnostic Test	Accuracy	Other Tests	Additional Tests
Demodex canis	Deep scrape	High	Biopsies may be needed with extremely thickened lesions	
Demodex cati	Deep scrape	High		
Demodex gatoi	Superficial scrape	Low Mites may be difficult to find	Lime sulfur dip trial, response to treatment	
Sarcoptes	Superficial scrape	Low (only 20%)	Respond to treatment	Pinnal-pedal reflex (80%)
Otodectes	Otic mineral oil prep, superficial scrape	High		
Cheyletiella	Flea comb, tape prep, superficial scrape, vacuum	Moderate	Vacuum collection techniques are preferred by some veterinarians	Possible identification of mites by fecal flotation
Lice	Tape prep (usually grossly visible)	High		
Notoedres cati	Superficial scrape	High		
Trombiculosis	Targeted scrape on focal lesion	Moderate		

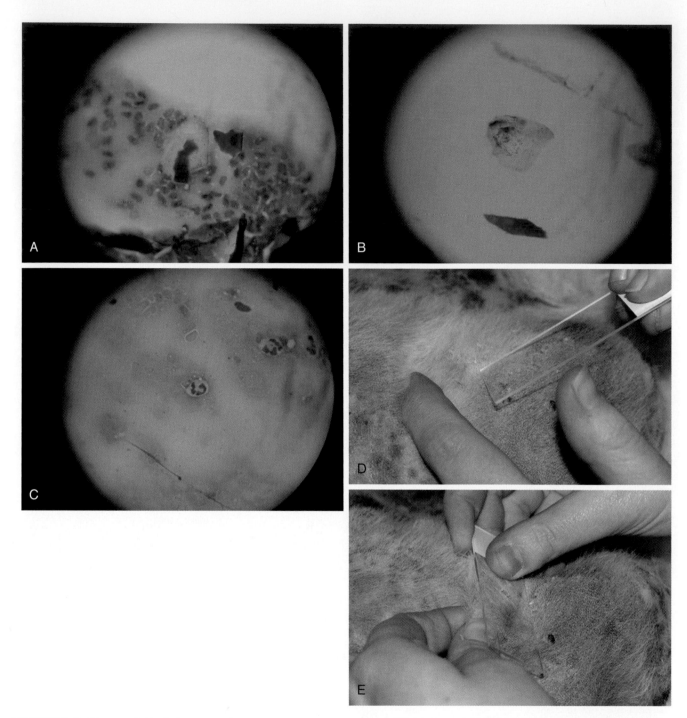

FIGURE 2-2 Diagnostic Techniques. A, This microscopic image (10× objective) demonstrates the typical angular shape of a normal, mature keratinocyte. Note the absence of a nucleus and and the small melanin granules (often mistaken for bacteria but pigmented brown). **B,** This microscopic image (10× objective) reveals the brown pigmented melanin granules within the anuclear keratinocyte with typical angular cell walls. Note the dark blue structure, which is likely a rolled-up keratinocyte. **C,** This microscopic image demonstrates the typical appearance of a neutrophil at 10× magnification. **D,** To collect a sample ideal for cytologic evaluation, the superficial crust should be gently scraped away and the glass slide applied firmly to the skin. **E,** To collect a sample ideal for cytologic evaluation, the superficial crust should be gently scraped away and the glass slide applied firmly to the skin. *Note:* It may be easier to collect the sample if the skin is slightly elevated by pinching or rolling the skin into a mound.

mites, but the accuracy of this technique compared with skin scrapes is unknown.

Regardless of the collection technique used, the entire slide should be searched for mites with the use of low power (usually a 10× objective). A search of the entire slide ensures that if only one or two mites are present (as is typical of scabies infection), the user will likely find them. It may be helpful to lower the microscope condenser; this provides greater contrast to the mites, thereby enhancing their visibility. (One must be

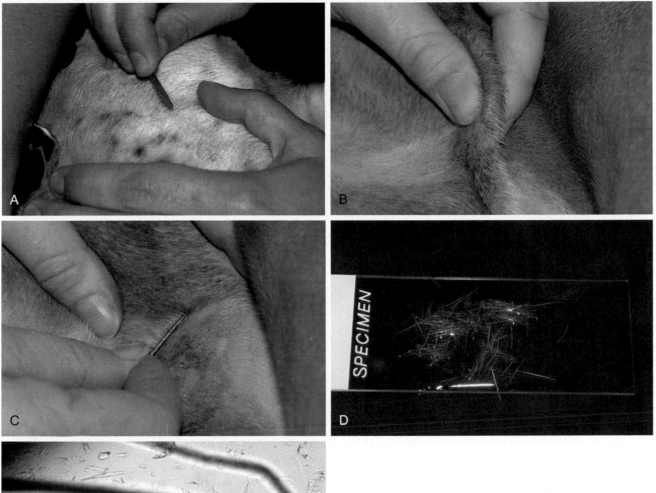

FIGURE 2-3 **Skin Scrape. A,** A new, dulled scalpel blade is used to scrape in the direction of hair growth. **B,** For deep skin scrapes, once capillary oozing is initiated, the skin is usually squeezed before a final scrape is performed to collect the material. **C,** Capillary oozing is apparent as the sample material is collected. **D,** The collected sample is evenly distributed in mineral oil on a glass slide. **E,** Microscopic image of the *Demodex* mite as seen with a 10× objective.

sure to raise the condenser before looking for cells or bacteria on stained slides.)

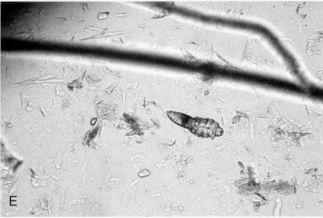

Cutaneous Cytology

Cutaneous cytology is the second most frequently employed dermatologic diagnostic technique (slide #2 in the 3-slide technique). Its purpose is to help the practitioner to identify bacterial or fungal organisms (yeast) and assess the infiltrating cell types, neoplastic cells, or acantholytic cells (typical of pemphigus complex).

Procedure

Direct Impression Smear. Moist exudate is collected from pustules, erosions, ulcers, or draining lesions. Alternatively, crusts can be lifted, revealing a moist undersurface. Papular lesions may be traumatized by the corner of a glass slide or a needle, then squeezed to express fluid. Yeast dermatitis can be sampled by repeated sticking of the slide onto lichenified lesions, or through the use of a dry scalpel blade to collect material that is then smeared onto a dry slide. Regardless of which technique is used, the moist exudate collected on the slide is allowed to dry. The slide is then stained with a commercially available cytology stain (e.g., modified Wright's stain [Diff-Quik is the most common]), and it is gently rinsed. A low-power objective is used to scan the slide to allow selection of ideal areas for closer examination. A high-power (40× or, preferably, 100× oil) objective is used to identify individual cell types, as well as bacterial or fungal organisms.

Fine Needle Aspirate Method. A needle (22–25 gauge) and a 6-mL syringe should be used to aspirate the mass. The area should be cleaned if necessary with alcohol or chlorhexidine. The lesion is then immobilized. The practitioner should insert the needle into the nodule while aiming for the center of the lesion, pull back on the plunger to apply suction, release and redirect, pull back on the plunger again, and stop if any blood is visible in the hub of the needle, as this will dilute the cellular sample. Negative pressure should be released before the needle is removed from the lesion. An alternative technique involves repeated insertion of the needle without the syringe into the lesion, while redirecting several times. This latter technique (without negative pressure), which decreases the frequency of inadvertent dilution of the sample with blood, works best for soft masses. Once the sample has been collected, the material is expressed onto a microscope slide by blowing a syringe-full of air through the needle to spray the cells onto the slide. The material is smeared gently to thin the clumps of cells stained with cytology stain. The slide should be scanned with low power (4×–10×) to reveal a suitable area for closer examination. A high-power (40×) objective may be used to reveal the infiltrating cell type and the cellular atypia.

Acetate Tape Preparations

Tape preps are used to evaluate a variety of different conditions. The basic technique involves the use of crystal clear tape (single- or double-sided) to collect a sample of hair or superficial skin debris.

> **Author's Note**
>
> The infections are always secondary to a primary disease; however, all too often, the patient is not evaluated or treated for the primary disease for three major reasons:
> 1. Only the secondary infections are treated over and over again.
> 2. The nature of the allergy is confusing.
> 3. Cheap steroids that have delayed repercussions are available.

Tape Preps for Mites

Tape preps can be an effective method of collecting and restraining *Cheyletiella* and lice for microscopic examination. The mites are usually large enough to be seen, so a piece of tape can be used to capture a specimen. The tape prevents the creatures from escaping.

Tape Preps for Hair (trichogram)

Tape is used to secure the hair sample in position on a glass slide. The sample is examined under low power (4×–10× objective). (See "Trichogram" section for more information on analysis techniques.) Oil may be a better medium for use with trichograms.

Tape Preps for Yeast

Tape preps for yeast dermatitis are some of the most efficient and effective methods of identifying *Malassezia* skin infections. Although they are not as reliable and quantitative as impression cultures that use Sabouraud's media, the speed and ease of tape preps for yeast make them the techniques most commonly employed for identifying *Malassezia*. The lichenified lesion (elephant skin on the ventral neck or ventrum) is sampled by repeated application of the sticky side of the tape onto the lesion. The tape is then adhered to a glass slide and is stained with a cytology stain (while the first alcohol stain solution is admitted). The tape serves as a coverslip and can be examined under high power (100× oil immersion) for visualization of *Malassezia* organisms. This technique is useful, but false-negative results are common with all yeast collection techniques.

Otic Swabs

Screening

Otic swabs are useful for determining whether a normal-appearing ear canal actually has exudate deep within the ear (slide #3 in the 3-slide technique). If a cotton swab is used to gently collect a sample, and if it is relatively clean, then the ear most likely is normal. If the sample demonstrates a black waxy exudate, then a mineral oil prep should be performed for identification of any mites (e.g., *Otodectes*, *Demodex*). If the sample is light brown or demonstrates a purulent exudate, cytology should be performed for identification of bacteria or yeast.

Mites

Mineral oil can be used to dissolve the black waxy material collected from an otic swab. The swab should be stirred in the oil to remove the exudate and to make the sample suitable for examination. The entire slide should be examined under low power (4× or 10× objective) for identification of any mites. Usually, *Otodectes* mites are easy to visualize, but dropping the condenser and scanning the entire slide may make the practitioner more certain of the diagnosis.

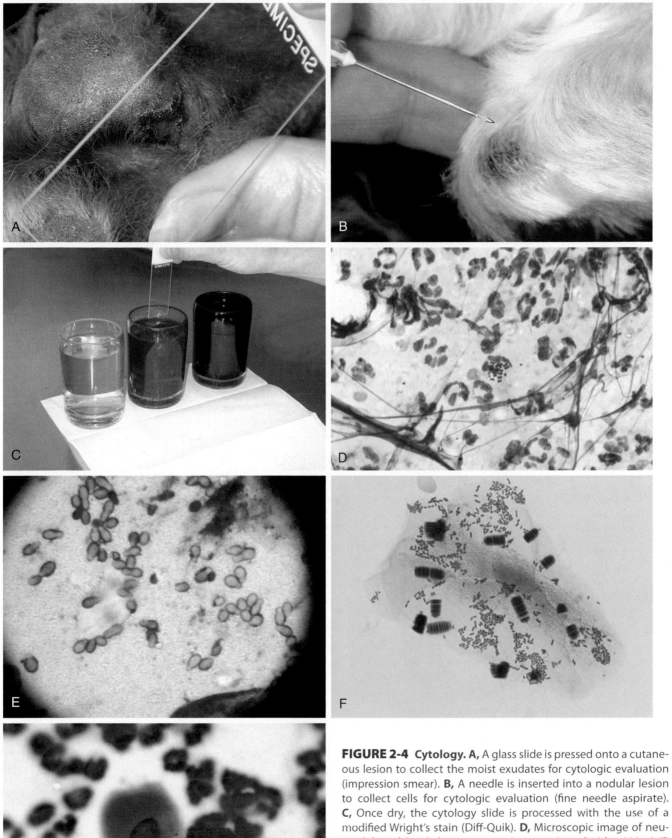

FIGURE 2-4 **Cytology. A,** A glass slide is pressed onto a cutaneous lesion to collect the moist exudates for cytologic evaluation (impression smear). **B,** A needle is inserted into a nodular lesion to collect cells for cytologic evaluation (fine needle aspirate). **C,** Once dry, the cytology slide is processed with the use of a modified Wright's stain (Diff-Quik). **D,** Microscopic image of neutrophils and *Staphylococcus* organisms, as viewed with a 100× (oil) objective. **E,** Microscopic image of *Malassezia* yeast, as viewed with a 100× (oil) objective. **F,** Microscopic image of a keratinocyte, melanin granules, and *Simonsiella* organisms, as viewed with a 100× (oil) objective. *Simonsiella* is a common oral bacterium; its presence suggests that the patient has been licking (pruritus). **G,** Microscopic image of neutrophils and acantholytic cells, as viewed with a 100× (oil) objective. Acantholytic cells are suggestive of pemphigus.

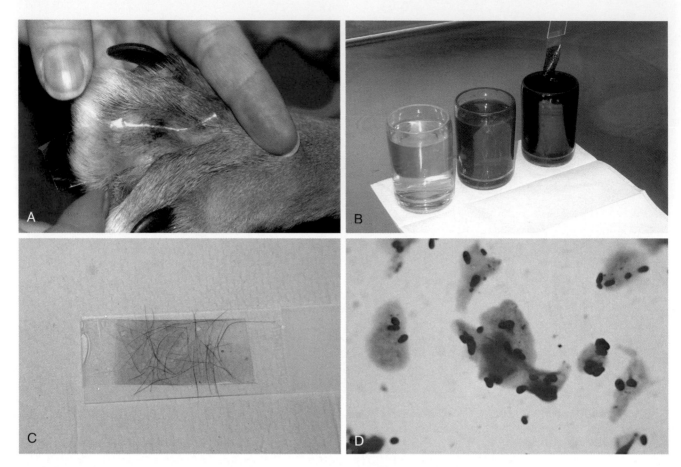

FIGURE 2-5 Tape Preps. A, Clear acetate tape is pressured repeatedly into the interdigital space for collection of a superficial sample. **B,** The tape is processed with a modified Wright's stain (Diff-Quik) with omission of the first light blue alcohol solution, which dissolves the tape adhesive. **C,** After processing has been completed, the sample material is easily visible under the tape. **D,** Microscopic image of *Malassezia* organisms and keratinocytes, as viewed with a 100× (oil) objective.

Bacteria and Yeast

Otic cytology is used to identify secondary yeast and bacterial otitis externa. Debris is collected with a cotton swab. An easy and quick technique is to roll the swab from the right ear onto the right side of the slide, and the swab from the left ear onto the left side of the slide, assuming that the slide has markings by which to identify which direction is up. If the material is very waxy, the end of the slide should be heated to help melt the wax and allow the stain to penetrate the sample. The sample should be stained with cytology stain (modified Wright's stain [Diff-Quik]), then examined under low power (10× objectives), so that a cellular area likely to include organisms can be identified. Then, the high-power objective (40× or 100× oil immersion) should be used to identify the organisms that are causing the secondary otitis.

Dermatophyte Test Medium Fungal Cultures

Dermatophyte test medium (DTM) fungal cultures are used to isolate and identify dermatophyte organisms. DTM is made with special ingredients that inhibit

Author's Note

When an owner brings the pet into the clinic for a small hairless spot, it would be appropriate to question the necessity for an otic cytology when the hairless spot is the problem. However, the 3-Slide Technique is most helpful in these exact types of cases. If focal pruritus occurs in a dog and the patient has a secondary otitis (which the technician identified during the infection screen), the veterinarian should more aggressively discuss and work up the patient for possible allergy. If the patient did not have otitis, the skin pruritus could be minimized in the hope that it was a short-term problem that may self-resolve.

Author's Note

Otic cytology is necessary for identifying the type of secondary infection present, so that the best medical therapy can be selected. Additionally, otic cytology is useful for evaluating a patient's response to treatment, especially when the otitis has not completely resolved. In these cases, otic cytology can be used to determine whether the number and the mixture of organisms are improving. This determination is crucial for preventing premature discontinuation or switching of treatments, which may lead to increased antimicrobial resistance.

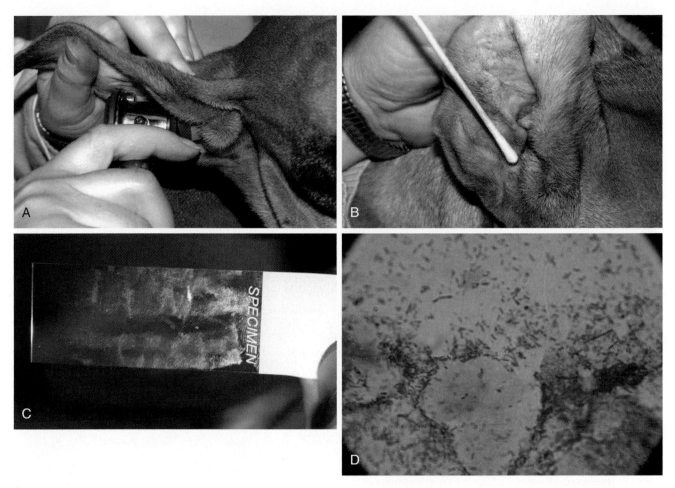

FIGURE 2-6 **Otic Cytology. A,** Before an otic sample is obtained for cytologic evaluation, the ear canal and the tympanic membrane should be evaluated visually. **B,** A cotton swab is used to obtain a sample of exudates from the ear canal. **C,** The exudates collected on the swab are smeared onto the slide. The left ear sample has been smeared onto the left half of the slide, and the right ear sample onto the right side of the slide. **D,** Microscopic image of otic cytology demonstrating numerous neutrophils and mixed bacteria, as viewed with a 10× objective.

bacterial growth and turn red when dermatophytes grow. Alternatively, proprietary media plates that have unique attributes are available; however, DTM cultures remain the customary technique.

Procedure

The area to be sampled is usually cleaned by gentle application of alcohol to the hair and skin. The alcohol should dry before the specimen is collected. Samples of hair, crust, or scale are collected from lesional skin with the use of a sterile forceps. Use of a Wood's lamp to collect fluorescing hairs may enhance diagnostic accuracy. The collected material should be gently applied to DTM, with care taken not to bury the sample within the medium. Bringing the medium to room temperature before the sample is placed on it helps to hasten fungal growth. Fungal culture plates with a large removable or flip-up lid (e.g., standard petri dish or Bactilabs culture plates) make sample deposition much easier. For animals with no lesions (i.e., those with resolving infection, or subclinical carriers), a new toothbrush can be used to brush the entire hair coat. The collected sample is then distributed onto the culture plate. Claws can be cultured by clipping an affected nail and grinding or shaving its surface to produce small particles that are deposited onto the medium. Dermatophytes grow within the keratin structure of the claw, causing distinctive onychodystrophy.

The DTM culture plates should be examined daily for 2 to 3 weeks. With dermatophytes, the medium will change color as soon as a white/buff-colored fluffy colony becomes visible on the medium. Some contaminants (usually black, gray, and green) will be able to change the medium to red but only after growing for several days. If the culture plate has not been evaluated daily, it will be impossible to determine when the color change occurred in relation to the appearance of fungal colony growth.

Once the fungal colony has been growing for several days, it begins to produce macroconidia. Keeping the culture warm in a humid environment facilitates the formation of conidia. The macroconidia should be sampled and microscopically examined so that the dermatophyte species can be identified. Clear acetate tape is touched to the surface of the fungal colony to be evaluated. The tape is then adhered to a glass slide, and a drop of cytology stain is applied. The macroconidia are usually apparent under a low-power (10×) objective. This is especially important in dogs because the identification of *Microsporum canis* may indicate the presence of an infected asymptomatic cat in the immediate environment. Identification of *Trichophyton* or *Microsporum gypseum* suggests an environmental source for the dermatophyte infection (other than an infected cat).

Some fungal species that cause deep infection/cellulitis (e.g., blastomycosis, pythiosis, histoplasmosis, coccidioidomycosis) represent a zoonotic hazard when grown as in-house cultures. If such species are suspected, swab samples and tissue specimens should be submitted to and cultured by well-equipped microbiology laboratories.

Trichogram

A trichogram is used to visualize the hair for evidence of pruritus, fungal infection, and pigmentation defects, and to assess the growth phase (for evaluation of hair tips, roots, and shafts).

Procedure

A small amount of hair to be examined is epilated. Tape or mineral oil is used to secure the hair sample in position on a glass slide. The sample is examined under a low-power (4× or 10×) objective.

Hair Tips.   Hair tips are usually evaluated to determine whether the patient is pruritic (especially cats), or if the cause of hair loss is nontraumatic (e.g., endocrine disease, follicular dysplasia). Pruritic animals break the tips off the hairs, leaving a broken end that can be detected easily. This determination is especially useful

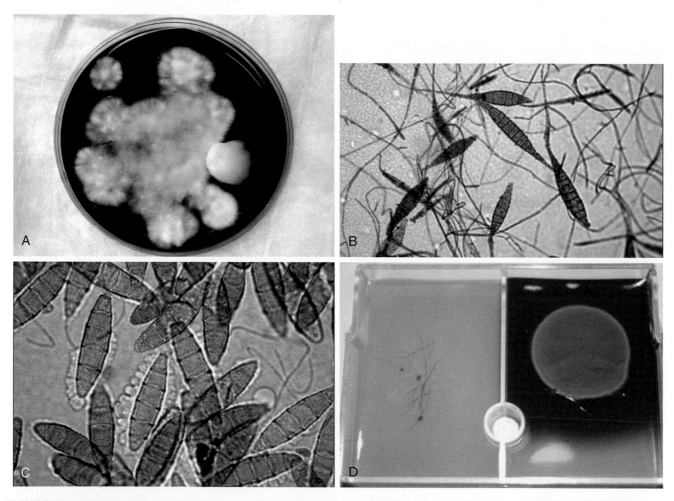

FIGURE 2-7 Dermatophyte Test Medium (DTM) Fungal Culture. A, *Microsporum canis* demonstrating the typical white, fluffy colony growth and red color change. The red color should develop as soon as colony growth becomes visible. **B,** Microscopic image of *M. canis* organisms, as viewed with a 10× objective. Note the six or more cell divisions. **C,** Microscopic image of *M gypsum*, as viewed with a 10× objective. Note the six or fewer cell divisions. **D,** Fungal contaminant growing on DTM medium. The pigmented colony rules out dermatophyte infection. The red color change occurred well after the pigmented colony had been growing for several days. Dermatophytes cause the red color change as soon as colony growth becomes visible.

in feline patients when owners are not convinced that the patient is pruritic because of its secretive nature (noted in some cats).

Hair Roots. Hair roots may be examined for identification of anagen and telogen hairs in an attempt to determine whether hair follicles are cycling normally. In most breeds, the greatest number of hairs will be found in the telogen stage, but some anagen hairs should be identifiable. In breeds with prolonged growth periods (Poodles), most of the hairs may be in anagen, with relatively few hairs in the telogen stage. During telogen defluxion, all of the epilated hairs are observed to be in telogen.

Hair Shafts. Dermatophyte ectothrix sometimes can be visualized in patients with dermatophytosis. Identification of ectothrix can be difficult, and potassium hydroxide (KOH) and cytology stain may be required to help dissolve the excessive keratin. With ectothrix, the cortex of the hair appears swollen and damaged, and, if broken, the ends appear frayed (like a broom). The organisms (small spherical structures) may be clumped around the damaged region of the hair shaft. Hair shafts can be examined for pigmentary clumping, which is suggestive of color dilution alopecia and follicular dysplasia. Ectoparasite eggs attached to the hair shaft may be visible with pediculosis and cheyletiellosis. Other hair shaft abnormalities have been reported but are extremely rare.

Wood's Lamp Examination

A Wood's lamp is a special ultraviolet (UV) light source that uses a wavelength of 340 to 450 mm (UVA spectrum that does not hurt the skin or eyes). This unique combination causes tryptophan metabolites produced by some strains of *M. canis* to fluoresce a bright apple green color. Unfortunately, not all *Microsporum* strains produce this cell product, making the Wood's lamp useful in only approximately 50% of cases of *M. canis* infection. This technique cannot be used to identify *Trichophyton* species or *M. gypseum*.

It is important that the light source be allowed to warm up, so the appropriate wavelength of light is produced. Many false-positives may be observed because of the fluorescence of the scale and certain topical medications. A true dermatophyte infection reveals an apple green fluorescence on the roots of the hair shafts. All dermatophyte infections should be confirmed by means of fungal culture.

Biopsy

Cutaneous biopsy evaluation can be frustrating for the practitioner and the pathologist. The practitioner can improve the diagnostic reliability of skin biopsies by properly selecting lesions for biopsy, by using the services of a dermatopathologist, and by providing the pathologist with a complete clinical differential diagnosis list.

Cutaneous biopsy has the potential to provide the greatest amount of information in the shortest period of time. Even if cutaneous histopathology cannot identify the exact cause of the lesion, the pathologist should be able to classify cutaneous changes into one of six general categories:

1. Neoplasia.
2. Infection (e.g., folliculitis, cellulitis).
3. Immune-mediated event (e.g., autoimmune disease, vasculitis, drug reaction).
4. Endocrine-like disorder (e.g., hypothyroidism, Cushing's disease, follicular dysplasia).
5. Keratinization defect (e.g., primary seborrhea, sebaceous adenitis, ichthyosis).
6. Allergy.

Practitioners can improve the diagnostic efficiency of cutaneous biopsies by doing the following:

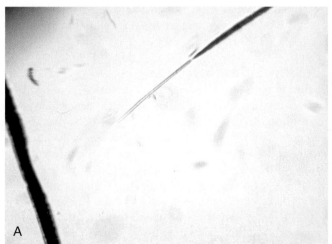
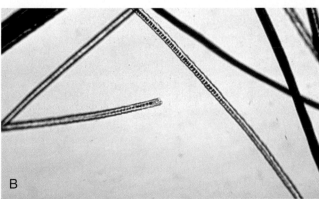

FIGURE 2-8 **Trichogram. A,** Microscopic image of a normally tapered hair tip, as viewed with a 10× objective. **B,** Microscopic image of a broken hair tip (indicating pruritus), as viewed with a 10× objective. *Continued*

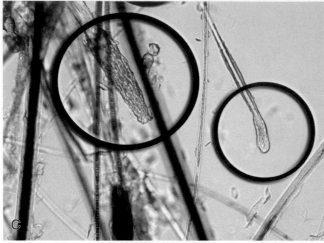

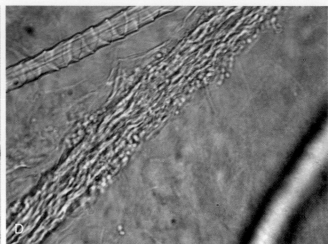

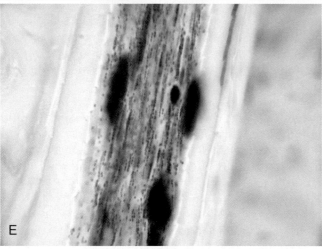

FIGURE 2-8, cont'd **C,** Microscopic image of a telogen hair root (*left*, spearhead-shaped root) and an anagen hair root (*right*, bent knob-shaped root), as viewed with a 10× objective. **D,** Microscopic image of a dermatophyte-infected hair. Misshapen hair with beadlike ectothrix organisms, as viewed with a 100× (oil) objective. **E,** Microscopic image of pigmentary clumping (as seen in color dilution alopecia or black hair follicle dysplasia), as viewed with a 100× (oil) objective.

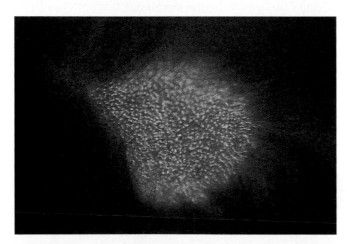

FIGURE 2-9 Wood's Lamp. Wood's lamp examination of dermatophyte-infected hairs demonstrating typical apple green fluorescence. Only *Microsporum canis* fluoresces and in only about half of cases.

1. Obtaining several skin biopsies from different representative lesions. A biopsy sample should be taken from everything that looks different.
2. Providing the pathologist with a detailed list of differential diagnoses based on clinical lesions, patterns, and responses to treatment.

3. Insisting on a histopathology report that includes a thorough description of skin sections, as well as a discussion of how these findings rule in or rule out the differential diagnoses provided by the submitting veterinarian.
4. Using a dermatopathology service to take advantage of the special interests and training of pathologists who provide these services (lists available at itchnot. com or VIN).

Lesion Selection

Primary cutaneous lesions (i.e., pustules, vesicles, petechiae, erythematous macules, papules) are preferred for sampling. Secondary lesions (e.g., crust, alopecia, scale, ulcers, erosions) may be useful but typically have less diagnostic impact. A good strategy is to sample several sites (at least three), while making sure to get a range of lesion types. Generally, biopsy samples should be obtained from every area that appears different.

The nose and the footpads are particularly painful areas from which to collect biopsy specimens; however, these areas very often are affected by autoimmune skin disease and should be sampled. Heavy sedation or general anesthesia may be required for collection of biopsy specimens from the nose or the footpads.

Procedure

Once the areas to be submitted for biopsy have been selected, the lesions should be left untraumatized. Target areas should not be cleaned or prepped because these processes would remove the superficial crust and scale that may be essential for determining the diagnosis. A local anesthetic (e.g., septocaine, lidocaine, articaine, novocaine) may be injected into the subcutaneous tissue, with care taken not to inject too superficially. Lidocaine may decrease the viability of some infectious organisms; therefore, its use in biopsy samples destined for minced tissue culture should be avoided.

A disposable Baker's punch (4–8 mm) should be used to perform the biopsy. The biopsy punch is placed on the lesion, and moderate pressure is applied while the biopsy punch is twisted. Once it has penetrated the full thickness of the skin, the punch is removed, leaving the skin sample attached to the subcutaneous fat. With great care taken not to traumatize the skin sample, forceps should be used to grasp the sample by the deep fat (this prevents forceps marks in the epidermis, which decrease the diagnostic potential of the sample). The subcutaneous fat can be cut to release the skin biopsy sample. If the skin is thin, or if it is critical that the pathologist be able to orient the sections, the sample should be placed on a firm substrate (a piece of index card or a tongue depressor). The sample should be submitted in 10% formalin.

An alternate method requires that a scalpel be used to obtain an excisional biopsy sample through a classic elliptical excision approach. This is the preferred technique for large lesions.

Nails can be sampled for biopsy by using one of two techniques. If the nail is soft, an 8-mm Baker's punch can be used to collect a sample from a lateral portion of the nail, nail bed, and nail base. This technique works only when the nail is soft enough to be sectioned. When the nail is hard (a more normal state), amputation of the third phalanx is required. Obviously, this is not the ideal sample collection technique in that many owners are extremely reluctant to permit digital amputation. Often, a dewclaw can be harvested to minimize the impact of diagnostic amputation.

Once the sample has been removed, the wound should be closed with suture or cutaneous staples.

Cultures

Bacterial and fungal cultures are an important part of diagnostics in dermatology. Any deep cellulitis-like lesions, especially those with draining tracts, should be cultured for bacterial and fungal organisms. Nodules and tumors should be cultured when infectious causes are included on the differential list.

Procedure

Culturette swabs are useful for collecting moist exudates for culture. All superficial purulent exudate should be removed and the lesion cleaned with nonpreserved saline or water. Fresh exudate then can be expressed and collected with the swab for submission to the microbiology laboratory. This cleaning technique helps reduce the number of contaminant organisms in the sample.

Otic cultures should be obtained before any lavage or cleaning procedures are performed.

For deep skin cultures, the preferred technique involves use of a sterile biopsy procedure to collect a piece of skin for submission to the microbiology laboratory. The skin should be surgically prepped and rinsed well with nonpreserved saline or water. This prevents the disinfectant solution from killing the pathologic organisms. Once the skin sample has been harvested, it should be placed in a culture swab or sterile container (with a drop of nonpreserved saline), refrigerated, and shipped overnight. Caution should be taken to avoid freezing the skin samples intended for culture because this will decrease the accuracy of the culture. The laboratory then should perform a minced tissue culture to isolate the organisms within the dermis.

Polymerase Chain Reaction Assays

Polymerase chain reaction (PCR) assays use laboratory methods to amplify DNA within a sample. PCR is many times more sensitive and specific than other diagnostic tests for the identification of viral, bacterial, and fungal organisms. In the future, PCR will become a powerful tool for the diagnosis of most cutaneous infections. At this writing, most diagnostic laboratories provide testing for mycobacteria and some deep fungal organisms. Because this technology is evolving extremely rapidly, it may be helpful for the practitioner to contact the diagnostic laboratory for testing availability and sample requirements.

Serology

The detection of antibodies for select infectious agents may provide useful information regarding patient exposure, active infection, and resolution of some fungal, rickettsial, and protozoal diseases. This diagnostic test may be most useful for identifying rickettsial diseases and *Cryptococcus*.

Immunostaining Techniques

Direct immunofluorescence provides a unique method for the diagnosis of autoimmune skin diseases. Direct immunofluorescence has been used in veterinary dermatology for longer than 30 years, but the accuracy and repeatability of this diagnostic test have been questioned. The body region selected for testing can greatly influence the results of direct immunofluorescence; 11% to 78% of normal footpad or nasal samples demonstrate false-positive results. Additionally, diagnostic laboratories can demonstrate poor reproducibility with

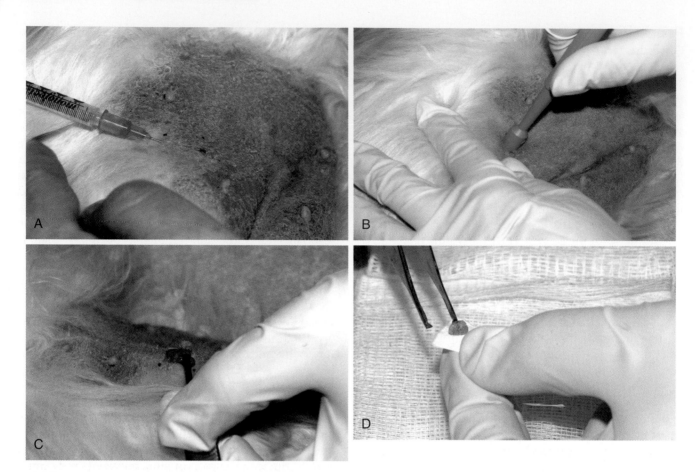

FIGURE 2-10 Biopsy. A, A local anesthetic is injected into the subcutaneous tissue below the biopsy site. The skin is not scrubbed or surgically prepared; this would remove potentially diagnostic crusts or other superficial lesions. **B,** A disposable Baker's biopsy punch is twisted with moderate pressure to obtain the sample. **C,** The practitioner detached the skin sample from the subcutaneous tissue by grasping the subcutaneous tissue, retracting the sample, and cutting the subcutaneous fat. The skin itself should not be grasped because this damages epidermal structures. **D,** Once separated, the skin sample is placed onto a rigid surface (e.g., piece of tongue depressor, index card, cardboard) to prevent curling; it is placed in formalin.

duplicate samples. More recently developed techniques, including immunoperoxidase and monoclonal antibodies, seem to provide more accurate results; however, their use is limited.

Procedure

Skin samples are collected through traditional biopsy techniques. If immunofluorescence will be used, Michel's preservative is required. The need for special media has caused immunofluorescence to be less favored by many practitioners and diagnostic laboratories. Immunoperoxidase offers the same diagnostic value but can be performed on formalin-fixed tissue, eliminating the need for additional biopsy samples preserved in Michel's preservative. The diagnostic laboratory should be contacted in advance for testing availability and sample requirements.

Diascopy

Diascopy is a simple technique that involves placing a glass slide over an erythematous lesion and applying moderate pressure. The skin under the slide blanches (i.e., turns white as the blood is squeezed out) or remains erythematous. This test is useful for differentiating vasodilatation from ecchymosis. Urticarial lesions are caused by dilated blood vessels that leak fluid but not red cells; therefore, these red lesions blanch when pressure is applied. Ecchymosis (typical of vasculitis) is caused by red blood cells leaking out of the vessels. These erythematous lesions do not blanch because the cells are located within the dermis.

Allergy Testing

Serologic Testing

Serum immunoglobulin levels rise in allergic dogs, making it possible for the pathologist to identify and measure antigen-specific antibody levels. Tests are readily available from several different companies and can be easily performed in any practice environment. In general, the patient does not have to be withdrawn from medications that would interfere with traditional intradermal allergy testing; however, because these tests do

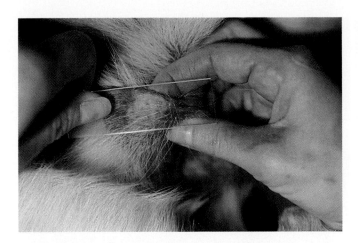

FIGURE 2-11 **Diascopy.** A glass slide is used to apply pressure to an erythematous lesion. If the lesion is caused by vasodilatation (urticaria), it will blanch (turn white). If the lesions are petechial or ecchymotic (caused by blood leaking from the vessel [vasculitis]), they will remain erythematous (i.e., they will not blanch).

measure a component of the immune response, antiinflammatory medications may alter the results. Discontinuation of all steroid-containing medications, as would be required before intradermal allergy testing, should be considered before the patient's serum sample is acquired. Some companies include steroid withdrawal in their patient preparation requirements.

Skin Testing

For many years, intradermal allergy testing has been considered the gold standard for diagnosing and treating canine atopy, and it remains the primary testing method used by most veterinary dermatologists. Intradermal allergy testing permits skin testing at the place where the allergic response is occurring. Most animals tolerate the procedure well, and results are immediately available. Animals should be sedated to minimize anxiety or stress; they should be withdrawn from antihistamines for 10 to 14 days and from all steroid-containing medications for at least 4 weeks. The antigens used should be carefully stored and maintained to ensure high-quality testing materials and appropriate antigen stock for immunotherapy vaccine formulation. Generally, at least 40 allergens should be included so that a large enough spectrum of regional allergens has been incorporated into the test.

Procedure

The patient is withdrawn from all medications that contain steroids or antihistamines. The patient is sedated to avoid excess stress and cortisol release. An area on the lateral thorax is clipped with a #40 blade. The skin should not be traumatized or cleaned. A permanent marker is used to indicate sites for injection. A special syringe is used to administer 0.05 to 0.1 mL of each allergen that has been prediluted to 1000 to 1500 protein nitrogen units (PNUs) (for most allergens). The test should be completed within a 30-minute window; after this time, initial injections should be ready to be read. Each injection site is evaluated for erythema and swelling. Histamine and saline controls are used to help determine the range of reactivity, and a 0 to 4 scale is used to assign the relative reactivity of each injection site. A good positive should look like a bee sting with a sharp ridge at the peripheral margin of the reaction. Negative reactions may have some noticeable swelling caused by the injected volume of fluid, but erythema and a distinctive sharp ridge on palpation are absent.

Which Is the Better Test?

Few clinical studies have directly compared patient response rates to immunotherapy based on each of the allergy testing methods. The limited information that is available suggests that the average response rate to immunotherapy vaccine based on serologic allergy testing is about 60% (55%–60% of treated dogs show good to excellent response); however, if the immunotherapy vaccine is based on intradermal allergy testing, about 68% (50%–86%) of treated dogs demonstrate good to excellent response. Perhaps the ideal allergy test would combine the information provided from intradermal and serologic allergy testing to render a more complete representation of the dog's allergic condition. Indeed, some veterinary dermatologists have started performing both tests in every animal that they evaluate for atopy.

Patch Testing

Patch testing is the method of choice for identifying allergens in humans; however, because of the limitations of veterinary species and the artificial dermatitis created by the occlusive bandaging needed, patch testing of animals is extremely problematic and unreliable.

Therapeutic Trials

Therapeutic trials are often needed to eliminate some causes of a patient's lesions.

Fleas

Flea allergy dermatitis is one of the most common skin diseases in animals. Many pet owners are extremely effective at removing fleas and flea dirt through grooming, making it difficult for the practitioner to prove the existence of a flea infestation. Therefore, dogs with lumbar dermatitis and all pruritic cats should be treated aggressively for possible flea allergy dermatitis. As of this writing, the only product that can kill adult fleas rapidly enough to stop flea allergy reaction in the treated

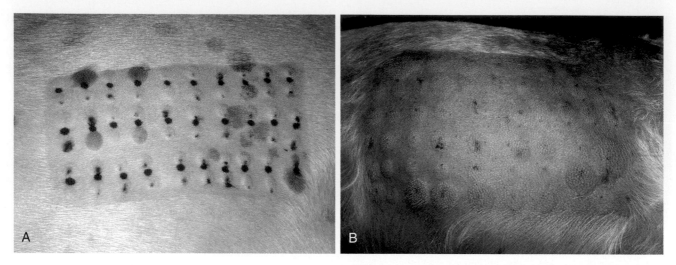

FIGURE 2-12 **Allergy Skin Test. A,** A reactive allergy skin test. The positive reactions are well-demarcated erythematous wheals, which have the appearance of bee stings. **B,** Note that the lesions are less apparent on pigmented skin.

patient is nitenpyram (Capstar) administered every 24 to 48 hours for 1 month. Because nitenpyram kills only fleas and maggots, any improvement in the patient's dermatitis would result from the prevention of flea saliva injection. Other adulticides like Fipronil, imidicloprid, and selamectin work well but may take several months to produce significant improvement and require all animals to be treated aggressively. Because of grooming and the limitations of each product, treatments should be applied every 2 to 3 weeks in flea-allergic animals. In heavily infested environments, it may take several weeks to reduce the number of emerging fleas. Owners may perceive this as lack of efficacy, when, in fact, it is caused by the presence of large numbers of fleas in the pupal stage.

Feline *Demodex*

Feline demodicosis caused by *D. gatoi* is emerging as a contagious, pruritic feline alopecic dermatosis, especially in the southern part of the United States. *D. gatoi* may be difficult to find. Therefore, a therapeutic trial consisting of lime sulfur dips applied weekly for 4 to 6 weeks is needed to eliminate *D. gatoi* as a possible cause. Alternative treatments do not seem to be efficacious for this parasite.

Scabies

Sarcoptiform mites (e.g., scabies, *Notoedres*, *Cheyletiella*) are uncommon but demonstrate regional variation in infection rates. Most mites are readily found on skin scrapes; however, in some cases, mites may be difficult to find. A therapeutic trial with an effective miticide serves to eliminate this cause as a differential.

Food Trials

Currently, a food allergy dietary trial is the only way to confirm or eliminate food allergy dermatitis as a cause of pruritus. No in vitro testing methods correlate with clinical disease. Limited-ingredient commercial diets offer the benefit of being balanced and suitable for long-term management. If the patient refuses to eat a variety of commercially available diets, a home-cooked diet can often be used successfully. During the 12-week trial phase, the patient should be fed a simple diet that consists of one or two ingredients. It is important that the patient not receive any additional treats or be allowed access to wild game (hunting). After the 12-week trial has been completed, the patient should be assessed for overall improvement. It is usually best to definitively confirm or rule out food allergy by challenging the patient with its previous diet. A food-allergic patient should demonstrate improvement during the 12-week food trial and should relapse within hours to days of exposure to its previous diet. Once it has been determined that the patient is allergic to a particular food, the patient should be transitioned to a balanced diet for long-term control. A balanced diet can be achieved by adding supplements to a home-cooked diet or by selecting a commercially prepared diet with ingredients that have been successfully used to control the allergy.

If the client and the patient cannot follow a strict limited-ingredient diet for 12 weeks, simply restricting the dog's diet to avoid all beef and all dairy ingredients may result in significant improvement without the extreme difficulty involved in providing a strict elimination diet.

CHAPTER 3

Bacterial Skin Diseases

- Pyotraumatic Dermatitis (acute moist dermatitis, hot spots)
- Impetigo (superficial pustular dermatitis)
- Superficial Pyoderma (superficial bacterial folliculitis)
- Deep Pyoderma
- Chin Pyoderma (canine acne)
- Skin Fold Dermatitis (intertrigo, skin fold pyoderma)
- Mucocutaneous Pyoderma
- Nasal Pyoderma (nasal folliculitis and furunculosis)
- Bacterial Pododermatitis
- Canine Pedal Furunculosis (interdigital bullae, interdigital pyogranuloma)
- Subcutaneous Abscess (cat and dog fight/bite abscess)

- Botryomycosis (bacterial pseudomycetoma, cutaneous bacterial granuloma)
- L-Form Infection
- Actinomycosis
- Nocardiosis
- Opportunistic Mycobacteriosis (atypical mycobacterial granuloma, mycobacterial panniculitis)
- Feline Leprosy Syndrome
- Canine Leproid Granuloma Syndrome (canine leprosy)
- Tuberculosis
- Plague

Pyotraumatic Dermatitis (acute moist dermatitis, hot spots)

Features

Pyotraumatic dermatitis is an acute and rapidly developing surface bacterial skin infection that occurs secondary to self-inflicted trauma. A lesion is created when the patient licks, chews, scratches, or rubs a focal area on its body in response to a pruritic or painful stimulus (Box 3-1). This usually is a seasonal problem that becomes more common when the weather is hot and humid. Fleas are the most common initiating stimulus. Pyotraumatic dermatitis is common in dogs, especially in thick-coated, long-haired breeds. It is rarely seen in cats.

Pyotraumatic dermatitis is an acutely pruritic, rapidly enlarging area of erythema, alopecia, and weepy, eroded skin with well-demarcated margins. Lesions are usually single, but they may be multiple and often are painful. They occur most frequently on the trunk, tail base, lateral thigh, neck, and face. A spreading superficial pyoderma is often present.

Top Differentials

Differentials include superficial pyoderma, demodicosis, and dermatophytosis.

37

Pyotraumatic Dermatitis—*cont'd*

BOX 3-1 Causes of Pyotraumatic Dermatitis

- Fleas
- Other parasites (e.g., pediculosis, cheyletiellosis, scabies)
- Hypersensitivity (e.g., atopy, food, flea bite)
- Anal sac disease
- Otitis externa
- Folliculitis (e.g., bacterial, *Demodex* sp., dermatophytic)
- Trauma (e.g., minor wounds, foreign body)
- Contact dermatitis

Diagnosis

1. History, clinical findings; rule out other differentials.
2. Cytology (impression smears): suppurative inflammation and mixed bacteria.

Treatment and Prognosis

1. The underlying cause (see Box 3-1) should be identified and treated.
2. Aggressive flea control should be provided.
3. The lesion should be clipped and cleaned, with the patient under sedation if necessary.
4. A topical drying agent or astringent (e.g., 5% aluminum acetate) should be applied every 8 to 12 hours for 2 to 7 days. Alcohol-containing products should be avoided.
5. If pruritus is mild, a topical analgesic (e.g., lidocaine, pramoxine hydrochloride) or corticosteroid-containing cream or solution should also be applied every 8 to 12 hours for 5 to 10 days.
6. If pruritus is severe, short-term steroids, such as injectable dexamethasone sodium phosphate (up to 0.1 mg/kg SQ or IM) or prednisone (0.5–1.0 mg/kg PO should be administered every 24 hours for 5 to 10 days), may be helpful.
7. If the central lesion is surrounded by papules or pustules, systemic antibiotic therapy should also be instituted and continued for 3 to 4 weeks (Box 3-2).
8. The prognosis is good if the underlying cause can be corrected or controlled.

BOX 3-2 Antibiotics for Bacterial Skin Infection*

Antibiotic and Dose
First-Line Drugs
- Cefadroxil 22 mg/kg q 8–12 hours
- **Cefpodoxime** 5–10 mg/kg q 12–24 hours
- **Cefovecin** sodium (Convenia) 8 mg/kg SQ
- Cephalexin 22 mg/kg q 8 hours, or 30 mg/kg q 12 hours
- Cephradine 22 mg/kg q 8 hours
- Clavulanated amoxicillin 12.5 mg/kg q 8 hours or 22 mg/kg q 12 hours
- **Ormetoprim/sulfadimethoxine** (Primor) 55 mg/kg once on day 1, then 27.5 mg/kg q 24 hours
- Oxacillin 22 mg/kg q 8 hours
- Trimethoprim/sulfadiazine 22–30 mg/kg q 12 hours

Second-Line Drugs
- Chloramphenicol 30–50 mg/kg q 8 hours
- Clindamycin hydrochloride 11 mg/kg q 12 hours
- Erythromycin 10–15 mg/kg q 8 hours

*Antibiotics in bold are the author's preferred selections because of improved owner compliance.

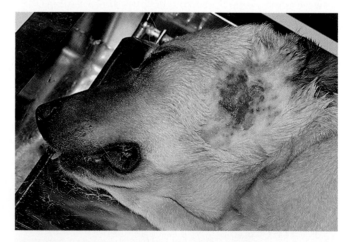

FIGURE 3-1 Pyotraumatic Dermatitis. This moist, erosive lesion on the base of the ear is characteristic of a hot spot.

Author's Note

Fluoroquinilone antibiotics may be indicated but likely increase the risk of methicillin resistance.

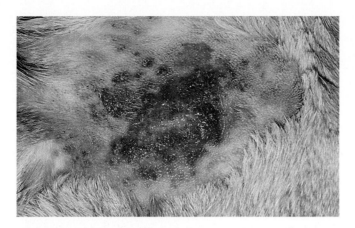

FIGURE 3-2 Pyotraumatic Dermatitis. Close-up of the dog in Figure 3-1. The moist, erosive surface of the lesion is apparent. The papular perimeter suggests an expanding superficial pyoderma.

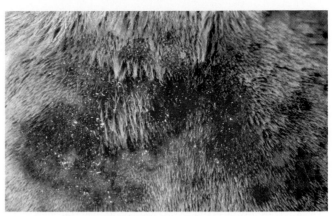

FIGURE 3-3 Pyotraumatic Dermatitis. Close-up of a hot spot demonstrating the erosive lesion with a moist serous exudate.

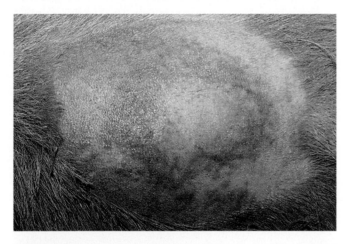

FIGURE 3-4 Pyotraumatic Dermatitis. An early superficial lesion (after clipping) on the lumbar region of a dog with flea allergy dermatitis. The papular perimeter suggests an expanding bacterial folliculitis.

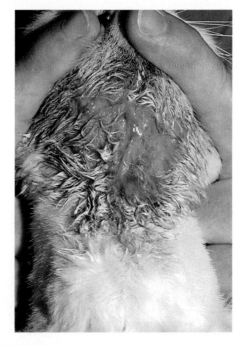

FIGURE 3-6 Pyotraumatic Dermatitis. A severe erosive lesion with exudate on the ventral neck of a food-allergic cat.

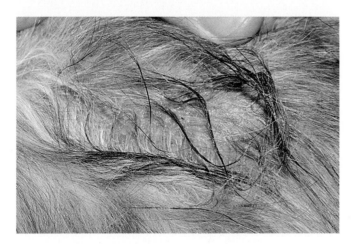

FIGURE 3-5 Pyotraumatic Dermatitis. This moist lesion developed acutely on the dorsum of this flea-allergic cat.

Impetigo (superficial pustular dermatitis)

Features

Impetigo is a superficial bacterial infection of nonhaired skin that may be associated with a predisposing disease or other underlying factors, such as endoparasitism, ectoparasitism, poor nutrition, or a dirty environment. It is commonly seen in young dogs before the time of puberty.

Impetigo is characterized by small, nonfollicular pustules, papules, and crusts that are limited to the inguinal and axillary skin. Lesions are not painful or pruritic.

Top Differentials

Differentials include demodicosis, superficial pyoderma, dermatophytosis, insect bites, and early scabies.

Diagnosis

1. Signalment, history, clinical findings; rule out other differentials.

2. Cytology (pustule): neutrophils and bacterial cocci.
3. Dermatohistopathology: nonfollicular subcorneal pustules that contain neutrophils and bacterial cocci.
4. Bacterial culture: *Staphylococcus* organisms.

Treatment and Prognosis

1. Any predisposing factors (poor hygiene and nutrition) should be identified and corrected.
2. Affected areas should be cleaned every 24 to 48 hours for 7 to 10 days with an antibacterial shampoo that contains chlorhexidine.
3. If lesions are few in number, topical mupirocin or neomycin ointment or cream should be applied every 12 hours for 7 to 10 days.
4. If lesions do not resolve with topical therapy, appropriate systemic antibiotics should be administered for 3 weeks, with treatment continued for 1 week beyond complete clinical resolution (see Box 3-2).
5. The prognosis is good.

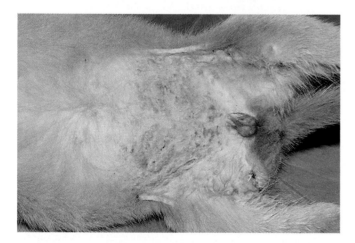

FIGURE 3-7 Impetigo. Numerous superficial pustules and crusts on the abdomen of this puppy are typical of this disease.

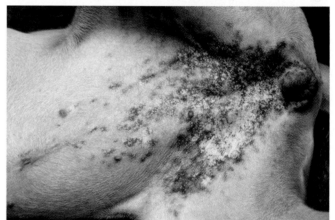

FIGURE 3-8 Impetigo. More chronic lesions demonstrated by hyperpigmented macules on the abdomen of a puppy. Note that the papular dermatitis is still apparent.

Superficial Pyoderma (superficial bacterial folliculitis)

Features

Superficial pyoderma is a superficial bacterial infection involving hair follicles and the adjacent epidermis. The infection is almost always secondary to an underlying cause; allergies and endocrine disease are the most common causes (Box 3-3). Superficial pyoderma is one of the most common skin diseases in dogs but is rare in cats.

Superficial pyoderma is characterized by focal, multifocal, or generalized areas of papules, pustules, crusts and scales, or epidermal collarettes, or circumscribed areas of erythema and alopecia, that may have hyperpigmented centers. Short-coated dogs often present with a "moth-eaten" patchy alopecia, small tufts of hair that stand up, or reddish brown discoloration of white hairs. In long-coated dogs, symptoms can be insidious and may include a dull, lusterless hair coat, scales, and excessive shedding. In both short- and long-coated breeds, primary skin lesions are often obscured by remaining hairs but can be readily appreciated if an affected area is clipped. Pruritus is variable, ranging from none to intense levels. Bacterial infection secondary to endocrine disease may cause pruritus, thereby mimicking allergic skin disease.

Staphylococcus pseudintermedius (previously *Staphylococcus intermedius*) is the most common bacterium isolated from canine pyoderma and is usually limited to dogs. *Staphylococcus schleiferi* is a bacterial species in dogs and humans that is emerging as a common canine isolate in patients with chronic infection and previous antibiotic exposure. Both *S. pseudintermedius* and *S. schleiferi* may develop methicillin resistance, especially if subtherapeutic doses of antibiotics or fluoroquinilone antibiotics have been used previously in the patient. Additionally, methicillin-resistant *Staphylococcus aureus* (human MRSA) is becoming more common among veterinary species. All three types of *Staphylococcus* may be zoonotic, moving from human to canine or from canine to human; immunosuppressed individuals are at greatest risk.

Top Differentials

Differentials include demodicosis, dermatophytosis, scabies, and autoimmune skin diseases.

Top Diagnosis

1. Rule out other differentials.
2. Cytology (pustule, skin impression): neutrophils and bacterial cocci.
3. Dermatohistopathology: epidermal microabscesses, nonspecific superficial dermatitis, perifolliculitis, and folliculitis. Intralesional bacteria may be difficult to find.
4. Bacterial culture: *Staphylococcus* species.

Top Treatment and Prognosis

1. The underlying cause must be identified and controlled.
2. Systemic antibiotics (minimum 3–4 weeks) should be administered and continued 1 week beyond complete clinical and cytologic resolution (see Box 3-2).
3. Concurrent bathing every 2 to 7 days with an antibacterial shampoo that contains chlorhexidine or benzoyl peroxide is helpful.
4. If lesions recur within 7 days of antibiotic discontinuation, the duration of therapy was inadequate and antibiotics should be reinstituted for a longer time period; better attempts to identify and control the underlying disease should be made.
5. If lesions do not completely resolve during antibiotic therapy, or if the antibiotics produce no response, antibiotic resistance should be assumed, and a bacterial culture and sensitivity submitted.
6. If antibiotic resistance is suspected or confirmed, frequent bathing (up to daily) and frequent application of topical chlorhexidine solutions, combined with simultaneous administration of two different classes of antibiotics at high doses, seem to produce the best results. Monitoring the infection with cytology and cultures with antibiotic sensitivities is important for determining when treatments can be stopped. Premature discontinuation of therapy, inability to completely control the primary disease, and the use of fluoroquinilone antibiotics will likely perpetuate the resistant infection.
7. The prognosis is good if the underlying cause can be identified and corrected or controlled.

BOX 3-3 Causes of Secondary Superficial and Deep Pyoderma

- Demodicosis, scabies, *Pelodera*
- Hypersensitivity (e.g., atopy, food, flea bite)
- Endocrinopathy (e.g., hypothyroidism, hyperadrenocorticism, sex hormone imbalance)
- Immunosuppressive therapy (e.g., glucocorticoids, progestational compounds, cytotoxic drugs)
- Autoimmune and immune-mediated disorders
- Trauma or bite wound
- Other skin diseases

Superficial Pyoderma—*cont'd*

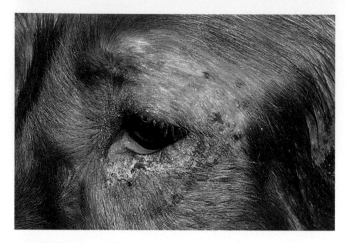

FIGURE 3-9 Superficial Pyoderma. Alopecia, papules, and crusts around the eye of this allergic Irish setter are typical of bacterial folliculitis.

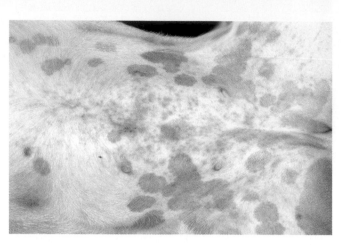

FIGURE 3-10 Superficial Pyoderma. Papular rash on the abdomen of an allergic dog caused by multidrug-resistant *Staphylococcus schleiferi*. The papular rash typical of pyoderma persisted despite high-dose antibiotic therapy, suggesting the antibiotic-resistant nature of the organism.

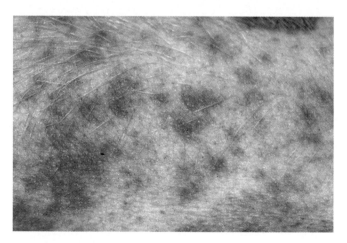

FIGURE 3-11 Superficial Pyoderma. Close-up of the papular rash in Figure 3-10.

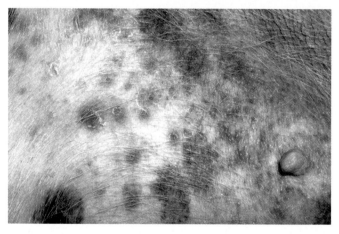

FIGURE 3-12 Superficial Pyoderma. This papular dermatitis forms coalescing lesions as demonstrated by the erythematous plaque. Note the early epidermal collarettes associated with some papules.

Author's Note

Superficial pyoderma is one of the most common skin diseases in dogs and almost always has an underlying cause (allergies or endocrine disease).

Cefpodoxime, ormetoprim/sulfadimethoxine (Primor), and Convenia provide the most consistent compliance; therefore they seem to help reduce the development of resistance when used at high doses.

Methicillin-resistant *Staphylococcus aureus* (MRSA), methicillin-resistant *S. schleiferi* (MRSS), methicillin-resistant *S. intermedius* (MRSI), and methicillin-resistant *S. pseudintermedius* (MRSP) are emerging problems in some regions of the United States.

The most likely risk factors include previous exposure to fluoroquinilone antibiotics, subtherapeutic antibiotic dosing, and concurrent steroid therapy.

Daily baths and topical treatments can be very beneficial in resolving the infection.

Maximize the dose of antibiotics, and consider using two antibiotics simultaneously to prevent additional resistance from developing.

Practice good hygiene (hand washing) to prevent zoonosis.

Consider screening dogs that visit the elderly or the sick to prevent zoonosis. Cultures from the nose, lips, ears, axilla, and perianal areas are best for screening patients for MRS.

Text continued on page 49.

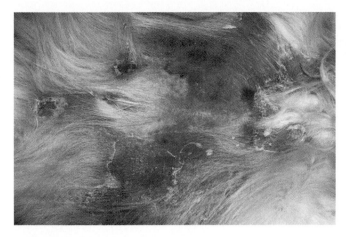

FIGURE 3-13 Superficial Pyoderma. Severe erythematous dermatitis with large epidermal collarettes caused by a multidrug-resistant infection.

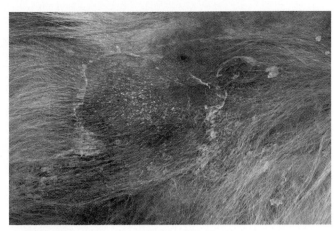

FIGURE 3-14 Superficial Pyoderma. Close-up of the dog in Figure 3-13. Erythematous dermatitis with epidermal collarettes formation is apparent.

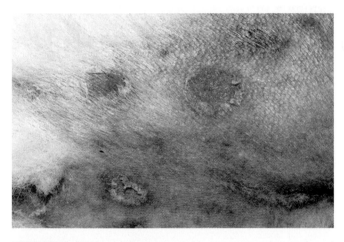

FIGURE 3-15 Superficial Pyoderma. More typical epidermal collarettes in a dog with resolving pyoderma.

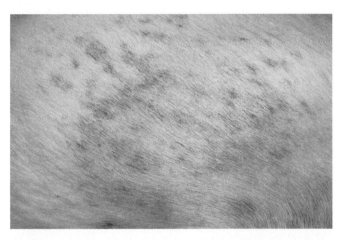

FIGURE 3-16 Superficial Pyoderma. This moth-eaten texture of the hair coat is a characteristic finding in short-coated breeds with pyoderma.

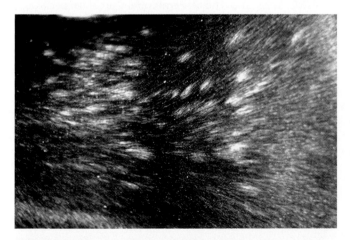

FIGURE 3-17 Superficial Pyoderma. The moth-eaten alopecia is typical of pyoderma in short-coated breeds.

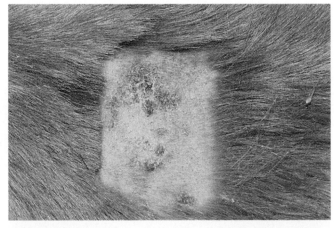

FIGURE 3-18 Superficial Pyoderma. Focal papules and crusts caused by pyoderma can be hidden by a dense fur coat. A window was clipped within the fur coat to reveal these lesions.

Superficial Pyoderma—*cont'd*

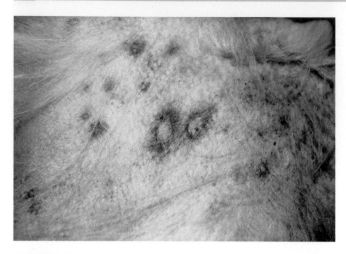

FIGURE 3-19 Superficial Pyoderma. Large pustules within an erythematous papular rash are an uncommon lesion in association with pyoderma. Pustules are easily ruptured, making them difficult to find.

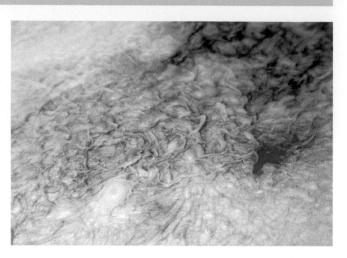

FIGURE 3-20 Superficial Pyoderma. Large coalescing pustules in a dog with underlying hyperadrenocorticism. Cushing's disease has altered the normal lesion development typically seen in pyoderma.

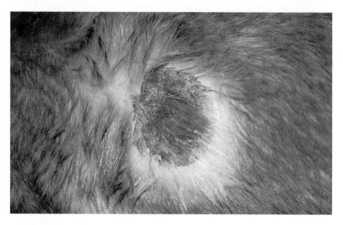

FIGURE 3-21 Superficial Pyoderma. This large focal area of alopecia, erythema, and hyperpigmentation with central regrowth of hair is often misdiagnosed as dermatophytosis.

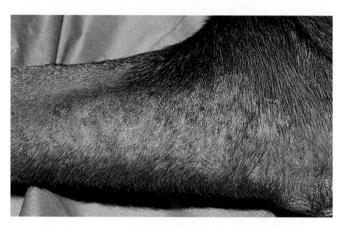

FIGURE 3-22 Superficial Pyoderma. Partial alopecia and mild papular rash on the foreleg of this dog were caused by secondary bacterial folliculitis associated with hypothyroidism.

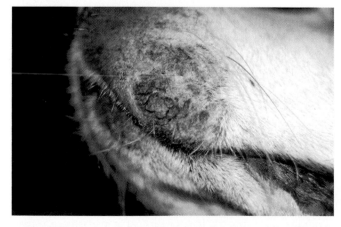

FIGURE 3-23 Superficial Pyoderma. This focal area of lichenification with adherent crust formation on the upper lip of a dog responded to topical mupirocin therapy. *(Courtesy L. Frank.)*

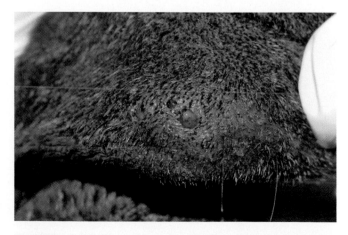

FIGURE 3-24 Superficial Pyoderma. Alopecic dermatitis with a purulent exudate on the lip of a dog. Note how the dog's normal pigmentation masks the papular dermatitis.

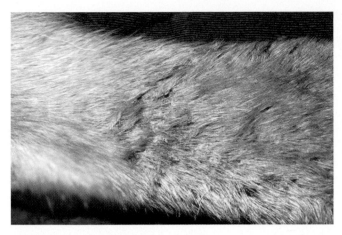

FIGURE 3-25 Superficial Pyoderma. Crusting papular dermatitis caused matting of the hair in this medium-haired dog. In thick-coated breeds, it may be difficult to see the underlying cutaneous lesions.

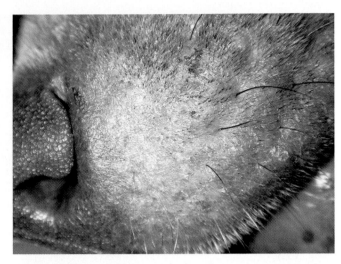

FIGURE 3-26 Superficial Pyoderma. Papular crusting dermatitis with alopecia on the muzzle of a dog.

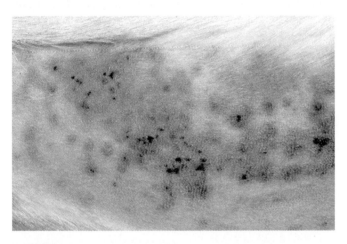

FIGURE 3-27 Superficial Pyoderma. Multifocal, punctate lesions on the dorsum are a typical feature of postbathing folliculitis and furunculosis.

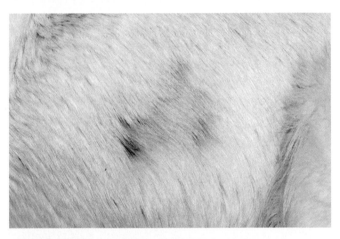

FIGURE 3-28 Superficial Pyoderma. Focal area of alopecia caused by folliculitis in an allergic dog. Cutaneous cytology is necessary.

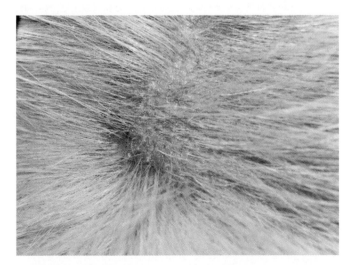

FIGURE 3-29 Superficial Pyoderma. Erythema caused by secondary infection in an allergic dog. The lesion is indistinguishable from a *Demodex*, dermatophyte, or yeast infection.

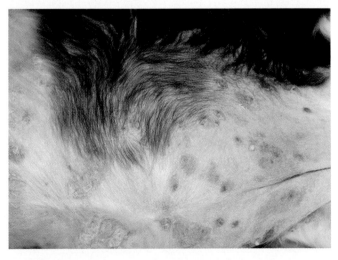

FIGURE 3-30 Superficial Pyoderma. Multiple papules, crusts, and epidermal collarettes in a dog with hypothyroidism.

Superficial Pyoderma—*cont'd*

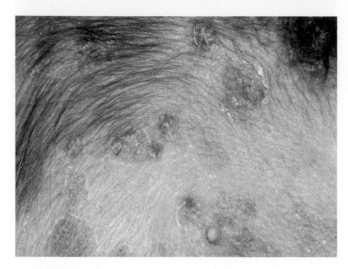

FIGURE 3-31 Superficial Pyoderma. Close-up of the dog in Figure 3-30. Papular rash with crusting is apparent.

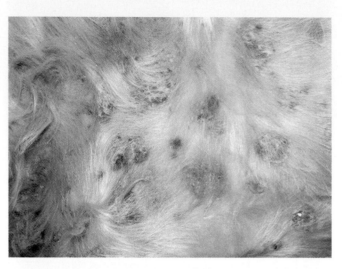

FIGURE 3-32 Superficial Pyoderma. Severe papular rash with crusting dermatitis in an allergic dog.

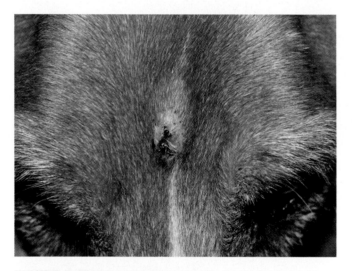

FIGURE 3-33 Superficial Pyoderma. An unusual pyoderma lesion on the head of a dog with allergies.

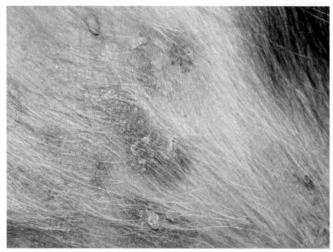

FIGURE 3-34 Superficial Pyoderma. Severe erythematous dermatitis without the typical papular, crusting rash, which is more typical of pyoderma.

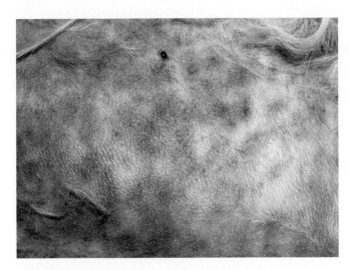

FIGURE 3-35 Superficial Pyoderma. Same dog as in Figure 3-34. Erythematous macular lesions without a papular rash are apparent.

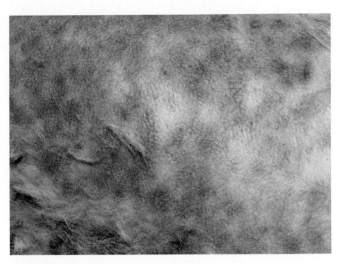

FIGURE 3-36 Superficial Pyoderma. Same dog as in Figure 3-34. Erythematous macular lesions without a papular rash are apparent.

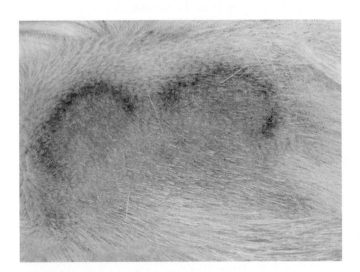

FIGURE 3-37 Superficial Pyoderma. Atypically shaped erythematous lesions in an allergic dog. Cutaneous cytology identified cocci, and the patient responded to oral antibiotics administered for 3 weeks.

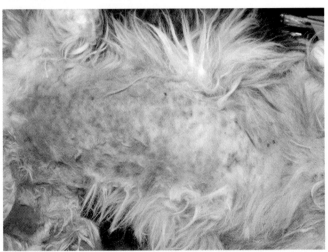

FIGURE 3-38 Superficial Pyoderma. Generalized dermatitis in an allergic dog. The severe inflammation is similar to staphylococcal scalded skin syndrome in humans.

Superficial Pyoderma—*cont'd*

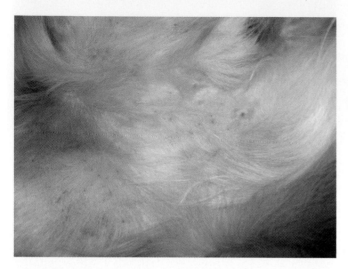

FIGURE 3-39 Superficial Pyoderma. Mild erythema and crusting papules on the abdomen of a male dog. Cytology identified cocci and ruled out demodicosis.

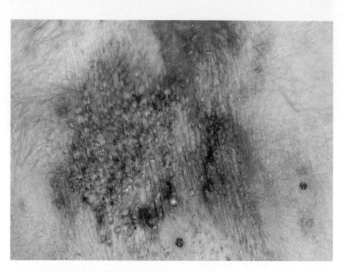

FIGURE 3-40 Superficial Pyoderma. Severe inflammation caused by secondary bacterial infection. Comedones and pustules are visible.

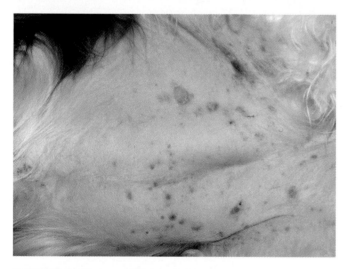

FIGURE 3-41 Superficial Pyoderma. Papular rash and epidermal collarettes are classic lesions caused by folliculitis. Cutaneous cytology is necessary to determine whether the cause is a bacterium, *Demodex*, or a dermatophyte.

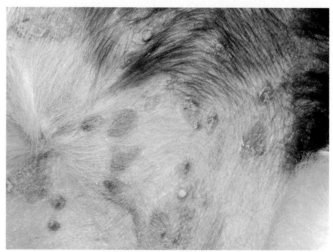

FIGURE 3-42 Superficial Pyoderma. Papular rash with epidermal collarettes typical of folliculitis in an allergic dog.

Deep Pyoderma

Features

Deep pyoderma is a surface or follicular bacterial infection that breaks through hair follicles to produce furunculosis and cellulitis. Its development is often preceded by a history of chronic superficial skin disease, and it is almost always associated with some predisposing factor (see Box 3-3). Deep pyoderma is common in dogs and rare in cats.

Staphylococcus pseudintermedius (previously *Staphylococcus intermedius*) is the most common bacterium isolated from canine pyoderma and is usually limited to dogs. *Staphylococcus schleiferi* is a bacterial species in dogs and humans that is emerging as a common canine isolate in patients with chronic infection and previous antibiotic exposure. Both *S. pseudintermedius* and *S. schleiferi* may develop methicillin resistance, especially if subtherapeutic doses of antibiotics or fluoroquinilone antibiotics have been used previously in the patient. Additionally, methicillin-resistant *Staphylococcus aureus* (human MRSA) is becoming more common among veterinary species. All three types of *Staphylococcus* may be zoonotic, moving from human to canine or from canine to human; immunosuppressed individuals are at greatest risk.

Deep pyoderma manifests as focal, multifocal, or generalized skin lesions characterized by papules, pustules, cellulitis, tissue discoloration, alopecia, hemorrhagic bullae, erosions, ulcers, and crusts, as well as serosanguineous to purulent draining fistulous tracts. Lesions are often pruritic or painful. They most often involve the trunk and pressure points but can appear anywhere on the body. Lymphadenomegaly is common. If the animal is also septic, other symptoms include fever, anorexia, and depression.

Top Differentials

Differentials include demodicosis, fungal infection, actinomycosis, nocardiosis, mycobacteriosis, neoplasia, and autoimmune skin disorders.

Diagnosis

1. Rule out other differentials.
2. Cytology (impression smears, exudate): suppurative to pyogranulomatous inflammation with bacterial cocci or rods.
3. Dermatohistopathology: deep suppurative to pyogranulomatous folliculitis, furunculosis, cellulitis, and panniculitis. Intralesional bacteria may be difficult to find.
4. Bacterial culture: primary pathogen is usually *Staphylococcus*, but occasionally, *Pseudomonas* is isolated. Mixed gram-positive and gram-negative bacterial infections are also common.

Treatment and Prognosis

1. Any underlying cause should be identified and corrected (see Box 3-3).
2. Crusts should be loosened and exudate removed with daily warm water soaks or whirlpool baths that contain a chlorhexidine solution. If tub soaks are not possible, shampoo therapy may be effective.
3. Systemic antibiotics should be administered over the long term (minimum 6–8 weeks) and should be continued 2 weeks beyond complete clinical resolution (see Box 3-2). Antibiotics should be selected on the basis of in vitro sensitivity results because resistance is common.
4. If lesions do not completely resolve during antibiotic therapy, or if the antibiotics produce no response, antibiotic resistance should be assumed, and a bacterial culture and sensitivity submitted.
5. If antibiotic resistance is suspected or confirmed, frequent bathing (up to daily) and frequent application of topical chlorhexidine solutions, combined with simultaneous administration of two different classes of antibiotics at high doses, seem to produce the best results. Monitoring the infection with cytology and cultures with antibiotic sensitivities is important for determining when treatments can be stopped. Premature discontinuation of therapy, inability to completely control the primary disease, and use of fluoroquinilone antibiotics will likely perpetuate the resistant infection.
6. The prognosis is good, but in severe or chronic cases, fibrosis, scarring, and alopecia may be permanent sequelae.

Deep Pyoderma—*cont'd*

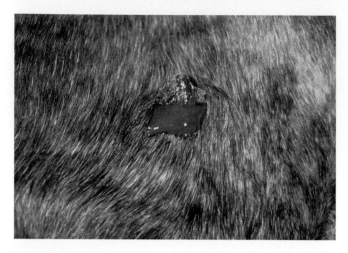

FIGURE 3-43 Deep Pyoderma. Purulent exudate from a deep ulcerative lesion and draining tract.

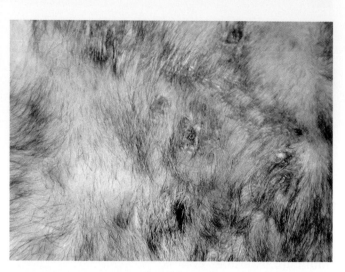

FIGURE 3-44 Deep Pyoderma. Patchy alopecia with focal crusted lesions covering ulcers and draining tracts. Note that deep pyoderma (cellulitis) affects a large region of skin, rather than discrete papules or pustules typical of superficial pyoderma.

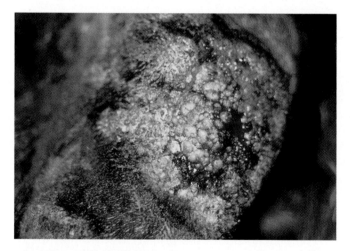

FIGURE 3-45 Deep Pyoderma. This focal area of alopecia and lichenification demonstrates an ulcer and draining tract typical of deep pyoderma. Note that lichenification is caused by the chronicity of the lesion.

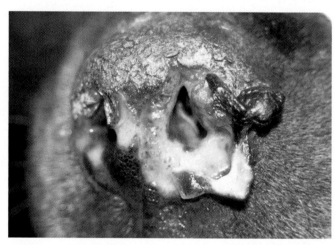

FIGURE 3-46 Deep Pyoderma. This aggressive bacterial infection was causing necrosis of large sections of skin, suggestive of necrotizing fasciitis. Numerous bacterial species, including methicillin-resistant *Staphylococcus aureus*, were isolated on culture.

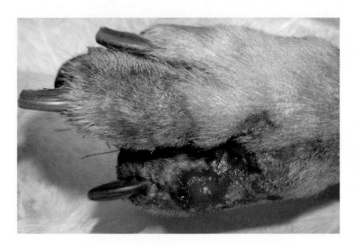

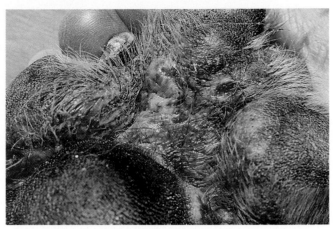

FIGURE 3-47 **Deep Pyoderma.** Diffuse erythematous dermatitis of the foot. The medial digit is the site of previous surgery; it subsequently became infected with *Pseudomonas*. Note that dermatitis of surrounding tissue is caused by opportunistic infection at the surgical site.

FIGURE 3-48 **Deep Pyoderma.** Severe interdigital dermatitis (alopecia, erythema, lichenification) with a moist exudate and draining tract typical of deep pyoderma.

Chin Pyoderma (canine acne)

Features

Chin pyoderma is a bacterial infection that is not true acne, but rather is a traumatic furunculosis. Short, stiff hairs are forced backward through the hair follicle, creating a sterile foreign body reaction that may become subsequently infected. This may be induced by trauma to the chin (e.g., caused by lying on hard floors, friction from chew toys). Chin pyoderma is common in short-coated breed dogs, especially when young (3- to 12-month-old).

Chin pyoderma manifests as nonpainful and nonpruritic comedones, papules, pustules, and bullae, or as ulcerative draining tracts with serosanguineous discharge, on the chin or muzzle. Often hair can be expressed from the lesions when gently squeezed.

Top Differentials

Differentials include demodicosis, dermatophytosis, early juvenile cellulitis, and contact dermatitis.

Diagnosis

1. Signalment, history, clinical findings; rule out other differentials.
2. Cytology (pustules, exudate, skin impression smear): suppurative inflammation and bacterial cocci.
3. Dermatohistopathology: follicular hyperkeratosis, folliculitis, or furunculosis. Intralesional bacteria may be difficult to find.
4. Bacterial culture: primary pathogen is usually *Staphylococcus*. Mixed bacterial infections are possible.

Treatment and Prognosis

1. Trauma and pressure to the chin should be minimized.
2. For mild lesions, the area should be scrubbed with benzoyl peroxide or chlorhexidine shampoo in the direction of hair growth. This mechanical scrubbing to remove "ingrown" hairs is important for preventing future lesions and speeding resolution.
3. Mupirocin ointment or benzoyl peroxide gel should be applied every 24 hours until lesions resolve, then every 3 to 7 days, as needed for control.
4. For moderate to severe lesions, in addition to topical treatment, systemic antibiotics should be administered (minimum 4–6 weeks) and continued 2 weeks beyond complete clinical and cytologic resolution (see Box 3-2).
5. Adhesive tape (Elasticon) can be used to tape strip the "ingrown" hairs, making hair removal both easy and fun.
6. The prognosis is good. In many dogs, the lesions resolve permanently; however, some dogs require lifelong routine topical therapy for control.

Author's Note

The cause of chin pyoderma is unknown, but focusing on removing the "ingrown" hairs seems to work well in preventing recurrence; however, active infections should be treated both topically and orally. Interdigital bullae may have a similar underlying pathology.

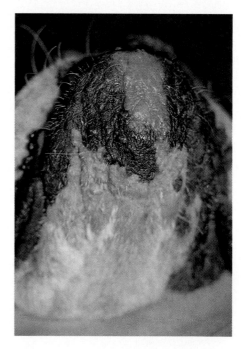

FIGURE 3-49 Chin Pyoderma. Erythematous papular lesions with alopecia on the chin of an English bulldog.

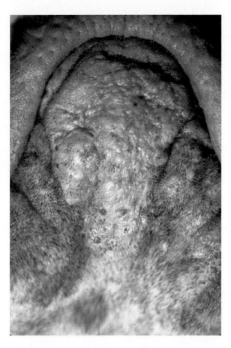

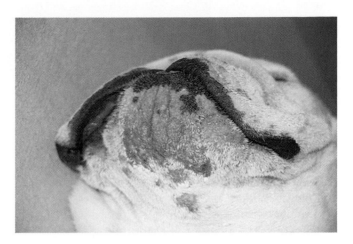

FIGURE 3-51 Chin Pyoderma. Mild erythematous papular lesions with alopecia on the chin of an English bulldog.

FIGURE 3-50 Chin Pyoderma. Alopecic papular dermatitis on the chin. Note the large dilated follicles associated with each papule.

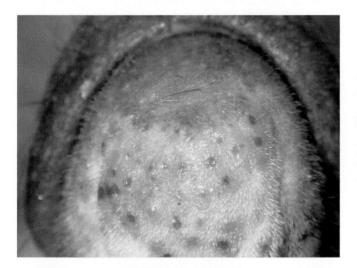

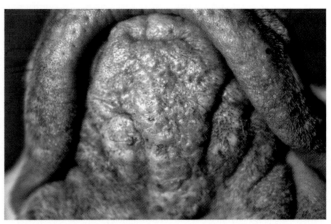

FIGURE 3-53 Chin Pyoderma. Severe papular dermatitis with alopecia on the chin and upper lip.

FIGURE 3-52 Chin Pyoderma. Severe papular crusting dermatitis with alopecia. Note that the purulent exudate suggests a deep infection.

Skin Fold Dermatitis (intertrigo, skin fold pyoderma)

Features

Skin fold dermatitis is a common bacterial surface skin infection that occurs in dogs with excessive skin folds. Infection involves the facial folds of brachycephalic breeds, the lip folds of dogs with large lip flaps, the tail folds of brachycephalic breeds with "corkscrew" tails, the vulvar folds of females with small recessed vulvas, and the body folds of dogs with excessive trunk or leg folds. Obesity is a common contributing factor; when addressed, the severity and recurrence of skin fold dermatitis are often improved.

Facial fold dermatitis: nonpainful, nonpruritic, erythematous facial folds that may also be malodorous. Concurrent traumatic keratitis or corneal ulceration is common.

Lip fold dermatitis: fetid breath caused by saliva accumulating in macerated, erythematous lower lip fold(s) is usually the presenting complaint. Concurrent dental calculi, gingivitis, and excessive salivation may contribute to the halitosis.

Tail fold dermatitis: skin under the tail is macerated, erythematous, and malodorous.

Vulvar fold dermatitis: symptoms include erythematous, macerated, and malodorous vulvar folds, excessive vulvar licking, and painful urination. A secondary urinary tract infection may be present, causing the skin fold infection (descending) or resulting from the urinary tract infection (ascending).

Body fold dermatitis: erythematous, seborrheic, often malodorous and sometimes mildly pruritic truncal or leg folds.

Top Differentials

Differentials include superficial pyoderma, *Malassezia* dermatitis, demodicosis, and dermatophytosis. Vulvar fold dermatitis also includes urine scald or primary cystitis or vaginitis.

Diagnosis

1. Signalment, history, clinical findings; rule out other differentials.
2. Cytology (impression smears): presence of mixed bacteria and possibly yeast.
3. Urinalysis (cystocentesis): bacteriuria in dogs with vulvar fold dermatitis that have a secondary urinary tract infection.

Treatment and Prognosis

1. A weight reduction program should be initiated if the dog is obese.
2. Cleansing wipes (i.e., alcohol-free acne pads, baby wipes, chlorhexidine-containing pledgets, other antimicrobial wipes) used every 12 to 72 hours work very well.
3. Alternatively, routine topical therapy can be used to control the skin problem. For facial, tail, lip, or vulvar fold dermatitis, the affected area should be cleaned every 1 to 3 days as needed with an antibacterial shampoo that contains chlorhexidine, benzoyl peroxide, or ethyl lactate.
4. Topical application of an antibiotic ointment, solution, or spray every 24 hours for the first 5 to 7 days of therapy may be helpful.
5. Any concurrent disease (e.g., corneal ulcers, dental disease, gingivitis, urinary tract infection) should be treated.
6. Surgical excision of excess facial, lip, or vulvar folds or tail amputation for tail fold dermatitis is usually curative.
7. Prognosis is good, but lifelong topical maintenance therapy may be needed if surgical correction is not performed.

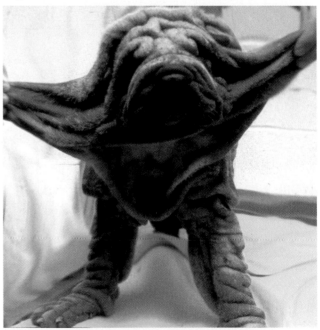

FIGURE 3-54 Skin Fold Dermatitis. A Shar pei with its distinctive wrinkles that predispose this breed to skin fold dermatitis.

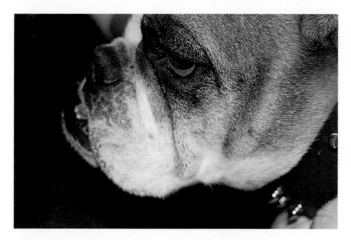

FIGURE 3-55 **Skin Fold Dermatitis.** A mature Boxer with a deep facial skin fold. Dermatitis was not apparent until the skin fold was examined.

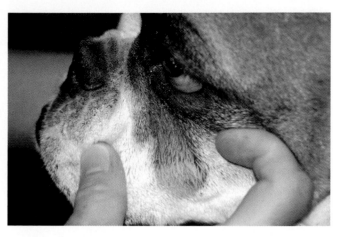

FIGURE 3-56 **Skin Fold Dermatitis.** Close-up of the dog in Figure 3-55. The skin fold was retracted, revealing a moist, erythematous dermatitis.

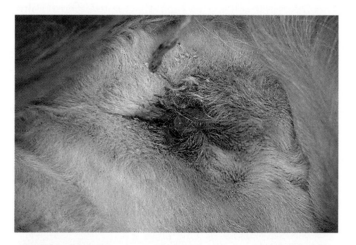

FIGURE 3-57 **Skin Fold Dermatitis.** A mature Golden retriever with vulvar fold dermatitis. Dermatitis was not apparent until the skin fold was retracted.

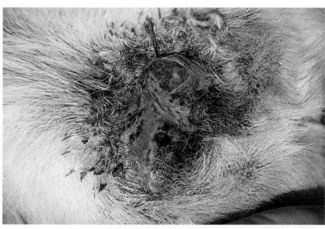

FIGURE 3-58 **Skin Fold Dermatitis.** Close-up of the dog in Figure 3-57. The skin fold was retracted, revealing a moist, severely erosive dermatitis.

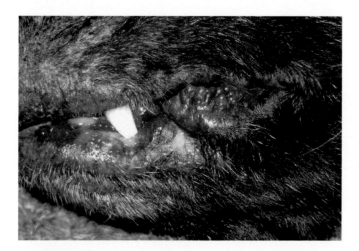

FIGURE 3-59 **Skin Fold Dermatitis.** Lip fold dermatitis. The inflamed lesion is not apparent until the fold is retracted.

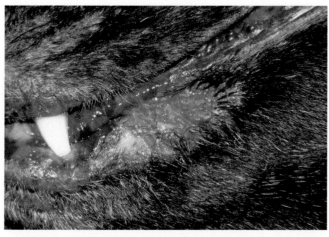

FIGURE 3-60 **Skin Fold Dermatitis.** Same dog as in Figure 3-59. The lip fold has been retracted, revealing moist, erosive dermatitis caused by the superficial bacterial infection.

Skin Fold Dermatitis—*cont'd*

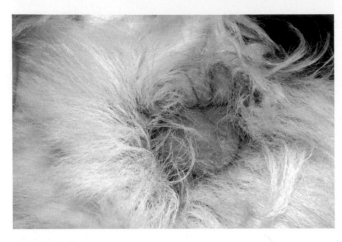

FIGURE 3-61 Skin Fold Dermatitis. Perivulvar dermatitis caused by superficial bacteria and yeast.

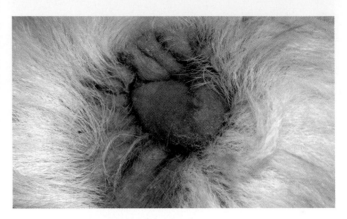

FIGURE 3-62 Skin Fold Dermatitis. Same dog as in Figure 3-61. The perivulvar tissue has been retracted, revealing the large area of alopecic, erythematous, lichenified skin. This dermatitis was caused by superficial bacterial and yeast infection.

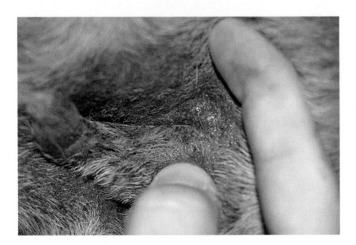

FIGURE 3-63 Skin Fold Dermatitis. A mature English bulldog with tail fold dermatitis. The deep skin folds associated with the tail of this breed are common sites for infection.

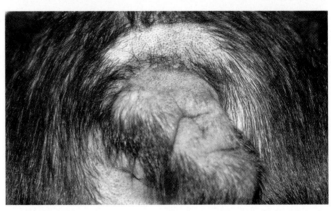

FIGURE 3-64 Skin Fold Dermatitis. Tail fold dermatitis.

Mucocutaneous Pyoderma

Features

Mucocutaneous pyoderma is a bacterial infection of mucocutaneous junctions. It is uncommon in dogs; German shepherds and their crosses are possibly predisposed, indicating possible association with the ulcerative syndromes of German shepherds (mucocutaneous pyoderma, perianal fistula, metatarsal ulceration).

Lesions are characterized by mucocutaneous swelling, erythema, and crusting, often bilateral and sometimes symmetrical. Affected areas may be painful or pruritic and self-traumatized; they may become exudative, eroded, ulcerated, fissured, and depigmented. The margins of the lips, especially at the commissures, are most frequently affected.

Top Differentials

Differentials include superficial pyoderma, lip fold dermatitis, autoimmune skin disorders, demodicosis, dermatophytosis, *Malassezia* dermatitis, candidiasis, and epitheliotropic lymphoma.

Diagnosis

1. History, clinical findings; rule out other differentials.

2. Cytology (impression smear): bacterial cocci or rods.
3. Dermatohistopathology: epidermal hyperplasia, superficial epidermal pustules, crusting, and lichenoid dermatitis with preservation of basement membrane. Dermal infiltrates often are predominantly composed of plasma cells, with varying numbers of lymphocytes, neutrophils, and macrophages.

Treatment and Prognosis

1. For mild to moderate lesions, affected areas should be clipped and cleaned with shampoo that contains chlorhexidine.
2. Topical mupirocin ointment or cream should be applied every 12 to 24 hours for 1 week, then every 3 to 7 days for maintenance therapy, as needed.
3. For severe lesions, in addition to topical therapy, appropriate systemic antibiotics should be administered for 3 weeks (see Box 3-2).
4. Prognosis is good if an underlying primary disease (e.g., allergy, endocrinopathy) can be identified and controlled, but lifelong maintenance therapy is often needed. If regularly applied, topical antibiotics may maintain remission.

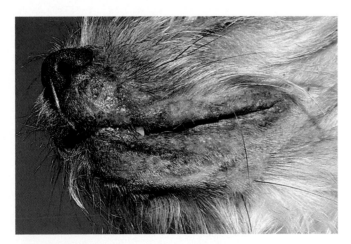

FIGURE 3-65 Mucocutaneous Pyoderma. The acute perioral dermatitis in this terrier was intensely pruritic. Alopecia, erythema, and erosions are visible around the mucocutaneous junction.

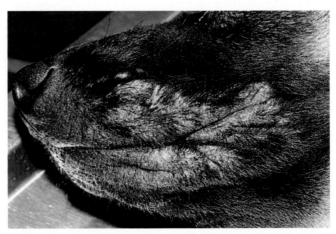

FIGURE 3-66 Mucocutaneous Pyoderma. Alopecia is the principal lesion in this German shepherd with perioral dermatitis.

Mucocutaneous Pyoderma—*cont'd*

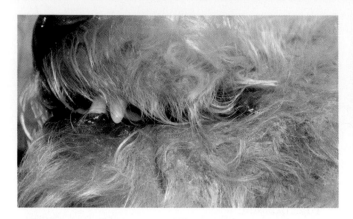

FIGURE 3-67 Mucocutaneous Pyoderma. This erythematous dermatitis with crusts was caused by a concurrent bacterial and *Malassezia* dermatitis.

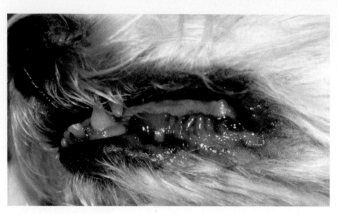

FIGURE 3-68 Mucocutaneous Pyoderma. Erythematous, alopecic dermatitis with a moist exudate predominantly on the lower lip.

Nasal Pyoderma (nasal folliculitis and furunculosis)

Features

Nasal pyoderma is a facial bacterial skin infection that may occur secondary to trauma or insect bites. This disease may be closely associated with eosinophilic furunculosis in that both disorders have very similar clinical progression and appearance. It is uncommon in dogs and rare in cats.

Nasal pyoderma appears as papules, pustules, erythema, alopecia, crusting, swelling, erosions, or ulcerative fistulae that develop over the bridge of the nose. Lesions may be painful.

Top Differentials

Differentials include eosinophilic furunculosis of the face (dog), demodicosis, dermatophytosis, autoimmune skin disorders, dermatomyositis, nasal solar dermatitis, and mosquito bite hypersensitivity (cat).

Diagnosis

1. Rule out other differentials.
2. Cytology (exudate, impression smear): suppurative inflammation with bacterial cocci or rods.
3. Dermatohistopathology: perifolliculitis, folliculitis, furunculosis, or cellulitis. Intralesional bacteria may be difficult to find.
4. Bacterial culture: primary pathogen is usually *Staphylococcus*, but mixed bacterial infections are also common.

Treatment and Prognosis

1. Gentle, topical, warm water soaks with a chlorhexidine shampoo should be used every 24 hours for 7 to 10 days to remove crusts.
2. Systemic antibiotics should be administered (minimum 3–4 weeks) and continued 2 weeks beyond complete clinical resolution (see Box 3-2).
3. The prognosis is good, but scarring may be a permanent sequela in some dogs.

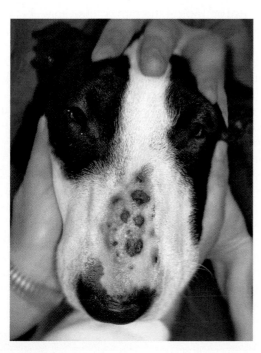

FIGURE 3-69 Nasal Pyoderma. Erythematous papular rash with alopecia on the dorsal nose. Note that the lesions are on haired skin, unlike autoimmune skin disease, which affects the nasal planum.

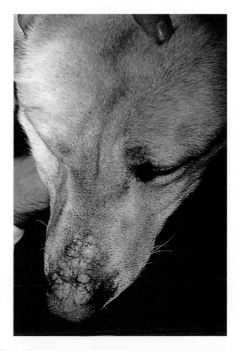

FIGURE 3-70 Nasal Pyoderma. Alopecia, erythema, and papular swelling on the bridge of a dog's nose. Note the similarity to eosinophilic furunculosis of the face. *(Courtesy D. Angarano.)*

Bacterial Pododermatitis

Features

Bacterial pododermatitis is a deep bacterial infection of the feet that almost always occurs secondary to some underlying factor (Box 3-4). It is common in dogs and rare in cats.

One or more feet may be affected by interdigital erythema, pustules, papules, nodules, hemorrhagic bullae, fistulae, ulcers, alopecia, or swelling. Pruritus (licking, chewing), pain, or lameness may be present. Regional lymphadenomegaly is common. Occasionally, pitting edema of the associated metatarsus or metacarpus is seen. Lesions spontaneously resolve, wax and wane, or persist indefinitely.

Top Differentials

Differentials include demodicosis, *Malassezia* pododermatitis, dermatophytosis, actinomycosis, nocardiosis, mycobacteriosis, deep fungal infection, autoimmune skin disorders, canine pedal furunculosis, and neoplasia.

Diagnosis

1. Rule out other differentials.
2. Cytology (impression smear, exudate): suppurative to pyogranulomatous inflammation with bacterial cocci or rods.
3. Dermatohistopathology: suppurative to pyogranulomatous perifolliculitis, folliculitis, furunculosis, and nodular to diffuse pyogranulomatous dermatitis. Intralesional bacteria may be difficult to find.
4. Bacterial culture: primary pathogen is usually *Staphylococcus*. Mixed bacterial infections are also common.

> **BOX 3-4 Causes of Secondary Bacterial Pododermatitis**
>
> - Foreign body (e.g., plant awn, wood splinter, thorn)
> - Parasite (e.g., demodicosis, ticks, *Pelodera*, hookworm dermatitis)
> - Fungus
> - Hypersensitivity (e.g., food, atopy)
> - Endocrinopathy (e.g., hypothyroidism, hyperadrenocorticism)
> - Trauma (e.g., stones, stubble, briars, wire floors, burns)
> - Autoimmune and immune-mediated skin disorders

Treatment and Prognosis

1. Any underlying cause should be identified and corrected (see Box 3-4).
2. Systemic antibiotics should be administered over the long term and continued 2 weeks beyond complete clinical resolution. The antibiotic should be selected on the basis of in vitro sensitivity results because resistance is common (see Box 3-2).
3. Cleansing wipes (alcohol-free acne pads, baby wipes, chlorhexidine-containing pledgets, or other antimicrobial wipes) used every 12 to 72 hours work very well.
4. For interdigital bullae, surgical removal of the ruptured hair follicle and "ingrown" hair with a biopsy punch or laser speeds resolution. For developing bullae, topical dimethyl sulfoxide (DMSO) combined with enrofloxacin (to make a 10-mg/mL solution) and steroid (dexamethasone or fluocinolone) should be applied every 12 to 72 hours until lesions resolve. To prevent recurrence, the feet should be wiped or scrubbed in the direction of hair growth to remove any "ingrown" hairs.
5. Adjunctive topical therapies that may be helpful include daily foot soaks for 10 to 15 minutes in 0.025% chlorhexidine solution, 0.4% povidone-iodine solution, or magnesium sulfate (30 mg/L water) for the first 5 to 7 days. Alternatively, foot scrubs with antibacterial shampoo or surgical scrub provided every 1 to 7 days as needed may be useful.
6. Foot trauma should be minimized by having the dog confined indoors, leash-walked, and kept away from rough surfaces.
7. Fusion podoplasty, whereby all diseased tissue is removed and digits are fused together, is a radical surgical alternative that is available for severe cases.
8. The prognosis is good to guarded, depending on whether the underlying cause can be identified and corrected. In severe and chronic cases, permanent fibrosis and scarring may contribute to future relapses by predisposing feet to traumatic injury.

> **Author's Note**
>
> Interdigital bullae are a common disorder of short-coated breeds.
>
> Active lesions should be removed and the patient treated for infection based on cytology and possible cultures.
>
> New bullae can be prevented with frequent wiping or scrubbing to the interdigital space in the direction of hair growth to remove and prevent "ingrown" hairs.
>
> Patients with interdigital bullae often have concurrent chin pyoderma, which is likely caused by a similar mechanism.

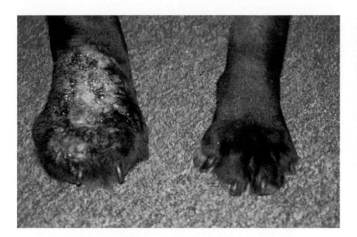

FIGURE 3-71 Bacterial Pododermatitis. Severe swelling with alopecia, ulcers, and draining lesions affecting only one foot. The infection had progressively worsened once over the previous several weeks.

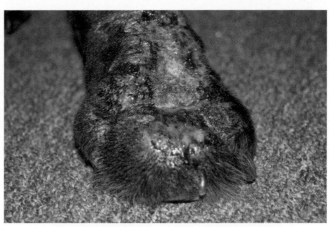

FIGURE 3-72 Bacterial Pododermatitis. Close-up of the dog in Figure 3-71. Profound tissue swelling and drainage with alopecia and crusting ulcers are apparent.

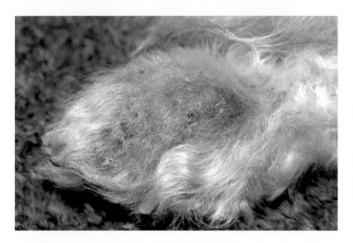

FIGURE 3-73 Bacterial Pododermatitis. Alopecia and crusting papular dermatitis that originated in the interdigital space progressing onto the dorsal surface of the foot. This bacterial infection occurred secondary to an underlying allergy. Note the lesion's similarity to yeast dermatitis.

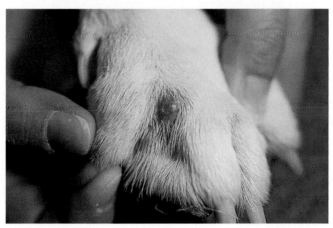

FIGURE 3-74 Bacterial Pododermatitis. This interdigital bulla (pedal furunculosis) was apparent only when the toes were separated and the interdigital space examined.

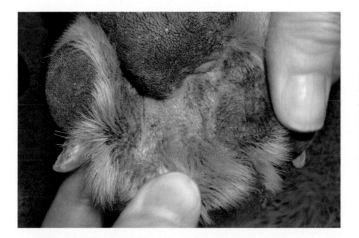

FIGURE 3-75 Bacterial Pododermatitis. Interdigital erythema and alopecia in an allergic dog. The bacterial infection is secondary to an underlying allergy and subsequent foot licking that created a persistently moist environment.

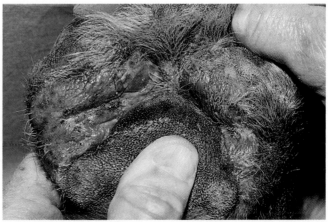

FIGURE 3-76 Bacterial Pododermatitis. Severe swelling with alopecia, erythema, and erosions. The infection occurred secondary to allergic dermatitis.

Bacterial Pododermatitis—*cont'd*

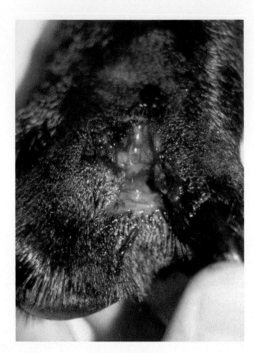

FIGURE 3-77 Bacterial Pododermatitis. This chronic interdigital fistula and draining tract (pedal furunculosis) were caused by a penetrating plant foreign body.

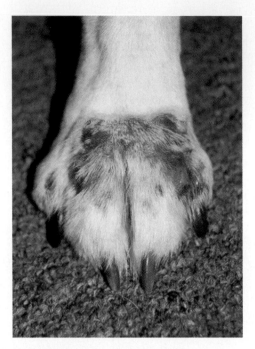

FIGURE 3-78 Bacterial Pododermatitis. Diffuse alopecia, erythema, and swelling affected most of the cutaneous surface. This severe case also had multiple erosions and draining lesions around the nail bed and in the interdigital space.

Canine Pedal Furunculosis (interdigital bullae, interdigital pyogranuloma)

Features

The etiopathogenesis is unclear, but one hypothesis is that sterile pedal furunculosis is a persistent, immune-mediated, inflammatory response to keratin and triglycerides liberated from ruptured hair follicles, sebaceous glands, and the panniculus. The condition is thought to develop after the initiating case of furunculosis (e.g., mechanical, infectious, parasitic, allergic) has been resolved. It is uncommon in dogs, with short-coated breeds possibly predisposed.

Canine pedal furunculosis manifests as single to multiple, erythematous papules; firm to fluctuant nodules; or bullae of one or more feet that appear in the interdigital areas. The lesions may be painful or pruritic, may ulcerate, may develop draining tracts with serosanguineous or purulent exudates, and, with chronicity, may become fibrotic. Lesions spontaneously resolve, wax and wane, or persist indefinitely. Regional lymphadenopathy is common, but no systemic signs of illness are noted. Secondary bacterial and yeast infections are common.

Interdigital bullae are a common problem in short-coated breeds. Their severity and recurrence are often worsened by underlying pruritic disease like atopy. Although the cause is unknown, short hairs that are forced through the follicle, creating a sterile furuncle, which subsequently becomes secondarily infected, seem to be an important component of the disease. "Ingrown" hairs are a key feature in the development of interdigital bullae.

Top Differentials

Differentials include bacterial pododermatitis, demodicosis, dermatophytosis, deep bacterial and fungal infections (cellulitis), autoimmune skin disorders, and neoplasia.

Diagnosis

1. Based on history, clinical findings; rule out other differentials.
2. Cytology (aspirate of nodule or nonruptured bulla): (pyo)granulomatous inflammation with no microorganisms unless secondary infections are present.
3. Dermatohistopathology: multifocal, nodular to diffuse, (pyo)granulomatous dermatitis. Special stains do not reveal infectious agents unless secondary infections are present.
4. Microbial cultures (biopsy specimens): negative for bacteria, mycobacteria, and fungi.

Treatment and Prognosis

1. The clinician should make sure that the initiating cause of the furunculosis (e.g., food allergy, wet environment, dirt kennels, friction in short-coated breeds) has been identified and corrected.
2. If draining lesions are secondarily infected, appropriate antibiotics or antifungal medications should be administered for a minimum of 4 to 6 weeks.
3. For solitary lesions, surgical excision or laser ablation may be curative.
4. Cleansing wipes (alcohol-free acne pads, baby wipes, chlorhexidine-containing pledgets, or other antimicrobial wipes) used every 12 to 72 hours work very well. For interdigital bullae, surgical removal of the ruptured hair follicle and "ingrown" hair with a biopsy punch or laser speeds resolution. For developing bullae, topical dimethyl sulfoxide (DMSO) combined with enrofloxacin (to make a 10-mg/mL solution) and steroid (dexamethasone or fluocinolone) should be applied every 12 to 72 hours until lesions resolve. To prevent recurrence, the feet should be wiped or scrubbed in the direction of hair growth to remove any "ingrown" hairs.
5. Alternatively, treatment with combination tetracycline and niacinamide may be effective in some dogs. A beneficial response should be seen within 6 weeks of treatment initiation. Administer 500 mg of each drug (dogs >10 kg) or 250 mg of each drug (dogs ≤10 kg) PO every 8 hours until lesions have resolved (approximately 2–3 months) (see Table 8-2). Then, administer each drug every 12 hours for 4 to 6 weeks, subsequently attempting to decrease frequency to every 24 hours for maintenance. Anecdotal reports suggest that doxycycline 10 mg/kg should be administered every 12 hours until response occurs, then tapered to the lowest effective dose (doxycycline may be substituted for tetracycline).
6. Anecdotal reports suggest that treatment with cyclosporine 5 mg/kg PO administered every 24 hours may be effective in some dogs. Once clinical resolution is achieved (usually within 6 weeks), cyclosporine should be gradually tapered to the lowest possible daily or alternate-day dose that maintains remission. Addition of ketoconazole (5–11 mg/kg/day PO with food) to the regimen may allow for further reduction in the cyclosporine dosage.
7. For severe, nonsurgical, or multiple lesions, treatment with glucocorticosteroids may be effective. Prednisone or prednisolone 2–4 mg/kg PO should be administered every 24 hours. Significant improvement should be seen within 1 to 2 weeks. After lesions have resolved (approximately 2–3 weeks),

Canine Pedal Furunculosis—*cont'd*

the steroid dose should be gradually tapered to the lowest alternate-day dose that maintains remission. In some dogs, steroid therapy can eventually be discontinued. Secondary infections are common and should be treated aggressively.

8. The prognosis is good to fair. Lifelong medical therapy may be needed to maintain remission, and interdigital fibrosis may be a permanent sequela in chronic cases.

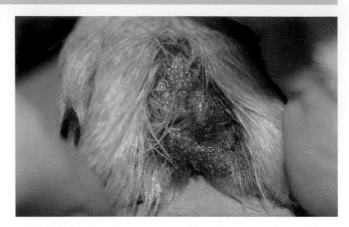

FIGURE 3-81 Pedal Furunculosis. Interdigital bulla with a moist exudate and bruising of the surrounding tissue.

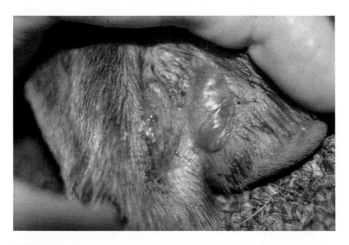

FIGURE 3-79 Pedal Furunculosis. The large, flaccid bulla in the interdigital space is typical of this disease.

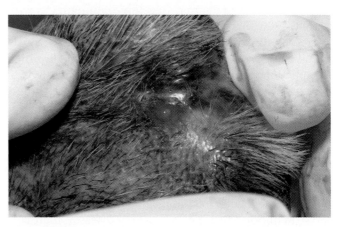

FIGURE 3-82 Pedal Furunculosis. The toes have been separated, revealing the interdigital space, which appears bruised. The skin seems thin, with a focal area of exudate identifying a focal abscess.

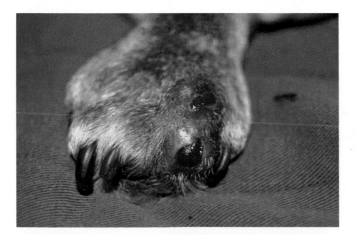

FIGURE 3-80 Pedal Furunculosis. Severe interdigital tissue swelling with ulceration was caused by traumatic furunculosis and subsequent recurrent bacterial infections.

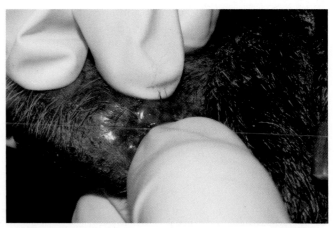

FIGURE 3-83 Pedal Furunculosis. The clinician is applying gentle pressure to the lateral aspects of the lesion to demonstrate the presence of hair within the abscess. This technique is not recommended because rupturing the lesion internally could worsen cellulitis and scarring.

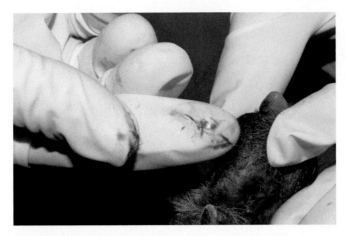

FIGURE 3-84 Pedal Furunculosis. Expressed material includes an exudate with numerous hairs. These hairs act as a foreign body and a nidus for recurrent secondary infections.

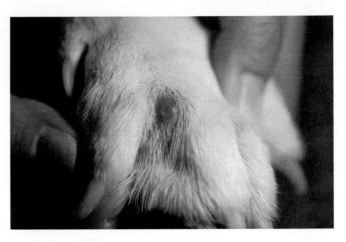

FIGURE 3-85 Pedal Furunculosis. A small interdigital bulla.

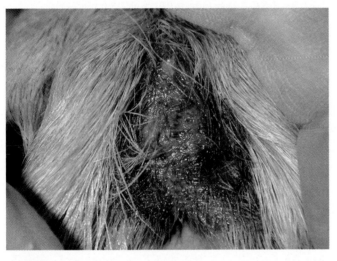

FIGURE 3-86 Pedal Furunculosis. The interdigital tissue is affected by a severe pyogranulomatous infiltrate that results in cellulitis.

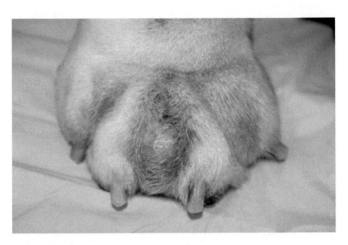

FIGURE 3-87 Pedal Furunculosis. Severe swelling of the interdigital space caused by chronic inflammation.

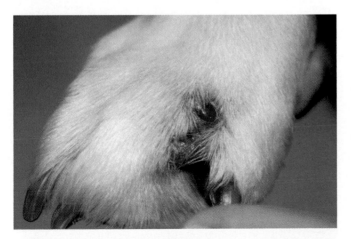

FIGURE 3-88 Pedal Furunculosis. A focal interdigital bulla that has ruptured and is draining a purulent exudate.

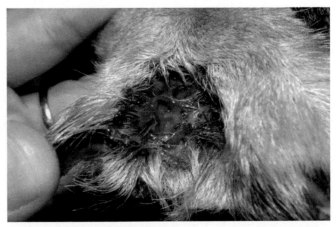

FIGURE 3-89 Pedal Furunculosis. Severe interdigital cellulitis with a deep ulcerative tract.

Subcutaneous Abscess (cat and dog fight/bite abscess)

Features

Disease occurs when normal oral bacterial microflorae are inoculated into the skin through puncture wounds. A history of a recent cat or dog fight can usually be documented. Subcutaneous abscesses are common in dogs and cats, especially among intact male cats.

Subcutaneous abscesses are characterized by localized, often painful, swelling or abscess with a crusted-over puncture wound from which a purulent material may drain. Lesions are most commonly found on the tail base, shoulder, neck, face, or leg. Regional lymphadenomegaly is common. Animals may be febrile, anorexic, and depressed.

Top Differentials

Differentials include abscess caused by a foreign body, other bacteria (e.g., actinomycosis, nocardiosis, mycobacteriosis), or neoplasia.

Diagnosis

1. History, clinical findings.
2. Cytology (exudate): suppurative inflammation with a mixed bacterial population.
3. Polymerase chain reaction (PCR) analysis, where available, may simplify the diagnosis.

Treatment and Prognosis

1. The abscess should be clipped, lanced, and cleaned with 0.025% chlorhexidine solution.
2. Systemic antibiotics should be administered for 7 to 10 days, or until lesions completely heal. Effective antibiotics include the following:
   - Amoxicillin 20 mg/kg PO, SQ, or IM q 8–12 hours (cats)
   - Clavulanated amoxicillin 22 mg/kg PO q 8–12 hours
   - Clindamycin 10 mg/kg PO or IM q 12 hours
   - Cefovecin sodium (Convenia) 8 mg/kg SQ
3. The prognosis is good. Castrating intact male cats is a helpful preventive measure.

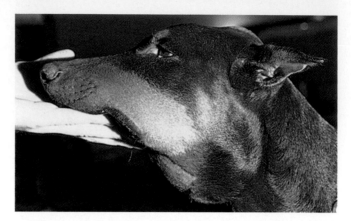

FIGURE 3-90 Subcutaneous Abscess. Submandibular swelling in this Doberman was caused by an extensive subcutaneous abscess. *(Courtesy D. Angarano.)*

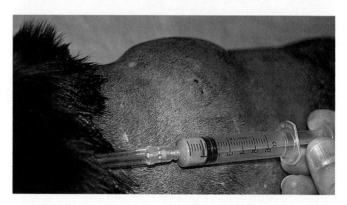

FIGURE 3-91 Subcutaneous Abscess. Feline abscess caused by a cat bite. The syringe contains purulent material aspirated from the abscess.

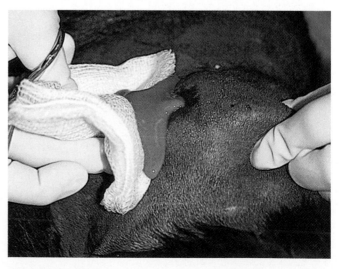

FIGURE 3-92 Subcutaneous Abscess. Same cat as in Figure 3-91. The abscess has been lanced, and purulent material is easily expressed.

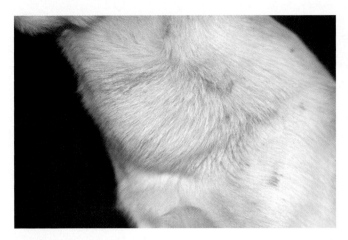

FIGURE 3-93 **Subcutaneous Abscess.** Large subcutaneous swelling on the neck, typical of an abscess.

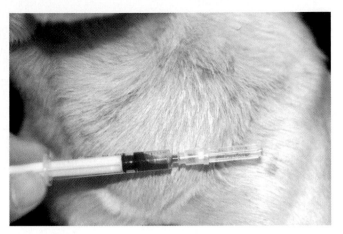

FIGURE 3-94 **Subcutaneous Abscess.** Same dog as in Figure 3-93. The syringe contains fluid aspirated from the mass. Note that the serosanguineous fluid is more typical of a seroma.

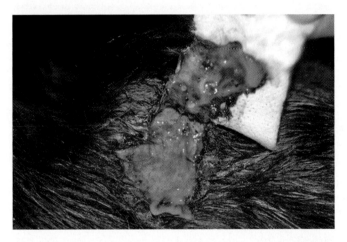

FIGURE 3-95 **Subcutaneous Abscess.** Purulent exudate covering a large ulcer on the dorsum of a cat. Necrotic skin covering the abscess has been debrided and is lying on the gauze pad.

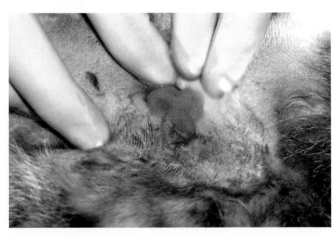

FIGURE 3-96 **Subcutaneous Abscess.** Purulent exudate being expressed from an abscess on the inguinal region of a cat.

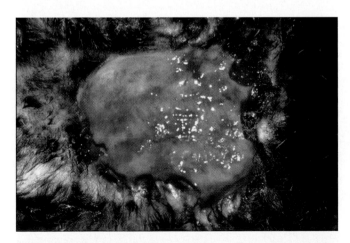

FIGURE 3-97 **Subcutaneous Abscess.** Large ulcer on the thorax of a cat covered with a purulent exudate. The overlying skin had necrosed and was removed.

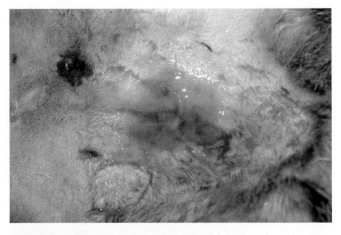

FIGURE 3-98 **Subcutaneous Abscess.** The abundance of purulent exudate is typical of feline abscesses.

Botryomycosis (bacterial pseudomycetoma, cutaneous bacterial granuloma)

Features

Botryomycosis is an unusual type of skin infection in which bacterial organisms form macroscopic or microscopic tissue granules. Infection may be a sequela to a penetrating injury, foreign body reaction, or bite wound. Botryomycosis is uncommon in dogs and cats.

Botryomycosis appears as single to multiple nonpainful, and usually nonpruritic, firm nodules with draining fistulae. Purulent discharge may contain small, white granules (macroscopic colonies of bacteria). Lesions develop slowly and may appear anywhere on the body.

Top Differentials

Differentials include actinomycosis, nocardiosis, mycobacteriosis, deep fungal infection, neoplasia, and foreign body reaction.

Diagnosis

1. Cytology (exudate): suppurative inflammation that may contain granules composed of dense bacterial colonies.
2. Dermatohistopathology: nodular to diffuse (pyo) granulomatous dermatitis and panniculitis with tissue granules composed of bacteria.
3. Bacterial culture: causative organism is usually *Staphylococcus*, but occasionally other bacteria such as *Pseudomonas* or *Proteus* are isolated.
4. PCR analysis, where available, may simplify the diagnosis.

Treatment and Prognosis

1. Nodules should be surgically excised; systemic antibiotics should be administered over the long term (minimum 4 weeks) based on in vitro sensitivity results. Without surgery, antibiotic therapy alone is rarely effective.
2. The prognosis is good with combined surgical and medical therapy.

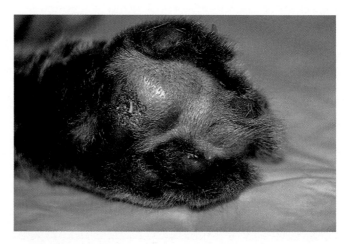

FIGURE 3-100 Botryomycosis. The swelling of this cat's foot was associated with moderate pain and lameness. The crust was covering a deep tract that periodically drained a purulent exudate.

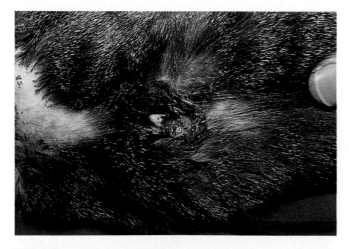

FIGURE 3-99 Botryomycosis. Deep draining lesion with superficial crust formation on the dorsum of a cat.

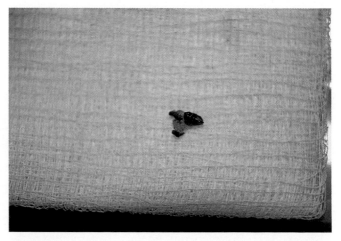

FIGURE 3-101 Botryomycosis. Tissue grain dissected from the foot of the cat shown in Figure 3-100.

L-Form Infection

Features

L-form infection is a skin infection caused by cell wall–deficient bacteria that contaminate bite wounds or surgical incisions. It is uncommon in cats and rare in dogs.

L-form infection is characterized by persistently spreading and draining cellulitis and synovitis that usually begin on the extremities. Concurrent fever is present. Polyarthritis may also be seen.

Top Differentials

Differentials include other bacterial (e.g., actinomycosis, nocardiosis, mycobacteriosis) and deep fungal infections and neoplasia.

Diagnosis

1. Rule out other differentials.
2. Cytology (exudate): pyogranulomatous inflammation. L-forms cannot be visualized, but contaminating bacterial cocci and rods may be present.
3. Dermatohistopathology (nondiagnostic): pyogranulomatous dermatitis.
4. Radiography: periarticular soft tissue swelling and periosteal proliferation.
5. Bacterial culture: L-forms cannot be cultured unless special L-form medium is used. Contaminant bacteria are often isolated.
6. Electron microscopy (biopsy specimens): pleomorphic cell wall–deficient organisms are found in phagocytes.
7. PCR analysis, where available, may simplify the diagnosis.

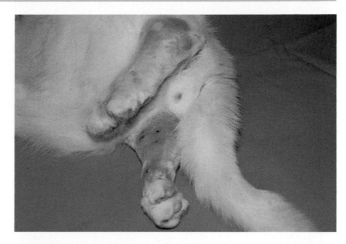

FIGURE 3-102 L-forms Infection. Diffuse cellulitis with multiple draining tracts. Confirming this diagnosis may be difficult and may require special laboratory techniques. *(Courtesy University of Florida; case material.)*

Treatment and Prognosis

1. Antibiotics typically used to treat other bacterial infections are not effective.
2. Tetracycline 22 mg/kg PO should be administered every 8 hours, or doxycycline 5–10 mg/kg PO every 12 hours. Treatment should be continued at least 1 week beyond complete clinical resolution.
3. The prognosis is good. In severe cases, however, chronic arthritis may be a permanent sequela.

Actinomycosis

Features

Actinomycosis is a disease that occurs when *Actinomyces*, a normally nonpathogenic bacterium found in the oral cavity, is inadvertently inoculated into tissue. A previous history of bite wound or penetrating injury at the site of infection can usually be documented. Actinomycosis is an uncommon cause of skin disease in cats and dogs; the greatest incidence is noted in outdoor and hunting dogs.

Dogs

Actinomycosis appears as subcutaneous, firm to fluctuant swellings and abscesses that may fistulate or ulcerate. Drainage is serosanguineous to purulent and often malodorous, and may contain yellow-tan granules (macroscopic colonies of Actinomycetes). The ventral and lateral cervical, mandibular, and submandibular areas are most often affected. Chronic progressive weight loss and fever suggest concurrent thoracic or abdominal cavity involvement.

Cats

Pyothorax and subcutaneous abscesses that contain a malodorous, serosanguineous to purulent exudate are the most common presentations of actinomycosis in cats.

Top Differentials

Differentials include other bacterial and deep fungal infections and neoplasia.

Diagnosis

1. Rule out other differentials.
2. Cytology (exudate): suppurative to pyogranulomatous inflammation with a mixed population of bacteria that includes *Actinomyces* organisms. Actinomycetes appear individually or in aggregate as gram-positive, non–acid-fast, beaded, filamentous organisms with occasional branching. The organisms may be difficult to find.
3. Dermatohistopathology: nodular to diffuse suppurative or pyogranulomatous dermatitis and panniculitis that may contain tissue grains composed of gram-positive, non–acid-fast, filamentous organisms. The organisms may be difficult to find.
4. Anaerobic bacterial culture (deep percutaneous aspirate or biopsy specimen directly inoculated into anaerobic transport medium [refrigeration should be avoided]): often, a mixed bacterial population is isolated that may not include *Actinomyces* because *Actinomyces* have fastidious growth requirements and are difficult to culture.
5. PCR analysis, where available, may simplify the diagnosis.

Treatment and Prognosis

1. Wide surgical excision and tissue debulking should be performed to remove as much diseased tissue as possible. Surgery may spread the infection along tissue planes.
2. Systemic antibiotics should be administered over the long term (several months) and continued several weeks beyond complete clinical resolution.
3. The antibiotic of choice is penicillin G potassium (PO, SQ, IM, IV) or penicillin V potassium (PO); recommended dosage is at least 60,000 U/kg every 8 hours.
4. Alternative drugs that may be effective include the following:
   - Clindamycin 5–10 mg/kg SQ q 12 hours
   - Erythromycin 10 mg/kg PO q 8 hours
   - Minocycline 5–25 mg/kg IV or PO q 12 hours
   - Amoxicillin 20–40 mg/kg IM, SQ, or PO q 6 hours
5. The prognosis for cure is guarded. This disease is not considered contagious to other animals or to humans.

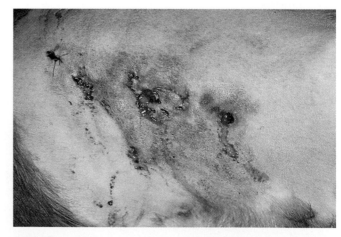

FIGURE 3-103 Actinomycosis. Diffuse cellulitis with multiple draining tracts on the lumbar region of this dog had persisted for several months.

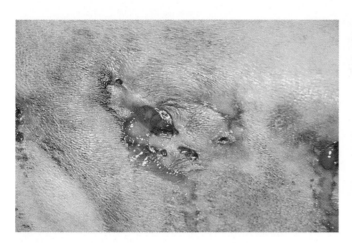

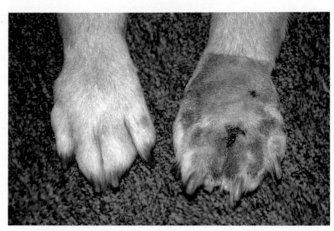

FIGURE 3-104 **Actinomycosis.** Close-up of the dog in Figure 3-103. Deep draining tracts with tissue discoloration typical of cellulitis are apparent.

FIGURE 3-105 **Actinomycosis.** Severe swelling with erythema and a draining tract on the foot of an adult dog. Note that the skin and subcutaneous tissue have been sampled for histopathology and minced tissue culture (bacterial and fungal cultures).

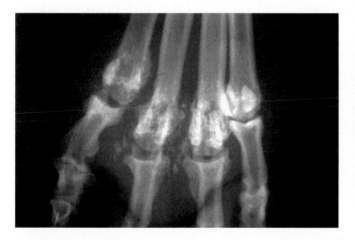

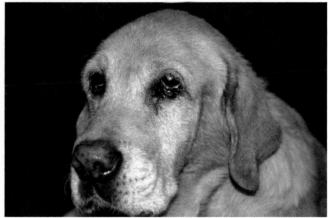

FIGURE 3-106 **Actinomycosis.** Same dog as in Figure 3-105. A radiograph of the foot demonstrated bony changes consistent with cellulitis and osteomyelitis.

FIGURE 3-107 **Actinomycosis.** Same dog as in Figure 3-105. The tragic facial expression was caused by underlying hypothyroidism, which likely predisposed the dog to developing actinomycosis.

Nocardiosis

Features

Nocardiosis is a cutaneous disease that occurs when *Nocardia*, a soil saprophyte, is inadvertently inoculated into a skin puncture wound. It is uncommon in dogs and cats.

Nocardiosis manifests as localized nodules, cellulitis, and abscesses, with ulcerations and fistulous tracts that drain a serosanguineous discharge. Lesions usually occur on the limbs, feet, or abdomen. Peripheral lymphadenomegaly is common.

Top Differentials

Differentials include other bacterial and deep fungal infections and neoplasia.

Diagnosis

1. Rule out other differentials.
2. Cytology (exudate): suppurative to pyogranulomatous inflammation with individual or loose aggregates of gram-positive, partially acid-fast, beaded, branching filamentous organisms.
3. Dermatohistopathology: nodular to diffuse pyogranulomatous dermatitis and panniculitis, with intralesional gram-positive, partially acid-fast, branching, beaded organisms that may form tissue grains.
4. Bacterial culture: *Nocardia*.
5. PCR analysis, where available, may simplify the diagnosis.

Treatment and Prognosis

1. The practitioner should surgically drain, debulk, and excise as much diseased tissue as possible. Surgery may spread the infection along tissue planes.
2. Systemic antibiotics should be administered over the long term (weeks to months) and continued at least 4 weeks beyond complete clinical resolution. Antibiotic selection should be based on in vitro susceptibility results, if possible.
3. Antibiotics that may be effective empirically include the following:
   - Sulfadiazine 80 mg/kg PO q 8 hours, or 110 mg/kg PO q 12 hours
   - Sulfamethizole 50 mg/kg PO q 8 hours
   - Sulfisoxazole 50 mg/kg PO q 8 hours
   - Trimethoprim-sulfadiazine 15–30 mg/kg PO or SQ q 12 hours
   - Ampicillin 20–40 mg/kg IV, IM, SQ, or PO q 6 hours
   - Erythromycin 10 mg/kg PO q 8 hours
   - Minocycline 5–25 mg/kg PO or IV q 12 hours
4. The prognosis for cure is guarded. This disease is not contagious to other animals or to humans.

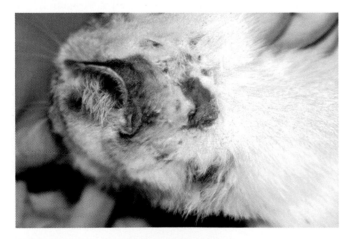

FIGURE 3-108 Nocardiosis. Ulcerative crusting lesions with a purulent exudate on the head and base of the ear of an adult cat.

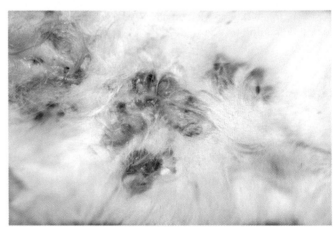

FIGURE 3-109 Nocardiosis. Same cat as in Figure 3-108. Multiple ulcerative draining lesions on the abdomen. Note the similarity of the lesions and the location with opportunistic mycobacteriosis in cats.

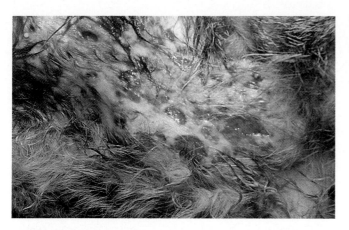

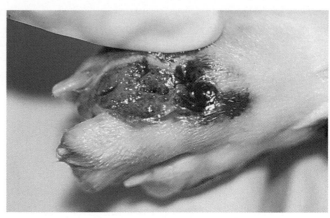

FIGURE 3-110 Nocardiosis. Numerous ulcerative draining lesions on the abdomen of an adult cat. The lesions and location are typical for nocardiosis and opportunistic mycobacteriosis in cats.

FIGURE 3-111 Nocardiosis. The deep ulcerative lesion on the dorsal surface of this dog's foot developed over several months. Deep tracts with tissue proliferation can be seen with any aggressive bacterial or fungal infection.

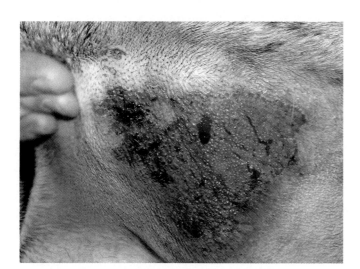

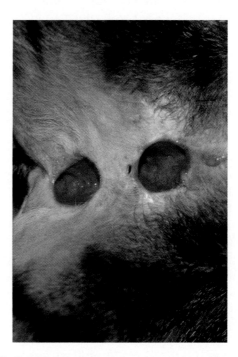

FIGURE 3-112 Nocardiosis. Focal area of erosive dermatitis with draining lesions on the inguinal area of an adult Great Dane. Gloves should be worn when any draining lesion is examined.

FIGURE 3-113 Nocardiosis. Large open ulcers on the abdomen. *(Courtesy L. Schmeitzel.)*

Opportunistic Mycobacteriosis (atypical mycobacterial granuloma, mycobacterial panniculitis)

Features

Opportunistic mycobacteriosis is a deep-seated skin infection that occurs when saprophytic mycobacteria, normally found in soil and water, are inadvertently inoculated into the skin through puncture wounds. Most cases are caused by mycobacteria that grow rapidly on culture medium. Opportunistic mycobacteriosis is uncommon in cats and rare in dogs; obese animals may be predisposed.

Opportunistic mycobacteriosis appears as chronic, nonhealing, slowly developing, alopecic subcutaneous nodules, abscesses, and cellulites, with focal purple depressions intermingled with punctate ulcers and fistulae that drain a serosanguineous or purulent discharge. Lesions may appear anywhere on the body, but in cats, the adipose tissue of the inguinal and caudal abdominal area is most often involved. The infected area gradually increases in size and depth and may eventually involve the entire ventral abdomen and adjacent flanks or limbs. Regional lymphadenomegaly may be present. Affected cats may become depressed, pyrexic, or anorexic; they may lose weight and become reluctant to move. Widespread dissemination to internal organs and lymph nodes is rare.

Top Differentials

Differentials include other bacterial or deep fungal infections and neoplasia.

Diagnosis

1. Rule out other differentials.
2. Cytology (exudate): neutrophils and macrophages. Intracellular acid-fast bacilli that stain poorly or not at all with routine stains may be seen but are often difficult to find.
3. Dermatohistopathology: nodular to diffuse pyogranulomatous dermatitis and panniculitis. Intralesional acid-fast bacilli may be difficult to find.
4. Mycobacterial culture: causative organisms include *M. fortuitum*, *M. chelonei*, *M. smegmatis*, *M. phlei*, *M.*

xenopi, *M. thermoresistible*, and *M. visibilis*. These organisms are easily cultured, unlike those that cause feline and canine leprosy, but cultures often may be negative.

5. PCR analysis, where available, may simplify the diagnosis.

Treatment and Prognosis

1. Radical surgical excision or extensive debridement of infected tissues followed by wound reconstruction should be performed, if possible. Surgery may spread the infection along tissue planes.
2. Systemic antimicrobial therapy should be administered over the long term (3–6 months) and continued 1 to 2 months beyond complete clinical resolution. Antimicrobial selection should be based on in vitro susceptibility results, if possible.
3. Drugs that may be effective empirically include the following:
   - Doxycycline or minocycline, 5–12.5 mg/kg PO q 12 hours, or 25–50 mg/cat PO q 8–12 hours immediately before meals
   - Marbofloxacin 2.75–5.5 mg/kg PO q 12 hours
   - Enrofloxacin 5–15 mg/kg PO q 12 hours, or 25–75 mg/cat PO q 24 hours (may cause retinal toxicity in cats)
   - Ciprofloxacin 62.5–125 mg/cat PO q 12 hours
   - Clarithromycin 5–10 mg/kg PO q 12 hours
   - Clofazimine 8 mg/kg PO q 24 hours
4. Topical DMSO with enrofloxacin (to make a 10-mg/mL solution) applied every 12 to 24 hours may be effective.
5. Doxycycline should be used prophylactically after penetrating injuries in obese cats and dogs are treated, to help prevent secondary mycobacterial infection.
6. The prognosis for complete cure is fair to guarded, although long-term medical therapy usually confines the infection sufficiently to enable the animal to lead a normal life. This disease is not considered contagious to other animals or to humans.

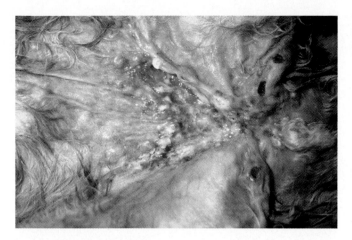

FIGURE 3-114 Opportunistic Mycobacteriosis. Numerous ulcers and draining tracts on the abdomen of a cat. Multiple nodules and an adherent purulent exudate can be seen. The nodules can act as a residual nidus for recurrence of the infection. Note the similarity to nocardiosis.

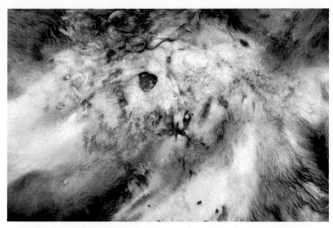

FIGURE 3-115 Opportunistic Mycobacteriosis. Multiple ulcerative lesions on the abdomen of an adult cat.

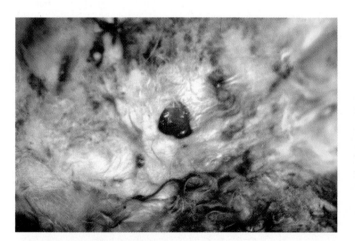

FIGURE 3-116 Opportunistic Mycobacteriosis. Large non-healing ulcer with purulent exudate and a deep tract.

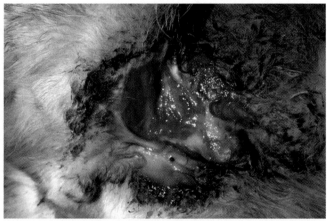

FIGURE 3-117 Opportunistic Mycobacteriosis. Close-up of the cat in Figure 3-116. Ulcerative lesions are apparent.

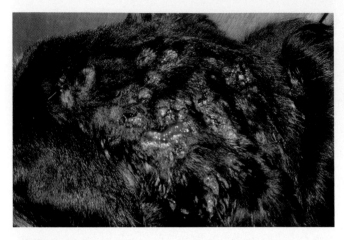

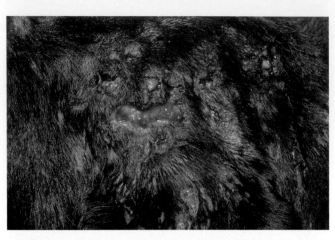

FIGURE 3-118 Opportunistic Mycobacteriosis. Severe cellulitis resulting in ulceration and crust formation on the head of an adult dog.

FIGURE 3-119 Opportunistic Mycobacteriosis. Same dog as in Figure 3-118. Deep ulceration resulting from the cellulitis is more apparent.

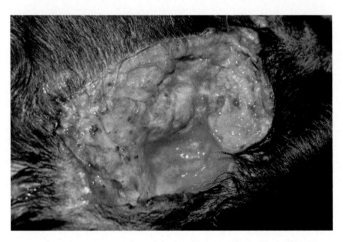

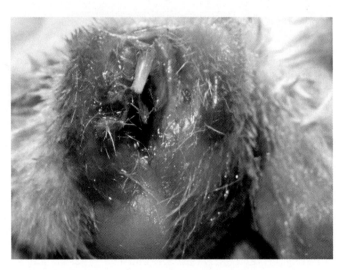

FIGURE 3-120 Opportunistic Mycobacteriosis. A deep, open, nonhealing ulcer is the result of a long-standing infection. Note the similarity to neoplasia.

FIGURE 3-121 Opportunistic Mycobacteriosis. Severe cellulitis affecting the nail bed. Swelling and severe bruising indicate the depth and severity of the infection.

Feline Leprosy Syndrome

Features

Feline leprosy is thought to be caused by two different mycobacterial species—*Mycobacterium lepraemurium* and another mycobacterial species that has not yet been named. *M. lepraemurium*, the agent of rat leprosy, is presumably transmitted to cats through the bites of infected rats. The environmental niche of novel mycobacterial species, which is thought to be an opportunistic saprophyte, has not yet been determined. Feline leprosy has been reported in the western part of the United States, western Canada, the Netherlands, Australia, New Zealand, and Great Britain. Cases caused by *M. lepraemurium* have been primarily limited to temperate coastal areas and seaside cities, whereas infections caused by novel mycobacterial species tend to occur in rural and semirural areas. Feline leprosy syndrome is uncommon in cats; the highest incidence of *M. lepraemurium* has been noted in adult cats younger than 4 years of age. The highest incidence of novel mycobacterial infection has been documented in cats older than 9 years of age that are immunocompromised from an underlying disease, such as long-standing feline immunodeficiency (FIV) infection, chronic renal insufficiency, or old age.

M. lepraemurium infections are characterized by rapidly progressive, locally spreading, nonpainful, raised, fleshy, tumor-like cutaneous and subcutaneous nodules. Lesions range from a few millimeters to 4 cm in diameter, with larger lesions usually ulcerated. Lesions can occur anywhere on the body but usually begin as a single nodule or a group of nodules on the head or limbs. Widespread cutaneous involvement tends to occur within 2 months, and regional lymphadenomegaly may be present. Despite the rapid development of generalized skin lesions, dissemination to internal organs does not occur.

Infection with novel mycobacterial species typically begins with localized subcutaneous and cutaneous nodules on the head, tail, or limbs that are firm and nonpainful, and that do not ulcerate. These lesions slowly progress over months or years to become generalized, and dissemination to internal organs may occasionally occur.

Top Differentials

Differentials include other bacterial and deep fungal infections and neoplasia.

Diagnosis

1. Rule out other differentials.
2. Cytology (aspirate, tissue impression): neutrophils and macrophages, some with intracellular, acid-fast bacilli that do not stain with routine stains.
3. Dermatohistopathology: diffuse (pyo)granulomatous dermatitis and panniculitis with intracellular and extracellular acid-fast bacilli. Lesions caused by *M lepraemurium* tend to have regions of caseous necrosis that contain sparse to moderate numbers of acid-fast bacilli, whereas lesions caused by novel species lack caseous necrosis and contain large numbers of acid-fast bacilli.
4. PCR technique (skin biopsy): detection of *M. lepraemurium* or novel mycobacterial DNA.
5. Mycobacterial culture: usually negative because causal organisms are fastidious and difficult to grow.

Treatment and Prognosis

1. Complete surgical excision is the treatment of choice for *M. lepraemurium* infection. Surgery may spread the infection along tissue planes.
2. If complete excision is not possible, treatment with clofazimine 8–10 mg/kg PO every 24 hours (25 mg/cat PO q 24 hours), or 50 mg/cat PO every 48 hours, may be effective. Therapy is administered over the long term and is continued 2 to 3 months beyond complete clinical resolution.
3. Complete surgical excision is rarely possible for infections caused by novel mycobacterial species. The medical treatment of choice is combination clarithromycin 62.5 mg/cat PO every 12 hours and rifampin 10–15 mg/kg PO every 24 hours. Therapy should be continued for several months and should extend at least 2 months beyond complete clinical resolution.
4. The prognosis is best if lesions can be completely excised. Feline leprosy is not considered contagious to other animals or to humans.

Feline Leprosy Syndrome—*cont'd*

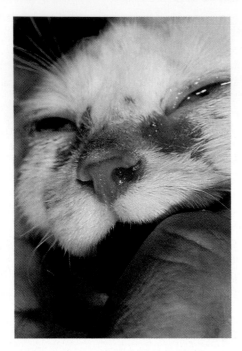

FIGURE 3-122 **Feline Leprosy.** Erosive lesions on the face of a cat infected with *Mycobacterium lepraemurium*. *(Courtesy A. Yu.)*

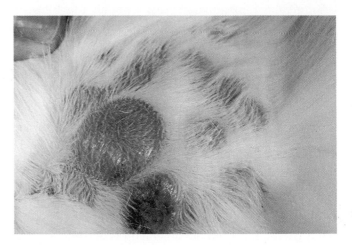

FIGURE 3-123 **Feline Leprosy.** Multiple alopecic, erythematous lesions on the body of a cat infected with *Mycobacterium lepraemurium*. *(Courtesy A. Yu.)*

Canine Leproid Granuloma Syndrome (canine leprosy)

Features

Canine leproid granuloma syndrome is a cutaneous mycobacterial disease of dogs. Its cause and pathogenesis have not been fully elucidated, but an unspeciated environmental mycobacterium is thought to be inoculated subcutaneously by biting insects. The most common mycobacterial disease of dogs in Australia, it has also been reported in New Zealand, Brazil, Zimbabwe, California, and Florida. Disease incidence is highest in short-coated dogs; Boxers and their crosses may be predisposed.

Canine leproid granuloma syndrome manifests as single to multiple well-circumscribed, firm subcutaneous nodules that range in diameter from 2 mm to 5 cm. The lesions are nonpainful and nonpruritic, sometimes alopecic, and they may become ulcerated if very large. The nodules are most commonly found on the head and dorsal ear folds but may appear anywhere on the body. Affected dogs are otherwise healthy and are not systemically ill.

Top Differentials

Differentials include other bacterial and deep fungal infections, noninfectious granuloma (e.g., suture left behind from ear cropping), and neoplasia.

Diagnosis

1. Rule out other differentials.
2. Cytology (aspirate): numerous macrophages with variable numbers of lymphocytes, plasma cells, and neutrophils. Few to moderate numbers of medium-length, acid-fast bacilli that do not stain with routine stains may be seen extracellularly or within macrophages.
3. Dermatohistopathology: pyogranulomatous dermatitis and panniculitis with intracellular and extracellular acid-fast bacilli.
4. PCR technique (skin biopsy): detection of a novel mycobacterial DNA sequence that has not been found in mycobacterial granulomas of any noncanine animals or humans.
5. Mycobacterial culture: negative because growth requirements for this fastidious organism have not yet been determined.

Treatment and Prognosis

1. Canine leproid granuloma syndrome is usually a self-limiting disease, with lesions typically regressing spontaneously within 3 to 4 weeks.
2. If lesions persist and are few in number, aggressive surgical excision is the treatment of choice.
3. For severe, refractory, chronic, disfiguring lesions, the medical treatment of choice is combination rifampin 10–15 mg/kg PO every 24 hours and clarithromycin 15–25 mg/kg PO, total daily dose divided every 8 to 12 hours. Treatment should be continued (minimum 4–8 weeks) until lesions have resolved.
4. Alternatively, combination rifampin 10–15 mg/kg PO every 24 hours and doxycycline 5–10 mg/kg PO every 12 hours may be effective.
5. Topically applied clofazimine ointment (prepared by mixing the extracted liquid dye from 40 crushed 50-mg clofazimine capsules with 100 g petroleum jelly) may be a helpful adjunct to systemic therapy.
6. The prognosis is good in that the disease tends to be self-limiting and usually spontaneously resolves. Small, hyperpigmented scars are possible sequelae at sites of the worst granulomas. This disease is not considered contagious to other animals or to humans.

Canine Leproid Granuloma Syndrome—*cont'd*

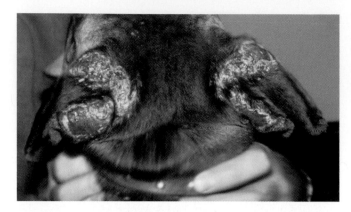

FIGURE 3-124 **Canine Leproid Granulomatous Syndrome.** Multiple alopecic, erosive granulomas on the ear pinnae of a dog. *(Courtesy R. Malik.)*

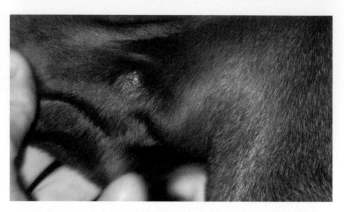

FIGURE 3-125 **Canine Leproid Granulomatous Syndrome.** A focal granuloma on the ear pinnae. *(Courtesy R. Malik.)*

Tuberculosis

Features

In tuberculosis (TB), tuberculous mycobacteria are transmitted to pets through close contact with infected owners or through consumption of contaminated milk or meat. TB occurs rarely in dogs and cats, with highest incidences reported in areas of endemic tuberculosis.

Tuberculosis manifests as single or multiple dermal nodules, plaques, abscesses, and nonhealing ulcers that drain a thick, purulent exudate. Lesions are found on the head, neck, and limbs. Concurrent symptoms of systemic involvement (e.g., fever, anorexia, depression, weight loss, lymphadenomegaly, cough, dyspnea, vomiting, diarrhea) are usually present.

Top Differentials

Differentials include other bacterial and deep fungal infections and neoplasia.

Diagnosis

1. Rule out other differentials.
2. Cytology (exudate): neutrophils and macrophages, some containing acid-fast bacilli that do not stain with routine stains.
3. Dermatohistopathology: nodular to diffuse pyogranulomatous dermatitis with few to many intracellular, acid-fast, positive bacilli.
4. Mycobacterial culture: causative organisms include *M. tuberculosis*, *M. bovis*, *M. tuberculosis–M. bovis* variant, and *M. avium* complex.
5. PCR analysis, where available, may simplify the diagnosis.

Treatment and Prognosis

1. Public health officials should be notified for guidance. The public health official will make recommendations based on the circumstances of the case.
2. If the owner refuses euthanasia, long-term (6–12 months) chemotherapy may be effective in some animals.
3. For *M. tuberculosis*, therapies that may be effective include the following:
   - For dogs and cats, combination isoniazid 10–20 mg/kg PO q 24 hours plus ethambutol 15 mg/kg IM q 24 hours
   - For dogs, combination pyrazinamide 15–40 mg/kg PO q 24 hours plus rifampin 10–20 mg/kg q 12–24 hours
4. For *M. bovis* in cats, localized lesions should be surgically excised, and the patient should be administered rifampin 4 mg/kg PO every 24 hours.
5. For *M. tuberculosis–M. bovis* variant in cats, combination rifampin 10–20 mg/kg PO administered every 24 hours, plus enrofloxacin 5–10 mg/kg PO administered every 12 to 24 hours, plus clarithromycin 5–10 mg/kg PO administered every 12 hours.
6. For *M. avium* complex in dogs and cats, combination doxycycline 10 mg/kg PO should be administered every 12 hours, or clofazimine 4 mg/kg PO should be administered every 24 hours, plus enrofloxacin 5–10 mg/kg PO administered every 12 to 24 hours, plus clarithromycin 5 mg/kg PO administered every 12 hours.
7. The prognosis is guarded. Tuberculosis is contagious to other animals and to humans.

Plague

Features

Plague is a zoonotic bacterial disease caused by *Yersinia pestis*. Dogs appear to be resistant, but cats are susceptible. Plague develops when cats eat infected rodents (natural reservoir) or are bitten by infected rodent fleas (vectors). Plague is uncommon in cats, with highest incidences reported in endemic areas of southwestern and western United States.

Plague occurs as an acute and often fatal disease that is characterized by fever, dehydration, lymphadenomegaly, and lymph node abscessation (bubo). The bubo may fistulate and may drain a thick, purulent exudate. The submandibular, retropharyngeal, and cervical lymph nodes are most often affected.

Top Differentials

Differentials include subcutaneous abscesses caused by other bacteria.

Diagnosis

1. Cytology (exudate, lymph node aspirate): suppurative inflammation with small, gram-negative, bipolar coccobacilli.
2. Serology: fourfold increase in the antibody titer against *Y. pestis* in serial serum samples taken 10 to 14 days apart.
3. Direct fluorescent antibody or PCR technique (exudate, lymph node aspirate): detection of *Y. pestis* antigen.
4. Bacterial culture: isolation of *Y. pestis*.
5. PCR analysis, where available, may simplify the diagnosis.

Treatment and Prognosis

1. Strict sanitation should be maintained because infected pus, saliva, tissue, and airborne respiratory droplets are highly contagious to humans and other animals. If possible, suspect animals should be caged in an isolation room. When handling suspect animals and specimens, the practitioner should wear gloves, gown, and surgical mask. Routine disinfectants should be used to clean tables and cages, and all contaminated materials (e.g., gauze pads) should be placed in a double plastic bag and incinerated.
2. Antibiotic therapy should be initiated immediately in all suspect cases. To minimize the likelihood that caregivers will contract infection by handling an infected animal, parenteral—not oral—administration is recommended. Treatment (minimum 3 weeks) should be continued well beyond complete clinical recovery.
3. The antibiotic of choice is gentamicin 2–4 mg/kg administered IM or SQ every 12 to 24 hours.
4. Alternative antibiotics that may be effective include the following:
   - Chloramphenicol 15 mg/kg SQ q 12 hours
   - Trimethoprim-sulfadiazine 15 mg/kg IM or IV q 12 hours
5. The animal should be treated with topical flea spray to quickly kill and prevent the spread of fleas (vectors). Aggressive flea control should be used for long-term avoidance.
6. Abscesses should be lanced and flushed with 0.025% chlorhexidine solution.
7. Asymptomatic, exposed animals should be treated prophylactically with tetracycline 20 mg/kg PO every 8 hours for 7 days.
8. The prognosis is poor unless antibiotic therapy is initiated early in the course of the disease. Plague is contagious to other animals and to humans.

CHAPTER 4

Fungal Skin Diseases

- Malasseziasis (*Malassezia* dermatitis)
- Candidiasis (candidosis, thrush)
- Dermatophytosis (ringworm)
- Dermatophytic Granulomas and Pseudomycetomas (Majocchi's granulomas)
- Phaeohyphomycosis (chromomycosis)
- Prototothecosis
- Pythiosis
- Zygomycosis (mucormycosis, entomophthoromycosis)
- Lagenidiosis
- Sporotrichosis
- Blastomycosis
- Coccidioidomycosis
- Cryptococcosis
- Histoplasmosis

Malasseziasis (*Malassezia* dermatitis)

Features

Malassezia pachydermatis is a yeast that is normally found in low numbers in the external ear canals, in perioral areas, in perianal regions, and in moist skin folds. Skin disease occurs in dogs when a hypersensitivity reaction to the organisms develops, or when cutaneous overgrowth occurs. In dogs, *Malassezia* overgrowth is almost always associated with an underlying cause, such as atopy, food allergy, endocrinopathy, keratinization disorder, metabolic disease, or prolonged therapy with corticosteroids. In cats, skin disease is caused by *Malassezia* overgrowth that may occur secondary to an underlying disease (e.g., feline immunodeficiency virus, diabetes mellitus, an internal malignancy). In particular, generalized *Malassezia* dermatitis may occur in cats with thymoma-associated dermatosis or paraneoplastic alopecia. Malasseziasis is common in dogs, especially among West Highland White terriers, Dachshunds, English setters, Basset hounds, American cocker spaniels, Shih tzus, Springer spaniels, and German shepherds. These breeds may be predisposed. Malasseziasis is rare in cats.

Dogs

Moderate to severe pruritus is seen, with regional or generalized alopecia, excoriations, erythema, and seborrhea. With chronicity, affected skin may become lichenified, hyperpigmented, and hyperkeratotic (leathery or elephant-like skin). An unpleasant body odor is usually present. Lesions may involve the interdigital spaces, ventral neck, axillae, perineal region, or leg folds. Paronychia with dark brown nail bed discharge may be present. Concurrent yeast otitis externa is common.

Cats

Symptoms include black, waxy otitis externa, chronic chin acne, alopecia, and multifocal to generalized erythema and seborrhea.

Top Differentials

Differentials include other causes of pruritus and seborrhea, such as demodicosis, superficial pyoderma, dermatophytosis, ectoparasites, and allergies.

83

Malasseziasis—cont'd

Diagnosis

1. Rule out other differentials.
2. Cytology (tape preparation, impression smear): yeast overgrowth is confirmed by the finding of round to oval budding yeasts (100×). In yeast hypersensitivity, organisms may be difficult to find.
3. Dermatohistopathology: superficial perivascular to interstitial lymphohistiocytic dermatitis with yeasts and occasionally pseudohyphae in keratin. Organisms may be few in number and difficult to find.
4. Fungal culture: *M. pachydermatis.*
5. Allergy test demonstrating a hypersensitivity to *Malassezia.*

Treatment and Prognosis

1. Any underlying cause (allergies, endocrinopathy, keratinization defect) must be identified and corrected.
2. For mild cases, topical therapy alone is often effective. The patient should be bathed every 2 to 3 days with shampoo that contains 2% ketoconazole, 1% ketoconazole/2% chlorhexidine, 2% miconazole, 2% to 4% chlorhexidine, or 1% selenium sulfide (dogs only). Shampoos that have two active ingredients provide better efficacy. Treatment should be continued until the lesions resolve and follow-up skin cytology reveals no organisms (approximately 4 weeks).
3. The treatment of choice for moderate to severe cases is ketoconazole (dogs) or fluconazole 10 mg/kg PO with food every 24 hours, Treatment should be continued until lesions resolve and follow-up skin cytology reveals no organisms (approximately 4 weeks).
4. Alternatively, treatment with terbinafine 5–40 mg/kg PO every 24 hours or itraconazole (Sporanox) 5–10 mg/kg every 24 hours for 4 weeks may be effective.
5. Pulse therapy protocols using several drugs and a variety of schedules have been published; however, these often take longer to resolve the active infection.
6. The prognosis is good if the underlying cause can be identified and corrected. Otherwise, regular once- or twice-weekly antiyeast shampoo baths may be needed to prevent relapse. This disease is not considered contagious to other animals or to humans, except for immunocompromised individuals.

Text continued on page 91.

Author's Note

Yeast dermatitis is currently the most commonly missed diagnosis in U.S. general practices. Any patient with leathery, elephant skin–like lesions on the ventrum should be suspected of having Malassezia dermatitis.

Cutaneous cytology is not always successful for finding Malassezia organisms, requiring the clinician to rely on clinical lesion patterns to make a tentative diagnosis.

Yeast dermatitis is severely pruritic, with owners reporting an itch level of 10 on a 0 to 10 visual analog scale.

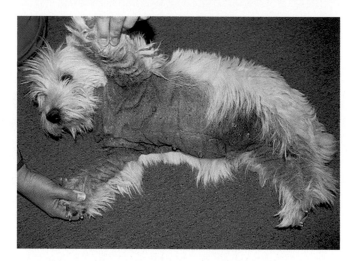

FIGURE 4-1 Malasseziasis. Severe alopecia, lichenification, and hyperpigmentation on the entire ventrum of a West Highland White Terrier. The yeast infection was secondary to allergic dermatitis.

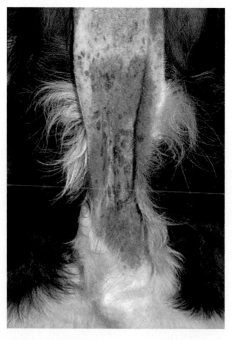

FIGURE 4-2 Malasseziasis. Alopecia, erythema, and lichenification on the ventral neck of an allergic dog.

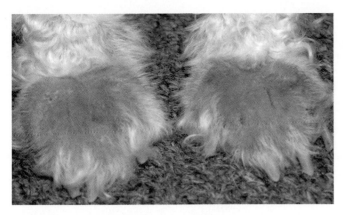

FIGURE 4-3 Malasseziasis. Pododermatitis caused by a secondary yeast infection demonstrates the alopecia and lichenification typical of *Malassezia* dermatitis.

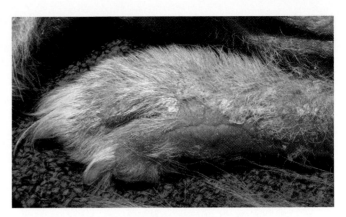

FIGURE 4-4 Malasseziasis. Severe pododermatitis demonstrating the intense inflammatory response caused by the hypersensitivity reaction to the *Malassezia* organisms. Severe erythema, alopecia, and lichenification are apparent.

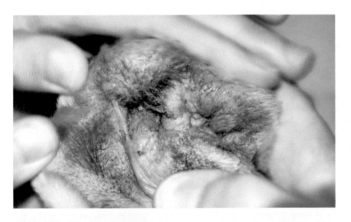

FIGURE 4-5 Malasseziasis. The interdigital dermatitis in this patient was caused by the secondary *Malassezia* infection. The greasy, alopecic, inflamed skin in between the footpads is typical of yeast pododermatitis.

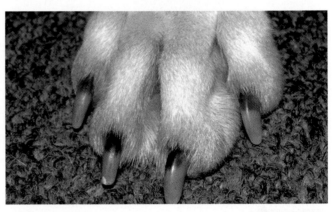

FIGURE 4-6 Malasseziasis. The brown discoloration around the base of the nails is a unique change typical of secondary *Malassezia* infections.

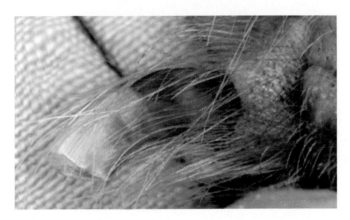

FIGURE 4-7 Malasseziasis. The brown discoloration caused by the yeast infection is more pronounced at the base of the nail and can be differentiated from normal pigmentation of the nail by its splotchy and interrupted pattern.

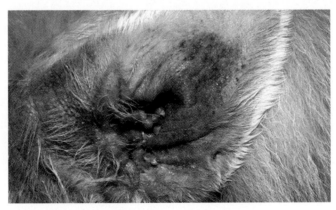

FIGURE 4-8 Malasseziasis. Secondary yeast otitis is a common finding in patients with an underlying primary allergy or endocrine disease. The ear canal and pinnae demonstrate the alopecia, intense erythema, and lichenification typical of *Malassezia* dermatitis.

Malasseziasis—*cont'd*

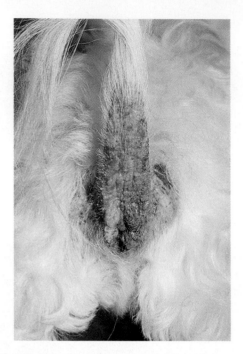

FIGURE 4-9 Malasseziasis. Perianal dermatitis caused by a secondary yeast infection in a food-allergic dog. The alopecia, erythema, and lichenification are characteristic of *Malassezia* dermatitis.

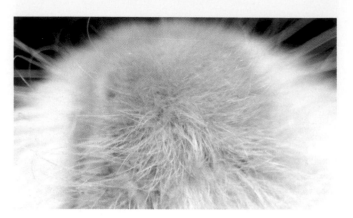

FIGURE 4-10 Malasseziasis. Yeast dermatitis can cause lesions typical of feline acne. Alopecia with brown discoloration and comedones is apparent.

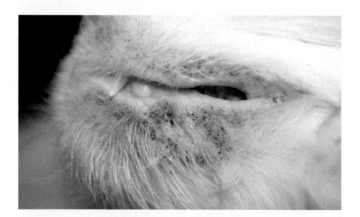

FIGURE 4-11 Malasseziasis. The perioral dermatitis in this cat was caused by a secondary *Malassezia* infection.

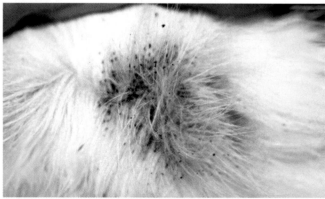

FIGURE 4-12 Malasseziasis. The secondary yeast infection can cause a seborrhea oleosa in cats. The waxy exudate clumping the base of this cat's hairs is typical of *Malassezia* dermatitis in cats.

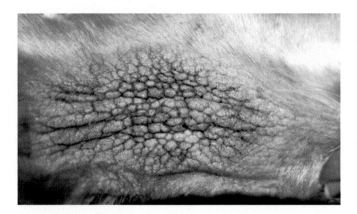

FIGURE 4-13 Malasseziasis. Typical "elephant skin" lesion demonstrating the alopecia, erythema, hyperpigmentation, and lichenification caused by *Malassezia* dermatitis.

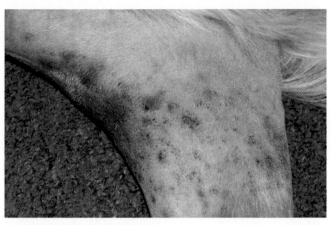

FIGURE 4-14 Malasseziasis. This papular dermatitis on the forearm of an allergic dog was caused by a secondary yeast infection. The papular dermatitis represents an unusual lesion pattern associated with *Malassezia* dermatitis and is more typical of bacterial *Pyoderma*.

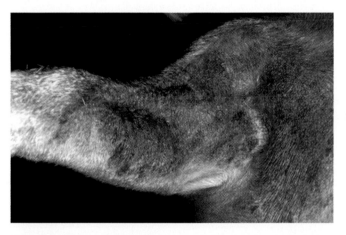

FIGURE 4-15 Malasseziasis. More typical yeast dermatitis of the forearm compared with Figure 4-14. The alopecia, hyperpigmentation, and lichenification ("elephant skin") are highly characteristic of yeast dermatitis.

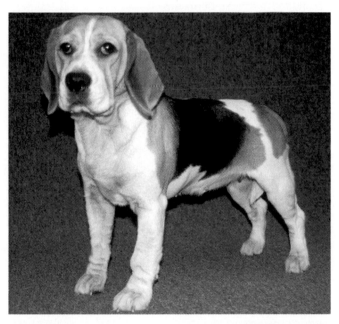

FIGURE 4-16 Malasseziasis. This young Beagle demonstrates brown discoloration of the hair on his feet and ventrum. The hair and skin are greasy with a rancid fat odor typical of a yeast infection.

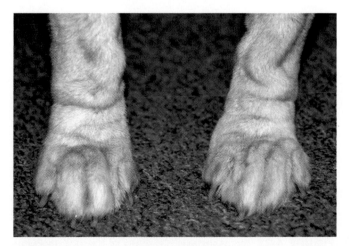

FIGURE 4-17 Malasseziasis. Close-up of the dog in Figure 4-16. Brown discoloration of the feet is apparent and represents an early change caused by the *Malassezia* infection.

Malasseziasis—cont'd

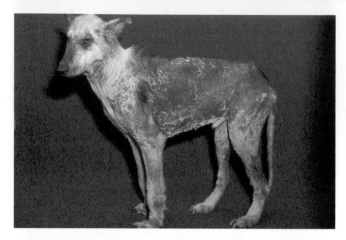

FIGURE 4-18 Malasseziasis. Generalized alopecia and lichenification in an adult Collie. The yeast infection was secondary to allergic dermatitis.

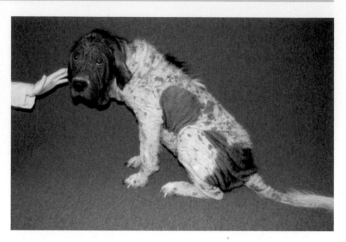

FIGURE 4-19 Malasseziasis. Generalized alopecia and lichenification ("elephant skin") typical of *Malassezia* dermatitis in a dog with primary idiopathic seborrhea.

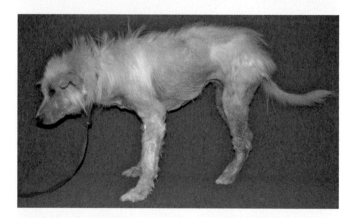

FIGURE 4-20 Malasseziasis. Generalized alopecia with intense erythema caused by a hypersensitivity reaction to the yeast organisms in a dog with severe *Malassezia* dermatitis secondary to allergy.

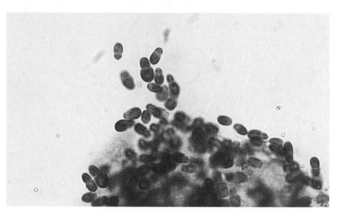

FIGURE 4-21 Malasseziasis. Cytology of *Malassezia* organisms, as viewed with a 100× (oil) objective.

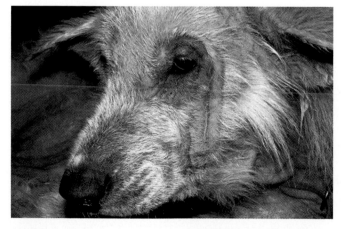

FIGURE 4-22 Malasseziasis. Close-up of the dog in Figure 4-20. Intense erythema and alopecia, with early lichenification caused by the hypersensitivity reaction to the yeast, are apparent.

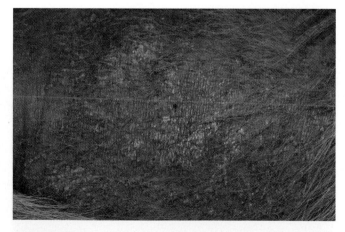

FIGURE 4-23 Malasseziasis. Close-up of the dog in Figure 4-20. Intense erythema and alopecia caused by the hypersensitivity reaction to yeast can be seen on the thorax. *Note:* The skin is beginning to become lichenified, typical of *Malassezia* dermatitis.

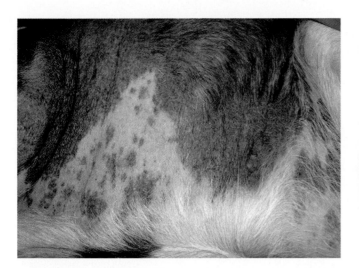

FIGURE 4-24 Malasseziasis. Severe alopecia and lichenification typical of yeast dermatitis on the ventrum of an allergic dog.

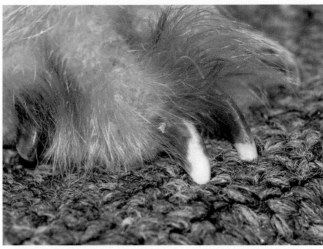

FIGURE 4-25 Brown splotchy discoloration of the nails is a unique symptom of yeast dermatitis.

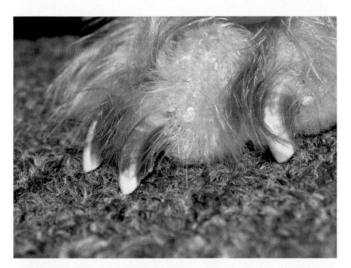

FIGURE 4-26 Malasseziasis. Brown discoloration of the nails is a characteristic of yeast dermatitis. If the color was natural pigmentation, the color would extend the entire length of the nail.

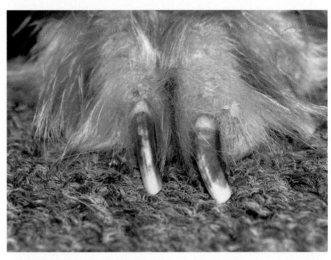

FIGURE 4-27 Malasseziasis. Brown splotchy discoloration of the nails is a unique symptom of yeast dermatitis.

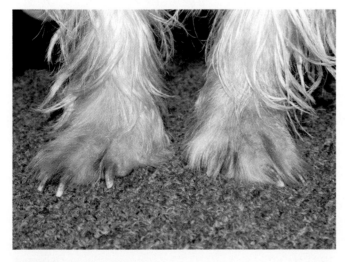

FIGURE 4-28 Malasseziasis. Severe pododermatitis in a dog with atopy. *Note:* The yeast infection affects the skin and nails in this dog.

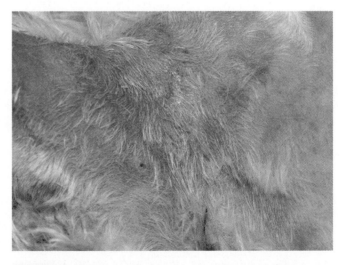

FIGURE 4-29 Malasseziasis. Severe erythema and alopecia in the axilla of a dog. Note the moist exudate starting to form.

Malasseziasis—_cont'd_

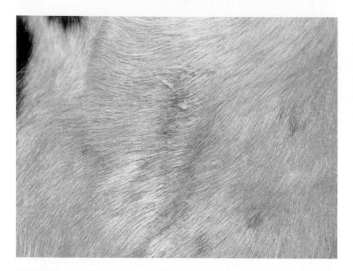

FIGURE 4-30 **Malasseziasis.** This papular rash with scaling is more typical of folliculitis, demonstrating the need for routine skin cytology to differentiate the cause of infection.

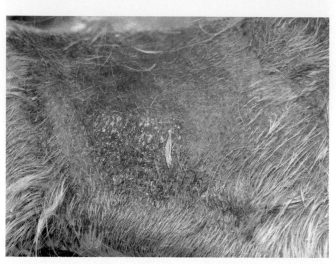

FIGURE 4-31 **Malasseziasis.** Severe erythema and alopecia with erosion formation. This deep lesion is not typical of yeast infections but was diagnosed through cutaneous cytology.

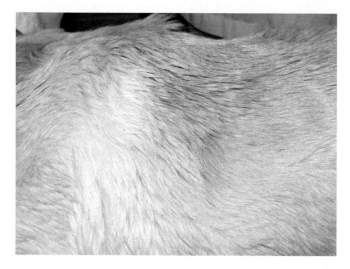

FIGURE 4-32 **Malasseziasis.** Generalized seborrhea oleosa (greasiness) of the skin and hair coat is a common symptom of yeast infection.

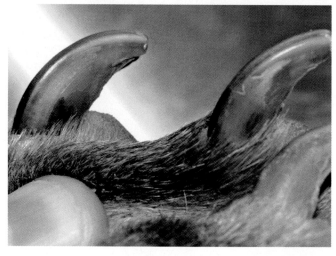

FIGURE 4-33 **Malasseziasis.** Brown, splotchy discoloration of the nails is a unique symptom of yeast dermatitis.

Candidiasis (candidosis, thrush)

Features

Candidiasis is an opportunistic cutaneous infection that results from overgrowth of *Candida*, a dimorphic fungus that is a normal mucosal inhabitant. Cutaneous overgrowth is usually facilitated by an underlying factor, such as skin damage caused by chronic trauma or moisture, an immunosuppressive disease, or long-term use of cytotoxic drugs or broad-spectrum antibiotics. Candidiasis occurs only rarely in dogs and cats.

Mucosal involvement is characterized by eroded or shallowly ulcerated mucocutaneous junctions, or by single to multiple nonhealing mucosal ulcers covered by grayish white plaques with erythematous margins. Cutaneous involvement is characterized by nonhealing, erythematous, moist, eroded, exudative, and crusty skin or nail bed lesions.

Top Differentials

Differentials include demodicosis, pyotraumatic dermatitis, superficial pyoderma, mucocutaneous pyoderma, other fungal infections, autoimmune disorders, vasculitis, cutaneous drug reactions, and cutaneous lymphosarcoma.

Diagnosis

1. Rule out other differentials.
2. Cytology (impression smear, exudate): suppurative inflammation with numerous budding yeasts and rare pseudohyphae.
3. Dermatohistopathology: superficial epidermitis, parakeratotic hyperkeratosis, and budding yeasts, along with occasional pseudohyphae or true hyphae in keratin.
4. Fungal culture: *Candida* spp. Because *Candida* is a normal mucosal inhabitant, positive fungal culture results should be confirmed histologically.

Treatment and Prognosis

1. Any underlying cause must be identified and corrected.
2. For localized cutaneous or mucocutaneous lesions, the affected area should be clipped and cleaned. The patient should be bathed every 2 to 3 days with shampoo that contains 2% ketoconazole, 1% ketoconazole/2% chlorhexidine, 2% miconazole, or 2% to 4% chlorhexidine. Shampoos that have two active ingredients provide better efficacy.
3. A topical antifungal product should be applied until lesions have healed (approximately 1–4 weeks). Effective topical therapies include the following:
   - 1% to 2% miconazole cream, spray, or lotion q 12–24 hours
   - 1% clotrimazole cream, lotion, or solution q 6–8 hours
   - 2% ketoconazole cream q 12 hours
4. For oral or generalized lesions, systemic antifungal medications should be administered (minimum 4 weeks) and continued at least 1 week beyond complete clinical resolution. Effective therapies include the following:
   - Ketoconazole 10 mg/kg PO with food q 24 hours
   - Fluconazole 10 mg/kg PO q 24 hours
   - Terbinafine 30–40 mg/kg PO q 24 hours
   - Itraconazole (Sporanox) 5–10 mg/kg PO with food q 24 hours
5. The prognosis is good to fair, depending on whether the underlying cause can be corrected. Candidiasis is not contagious to other animals or to humans.

Candidiasis—*cont'd*

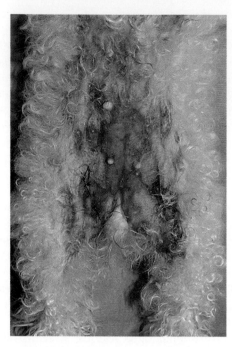

FIGURE 4-34 Candidiasis. Superficial moist, erosive lesions on the ventrum of the dog. *(Courtesy of A. Yu.)*

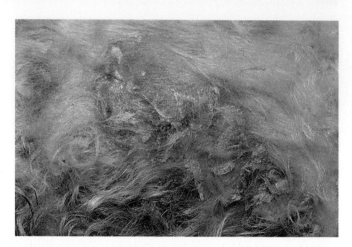

FIGURE 4-35 Candidiasis. Close-up of the dog in Figure 4-34. Erythema and crusting on the abdomen. *(Courtesy A. Yu.)*

Dermatophytosis (ringworm)

Features

Dermatophytosis is an infection of hair shafts and stratum corneum caused by keratinophilic fungi. It occurs commonly in dogs and cats, with highest incidences reported in kittens, puppies, immunocompromised animals, and long-haired cats. Persian cats and Yorkshire and Jack Russell terriers appear to be predisposed.

Skin involvement may be localized, multifocal, or generalized. Pruritus, if present, is usually minimal to mild but occasionally may be intense. Lesions usually include areas of circular, irregular, or diffuse alopecia with variable scaling. Remaining hairs may appear stubbled or broken off. Other symptoms in dogs and cats include erythema, papules, crusts, seborrhea, and paronychia or onychodystrophy of one or more digits. Rarely, cats present with miliary dermatitis or dermal nodules (see "Dermatophytic Granulomas and Pseudomycetomas"). Other cutaneous manifestations in dogs include facial folliculitis and furunculosis resembling nasal pyoderma, kerions (acutely developing, alopecic, and exudative nodules) on the limb or face, and truncal dermal nodules (see "Dermatophytic Granulomas and Pseudomycetomas"). Asymptomatic carrier states (subclinical infection) are common in cats, especially among long-haired breeds. Asymptomatic disease, although rare in dogs, has been reported in Yorkshire terriers.

Top Differentials

Dogs

Differentials in dogs include demodicosis and superficial pyoderma. If nodular, neoplasia and acral lick dermatitis should be included.

Cats

Differentials in cats include parasites, allergies, and feline psychogenic alopecia.

Diagnosis

1. Rule out other differentials.
2. Ultraviolet (Wood's lamp) examination: hairs fluoresce yellow-green with some *Microsporum canis* strains. This is an easy screening test, but false-negative and false-positive results are common.
3. Trichogram (hairs or scales in potassium hydroxide preparation): search for hair shafts infiltrated with hyphae and arthrospores. Fungal elements are often difficult to find.
4. Dermatohistopathology: variable findings may include perifolliculitis, folliculitis, furunculosis, superficial perivascular or interstitial dermatitis, epidermal and follicular orthokeratosis or parakeratosis, or suppurative epidermitis; fungal hyphae and arthrospores in stratum corneum or hair shafts.
5. Fungal culture: *Microsporum* or *Trichophyton* spp.
6. Polymerase chain reaction (PCR) analysis, where available, may simplify the diagnosis.

Treatment and Prognosis

1. If the lesion is focal, a wide margin should be clipped around it and topical antifungal medication applied every 12 hours until the lesion resolves. (Some dermatologists believe that clipping spreads lesions on the animal and further contaminates the environment.) Effective topicals for localized treatment include products that contain the following:
   - Terbinafine cream
   - Clotrimazole cream, lotion, or solution
   - Enilconazole cream
   - Ketoconazole cream
   - Miconazole cream, spray, or lotion
2. If response to localized treatment is poor, the animal should be treated for generalized dermatophytosis.
3. For generalized disease: Topical antifungal rinse or dip should be applied to the entire body one or two times per week (minimum 4–6 weeks) until follow-up fungal culture results are negative. Bathing the animal with a shampoo that contains chlorhexidine and miconazole (or ketoconazole) immediately preceding the antifungal dip may be helpful. Dogs with generalized dermatophytosis may be cured with topical therapy alone, whereas cats almost always require concurrent systemic therapy. Effective topical antifungal solutions include the following:
   - Enilconazole 0.2% solution
   - Lime sulfur 2% to 4% solution
4. For cats with dermatophytosis and dogs that are unresponsive to topical therapy alone, topical therapy for generalized infection should be combined with long-term systemic antifungal therapy and continued until 3 to 4 weeks beyond negative follow-up fungal culture results. The average duration of therapy is 8 to 12 weeks.
   Effective systemic antifungal drugs include the following:
   - Terbinafine 30–40 mg/kg PO q 24 hours
   - Ketoconazole 10 mg/kg PO q 24 hours with food (dogs)
   - Fluconazole 10 mg/kg PO q 24 hours with food

Dermatophytosis—*cont'd*

■ Itraconazole (Sporanox) 5–10 mg/kg PO q 24 hours with food
  Less effective systemic antifungal drugs include the following:
■ Microsized griseofulvin at least 50 mg/kg/day PO with fat-containing meal
■ Ultramicrosized griseofulvin 5–10 mg/kg/day PO with fat-containing meal

5. Alternatively, pulse therapy may be almost as effective, and multiple protocols have been published using various drugs. Pulse treatments should be continued until two consecutive follow-up fungal cultures taken 2 to 4 weeks apart are negative.

6. All infected animals, including asymptomatic carriers, should be identified and treated. Exposed, noninfected cats and dogs should be treated prophylactically with weekly topical antifungal rinse or dip for the duration of treatment of the infected animals.

7. The environment should be thoroughly cleaned by removing all contaminated materials, and the area should be disinfected with bleach (vacuums may further contaminate the environment).

8. For endemic infections involving multianimal homes, catteries, or animal facilities, treatment should be provided according to the recommendations outlined in Box 4-1.

9. Lufenuron has not demonstrated consistent efficacy in treating or preventing infection.

10. The prognosis is generally good, except for endemically infected multicat households and catteries. Animals with underlying immunosuppressive diseases also have a poorer prognosis for cure. Dermatophytosis is contagious to other animals and to humans.

BOX 4-1   Treating Dermatophytosis in Multianimal Homes, Catteries, and Animal Facilities

■ Culture all animals to determine the extent and location of animal infections.
■ Culture the environment (cages, counters, furniture, floors, fans, ventilation units, etc) to map infected areas to be disinfected.
■ Treat all infected animals with systemic antifungals until each animal has two negative fungal cultures taken at least 1 month apart.
■ Treat all infected and exposed animals with topical 2% to 4% lime sulfur solution every 3 to 7 days to prevent contagion and zoonosis. Continue until all animals have two negative fungal cultures taken at least 1 month apart. Do not clip cats, as this contaminates the clippers and facility and worsens the risk of contagion.
■ Dispose of all infected material. Remove clutter from animal facilities or other infected areas.
■ Clean and disinfect all surface areas every 3 days. Continue until all animals have two negative fungal cultures taken at least 1 month apart. Enilconazole (Clinafarm EC disinfectant, American Scientific Laboratories, Union, NJ) is a very effective environmental disinfectant, but it is licensed only for poultry farm use in the United States. Household chlorine laundry bleach (5% sodium hypochlorite) diluted 1:10 in water is an effective, inexpensive environmental disinfectant.

Author's Note

Microsporum canis is one of the most common zoonotic diseases in veterinary medicine.

Adopted kittens should be screened for infection during the first veterinary wellness visit.

Chronically infected animals likely have contaminated the home, requiring aggressive cleaning and disinfection of the environment.

Even long-standing and severe infections can be resolved with aggressive and persistent treatment.

Discontinuation of therapy MUST be based on negative cultures.

Text continued on page 102.

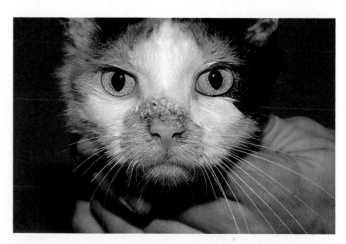

FIGURE 4-36 Dermatophytosis. Focal alopecia and crusting on the muzzle of a cat caused by *Microsporum canis*. *(Courtesy J. MacDonald.)*

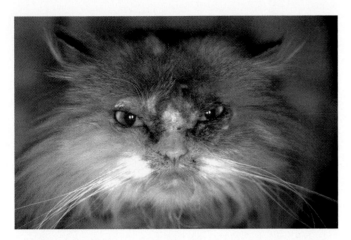

FIGURE 4-37 Dermatophytosis. Crusting alopecic dermatitis typical of dermatophytosis on the face of a cat.

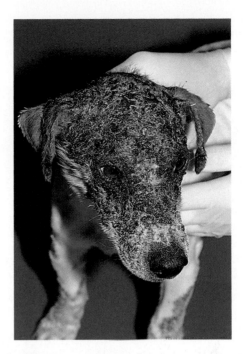

FIGURE 4-38 Dermatophytosis. Severe crusting on the entire head of this Jack Russell terrier was caused by a *Trichophyton* infection. Furunculosis resulted in severe cellulitis with subsequent scarring. *(Courtesy J. MacDonald.)*

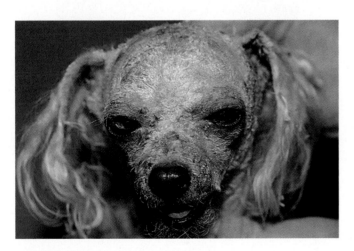

FIGURE 4-39 Dermatophytosis. Generalized alopecia, scale, and crust formation in a Toy Poodle.

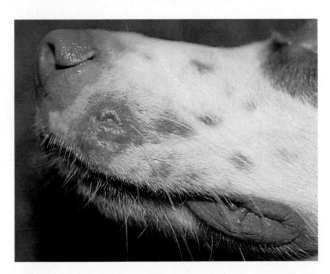

FIGURE 4-40 Dermatophytosis. Focal alopecia and erythema on the muzzle of a Brittany.

Dermatophytosis—*cont'd*

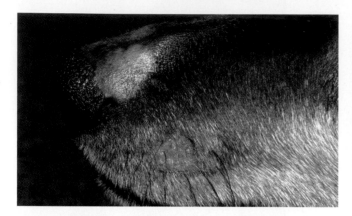

FIGURE 4-41 Dermatophytosis. Focal alopecia on the muzzle of a Dachshund. This is a typical location for dogs that frequently dig in soil.

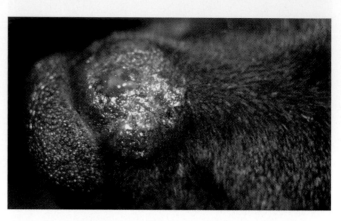

FIGURE 4-42 Dermatophytosis. This intense inflammatory reaction is typical of a kerion.

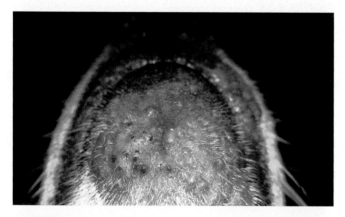

FIGURE 4-43 Dermatophytosis. Alopecia and erythema on the chin of a dog that frequently rooted in soil. Note the similarity to bacterial chin pyoderma.

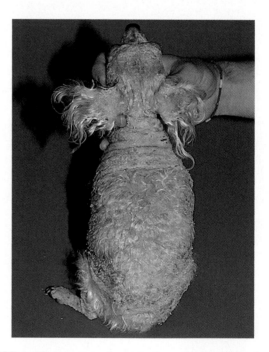

FIGURE 4-45 Dermatophytosis. Same dog as in Figure 4-39. Generalized alopecia and crusting on the entire dorsal cutaneous surface.

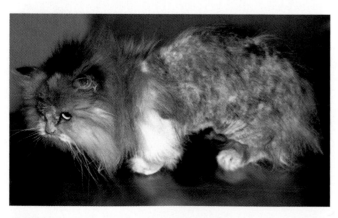

FIGURE 4-44 Dermatophytosis. Generalized alopecic, crusting dermatitis in a Persian with chronic dermatophytosis.

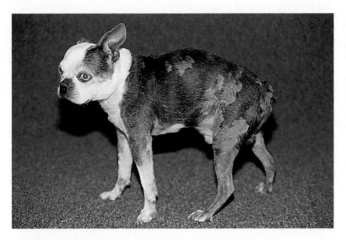

FIGURE 4-46 Dermatophytosis. Generalized alopecia and erythema in a Boston. The well-demarcated areas of dermatitis are typical of dermatophytosis.

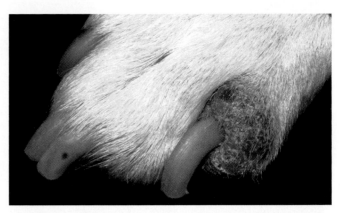

FIGURE 4-47 Dermatophytosis. Alopecia and erythema of the lateral digit are typical of nail bed infections caused by dermatophytes.

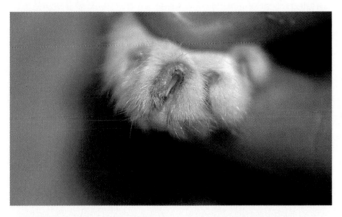

FIGURE 4-48 Dermatophytosis. Paronychia in a cat caused by *Microsporum canis*. The nail bed is erythematous and alopecic.

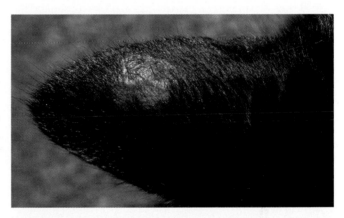

FIGURE 4-49 Dermatophytosis. A focal lesion of alopecia and erythema on the ear pinnae of a short-haired cat.

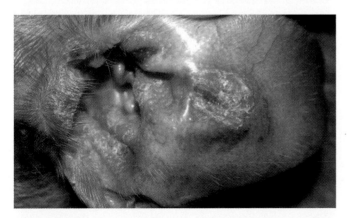

FIGURE 4-50 Dermatophytosis. Focal erythema with scaling on the pinnae and external ear canal of a dog. This could be confused with lesions typically seen with autoimmune skin disease.

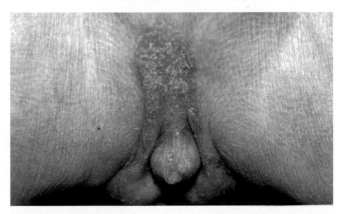

FIGURE 4-51 Dermatophytosis. Erythematous dermatitis in the skin fold of the vulva.

Dermatophytosis—cont'd

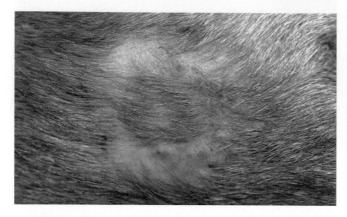

FIGURE 4-52 Dermatophytosis. This focal alopecic lesion was slowly expanding, with hair regrowth occurring in the central portion of the lesion. This "classic" ringworm lesion is unusual in our veterinary species.

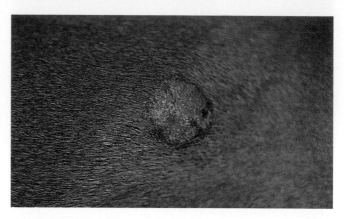

FIGURE 4-53 Dermatophytosis. This alopecic, erythematous nodule typical of a kerion occurred on the flank of a Boxer, and was caused by *Microsporum canis*.

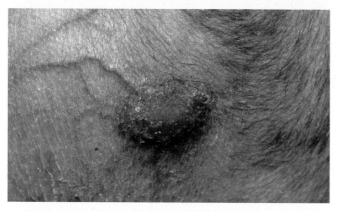

FIGURE 4-54 Dermatophytosis. Marked erythema associated with this focal dermatitis is caused by an intense immune reaction.

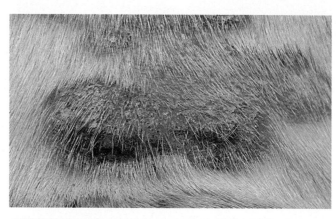

FIGURE 4-55 Dermatophytosis. Alopecia and erythema caused by *Microsporum canis* in a dog. Note the intense erythema and demarcation typical of dermatophytosis.

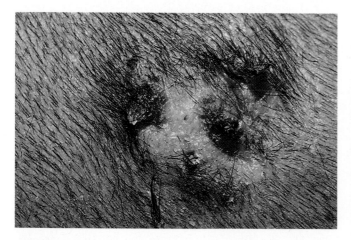

FIGURE 4-56 Dermatophytosis. A focal nodule with alopecia and crusting caused by *Trichophyton* mentagrophytes.

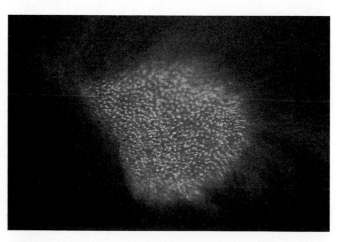

FIGURE 4-57 Dermatophytosis. Positive Wood's lamp examination of a cat with *Microsporum canis*. Note the apple green glow associated with the root of each hair.

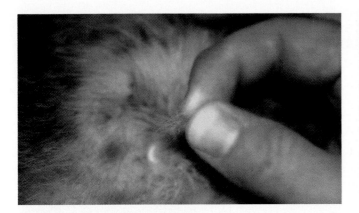

FIGURE 4-58 Dermatophytosis. Hair is easily epilated from folliculitis lesions. *Note:* The individual should be wearing gloves when dealing with a zoonotic infection.

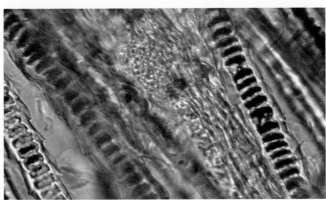

FIGURE 4-59 Dermatophytosis. Microscopic examination of a trichogram demonstrating an infected hair with fungal ectothrix, as seen with a 10× objective.

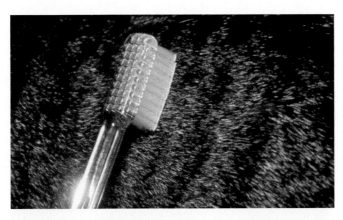

FIGURE 4-60 Dermatophytosis. A new toothbrush can be used to collect hairs from a patient without cutaneous lesions (McKinsey's toothbrush technique). The hairs should then be dispersed onto dermatophyte test medium (DTM) culture.

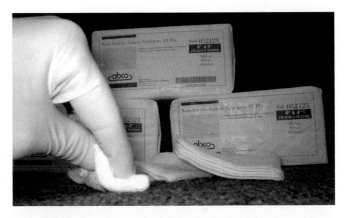

FIGURE 4-61 Dermatophytosis. Folded gauze can be used to wipe the fur of a patient or surface to collect material that then can be dispersed onto dermatophyte test medium (DTM) culture. *Note:* The individual learned the importance of wearing gloves when dealing with a zoonotic disease.

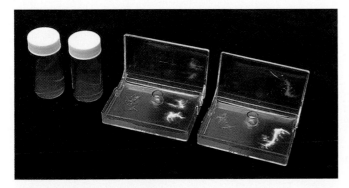

FIGURE 4-62 Dermatophytosis. Dermatophyte test medium (DTM) culture demonstrating the typical white colony growth associated with an immediate red color change.

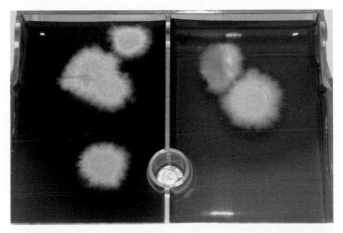

FIGURE 4-63 Dermatophytosis. Close-up of a dermatophyte test medium (DTM) fungal culture demonstrating typical white colony growth and red color change. This is suggestive of dermatophytosis, but microscopic examination should be performed to identify *Microsporum canis*.

Dermatophytosis—*cont'd*

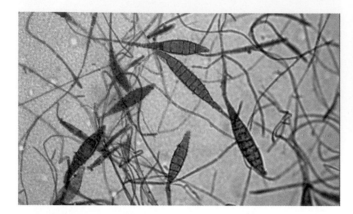

FIGURE 4-64 Dermatophytosis. *Microsporum canis* macroconidia as observed with a 10× objective. Note the pointed ends and six or more divisions.

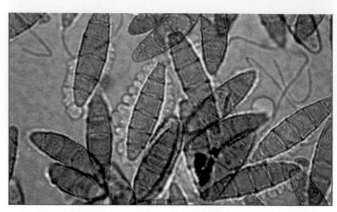

FIGURE 4-65 Dermatophytosis. *Microsporum gypseum* macroconidia as observed with a 40× objective. Note the more ovoid shape with six or fewer divisions.

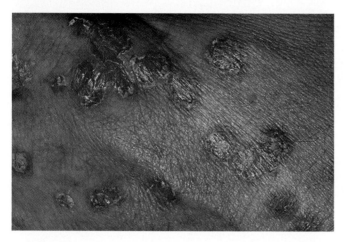

FIGURE 4-66 Dermatophytosis. *Microsporum canis* zoonosis. This person's hand demonstrates the typical intensely erythematous circular lesions caused by dermatophytes.

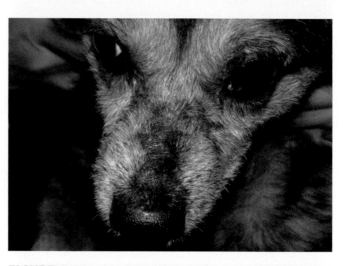

FIGURE 4-67 Dermatophytosis. Alopecia and hyperpigmentation on the face of a dog with chronic dermatophytosis.

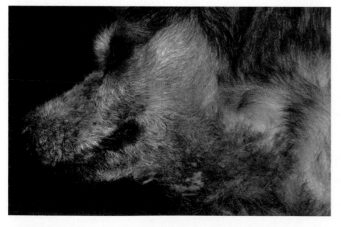

FIGURE 4-68 Dermatophytosis. Close-up of the dog in Figure 4-67. Hyperpigmented alopecia dermatitis was expanding down the dog's neck and extremities.

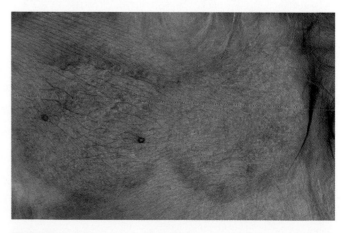

FIGURE 4-69 Dermatophytosis. Symmetrical areas of alopecia and erythema on the abdomen of a dog. The symmetrical lesion, a "kissing" lesion, is caused by contact of the skin on both sides of the ventral midline when the patient stands.

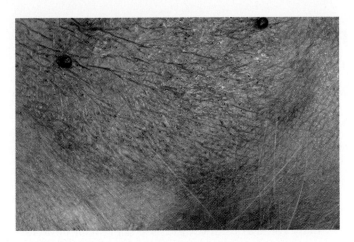

FIGURE 4-70 **Dermatophytosis.** Same dog as in Figure 4-69. A close-up of the lesion demonstrates the alopecia and erythema typical of a folliculitis.

Dermatophytic Granulomas and Pseudomycetomas

(Majocchi's granulomas)

Features

Dermatophytic granulomas and pseudomycetomas are unusual forms of dermatophytosis in which dermatophilic fungi form hyphae in dermal and subcutaneous tissue. These lesions are uncommon in cats, with reports limited to Persian cats. They are rare in dogs, with highest incidences reported in Yorkshire terriers. Nonpainful, nonpruritic, firm dermal or subcutaneous nodules and masses may ulcerate and form draining tracts. Lesions are most frequently found on the trunk, flanks, or tail. Concurrent superficial dermatophytosis is common. Peripheral lymphadenomegaly may be present.

Top Differentials

Differentials include other fungal and bacterial infections, foreign body reaction, and neoplasia.

Diagnosis

1. Cytology (exudate, aspirate): (pyo)granulomatous inflammation with fungal elements.
2. Dermatohistopathology: nodular to diffuse (pyo) granulomatous dermatitis and panniculitis with broad, hyaline, septate hyphae; chainlike pseudohyphae and chlamydospore-like cells (pseudomycetoma); or fungal hyphae scattered diffusely throughout the tissue (granuloma).
3. Fungal culture (exudate, aspirate, biopsy specimen): only *M. canis* has been isolated from cats. *M. canis* and *Trichophyton mentagrophytes* have been isolated from dogs.
4. PCR analysis, where available, may simplify the diagnosis.

Treatment and Prognosis

1. Lesions should be surgically excised, if possible.
2. Systemic antifungal therapy should be administered over the long term (weeks to months) and continued at least 1 month beyond complete clinical resolution.
3. Effective systemic antifungal drugs include the following:
   - Terbinafine 30–40 mg/kg PO q 24 hours
   - Ketoconazole 10 mg/kg PO q 24 hours with food (dogs)
   - Fluconazole 10 mg/kg PO q 24 hours with food
   - Itraconazole (Sporanox) 5–10 mg/kg PO q 24 hours with food
4. Combination surgical excision plus systemic antifungal therapy is more effective than either used alone.
5. The prognosis is fair to poor, with drug resistance and relapses common. Affected animals are potentially contagious and can cause superficial dermatophytosis in other animals and in humans.

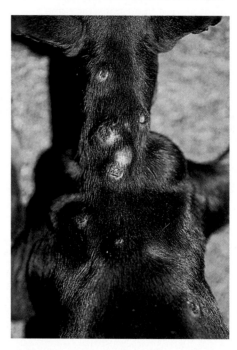

FIGURE 4-71 Dermatophyte Granuloma and Pseudomycetoma. Multiple nodules with draining tracts on the dorsum of a dog infected with *Trichophyton mentagrophytes*.

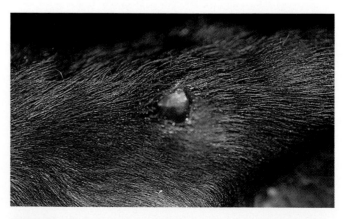

FIGURE 4-72 Dermatophyte Granuloma and Pseudomycetoma. Close-up of the dog in Figure 4-71. This nodular granuloma with a central ulcer periodically drained a purulent exudate.

Phaeohyphomycosis (chromomycosis)

Features

In phaeohyphomycosis, cutaneous lesions are caused by a variety of ubiquitous saprophytic fungi that live in soil but, when traumatically implanted into the skin, form pigmented hyphae without tissue granules. Phaeohyphomycosis is uncommon in cats and rare in dogs.

Cats

Usually, cats present with a solitary, firm to fluctuant subcutaneous nodule, abscess, or cystlike lesion that may ulcerate and drain. The lesion is most common on the distal extremities or the face. Dissemination is rare.

Dogs

Single to multiple poorly circumscribed subcutaneous nodules are often ulcerated and sometimes necrotic. Lesions are most common on the extremities and are often associated with underlying osteomyelitis. Dissemination may occur.

Top Differentials

Differentials include other fungal and bacterial infections, foreign body reaction, and neoplasia.

Diagnosis

1. Cytology (exudate, aspirate): (pyo)granulomatous inflammation. Pigmented fungal hyphae may be difficult to find.
2. Dermatohistopathology: nodular to diffuse (pyo) granulomatous dermatitis and panniculitis, with thick-walled, pigmented, septate, branched or non-branched hyphae of varying diameters with yeastlike swellings.
3. Fungal culture: causative organisms include *Alternaria, Bipolaris, Cladosporium (Xylohypha), Curvularia, Exophiala, Monilia, Ochroconis, Phialemonium, Phialophora, Pseudomicrodochium, Scolebasidium, Stemphilium,* and *Fonsecaea* species. Because these fungi are common environmental contaminants, positive fungal culture results should be confirmed histologically.
4. PCR analysis, where available, may simplify diagnosis.

Treatment and Prognosis

1. Wide surgical excision should be performed, if possible.
2. Systemic antifungal therapy should be administered over the long term (weeks to months) and continued at least 1 month beyond complete clinical resolution. Antifungal medication should be selected on the basis of in vitro sensitivity results, if available.
   Drugs to be considered include the following:
   - Terbinafine 30–40 mg/kg PO q 24 hours
   - Ketoconazole 10 mg/kg PO q 24 hours with food (dogs)
   - Fluconazole 10 mg/kg PO q 24 hours with food
   - Itraconazole (Sporanox) 5–10 mg/kg PO q 24 hours with food
3. The prognosis is good for local lesions and poor if disease is widespread or disseminated. It is not contagious to other animals or to humans.

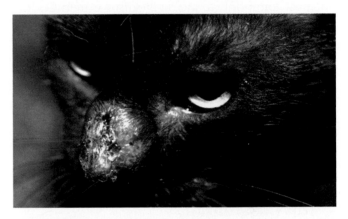

FIGURE 4-73 **Phaeohyphomycosis.** Swelling, alopecia, crusting, and purulent exudate on the nose of this cat were caused by a pigmented fungus. Note the similarity to *Cryptococcus* infections.

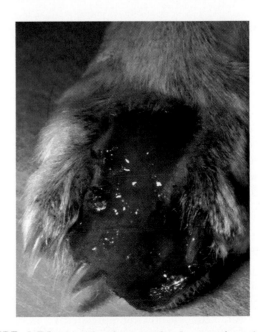

FIGURE 4-74 **Phaeohyphomycosis.** Severe ulceration and tissue destruction of a cat's foot. *(Courtesy D. Angarano.)*

Protothecosis

Features

Prototheca species are saprophytic, achlorophyllous algae found primarily in Europe, Asia, and North America (especially in southeastern United States). *Prototheca* species may cause infection via the gastrointestinal tract or through contact with injured skin or mucosa. Protothecosis is rare in dogs and cats, with highest incidences reported in immunosuppressed animals.

Cats

Infection appears as large, firm cutaneous nodules that are most commonly found on the distal extremities, the head, or the base of the tail.

Dogs

In dogs, infection manifests as a disseminated disease with multiorgan involvement. Signs may include protracted, bloody diarrhea; weight loss; central nervous system (CNS) signs; ocular lesions; and chronic nodules, draining ulcers, and crusty exudates on the trunk, on the extremities, and at mucocutaneous junctions.

Top Differentials

Differentials include other fungal and bacterial infections and neoplasia.

Diagnosis

1. Cytology (exudate, tissue aspirates): (pyo)granulomatous inflammation with numerous intracellular *Prototheca* organisms (round, oval, and polyhedral spherules that vary in size and often contain endospores).
2. Dermatohistopathology: nodular to diffuse (pyo)granulomatous dermatitis and panniculitis, with large numbers of *Prototheca* organisms.
3. Fungal culture: *Prototheca* species.
4. PCR analysis, where available, may simplify the diagnosis.

Treatment and Prognosis

1. Wide surgical excision of localized lesions is the treatment of choice.
2. Systemic antifungal therapy is usually ineffective; however, the following protocols have been proposed:

- Combination amphotericin B 0.25–0.5 mg/kg (dogs) or 0.25 mg/kg (cats) IV, three times per week until a cumulative dose of 8 mg/kg (dogs) or 4 mg/kg (cats) is reached, plus tetracycline 22 mg/kg PO q 8 hours
- Ketoconazole 10–15 mg/kg PO with food q 12–24 hours
- Fluconazole 10 mg/kg PO or IV q 12 hours
- Terbinafine 30–40 mg/kg PO q 24 hours
- Itraconazole (Sporanox) 5–10 mg/kg PO with food q 12 hours

3. The prognosis is poor if the disease is disseminated or the lesions are not surgically resectable. It is not contagious to other animals or to humans.

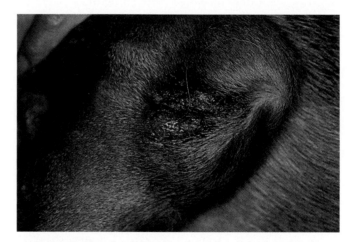

FIGURE 4-75 Protothecosis. Focal ulcerated draining lesions on the elbow of a mixed-breed dog. *(Courtesy K. Boyanowski.)*

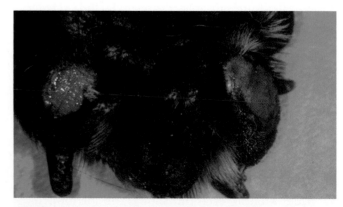

FIGURE 4-76 Protothecosis. Same dog as in Figure 4-75. Ulcerated footpads. *(Courtesy K. Boyanowski.)*

Pythiosis

Features

Pythium insidiosum is a protozoan with fungus-like features in tissue. This pathogenic aquatic organism causes disease when it enters damaged skin or mucosa. It is found in subtropical and tropical swamps of Asia, Australia, and Japan, and in parts of Central America and South America. In the United States, it is found primarily along the Gulf of Mexico in Alabama, Florida, Louisiana, and Texas. However, pythiosis has been described in animals living as far west as Arizona, and as far north as Indiana. Pythiosis is uncommon in dogs, with highest incidences reported in large-breed male dogs, especially hunting dogs and German shepherds. It is rare in cats, with young cats possibly predisposed.

Dogs

In dogs, pythiosis can manifest as a cutaneous or gastrointestinal disease. Skin lesions are variably pruritic nodules that converge to form large, spongy, proliferative, often rapidly expanding, locally invasive, fistulating, ulcerated masses. Draining exudate is serosanguineous or purulent. Lesions may appear anywhere on the body but are most common on the limbs, perineum, tail head, ventral neck, and head. Gastrointestinal disease is characterized by progressive weight loss, vomiting, regurgitation, or diarrhea resulting from infiltrative, granulomatous gastritis; esophagitis; or enteritis.

Cats

In cats, only a cutaneous disease is seen. Lesions are characterized by one or more, often highly locally invasive, draining nodules, ulcerated plaquelike lesions, or subcutaneous masses on the extremities, feet, inguinal area, tail head, or face.

Top Differentials

Differentials include foreign body reaction, neoplasia, deep bacterial infection, and other fungal infections (especially zygomycosis and lagenidiosis).

Diagnosis

1. Cytology (exudate): granulomatous inflammation that may contain eosinophils, but fungal elements are often not found.
2. Dermatohistopathology: nodular to diffuse granulomatous dermatitis and panniculitis, with foci of necrosis and accumulated eosinophils. Special fungal stains are often needed for visualization of the wide, occasionally septate, irregularly branching hyphae.
3. Immunohistochemistry (tissue specimen): detection of *P. insidiosum* antigens.
4. Enzyme-linked immunosorbent assay (ELISA) or Western immunoblot analysis for detection of anti–*P. insidiosum* serum antibodies.
5. PCR technique (tissue specimen) for detection of *P. insidiosum* DNA.
6. Fungal culture: *P. insidiosum*. *Note:* The organism may not grow unless special fungal medium is used.

Treatment and Prognosis

1. Complete, wide surgical excision or amputation of the affected limb is the traditional treatment of choice. To monitor for recurrence, serum anti–*P. insidiosum* antibody titers should be followed with the use of ELISA serology before and every 2 to 3 months after surgery for up to 1 year.
2. Immunotherapy with *P. insidiosum* vaccine may be effective in dogs with pythiosis of less than 2 months' duration. The vaccine is administered twice, with the first injection of 0.1 mL administered ID over one shoulder, and the second injection of 0.1 mL administered SC (not ID) over the other shoulder 2 weeks later. Lesion regression should be evident within 2 weeks of the first injection. At this writing, the vaccine is not yet commercially available, but it can be obtained from Dr. L. Mendoza at the Medical Technology Program, Department of Microbiology, Michigan State University, 322 N Kedzie Laboratories, East Lansing, MI 48824-1031, or by fax ordering at 517-432-2006.
3. Long-term (several months) systemic antifungal therapy based on in vitro sensitivity results can be attempted, but medical treatment is successful in less than 25% of cases. Treatment should be continued until follow-up ELISA anti-*Pythium* serum antibody titers normalize.
4. Itraconazole (Sporanox) 10 mg/kg PO should be administered with food every 24 hours for at least 3 to 6 months, or amphotericin B lipid complex should be administered in dogs at a dose of 2–3 mg/kg IV every 48 hours until a cumulative dose of 24–27 mg/kg is reached.
5. Alternatively, long-term combination itraconazole (Sporanox) (10 mg/kg PO with food q 24 hours) with terbinafine (30–40 mg/kg PO q 24 hours) may be more effective in dogs and cats than either itraconazole or amphotericin B alone.
6. The prognosis is poor if the disease is chronic and complete surgical excision is not possible. Pythiosis is not contagious to other animals or to humans.

Pythiosis—*cont'd*

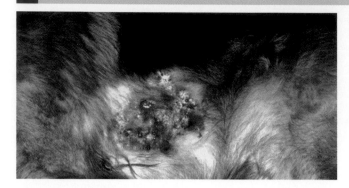

FIGURE 4-77 Pythiosis. Multiple nodular lesions with draining tracts on the lateral thorax of an adult German shepherd.

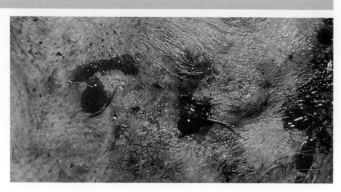

FIGURE 4-78 Pythiosis. Close-up of the dog in Figure 4-77. These draining nodular lesions are typical of infectious cellulitis.

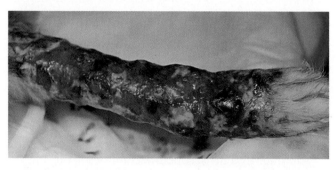

FIGURE 4-79 Pythiosis. Severe ulceration and cellulitis with multiple draining tracts on the entire distal limb of a dog. The infection had gradually progressed up the limb over several weeks. *(Courtesy M. Singer.)*

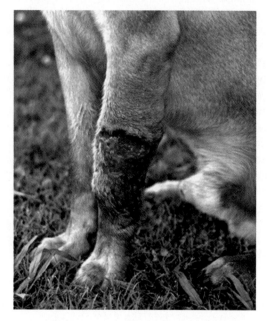

FIGURE 4-80 Pythiosis. Severe swelling with erosions and draining tracts on the distal extremity of a dog with pythiosis. *(Courtesy A. Grooters.)*

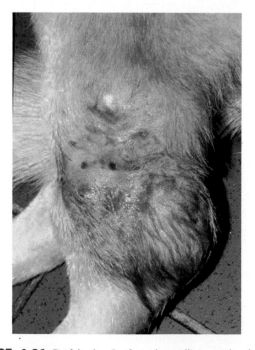

FIGURE 4-81 Pythiosis. Profound swelling with alopecia, papules, nodules, and multiple draining tracts on the proximal rear limb of a dog. *(Courtesy D. Angarano.)*

Zygomycosis (mucormycosis, entomophthoromycosis)

Features

Zygomycetes are ubiquitous, saprophytic, environmental fungi. Organisms may enter the body through the respiratory tract or the gastrointestinal (GI) tract or through wound inoculation. Zygomycosis is rare in dogs and cats.

This is often a fatal GI, respiratory, or disseminated disease. Skin lesions are characterized by ulcerated, draining nodules or by nonhealing wounds.

Top Differentials

Differentials include other fungal infections (especially pythiosis and lagenidiosis), deep bacterial infections, and neoplasia.

Diagnosis

1. Cytology (exudate): (pyo)granulomatous inflammation with fungal elements.
2. Dermatohistopathology: nodular to diffuse (pyo) granulomatous dermatitis and panniculitis, with numerous broad, occasionally septate, irregularly branching hyphae that have nonparallel sides.
3. Fungal culture: causative organisms include *Absidia*, *Basidiobolus*, *Conidiobolus*, *Mortierella*, *Mucor*, and *Rhizopus* species. Because these fungi are common environmental contaminants, positive fungal culture results should be confirmed histologically.

Treatment and Prognosis

1. Wide surgical excision or debulking is indicated.
2. Long-term (weeks to months) systemic antifungal therapy should be administered and continued at least 1 month beyond complete clinical resolution. Antifungal therapy should be selected on the basis of in vitro sensitivity results, if available.
3. Pending sensitivity results, treatment with amphotericin B 0.5 mg/kg (dogs) or 0.25 mg/kg (cats) IV should be administered three times per week until a cumulative dose of 8 to 12 mg/kg (dogs) or 4 to 6 mg/kg (cats) is reached.
4. Treatment with oral antifungals is usually ineffective:

   - Terbinafine 30–40 mg/kg PO q 24 hours
   - Ketoconazole 10 mg/kg PO q 24 hours with food (dogs)
   - Fluconazole 10 mg/kg PO q 24 hours with food
   - Itraconazole (Sporanox) 5–10 mg/kg PO q 24 hours with food

5. The prognosis is poor if complete surgical excision is not possible. This disease is not contagious to other animals or to humans.

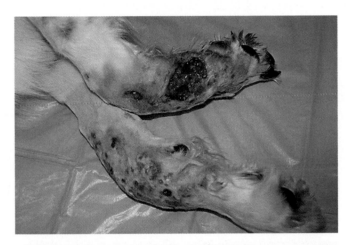

FIGURE 4-82 Zygomycosis. Severe swelling and ulceration with multiple draining lesions on the distal limbs of a dog infected with *Basidiobolus*.

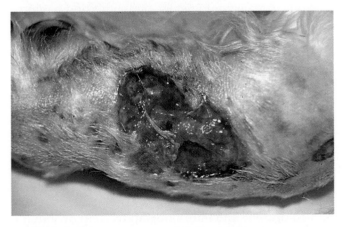

FIGURE 4-83 Zygomycosis. Close-up of the dog in Figure 4-82. Severe tissue destruction on the dorsal carpus.

Lagenidiosis

Features

Lagenidium species are aquatic oomycetes that normally parasitize other fungi, algae, nematodes, and crustaceans. Recently, *Lagenidium* species have been recognized to cause skin disease in dogs living in the southeastern United States. Lagenidiosis is rare in dogs, with highest incidences reported in young to middle-aged dogs that swim frequently in a lake or pond. Skin lesions are usually progressive and locally invasive, and are characterized by firm dermal to subcutaneous nodules, or ulcerated, edematous masses, with areas of necrosis and numerous fistulous tracts that drain a hemorrhagic, mucopurulent exudate. Lesions are most common on the extremities and the trunk. Regional lymphadenopathy is often present. Dissemination to distant sites such as great vessels, lungs, and mediastinum is common.

Top Differentials

Differentials include foreign body reaction, neoplasia, deep bacterial infection, and other fungal infections (especially pythiosis and zygomycosis).

Diagnosis

1. Cytology (exudate): granulomatous inflammation that may contain eosinophils and fungal elements.
2. Dermatohistopathology: nodular to diffuse eosinophilic (pyo)granulomatous dermatitis and panniculitis, with foci of necrosis and suppuration. Wide, occasionally septate, irregularly branching fungal hyphae are found intracellularly (within giant cells) and extracellularly (within areas of inflammation or necrosis).
3. Western immunoblot analysis: detection of anti-*Lagenidium* serum antibodies.
4. PCR technique (tissue specimens): detection of *Lagenidium* DNA.
5. Fungal culture: *Lagenidium* species. *Note:* The organism may not grow unless special fungal medium is used.
6. Radiography and ultrasonography: chest or abdominal lesions, if dissemination has occurred.

Treatment and Prognosis

1. Complete, wide surgical excision or amputation of the affected limb is the treatment of choice.
2. Long-term systemic antifungal therapy can be attempted, but treatments with itraconazole and amphotericin B are usually ineffective.
3. The prognosis is poor if complete surgical excision is not possible. Lagenidiosis is not contagious to other animals or to humans.

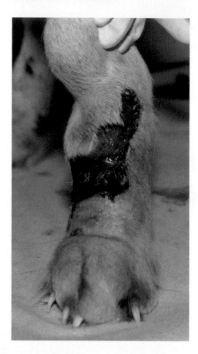

FIGURE 4-84 Lagenidiosis. Ulcerative dermatitis in a 1-year-old male Labrador retriever mix. *(Courtesy Grooters AM: Veterinary Clinics Small Animal Practice 33:695–720, 2003.)*

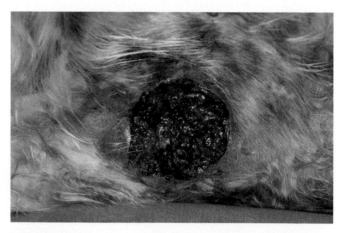

FIGURE 4-85 Lagenidiosis. A large (9 × 9 cm), raised, ulcerated, and exudative cutaneous lesion caused by *Lagenidium* species infection on the ventral abdomen of a 6-year-old female spayed Springer spaniel. *(Courtesy Grooters AM: Journal of Veterinary Internal Medicine 17:637–646, 2003.)*

Sporotrichosis

Features

Sporothrix schenkii is a dimorphic fungus and environmental saprophyte that can be found worldwide. Infection occurs when the organisms are inoculated into tissue through puncture wounds. Sporotrichosis is uncommon to rare in dogs and cats, with highest incidences reported in hunting dogs and intact male outdoor cats.

Dogs

Skin lesions are characterized by multiple nonpainful, nonpruritic, firm nodules that may ulcerate, drain purulent exudate, and crust over. Lesions are most commonly found on the head, trunk, or distal extremities. Nodules on the distal limbs may spread up ascending lymphatic vessels to form more ulcerated, draining nodules. Regional lymphadenomegaly is common. Dissemination is rare.

Cats

Skin lesions may include nonhealing puncture wounds, abscesses, cellulitis, crusted nodules, ulcerations, purulent draining tracts, and sometimes tissue necrosis. Lesions usually involve the head, distal limbs, or tail base. Concurrent lethargy, depression, anorexia, and fever may be present. Dissemination is common.

Top Differentials

Differentials include other fungal and bacterial infections and neoplasia.

Diagnosis

1. Cytology (exudate, tissue aspirate): suppurative or (pyo)granulomatous inflammation. Intracellular and extracellular round, oval, and cigar-shaped yeasts are usually easy to find in cats but are difficult to find in dogs.
2. Dermatohistopathology: nodular to diffuse suppurative or (pyo)granulomatous dermatitis. Yeasts that may resemble cryptococcal organisms are easily found in cats but are rarely found in dogs.
3. Immunofluorescent testing: detection of *Sporothrix* antigen in tissue or exudates.
4. Fungal culture: *S. schenckii* is easy to culture from infected cats but may be difficult to isolate from infected dogs (fungal cultures are highly infectious).
5. PCR analysis, where available, may simplify the diagnosis.

Treatment and Prognosis

1. Long-term (weeks to months) systemic antifungal therapy should be administered and continued at least 1 month beyond complete clinical resolution.
2. Treatments include the following:
   - Ketoconazole 5–15 mg/kg PO with food q 12 hours
   - Fluconazole 10 mg/kg PO with food q 24 hours
   - Terbinafine 30–40 mg/kg PO q 24 hours
   - Itraconazole (Sporanox) 5–10 mg/kg PO with food q 12–24 hours
   - In cats, the drug of choice is itraconazole (Sporanox).
3. Historic therapies include the following:
   - In dogs, the traditional treatment is supersaturated potassium iodide 40 mg/kg PO with food every 8 hours.
   - In cats, supersaturated potassium iodide 20 mg/kg PO with food q 12 hours
4. The prognosis is fair to good, but relapses can occur. No cases of disease transmission from dogs to humans have been reported, but infected cats are highly contagious to people. Good hygiene and gloves should be utilized when handling the patient.

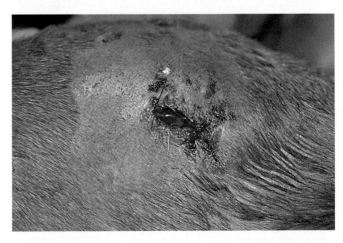

FIGURE 4-86 Sporotrichosis. Draining lesions with crusting on the swollen stifle of a dog.

Sporotrichosis—cont'd

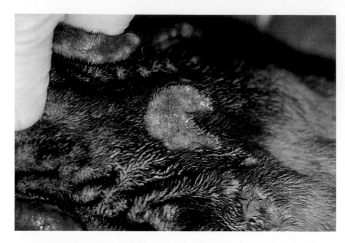

FIGURE 4-87 Sporotrichosis. Same dog as in Figure 4-86. Erosive lesion with purulent drainage on the ventral neck.

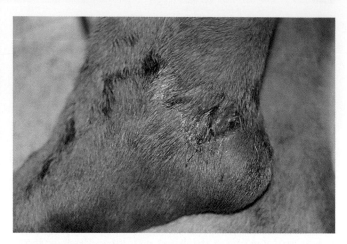

FIGURE 4-88 Sporotrichosis. Same dog as in Figure 4-86. These multiple crusting lesions on the hock periodically drained a purulent exudate.

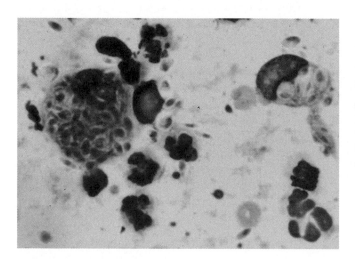

FIGURE 4-89 Sporotrichosis. Microscopic images of the *Sporothrix* organisms, as viewed with a 100× (oil) objective. Note the ovoid "cigar"-shaped intracellular organisms.

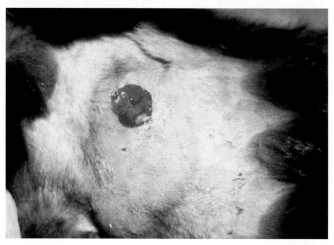

FIGURE 4-90 Sporotrichosis. A large fluctuant mass with a central ulcerative lesion on the lateral thorax of a cat. *(Courtesy D. Angarano.)*

Blastomycosis

Features

Blastomycosis is caused by inhaling the conidia of *Blastomyces dermatitidis*, a dimorphic fungus and environmental saprophyte. *B. dermatitidis* is found in moist, acidic, or sandy soil, primarily in North America along the Ohio, Mississippi, Missouri, St. Lawrence, and Tennessee Rivers; in southern Mid-Atlantic states; and in the southern Great Lakes region. After inhalation, a lung infection is established that disseminates to lymph nodes, eyes, skin, bones, and other organs. Rarely, direct inoculation may result in localized skin disease, but cutaneous blastomycosis is more commonly a sign of disseminated disease. Blastomycosis is rare in cats and uncommon in dogs, with highest incidences reported in young, male, large-breed outdoor dogs, especially hounds and sporting breeds.

Cutaneous lesions include discrete subcutaneous abscesses and firm, proliferative, ulcerated masses with fistulous tracts that drain a serosanguineous to purulent exudate. Lesions may be found anywhere on the body but are most common on the face, nasal planum, and nail beds. Nonspecific symptoms include anorexia, weight loss, and fever. Other symptoms, depending on the organ systems involved, may include exercise intolerance, cough, dyspnea, lymphadenomegaly, uveitis, retinal detachment, glaucoma, lameness, and CNS signs.

Top Differentials

Differentials include other fungal and bacterial infections, neoplasia, and foreign body reaction.

Diagnosis

1. Cytology (exudate, tissue aspirate): suppurative or pyogranulomatous inflammation with large, round, broad-based budding yeasts that have thick, refractile, double-contoured cell walls.
2. Dermatohistopathology: nodular to diffuse suppurative to (pyo)granulomatous dermatitis with large, thick, double-walled, broad-based budding yeasts.
3. Agar-gel immunodiffusion: detection of serum antibodies against *B. dermatitidis*; in early infection, test results may be negative.
4. Fungal culture (not needed to confirm diagnosis unless cytology and histopathology fail to reveal organism [submit to diagnostic laboratory because fungal cultures are highly infectious]): *B. dermatitidis.*
5. Radiography: pulmonary changes if lungs are involved; osteolytic lesions if long bones are involved.

6. PCR analysis, where available, may simplify the diagnosis.

Treatment and Prognosis

1. Long-term (minimum 2–3 months) systemic antifungal therapy should be administered and continued 1 month beyond complete clinical resolution.
2. The drug of choice is itraconazole (Sporanox). For cats, 5 mg/kg PO should be administered with food every 12 hours. For dogs, 5 mg/kg should be administered PO with food every 12 hours for 5 days, followed by 5 mg/kg PO with food every 24 hours.
3. Alternative therapies include the following:
   - Fluconazole 5–10 mg/kg PO or IV q 24 hours
   - Amphotericin B 0.5 mg/kg (dogs) or 0.25 mg/kg (cats) IV three times per week until a cumulative dose of 8–12 mg/kg (dogs) or 4–6 mg/kg (cats) is administered
   - Amphotericin B lipid complex (dogs) 1.0 mg/kg IV three times per week until a cumulative dose of 12 mg/kg is administered
4. The prognosis is good unless CNS or severe lung involvement is present. Regardless of the therapy used, approximately 20% of dogs relapse within 1 year of treatment because of premature discontinuation of therapy or the use of compounded medications; however, they usually respond to retreatment with itraconazole (Sporanox). Infected animals (yeast form) are not considered contagious to other animals or to humans, but fungal cultures (mycelial form) are highly infectious.

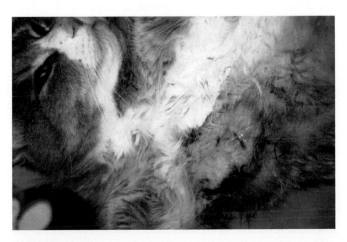

FIGURE 4-91 Blastomycosis. A large (3 cm) mass with multiple draining tracts in the axillary region of a cat.

Blastomycosis—cont'd

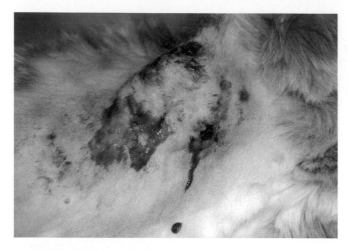

FIGURE 4-92 Blastomycosis. Close-up of the cat in Figure 4-91. Blood-tinged pus is exuding from multiple draining tracts of this cat's axillary mass.

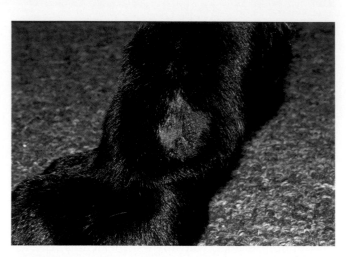

FIGURE 4-93 Blastomycosis. A small mass (2 cm) with alopecia and ulcerations on the carpus. Note the similarity to an acral lick granuloma.

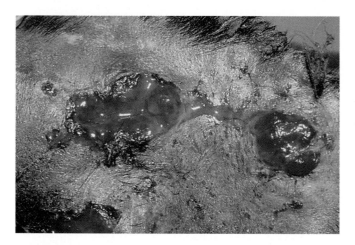

FIGURE 4-94 Blastomycosis. Cellulitis with draining tracts affecting the entire ear pinnae. *(Courtesy D. Angarano.)*

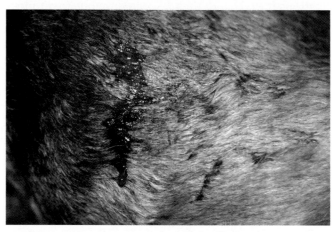

FIGURE 4-95 Blastomycosis. Multiple draining tracts on the flank of a dog with disseminated blastomycosis.

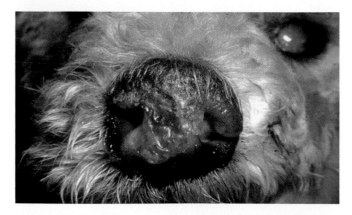

FIGURE 4-96 Blastomycosis. Severe swelling and ulceration of the nasal planum caused by blastomycosis. This could be mistaken for autoimmune skin disease. *(Courtesy L. Schmeitzel.)*

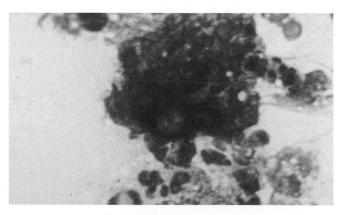

FIGURE 4-97 Blastomycosis. Microscopic image of blastomycosis organism, as viewed with a 100× (oil) objective. The large yeast with a thick cell wall and broad-based budding is visible within the clump of stained material.

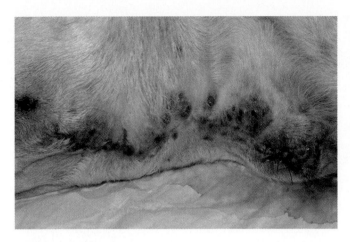

FIGURE 4-98 Blastomycosis. Deep cellulitis with purulent drainage on the ventrum is typical for deep fungal infection.

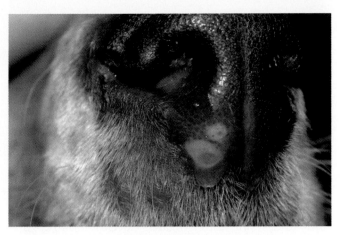

FIGURE 4-99 Blastomycosis. This focal area of depigmentation on the nasal planum could be confused with autoimmune skin disease; however, this is not the normal cobblestone appearance of unaffected regions of the nasal planum and focal swelling of the lesion, suggesting an infiltrative disease.

Coccidioidomycosis

Features

Coccidioides immitis is a dimorphic fungus and soil saprophyte that is endemic to desert areas in southwestern United States, Mexico, Central America, and parts of South America. Although primary cutaneous lesions from direct inoculation rarely occur, the organisms are more typically inhaled, and a lung infection is established that may disseminate to lymph nodes, eyes, skin, bones, and other organs. Coccidioidomycosis is rare in cats and uncommon in dogs, with highest incidences reported in young, medium- to large-breed outdoor dogs.

Skin lesions in dogs include ulcerated nodules, subcutaneous abscesses, and draining tracts over sites of long bone infection. Regional lymphadenomegaly is common. In cats, subcutaneous masses, abscesses, and draining lesions occur without underlying bone involvement. Regional lymphadenomegaly may be seen.

Other signs in dogs and cats include anorexia, weight loss, fever, and depression. Depending on the organs infected, cough, dyspnea, tachypnea, lameness from painful bone swellings, and ocular disease may be seen.

Top Differentials

Differentials include other fungal and bacterial infections, foreign body reaction, and neoplasia.

Diagnosis

1. Cytology (exudate, tissue aspirate): suppurative to (pyo)granulomatous inflammation. Fungal organisms are seldom found.
2. Dermatohistopathology: nodular to diffuse suppurative or (pyo)granulomatous dermatitis and panniculitis, with few to several large, round, double-walled structures (spherules) that contain endospores.
3. Serology: detection of antibodies against *C. immitis* by precipitin, complement fixation, latex agglutination, or ELISA testing. Both false-positive and false-negative results can occur (e.g., titers can be negative in early disease, and low-level titers are common among healthy animals living in endemic areas).
4. Fungal culture (submit to diagnostic laboratory because fungal cultures are highly infectious): *C. immitis.*

5. Radiography: pulmonary changes are common. Osteolytic lesions develop if bone is involved.
6. PCR analysis, where available, may simplify the diagnosis.

Treatment and Prognosis

1. Systemic antifungal therapy should be administered over the long term (minimum 1 year if disseminated) and continued at least 2 months beyond complete clinical and radiographic resolution of the lesions. Treatment should also be continued until follow-up serum *C. immitis* antibody titers are negative.
2. Effective therapies include the following:
   - Ketoconazole (dogs) 5–10 mg/kg PO with food q 12 hours
   - Itraconazole (Sporanox) 5–10 mg/kg PO with food q 12 hours
   - Fluconazole 10 mg/kg PO q 12 hours
   - Terbinafine 30–40 mg/kg PO q 24 hours may be effective.
3. The prognosis is unpredictable, and relapses are common. If relapse occurs, reinstitution of treatment until lesions resolve, followed by long-term low-dose therapy, may be needed to maintain remission. Infected animals (yeast form) are not considered contagious to other animals or to humans, but fungal cultures (mycelial form) are highly infectious.

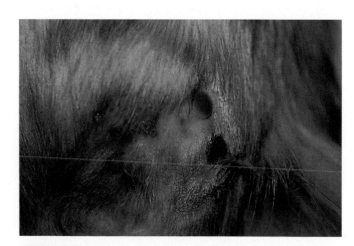

FIGURE 4-100 Coccidioidomycosis. Multiple draining tracts on the ischium of an infected cat. *(Courtesy A. Wolf.)*

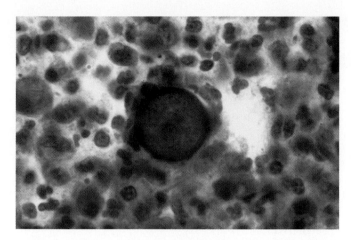

FIGURE 4-101 Coccidioidomycosis. Microscopic image of the *Coccidioides* organism, as viewed with a 100× (oil) objective. *(Courtesy A. Wolf.)*

Cryptococcosis

Features

Cryptococcus neoformans is an environmental saprophytic fungus that can be found worldwide. Cryptococcosis occurs when inhaled organisms establish an infection in the nasal cavity, paranasal sinuses, or lungs. Dissemination to skin, eyes, CNS, and other organs may follow. Cryptococcosis is uncommon in cats. It is rare in dogs, with highest incidences reported in young adults.

Cats

The upper respiratory tract is most commonly involved, with sneezing, snuffling, nasal discharge, nasal mass, or a firm, subcutaneous swelling over the bridge of the nose. Skin involvement is characterized by multiple nonpainful papules and nodules that may ulcerate. Regional lymphadenomegaly is common. Signs of CNS (variable neurologic signs) and ocular disease (fixed, dilated pupils; blindness) are also often seen.

Dogs

This is usually a neurologic or ophthalmic disease in dogs. The upper respiratory tract is also frequently involved. Occasionally, cutaneous ulcers occur, especially on the nose and lips, in the oral cavity, or around nail beds.

Top Differentials

Differentials include other fungal and bacterial infections and neoplasia.

Diagnosis

1. Cytology (exudate, tissue aspirates): (pyo)granulomatous inflammation with narrow, budding, thin-walled yeasts surrounded by variably sized, clear, refractile capsules.
2. Dermatohistopathology: nodular to diffuse (pyo) granulomatous dermatitis and panniculitis, with numerous organisms or vacuolated-appearing dermis and subcutis caused by large numbers of organisms.
3. ELISA or latex agglutination testing: detection of serum cryptococcal capsular antigen. In localized infections, test results may be negative.
4. Fungal culture: *C. neoformans*.
5. PCR analysis, where available, may simplify the diagnosis.

Treatment and Prognosis

1. Cutaneous lesions should be surgically excised, if possible.
2. Systemic antifungal therapy should be administered over the long term (several months) and continued at least 1 month beyond complete clinical resolution. Treatment should also be continued until follow-up serum cryptococcal antigen titers are negative.
3. Effective drugs include the following:
   - Itraconazole (Sporanox) 5–10 mg/kg PO should be administered with food every 12 to 24 hours.
   - Fluconazole 5–15 mg/kg PO should be administered every 12 to 24 hours.
   - Ketoconazole 5–10 mg/kg PO with food q 12–24 hours
   - Terbinafine 30–40 mg/kg PO q 24 hours
   - Amphotericin B 0.5–0.8 mg/kg (added to 0.45% saline/2.5% dextrose, 400 mL for cats, 500 mL for dogs <20 kg and 1000 mL for dogs >20 kg) SQ two to three times per week until a cumulative dose of 8–26 mg/kg is administered. Concentrations of amphotericin B >20 mg/L may cause local irritation.
4. The prognosis for cats is fair to good unless the CNS is involved. The prognosis for cats with CNS involvement and for dogs in general is poor. Infected animals and cultures are not considered contagious to other animals or to humans.

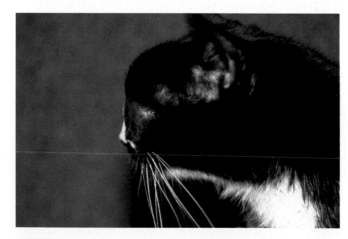

FIGURE 4-102 Cryptococcosis. Dramatic swelling of the bridge of the nose of this adult cat is typical of cryptococcal infections.

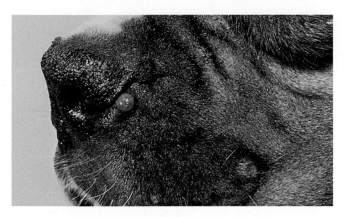

FIGURE 4-103 Cryptococcosis. This focal ulcerated nodule was caused by *Cryptococcus. (Courtesy D. Angarano.)*

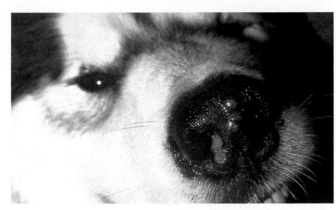

FIGURE 104 Cryptococcosis. Multiple nodules and ulcerated lesions on the nose. *(Courtesy L. Frank.)*

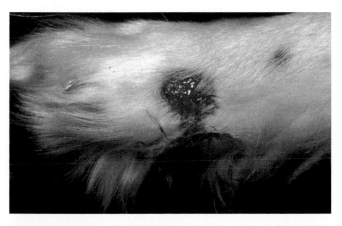

FIGURE 4-105 Cryptococcosis. An ulcerated lesion on the lateral digit with a draining tract. *(Courtesy L. Frank.)*

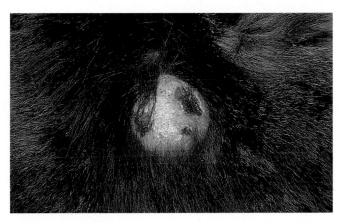

FIGURE 4-106 Cryptococcosis. Alopecic, ulcerated nodule on the head of an adult cat.

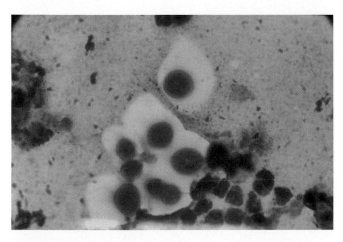

FIGURE 4-107 Cryptococcosis. Microscopic image of *Cryptococcus* organisms, as viewed with a 100× (oil) objective. *(Courtesy L. Frank.)*

Histoplasmosis

Features

Histoplasmosis is a systemic disease caused by *Histoplasma capsulatum*, a dimorphic fungus and soil saprophyte. After conidia are inhaled or ingested, an infection is established in the lungs or gastrointestinal (GI) tract that then disseminates elsewhere. *H. capsulatum* is found worldwide in temperate and subtropical areas. In the United States, the disease occurs most commonly along the Mississippi, Missouri, and Ohio Rivers. Histoplasmosis is rare in dogs and uncommon in cats, with highest incidences reported in young adult animals.

Skin involvement is rare, but multiple small nodules that ulcerate and drain or crust over have been reported. Nonspecific symptoms such as anorexia, depression, weight loss, and fever are typical. Other symptoms in dogs and cats may include dyspnea, tachypnea, and ocular disease. Lameness in cats and cough, diarrhea, icterus, and ascites in dogs may be seen.

Top Differentials

Differentials include other fungal and bacterial infections and neoplasia.

Diagnosis

1. Cytology (tissue aspirates): (pyo)granulomatous inflammation with numerous intracellular, small yeasts that have basophilic centers.
2. Dermatohistopathology: nodular to diffuse (pyo) granulomatous dermatitis with numerous intracellular yeasts. Special fungal stains may be needed for visualization of organisms.
3. Radiography: pulmonary lesions are often seen.
4. Fungal culture: submit to diagnostic laboratory because fungal cultures are highly infectious: *H. capsulatum*.
5. PCR analysis, where available, may simplify the diagnosis.

Treatment and Prognosis

1. Systemic antifungal therapy should be administered over the long term (minimum 4–6 months) and continued at least 2 months beyond complete clinical resolution.
2. Effective therapies include the following:
   - Ketoconazole (dogs) 5–10 mg/kg PO with food q 12 hours
   - Fluconazole 10 mg/kg PO q 12 hours
   - Terbinafine 30–40 mg/kg PO q 24 hours
   - Itraconazole (Sporanox) 10 mg/kg PO with food q 12 hours
3. For severe cases, a quicker response may be achieved by combining itraconazole (Sporanox) or fluconazole with amphotericin B 0.25 mg/kg (cats) or 0.5 mg/kg (dogs) IV three times per week, until a cumulative dose of 4–8 mg/kg (cats) or 5–10 mg/kg (dogs) is administered.
4. The prognosis is fair to good for most cats. The prognosis is poor for severely debilitated cats and for dogs with GI or severe signs of disseminated disease. Infected animals (yeast form) are not considered contagious to other animals or to humans, but fungal cultures (mycelial form) are highly infectious.

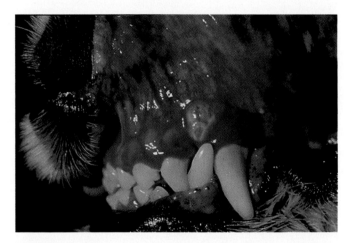

FIGURE 4-108 Histoplasmosis. Erosive lesion on the gingiva of an adult dog. *(Courtesy L. Schmeitzel.)*

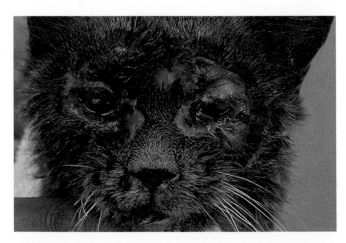

FIGURE 4-109 Histoplasmosis. Multiple erosive nodules and draining tracts on the face of an 11-year-old cat. *(Courtesy P. White.)*

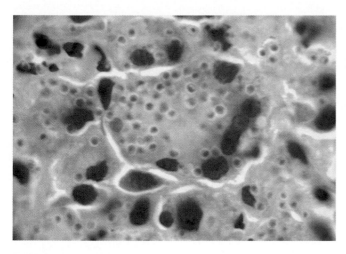

FIGURE 4-110 Histoplasmosis. Microscopic image of the intracellular organisms of histoplasmosis organisms within a giant cell, as viewed with a 100× (oil) objective.

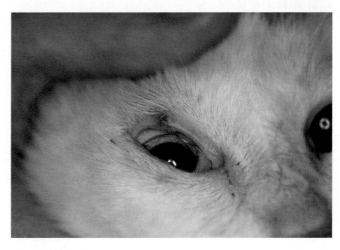

FIGURE 4-111 Histoplasmosis. Small nodule on the eyelid of a cat. *(Courtesy A. Grooters.)*

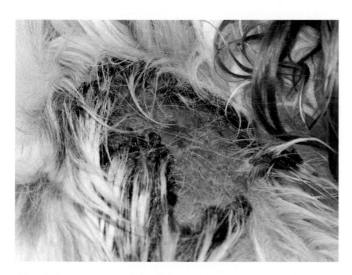

FIGURE 4-112 Histoplasmosis. Focal area of deep infection demonstrating cellulitis, alopecia, and crust formation.

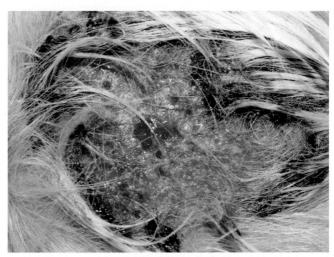

FIGURE 4-113 Histoplasmosis. Close-up of the dog in Figure 4-112. Cellulitis with drainage is apparent.

CHAPTER 5

Parasitic Skin Disorders

- **Ixodid Ticks (hard ticks)**
- **Spinous Ear Tick (*Otobius megnini*)**
- **Canine Localized Demodicosis**
- **Canine Generalized Demodicosis**
- **Feline Demodicosis**
- **Canine Scabies (sarcoptic mange)**
- **Feline Scabies (notoedric mange)**
- **Cheyletiellosis (walking dandruff)**
- **Ear Mites (*Otodectes cynotis*)**
- **Trombiculiasis (chiggers, harvest mites) and Straelensiosis**

- **Cat Fur Mite (*Lynxacarus radosky*)**
- **Fleas**
- **Pediculosis (lice)**
- ***Cuterebra***
- **Fly Bite Dermatitis**
- **Myiasis**
- **Hookworm Dermatitis (ancylostomiasis and uncinariasis)**
- **Dracunculiasis (dracunculosis)**

Ixodid Ticks (hard ticks)

Features

Ixodid ticks include the genera *Rhipicephalus* (i.e., brown dog tick), *Dermacentor* (i.e., American dog tick, Rocky Mountain wood tick, Pacific or West Coast tick), *Ixodes* (i.e., shoulder tick of North America, deer tick, British dog tick [Europe]), *Amblyomma* (i.e., black-legged tick, Lone Star tick), and *Haemophysalis* (i.e., yellow dog tick [Africa and Asia]). Ixodid ticks are more commonly found on dogs than on cats.

Symptoms of tick infestation include none (asymptomatic), inflamed nodule at the site of tick attachment, signs of tick-borne disease (e.g., ehrlichiosis, Rocky Mountain spotted fever, Lyme disease), and tick paralysis. Ticks are most commonly found on the ears or interdigitally, but they can be anywhere on the body.

Diagnosis

1. Direct visualization of ticks on the body.

Treatment and Prognosis

1. If infestation is mild, ticks should be carefully removed manually with forceps or fine-tipped tweezers. The tick should not be twisted or its mouth parts allowed to remain in the skin. Do not burn, puncture, squeeze, or crush the tick's body to kill it because its fluids may be infectious.
2. For severe infestations, topical insecticide labeled for use against ticks should be applied. Amitraz-containing collars, fipronil, and permethrins (dogs) seem to be most effective. New generation veterinary insecticides seem to provide variable efficacy against ticks with a wide range of safety.
3. Concurrent tick-borne disease, if present, should be treated. Products that repel or kill ticks rapidly enough to reduce the transmission of *Rickettsia* diseases are preferred.
4. Periodically, the premises should be treated with appropriately labeled insecticides (in homes and

kennels infested with *Rhipicephalus sanguineus* [brown dog tick]).

5. Spraying grassed and shrubbed areas every spring and midsummer with appropriately labeled pesticides may be helpful in controlling ticks.

6. The prognosis is good. Infected animals are sources of tick transmission to other animals and to humans.

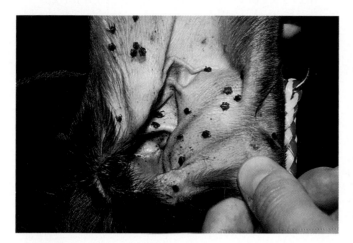

FIGURE 5-1 **Ixodid Ticks.** Multiple ticks attached to the inner ear pinnae. *(Courtesy D. Angarano.)*

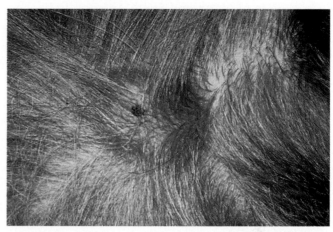

FIGURE 5-2 **Ixodid Ticks.** This erythematous lesion developed at the site of tick attachment. *(Courtesy D. Gram.)*

Spinous Ear Tick *(Otobius megnini)*

Features

Otobius megnini is a soft (argasid) tick primarily found in arid areas of North and South America, India, and southern Africa. Adult ticks are not parasitic, but larvae and nymphs infest external ear canals of animals. These ticks are uncommon in dogs and rare in cats.

The presence of *O. megnini* may be seen as acute onset of otitis externa with severe inflammation and waxy exudate, vigorous head shaking, and ear scratching.

Top Differentials

Differentials include other causes of otitis externa.

Diagnosis

1. Otoscopy: visualization of larval, nymph, and immature adult spinous ear ticks.

Treatment and Prognosis

1. Ticks should be manually removed with forceps.
2. The animal should be treated in topical insecticide labeled for use against ticks.
3. Any secondary ear infection should be treated with appropriate topical medication.
4. Adult ticks infest the animal's premises, so environmental treatment with insecticidal sprays is important.
5. The prognosis is good, but reinfestation can occur if adult ticks are not eliminated from the environment. Although these ticks are parasitic primarily on animals, they can also infest humans.

Canine Localized Demodicosis

Features

Skin lesions occur when there is a localized overpopulation of *Demodex canis*, a normal commensal inhabitant of canine skin. Demodectic overgrowth is often associated with a predisposing factor such as endoparasitism, poor nutrition, immunosuppressive drug therapy, or transient stress (e.g., estrus, pregnancy, surgery, boarding). Canine localized demodicosis is common in dogs, with highest incidence reported in puppies 3 to 6 months old.

Canine localized demodicosis may appear as one to five patchy areas of alopecia with variable erythema, hyperpigmentation, and scaling localized to one region of the body. Lesions are most common on the face, but they can be anywhere on the body. Lesions are not usually pruritic unless they are secondarily infected.

Top Differentials

Differentials include superficial pyoderma, dermatophytosis, and other causes of alopecia.

Diagnosis

1. Microscopy (deep skin scrapes): many *Demodex* sp. adults, nymphs, larvae, or ova.
2. Dermatohistopathology: intrafollicular demodectic mites with varying degrees of perifolliculitis, folliculitis, or furunculosis.

Treatment and Prognosis

1. Any predisposing factors and secondary pyoderma should be identified and treated.
2. Any secondary pyoderma should be treated with appropriate long-term (minimum 3–4 weeks) systemic antibiotics that are continued at least 1 week beyond clinical resolution of the pyoderma.
3. Most patients' conditions will be resolved with infection control and topical shampoo therapy using a 1% to 3% benzoyl peroxide shampoo every 3 to 7 days. Topical creams and ointments do not demonstrate any additional benefit when compared with shampoo therapy alone.
4. Miticidal treatment may not be necessary because many cases resolve spontaneously.
5. If the localized lesion persists, the patient should be neutered and given miticidal treatment. Effective miticidal therapies include the following:

   - Ivermectin 0.2–0.6 mg/kg PO every 24 hours is often effective. Initially, ivermectin 0.1 mg/kg PO is administered on day 1, then 0.2 mg/kg PO is administered on day 2, with oral daily increments of 0.1 mg/kg until 0.2–0.6 mg/kg/day is being administered, assuming that no signs of toxicity develop. The cure rate for 0.4 mg/kg/day ivermectin is 85% to 90%.
   - Milbemycin oxime, 0.5–2 mg/kg PO every 24 hours. The cure rate is 85% to 90%.
   - Doramectin 0.2–0.6 mg/kg SC once weekly. The cure rate is approximately 85%.
   - For dogs weighing less than 20 kg, the use of 9% amitraz collars may be effective. In small dogs, use of 9% amitraz collars alone may be as effective as ivermectin (0.6 mg/kg/day PO).
   - Topical application of Promeris (topical metaflumizone and amitraz solution) every 2 weeks has demonstrated good efficacy.
   - Topical moxidectin has demonstrated variable efficacy when applied every 2 to 4 weeks.
6. Historical (traditional miticidal) treatment includes the following:
   - Total body hair coat clip if dog is medium- to long-haired.
   - Weekly bath with 2.5% to 3% benzoyl peroxide shampoo, followed by a total body application of 0.03% to 0.05% amitraz solution. The cure rate ranges from 50% to 86%.
   - For demodectic pododermatitis, in addition to weekly amitraz dips, foot soaks in 0.125% amitraz solution should be performed every 1 to 3 days.
7. The prognosis is good. Most cases resolve within 4 to 8 weeks, but a few may progress to generalized demodicosis. Systemic therapy or total body dips should not be used in intact animals, as this may mask the development of generalized demodicosis, which is thought to be an inherited disease. *D. canis* is not considered contagious to other dogs (except for newborn puppies), to cats, or to humans.

Author's Note

Although localized demodicosis is not believed to be genetically predisposed, breeding of infected dogs should be discouraged.

Dogs with localized demodicosis may be more likely to develop adult-onset demodicosis if exposed to steroids later in life.

Canine Localized Demodicosis—*cont'd*

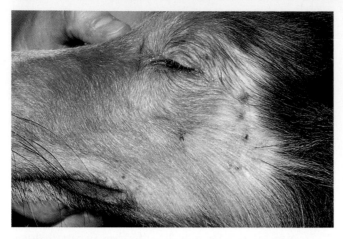

FIGURE 5-3 Canine Localized Demodicosis. Multiple alopecic papular lesions on the face of an adult Shetland Sheep dog. *(Courtesy D. Angarano.)*

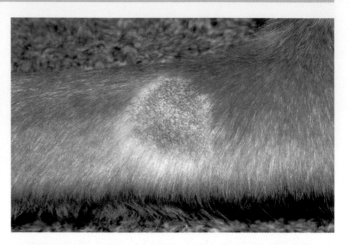

FIGURE 5-4 Canine Localized Demodicosis. Focal area of alopecia and hyperpigmentation typical of folliculitis.

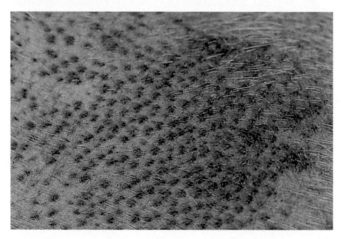

FIGURE 5-5 Canine Localized Demodicosis. Numerous comedones on the abdomen of a dog with hyperadrenocorticism. Comedones are often caused by demodicosis or Cushing's disease.

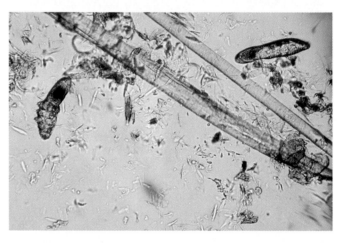

FIGURE 5-6 Canine Localized Demodicosis. Microscopic image of *Demodex* mites, as seen with a 10× objective.

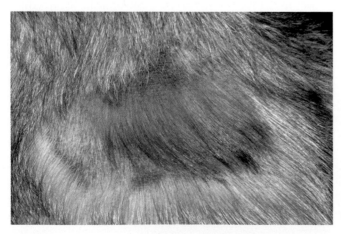

FIGURE 5-7 Canine Localized Demodicosis. This circular area of alopecia with central hair regrowth typical of folliculitis is often misdiagnosed as dermatophytosis.

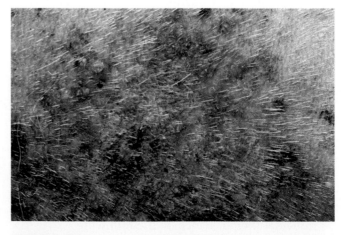

FIGURE 5-8 Canine Localized Demodicosis. Focal area of papular dermatitis caused by *Demodex*.

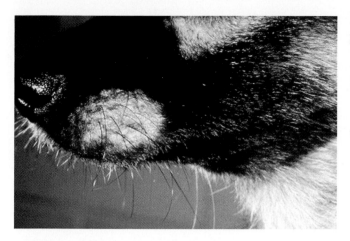

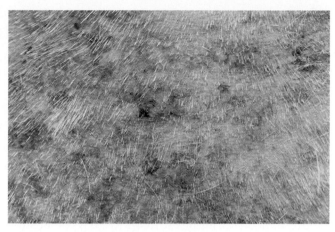

FIGURE 5-9 **Canine Localized Demodicosis.** Focal area of alopecia on the muzzle of a young dog. *(Courtesy D. Angarano.)*

FIGURE 5-10 **Canine Localized Demodicosis.** Papular dermatitis with hyperpigmentation typical of demodicosis.

Canine Generalized Demodicosis

Features

Canine generalized demodicosis may appear as a generalized skin disease that may have genetic tendencies and can be caused by three different species of demodectic mites: *D. canis*, *D. injai*, and an unnamed short-bodied *Demodex* mite. *D. canis*, a normal resident of the canine pilosebaceous unit (hair follicle, sebaceous duct, and sebaceous gland), is primarily transmitted from mother to neonate during the first 2 to 3 days of nursing, but adult-to-adult transmission may rarely occur. *D. injai*, a recently described, large, long-bodied *Demodex* mite, is also found in the pilosebaceous unit, but its mode of transmission is unknown. Mode of transmission is also unknown for the short-bodied unnamed *Demodex* mite, which, unlike the other two species, lives in the stratum corneum. Depending on the dog's age at onset, generalized demodicosis is classified as juvenile-onset or adult-onset. Both forms are common in dogs. Juvenile-onset generalized demodicosis may be caused by *D. canis* and the short-bodied unnamed *Demodex* mite. It occurs in young dogs, usually between 3 and 18 months of age, with highest incidence in medium-sized and large purebred dogs. Adult-onset generalized demodicosis can be caused by all three mite species and occurs in dogs older than 18 months of age, with highest incidence in middle-aged to older dogs that are immunocompromised because of an underlying condition such as endogenous or iatrogenic hyperadrenocorticism, hypothyroidism, immunosuppressive drug therapy, diabetes mellitus, or neoplasia. To date, only adult-onset disease has been reported with *D. injai*, with highest incidence noted in terriers.

Clinical signs of infestation with *D. canis* or the unnamed *Demodex* mite are variable. Generalized demodicosis is defined as five or more focal lesions, or two or more body regions affected. Usually, patchy, regional, multifocal, or diffuse alopecia is observed with variable erythema, silvery grayish scaling, papules, or pruritus. Affected skin may become lichenified, hyperpigmented, pustular, eroded, crusted, or ulcerated from secondary superficial or deep pyoderma. Lesions can be anywhere on the body, including the feet. Pododemodicosis is characterized by any combination of interdigital pruritus, pain, erythema, alopecia, hyperpigmentation, lichenification, scaling, swelling, crusts, pustules, bullae, and draining tracts. Peripheral lymphadenomegaly is common. Systemic signs (e.g., fever, depression, anorexia) may be seen if secondary bacterial sepsis develops.

D. injai infestations are typically characterized by focal areas of greasy seborrhea (seborrhea oleosa), especially over the dorsum of the trunk. Other skin lesions may include alopecia, erythema, hyperpigmentation, and comedones. Small breeds and terriers seem predisposed to *D. injai* infection.

Top Differentials

Differentials include pyoderma (superficial or deep), dermatophytosis, hypersensitivity (flea bite, food, atopy), and autoimmune skin disorders.

Diagnosis

1. Microscopy (deep skin scrapes): many demodectic adults, nymphs, larvae, and ova are typically found with *D. canis* and the short-bodied, unnamed demodectic mite, although *D. canis* may be difficult to find in fibrotic lesions and in feet. With *D. injai*, mites may be low in number and difficult to find, requiring skin biopsies.
2. Dermatohistopathology: minimal to mild suppurative perivascular dermatitis with mites in stratum corneum, or intrafollicular demodectic mites with varying degrees of perifolliculitis, folliculitis, or furunculosis.

Treatment and Prognosis

1. If adult-onset, any underlying conditions should be identified and corrected. All steroid-containing therapies should be discontinued, as steroid administration is the most common cause of adult-onset demodicosis.
2. Intact dogs, especially females, should be neutered. Estrus or pregnancy may trigger relapse.
3. Any secondary pyoderma should be treated with appropriate long-term (minimum 3–4 weeks) systemic antibiotics that are continued at least 1 week beyond clinical resolution of the pyoderma.
4. Topical shampoo therapy using a 1% to 3% benzoyl peroxide shampoo every 3 to 7 days will help speed resolution and will enhance miticidal treatments.
5. Effective miticidal therapies include the following:
   - Ivermectin 0.2–0.6 mg/kg PO every 24 hours is often effective against generalized demodicosis. Initially, ivermectin 0.1 mg/kg PO is administered on day 1, then 0.2 mg/kg PO is administered on day 2, with oral daily increments of 0.1 mg/kg until 0.2–0.6 mg/kg/day is being administered, assuming that no signs of toxicity develop. The cure rate for 0.4 mg/kg/day ivermectin is 85% to 90%.
   - Milbemycin oxime, 0.5–2 mg/kg PO every 24 hours. The cure rate is 85% to 90%.

- Doramectin 0.2–0.6 mg/kg SC once weekly. The cure rate is approximately 85%.
- For dogs ≤20 kg, the use of 9% amitraz collars may be effective. In small dogs, use of 9% amitraz collars alone may be as effective as ivermectin (0.6 mg/kg/day PO).
- Topical application of Promeris (topical metaflumizone and amitraz solution) every 2 weeks has demonstrated good efficacy.
- Topical moxidectin has demonstrated variable efficacy when applied every 2 to 4 weeks.

6. Historical (traditional miticidal) treatment includes the following:
   - Total body hair coat clip if dog is medium- to long-haired.
   - Weekly bath with 2.5% to 3% benzoyl peroxide shampoo, followed by a total body application of 0.03% to 0.05% amitraz solution. The cure rate ranges from 50% to 86%.
   - For demodectic pododermatitis, in addition to weekly amitraz dips, foot soaks in 0.125% amitraz solution should be performed every 1 to 3 days.
7. Regardless of the miticidal treatment chosen, therapy is administered over the long term (weeks to months). Treatments should be continued for at least 1 month beyond the time when the first follow-up skin scrapings become negative for mites (total of two negative skin scrapings).
8. The prognosis is good to fair. Relapses may occur, requiring periodic or lifelong treatment in some dogs. The use of glucocorticosteroids in any dog that has been diagnosed with demodicosis should be avoided. Because of its hereditary predisposition, neither female nor male dogs with juvenile-onset generalized demodicosis should be bred. *D. canis* is not considered contagious to cats or to humans. It is transmitted from bitch to newborn puppies during the first 2 to 3 days of nursing, and possibly between adult dogs that are close cohabitants. The mode of transmission for *D injai* and the unnamed short-bodied *Demodex* mite is unknown.

Author's Note

Steroids are the most common cause of adult-onset demodicosis.

Products containing amitraz tend to be the most toxic usually because of the product vehicle.

Aggressive treatment should be tried for up to 6 months before giving up.

One of the most common causes of treatment failure is that the patient will look greatly improved before negative skin scrapes are achieved. Many owners therefore will discontinue treatment prematurely, resulting in relapse.

The average time to achieve clinical improvement is 4 to 6 weeks; the first negative skin scrape usually occurs around 6 to 8 weeks; most patients need approximately 3 months of treatment to resolve the infection based on two negative skin scrapes at least 3 weeks apart.

Text continued on page 132.

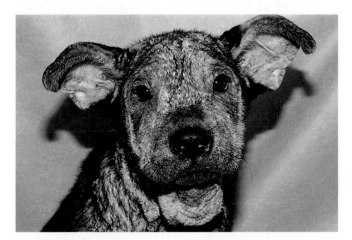

FIGURE 5-11 **Canine Generalized Demodicosis.** Generalized alopecia and papules with crusts and scales on the head and neck of a juvenile dog.

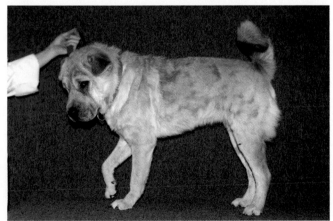

FIGURE 5-12 **Canine Generalized Demodicosis.** Multifocal alopecia over the head, trunk, and extremities of an adult dog with generalized demodicosis.

Canine Generalized Demodicosis—*cont'd*

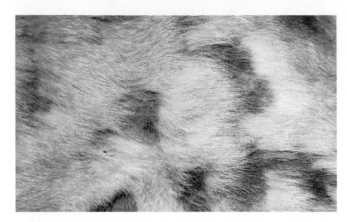

FIGURE 5-13 Canine Generalized Demodicosis. Close-up of the dog in Figure 5-12. Multifocal areas of alopecia with mild hyperpigmentation are apparent.

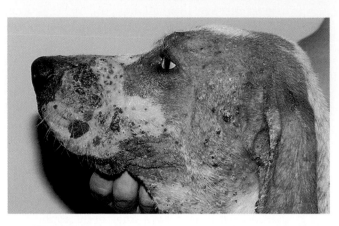

FIGURE 5-14 Canine Generalized Demodicosis. Diffuse alopecic, erythematous, crusting, papular lesions affecting the entire head and neck.

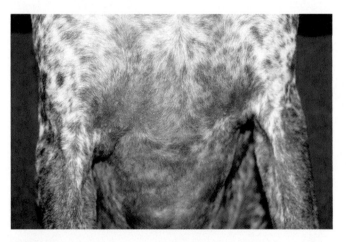

FIGURE 5-15 Canine Generalized Demodicosis. Alopecic, erythematous, papular dermatitis on the axilla and ventral trunk of an adult dog with iatrogenic hyperadrenocorticism.

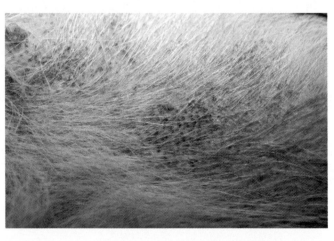

FIGURE 5-16 Canine Generalized Demodicosis. Multiple patches of comedones on the abdomen of a dog.

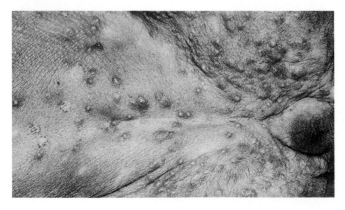

FIGURE 5-17 Close-up of the dog in Figure 5-11. Multiple pustules on the ventral abdomen can be seen.

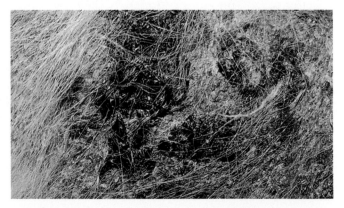

FIGURE 5-18 Canine Generalized Demodicosis. Alopecia, crusting, and papular lesions typically of folliculitis and furunculosis caused by *Demodex*.

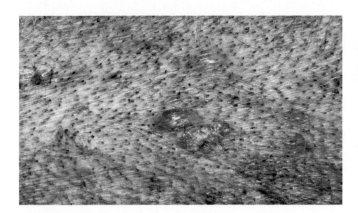

FIGURE 5-19 **Canine Generalized Demodicosis.** Numerous comedones, papules, and pustules on the abdomen of a dog. Note the similarity to superficial pyoderma.

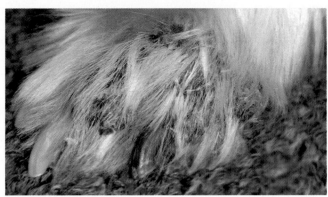

FIGURE 5-20 **Canine Generalized Demodicosis.** Matting of the hair associated with an underlying crusting papular dermatitis.

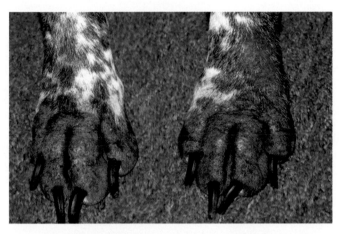

FIGURE 5-21 **Canine Generalized Demodicosis.** Severe alopecia, erythema, and hyperpigmentation with a papular rash on the feet of an adult dog with iatrogenic hyperadrenocorticism.

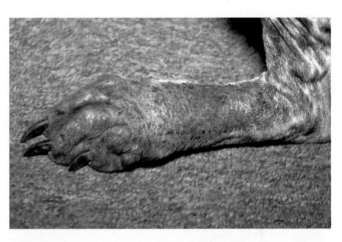

FIGURE 5-22 **Canine Generalized Demodicosis.** Alopecia and papular dermatitis with a large erosive lesion.

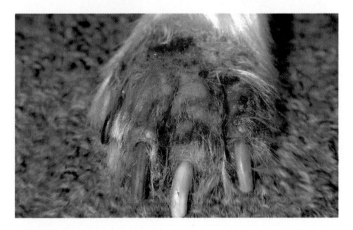

FIGURE 5-23 **Canine Generalized Demodicosis.** Alopecia, erythema, and crusting ulcerative lesions are typical of furunculosis caused by demodicosis.

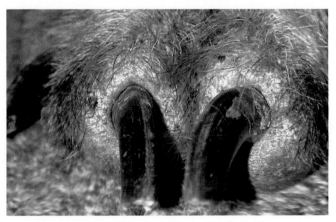

FIGURE 5-24 **Canine Generalized Demodicosis.** Alopecia and hyperpigmentation affecting the swollen nail beds (paronychia) of a dog with *Demodex*.

Canine Generalized Demodicosis—*cont'd*

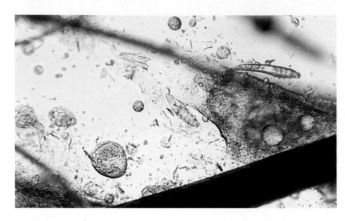

FIGURE 5-25 **Canine Generalized Demodicosis.** Microscopic image of *Demodex* mites, as seen with a 10× objective.

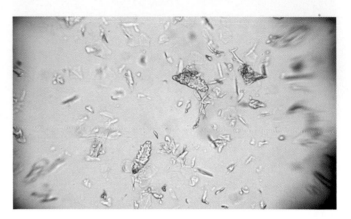

FIGURE 5-26 **Canine Generalized Demodicosis.** Microscopic image of *Demodex* mites, as seen with a 10× objective.

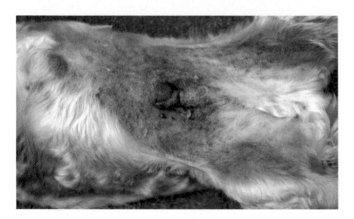

FIGURE 5-27 **Canine Generalized Demodicosis.** Diffuse papular dermatitis with hyperpigmentation on the abdomen of an adult Cocker spaniel.

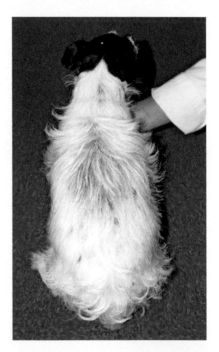

FIGURE 5-28 **Canine Generalized Demodicosis.** Focal area of alopecia and papular dermatitis on the dorsum of an adult dog with *Demodex injai*. Note the location and severe seborrhea oleosa that are characteristic of this species.

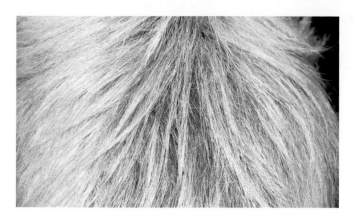

FIGURE 5-29 Canine Generalized Demodicosis. Same dog as in Figure 5-28. Clumping of the hair is caused by excessive sebaceous secretions.

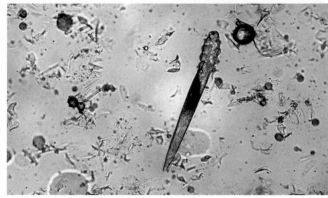

FIGURE 5-30 Canine Generalized Demodicosis. Microscopic image of *Demodex injai*, as seen with a 10× objective. The mite is larger than *Demodex canis*.

Feline Demodicosis

Features

Feline demodicosis is a skin disease that can be caused by two different species of demodectic mites—*D. cati* and *D. gatoi*, a short-bodied *Demodex* mite whose normal habitat is unknown. Skin disease may be localized or generalized. *D. gatoi* is contagious and usually causes pruritic skin disease. *D. cati* infections are often associated with an underlying immunosuppressive or metabolic disease such as feline immunodeficiency virus (FIV), feline leukemia virus (FeLV), toxoplasmosis, systemic lupus erythematosus, neoplasia, or diabetes mellitus. Localized or generalized demodicosis caused by *D. cati* infection is rare in cats. *D. gatoi* infections are emerging as a cause of pruritic skin disease in cats in the United States, especially in the southern United States.

Localized disease is characterized by a variably pruritic ceruminous otitis externa or by focal patchy alopecia and erythema that may be scaly or crusty. Localized skin lesions are most common around the eyes, on the head, or on the neck. Generalized disease is characterized by variably pruritic (none to extreme), multifocal, patchy, regional, or symmetrical alopecia, with or without erythema, scaling, crusts, macules, and hyperpigmentation. Lesions usually involve the head, neck, limbs, flanks, or ventrum. Ceruminous otitis externa and secondary pyoderma may be present.

Top Differentials

Differentials include dermatophytosis, other ectoparasites (*Cheyletiella*, *Notoedres*, ear mites), hypersensitivity (flea bite, food, atopy), psychogenic alopecia, and other causes of otitis externa.

Diagnosis

1. Microscopy (deep and superficial skin scrapings, ear swabs): demonstration of demodectic adults, nymphs, larvae, or ova. *D. gatoi* may be difficult to find.
2. *D. gatoi*: history, clinical signs, and response to weekly lime sulfur dips.
3. Dermatohistopathology: minimal to mild suppurative perivascular dermatitis with mites in stratum corneum, or intrafollicular mites with varying degrees of perifolliculitis and folliculitis.

Treatment and Prognosis

1. Any predisposing factors should be identified and corrected.
2. *D. gatoi* may be difficult to find on microscopy but respond well to lime sulfur dips.
   - 2% to 4% lime sulfur dips applied q 3–7 days for 4 to 8 weeks. Clinical improvement is often observed within 3 to 4 weeks, but therapy should be continued for a total of 6 to 8 weeks to resolve the infection.
   - All cats in close contact must be treated to prevent reinfection.
3. *D. cati*: localized lesions may resolve spontaneously without treatment.
   - For localized lesions, topical therapies (0.025%–0.03% amitraz solution) may be effective when applied q 24 hours.
   - For generalized lesions, treatments that may be effective include the following:
     - 2% to 4% lime sulfur solution applied to the entire body q 7 days
     - Doramectin 0.2–0.6 mg/kg SC once weekly
     - 0.015% to 0.025% amitraz solution applied to entire body q 1–2 weeks. *Note:* Cats are extremely sensitive to amitraz. Do not use amitraz on diabetic cats.
   - For both localized and generalized disease, treatments should be continued until lesions have resolved and two follow-up skin scrapings are negative for mites (approximately 3–4 weeks).
4. The prognosis for localized demodicosis is good. The prognosis for generalized demodicosis is good to guarded, depending on the underlying cause. *D. cati* is not considered contagious to other cats (except for newborn kittens), to dogs, or to humans. The mode of transmission for *D. gatoi* is unknown, but reports of unrelated household cats being simultaneously affected suggest that it may be contagious between adult cats.

Author's Note

Diagnosis and treatment of feline demodicosis can be extremely difficult and frustrating. If treatments for other allergic diseases fail, *Demodex gatoi* should be suspected.

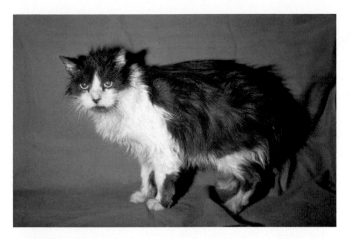

FIGURE 5-31 Feline Demodicosis. Generalized alopecic dermatitis caused the unkempt appearance of this cat's fur coat. *(Courtesy J. MacDonald.)*

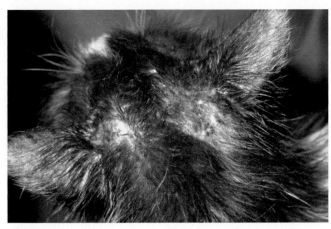

FIGURE 5-32 Feline Demodicosis. Close-up of the cat in Figure 5-31. Generalized alopecic, erythematous lesions on the head. *(Courtesy J. MacDonald.)*

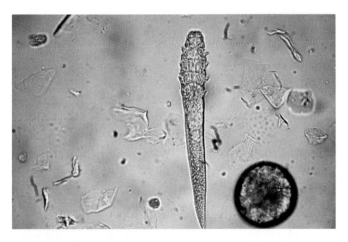

FIGURE 5-33 Feline Demodicosis. Microscopic image of *Demodex cati*, as seen with a 10× objective.

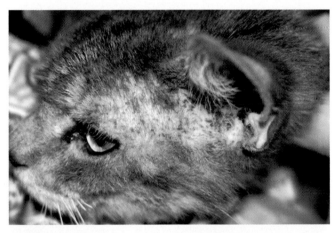

FIGURE 5-34 Feline Demodicosis. Papular crusting dermatitis (miliary dermatitis) on the preauricular area of a cat with *Demodex gatoi*.

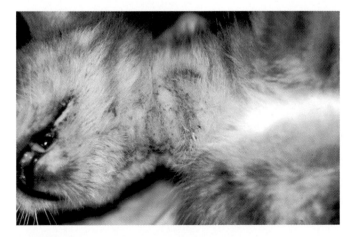

FIGURE 5-35 Feline Demodicosis. Same cat as in Figure 5-34. Alopecic crusting dermatitis on the ventral neck of this adult cat revealed numerous eosinophils on cytology.

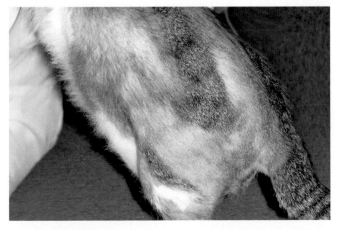

FIGURE 5-36 Feline Demodicosis. Symmetrical alopecia on the lumbar area and flanks of an adult cat with *Demodex gatoi*. Note the similarity to other allergic conditions, as well as to psychogenic alopecia.

Feline Demodicosis—*cont'd*

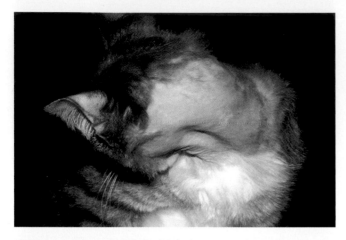

FIGURE 5-37 **Feline Demodicosis.** Complete alopecia on the dorsal neck of a cat with *Demodex gatoi*. Note that the general lack of primary lesions can be a common feature in cats with ectoparasitism or allergies.

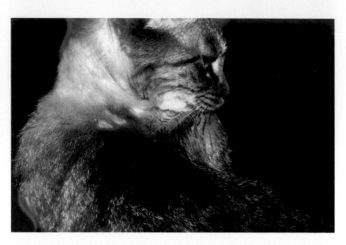

FIGURE 5-38 **Feline Demodicosis.** Same cat as in Figure 5-37. The cat would self-mutilate as soon as the protective collar was removed. This self-mutilation of the dorsal cervical region is a common feature of feline idiopathic ulcerative dermatitis but was caused by *Demodex gatoi* in this patient.

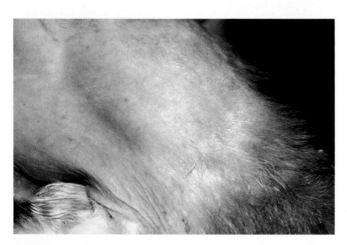

FIGURE 5-39 **Feline Demodicosis.** Close-up of the cat in Figure 5-37. A fine papular rash is apparent upon close examination.

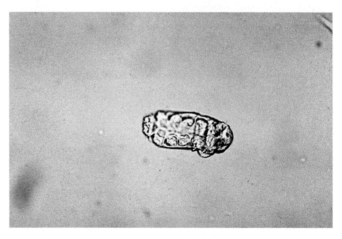

FIGURE 5-40 **Feline Demodicosis.** Microscopic image of *Demodex gatoi*, as seen when viewed with a 10× objective.

Canine Scabies (sarcoptic mange)

Features

Canine scabies manifests as a disease that is caused by *Sarcoptes scabiei* var. *canis*, a superficial burrowing skin mite. Mites secrete allergenic substances that elicit an intensely pruritic hypersensitivity reaction in sensitized dogs. Canine scabies is common in dogs. Affected dogs often have a previous history of being in an animal shelter, having contact with stray dogs, or visiting a grooming or boarding facility. Wildlife such as fox and coyotes are often the source of initial infection and possible repeated infections. In multiple-dog households, more than one dog is usually affected.

Canine scabies is a nonseasonal intense pruritus that responds only variably to corticosteroids. Lesions include papules, alopecia, erythema, crusts, and excoriations. Initially, less-hairy skin is involved, such as on the hocks, elbows, pinnal margins, and ventral abdomen and chest. With chronicity, lesions may spread over the body, but the dorsum of the back is usually spared. Peripheral lymphadenomegaly is often present. Secondary weight loss may occur. Heavily infested dogs may develop severe scaling and crusting. Some dogs may present with intense pruritus but no or minimal skin lesions. Although they are less common, asymptomatic carrier states are possible in dogs; however, in multiple-dog households, a range of symptoms (severe to nonpruritic) may exist.

Top Differentials

Differentials include hypersensitivity (food, atopy, flea), *Malassezia* dermatitis, pyoderma, demodicosis, dermatophytosis, and contact dermatitis.

Diagnosis

1. History, clinical findings, and response to scabicidal treatment.
2. Pinnal-pedal reflex: rubbing of the ear margin between thumb and forefinger may elicit a scratch reflex. This reflex is highly suggestive of a scabies infection with approximately 80% accuracy.
3. Microscopy (superficial skin scrapings): detection of sarcoptic mites, nymphs, larvae, or ova. False-negative results are common because mites are extremely difficult to find; approximately 20% accurate.
4. Serology (enzyme-linked immunosorbent assay [ELISA]): detection of circulating immunoglobulin (Ig)G antibodies against *Sarcoptes* antigens. This is a highly specific and sensitive test, but false-negative results can occur in young puppies and in dogs receiving corticosteroid therapy. Also, false-positive results may be seen in dogs that have been successfully treated for scabies because detectable antibodies may persist for several months after treatment cessation.
5. Dermatohistopathology (usually nondiagnostic): varying degrees of epidermal hyperplasia and superficial perivascular dermatitis with lymphocytes, mast cells, and eosinophils. Mite segments are rarely found within the stratum corneum.

Treatment and Prognosis

1. Affected and all in-contact dogs should be treated with a scabicide. Failure to treat all dogs results in reinfection and persistent pruritus.
2. Any secondary pyoderma should be treated with appropriate long-term (minimum 3–4 weeks) systemic antibiotics that are continued at least 1 week beyond clinical resolution of the pyoderma.
3. Topical shampoo therapy using a antimicrobial shampoo every 3 to 7 days will help speed resolution and will enhance miticidal treatment.
4. Systemic treatments are most effective because of accurate dosing and better compliance. Effective systemic treatments include the following:
   - Selamectin 6–12 mg/kg applied every 2 weeks (at least four times may be more effective)
   - Ivermectin 0.2–0.4 mg/kg PO q 7 days, or SC q 14 days, for 4 to 6 weeks
   - Doramectin 0.2–0.6 mg/kg SQ q 7 days for 4 to 6 weeks
   - Milbemycin oxime 0.75 mg/kg PO q 24 hours for 30 days, or 2 mg/kg PO q 7 days for 3 to 5 weeks
   - Topical moxidectin can be applied every 2 to 4 weeks for 4 to 6 weeks; frequent application may lead to increased adverse effects.
5. Topical treatments may be effective, but because of poorer compliance, treatment failures are more common. Effective topical products include the following:
   - 0.025% to 0.03% amitraz solution applied to the entire body three times at 2-week intervals, or once weekly for 2 to 6 weeks
   - Fipronil spray 3 mL/kg, applied as pump spray to the entire body three times at 2-week intervals, or 6 mL/kg applied as sponge-on once weekly for 4 to 6 weeks
   - 2% to 3% lime sulfur solution applied once a week for 4 to 6 weeks
   - Organophosphates (malathion, phosmet, mercaptomethyl phtalimide) are the most toxic and least effective therapies available.

Canine Scabies—*cont'd*

6. If the animal is severely pruritic and mites have been identified, steroids given the first 2 to 5 days of scabicidal treatment may be helpful. Use of steroids without the finding of mites makes it impossible for the practitioner to determine response to scabicidal therapy.

7. In kennel situations, bedding should be disposed of and the environment thoroughly cleaned and treated with parasiticidal sprays.

8. The prognosis is good. *S scabei* is a highly contagious parasite of dogs that can also transiently infest humans and, rarely, cats. Reinfection can occur, leading to chronic pruritic disease.

Author's Note

Scabies infections can very closely mimic food allergy and atopy.

The pinnal-pedal reflex (ear scratch test) is the easiest and most suggestive test for scabies.

If reinfection is suspected, long-term scabicidal therapy may be beneficial unless the source can be identified and treated.

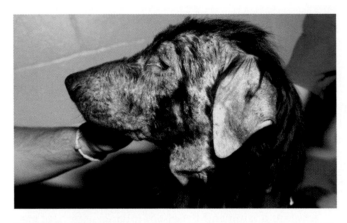

FIGURE 5-41 Canine Scabies. Generalized alopecia with crusting papular dermatitis affecting the head and neck of a young adult dog. Note that the ear margins are severely affected.

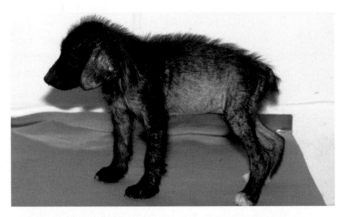

FIGURE 5-42 Canine Scabies. Generalized alopecia and crusts affecting a pruritic puppy. Alopecic ear pinnae are characteristic of scabies.

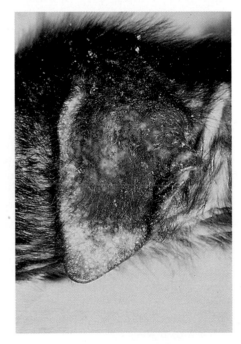

FIGURE 5-43 Canine Scabies. Alopecia and crusting dermatitis on the ear pinna margin of this dog are characteristic of scabies.

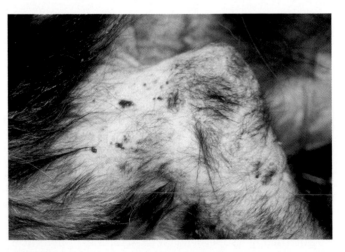

FIGURE 5-44 Canine Scabies. Alopecia and crusting on the lateral elbow of a dog with scabies.

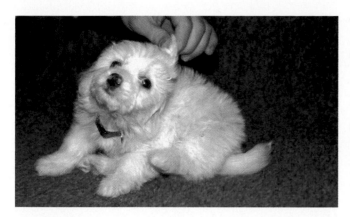

FIGURE 5-45 **Canine Scabies.** A positive pinnal-pedal reflex is highly suggestive of scabies.

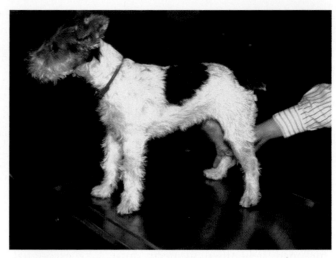

FIGURE 5-46 **Canine Scabies.** This pruritic 9-month-old Fox terrier had no cutaneous lesions other than diffuse erythema ("scabies incognito"). Note the similarity to allergic skin disease.

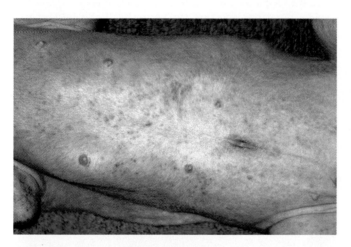

FIGURE 5-47 **Canine Scabies.** Diffuse papular rash with crust formation on the abdomen of a young dog with scabies. Note the similarity to superficial pyoderma.

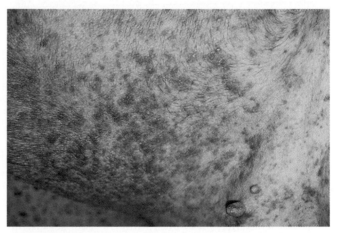

FIGURE 5-48 **Canine Scabies.** Generalized papular dermatitis affected almost the entire cutaneous surface of this dog.

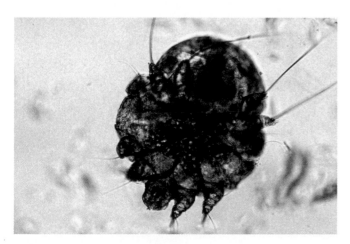

FIGURE 5-49 **Canine Scabies.** Microscopic image of scabies mite, as seen with a 40× objective.

Feline Scabies (notoedric mange)

Features

Feline scabies is a disease that is caused by *Notoedres cati*, a sarcoptic mite that burrows superficially in the skin. In multiple-cat households and catteries, more than one cat is usually affected. The condition is rare in cats.

Feline scabies is noted as intensely pruritic, dry, crusted lesions that usually first appear on the medial edges of ear pinnae, then spread rapidly over the ears, head, face, and neck. Lesions may subsequently spread to the feet and perineum. Infested skin becomes thickened, lichenified, alopecic, crusted, or excoriated. Peripheral lymphadenomegaly is common. If untreated, lesions may spread over large areas of the body, and anorexia, emaciation, and death may occur.

Top Differentials

Differentials include ear mites, dermatophytosis, demodicosis, hypersensitivity (flea bite, food, atopy), and autoimmune skin disorders.

Diagnosis

1. Microscopy (superficial skin scrapings): detection of notoedric mites, nymphs, larvae, or ova.
2. Dermatohistopathology: superficial perivascular or interstitial dermatitis with varying numbers of eosinophils and pronounced focal parakeratosis. Mite segments may be found in the superficial epidermis.

Treatment and Prognosis

1. Affected and all in-contact cats should be treated with a scabicide.
2. Traditional therapy is to bathe the animal with a mild antiseborrheic shampoo to loosen crusts, followed by total body application of 2% to 3% lime sulfur solution every 7 days until follow-up skin scrapings are negative for mites and lesions have resolved (approximately 4–8 weeks).
3. Alternative therapies include the following:
   - Ivermectin 0.2–0.3 mg/kg PO or SC every 1 to 2 weeks for three to four treatments
   - Doramectin 0.2–0.3 mg/kg SC every 1 to 2 weeks for treatments
4. The prognosis is good. *N. cati* is a highly contagious parasite of cats that can also transiently infest dogs, rabbits, and humans.

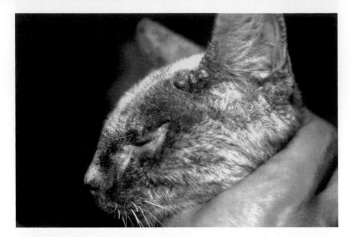

FIGURE 5-50 Feline Scabies. Severe alopecic, crusting, papular dermatitis affecting the entire head and neck of this adult cat. *(Courtesy G. Norsworthy.)*

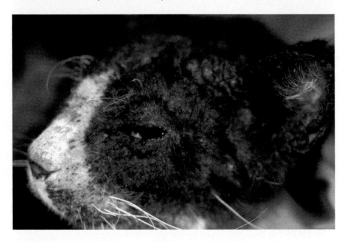

FIGURE 5-51 Feline Scabies. Generalized alopecia and crusting papular dermatitis on the head of an adult cat.

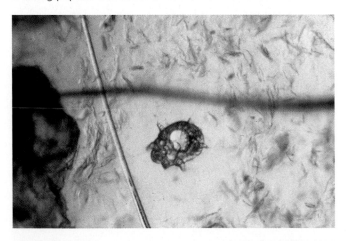

FIGURE 5-52 Feline Scabies. Microscopic image of *Notoedres cati* mite from a skin scraping, as seen with a 10× objective. *(Courtesy G. Norsworthy.)*

Cheyletiellosis (walking dandruff)

Features

Cheyletiellosis is a skin disease that is caused by *Cheyletiella* mites, which live on hair and fur, visiting the skin only to feed. All stages (larvae, nymphs, and adults) are parasitic. In a multiple-pet household, more than one animal is usually affected. Cheyletiellosis is uncommon in dogs and cats.

The most common symptom is excessive scaling (i.e., dandruff, scurf), which gives the hair coat a powdery or mealy appearance, especially over the dorsal midline of the back. Pruritus may be mild to severe. Papular, crusting eruptions (cats) or scabies-like lesions (dogs) are present. Other adult pets (dogs, cats, rabbits) in the household may be asymptomatic carriers.

Top Differentials

Differentials include other ectoparasites (pediculosis, scabies, demodicosis, hypersensitivities [flea bite, food, atopy]) and other causes of miliary dermatitis in cats.

Diagnosis

1. Rule out other differentials.
2. Direct visualization of mites: the procedure is to part the hair coat along the back over the sacrum, comb out dandruff onto dark paper, and observe for movement of mites in debris (may be difficult to find).
3. Microscopy (superficial skin scrapings, acetate tape impressions, flea-combed hairs and scales): detection of *Cheyletiella* mites, nymphs, larvae, or ova (may be difficult to find).
4. Fecal floatation: mites may be identified through standard fecal floatation procedures.
5. Dermatohistopathology (usually nondiagnostic): varying degrees of superficial perivascular dermatitis, with few to many eosinophils. Mite segments in the stratum corneum are rarely seen.

Treatment and Prognosis

1. All affected and in-contact animals (dogs, cats, rabbits) should be treated once weekly for 6 to 8 weeks.
2. Systemic treatments are generally more effective than topicals. Effective treatments include the following:
   - Ivermectin 0.2–0.3 mg/kg PO or SC 1 to 2 weeks apart for 4 to 6 weeks
   - Selamectin 6–15 mg/kg, applied topically at 1-month intervals; effectiveness may be enhanced when treatment is provided every 2 weeks for 4 to 6 weeks
   - Doramectin 0.2–0.4 mg/kg SQ every 7 days for 4 to 6 weeks
   - Topical moxidectin applied every 2 to 4 weeks for two to three applications. More frequent application of moxidectin may lead to increases in adverse effects.
3. Effective topical products for dogs include fipronil spray 6 mL/kg applied to entire body 2 weeks apart for 4 to 6 weeks. Other topical treatments for dogs include those containing 2% to 3% lime sulfur, pyrethrin, pyrethroid, carbamate, or an organophosphate. Effective topical products for cats include those containing 2% to 3% lime sulfur or a dilute water-based 0.2% pyrethrin.
4. The environment should be cleaned and treated with a flea insecticide.
5. The prognosis is good. *Cheyletiella* mites are highly contagious to cats, dogs, rabbits, and humans.

Author's Note

Cheyletiella infections seem to occur commonly in certain regions and may vary in frequency from year to year.

Cheyletiella may be difficult to find in some dogs and cats.

Cheyletiellosis—*cont'd*

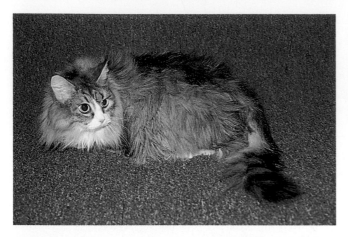

FIGURE 5-53 Cheyletiellosis. An unkempt fur coat in an adult cat.

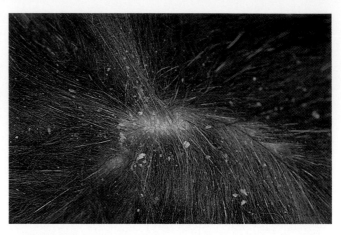

FIGURE 5-54 Cheyletiellosis. Close-up of the cat in Figure 5-53. Diffuse scaling and erythema are apparent upon close examination.

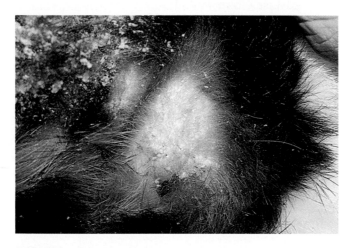

FIGURE 5-55 Cheyletiellosis. Alopecia with scale and crust.

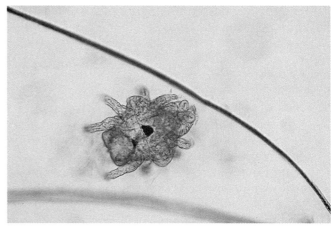

FIGURE 5-56 Cheyletiellosis. Microscopic image of a *Cheyletiella* mite from a skin scraping, as seen when viewed with a 10× objective. Note the hooked mouth parts used for piercing the skin.

Ear Mites (*Otodectes cynotis*)

Features

This disease is caused by infestation with *Otodectes cynotis*, a psoroptic mite that lives on the surface of skin and in ear canals. It occurs commonly in dogs and cats, with highest incidences noted in kittens. Adult cats are often asymptomatic carriers.

Typically, mild to marked accumulation of dark brown to black, waxy or crusty exudate is noted in the ear canals. The otic discharge becomes purulent if a secondary bacterial otitis develops. The ears are usually intensely pruritic, and scratching results in secondary alopecia and excoriations on the ears and head. Head shaking may result in aural hematoma. Occasionally, ectopic mites may cause a pruritic, papular, crusting skin eruption, especially on the neck, rump, or tail (otodectic acariasis).

Top Differentials

Differentials include other causes of otitis externa.

Diagnosis

1. Otoscopy: direct visualization of mites (moving white specks).
2. Positive pinnal-pedal reflex (cats): cat scratches with ipsilateral hindlimb when ear canal is swabbed.
3. Microscopy (ear swabs, superficial skin scrapings): detection of *O. cynotis* mites, nymphs, larvae, or ova.

Treatment and Prognosis

1. The ear canals of affected animals should be cleaned to remove accumulated debris.
2. Affected animals and all in-contact dogs and cats should be treated.
3. Traditional treatment is to instill a parasiticidal otic preparation at the dosage, frequency, and duration indicated on label instructions.
4. Other otic treatments effective against *Otodectes* include the following:
   - Milbemycin solution (Milbemite) instilled into each ear once is safe and effective.
   - Ivermectin topical solution (Acarex) instilled into each ear once is safe and effective.
   - Numerous additional treatments are available.
5. Effective systemic treatments include the following:
   - Selamectin 6–12 mg/kg applied topically once or twice 1 month apart for cats, and twice at a 1-month interval for dogs. Treatment effectiveness may be enhanced if administered every 2 weeks at least four times.
   - Ivermectin 0.3 mg/kg PO q 7 days for three or four treatments, or 0.3 mg/kg SC q 10–14 days for three treatments
6. Multimodal ear products may also provide benefit and eliminate the infection. Effective multimodal treatments include the following:
   - Neomycin-thiabendazole-dexamethasone (Tresaderm) 0.125–0.25 mL AU q 12 hours for 2 to 3 weeks
   - Gentamicin-clotrimazole-betamethasone 0.25–0.5 mL AU q 12 hours for 2 to 3 weeks
   - Gentamicin-clotrimazole-mometasone (Mometomax) 0.25–0.5 mL AU q 12 hours for 2 to 3 weeks
   - 10% fipronil solution 2 drops AU once or twice, 2 to 4 weeks apart
7. When otic treatments are used, they should be combined with whole body treatments with an appropriate acaricide to eliminate any ectopic mites. For whole body treatment, a pyrethrin spray, powder, or dip should be used once weekly for 4 weeks, or fipronil spray or spot-on can should be used two to three times 2 weeks apart.
8. The prognosis is good. However, ear mites are highly contagious to other cats and dogs.

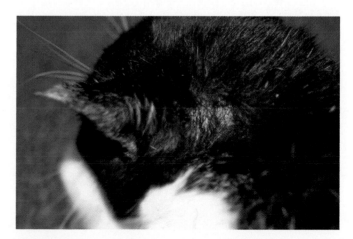

FIGURE 5-57 Ear Mites. Alopecic erythematous dermatitis caused by excoriations associated with a cat's otitis externa.

Ear Mites—*cont'd*

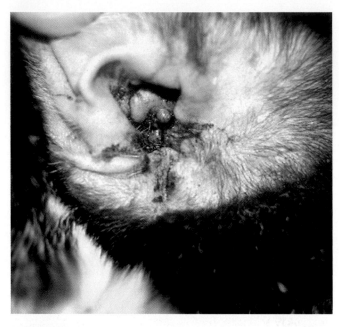

FIGURE 5-58 Ear Mites. Same cat as in Figure 5-57. The ear canal has a dark exudate typical of *Otodectes*.

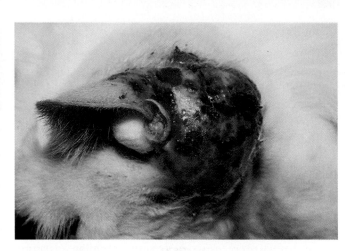

FIGURE 5-59 Ear Mites. Severe, erosive, crusting lesions on a cat's ear caused by intense pruritus associated with an ear mite infection.

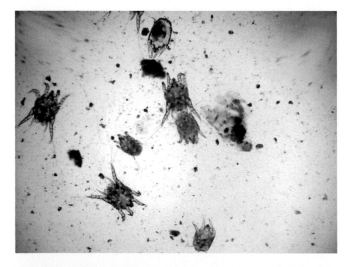

FIGURE 5-60 Ear Mites. Microscopic image of *Otodectes cynotis*, as viewed with a 4× objective.

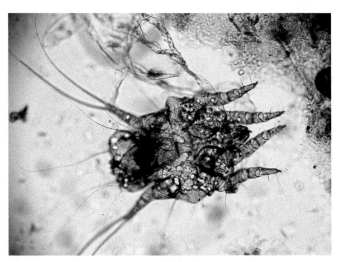

FIGURE 5-61 Ear Mites. Microscopic image of *Otodectes cynotis*, as viewed with a 40× objective.

Trombiculiasis (chiggers, harvest mites) and Straelensiosis

Features

Adults and nymphs of the genera *Neotrombicula* (harvest mites) and *Eutrombicula* (chiggers) are found worldwide in habitats ranging from semidesert to swamp. They are free living, or they may parasitize plants or other arthropods. Their larval stage feeds on vertebrate hosts, which are usually wild animals, although food-producing domestic animals, pets, and people may be infested accidentally. The larvae hatch from eggs laid in the soil and crawl up vegetation to attack birds and mammals that pass by. The skin disease that they cause is seasonal (summer-fall) in temperate climates and year round in warm regions. Trombiculiasis is rare to uncommon in dogs and cats.

Chiggers and Harvest Mites

Typically, these manifest as intensely pruritic wheals, papules, and vesicles that develop on skin that contacts the ground (e.g., limbs, feet, head, ears, ventrum). The larvae may be visible as tiny, pinpoint, bright red, orange, or yellow dots clustered on the papules. Occasionally, lesions are nonpruritic. Secondary scaling, crusts, excoriations, and alopecia from scratching may be present.

Top Differentials

Differentials include superficial pyoderma, other ectoparasites (e.g., insect stings/bites, scabies, demodicosis, *Pelodera*, hookworm dermatitis), and contact dermatitis.

Diagnosis

1. Microscopy (skin scrapings): for chiggers and harvest mites, intensely bright orange, ovoid trombiculid larvae (about 0.6 mm long) are seen, but sometimes, only the mouth parts (stylostomes) are present (the rest of the mite having been removed by the animal's scratching). For straelensiosis, skin scrapings are usually negative
2. Dermatohistopathology: for chiggers and harvest mites, histopathology is usually nondiagnostic, with superficial perivascular dermatitis that contains numerous eosinophils. Occasionally, mite stylostomes may be seen.

Treatment and Prognosis

1. Pets should be kept away from areas known to harbor large numbers of mites.
2. For chiggers and harvest mites, the affected animal should be treated with one or two applications (1–2 weeks apart) of a parasiticidal spray, spot-on, dip, or otic preparation. Recent studies suggest that 0.25% fipronil pump spray (dogs and cats) or combination permethrin-pyriproxyfen pump spray or spot-on (dogs only) is especially effective when used according to label instructions. In dogs, topically applied 0.25% fipronil spray 6 mL/kg administered every 2 to 4 weeks may also be effective in preventing reinfestations.
3. Appropriate systemic antibiotics should be administered for 2 to 4 weeks if secondary pyoderma is present.
4. The prognosis is good for chiggers and harvest mites. The mites are not contagious between animals or from animals to humans, but infested areas are a potential source of infestation for other dogs, cats, and humans.

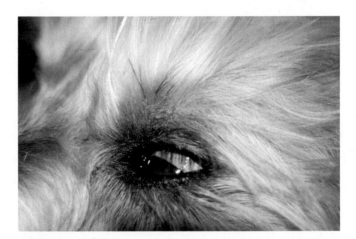

FIGURE 5-62 Trombiculiasis. Alopecic papular dermatitis around the eye. Small orange mites are barely visible.

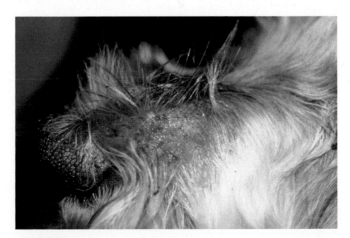

FIGURE 5-63 Trombiculiasis. Same dog as in Figure 5-62. Alopecic papular dermatitis on the bridge of the nose. The orange specks are the mites.

Trombiculiasis and Straelensiosis—*cont'd*

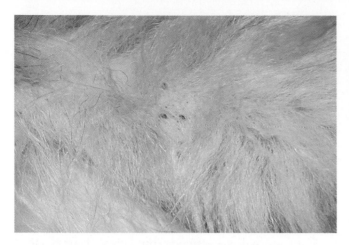

FIGURE 5-64 Trombiculiasis. Multiple papular lesions on the ventrum. Note the similarity to superficial pyoderma, demodicosis, and dermatophytosis.

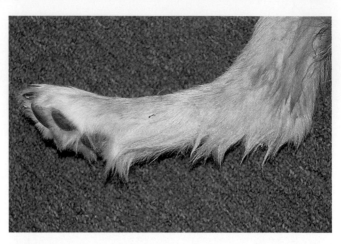

FIGURE 5-65 Trombiculiasis. Alopecia and erythema on the distal rear leg.

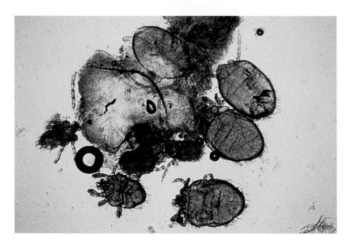

FIGURE 5-66 Trombiculiasis. Microscopic image of mites from a deep skin scrape, as seen with a 4× objective. *(Courtesy R. Malik.)*

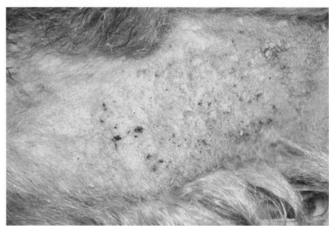

FIGURE 5-67 Trombiculiasis. Crusting papular lesions on the ventrum of an adult dog infected with chiggers. Note the similarity to folliculitis.

Cat Fur Mite (*Lynxacarus radosky*)

Features

The cat fur mite is a hair-clasping mite of cats primarily reported in Australia, Fiji, Hawaii, Puerto Rico, and Florida. It is rare in cats.

Hordes of mites on hairs give the coat a salt-and-pepper or scurfy appearance, especially over the dorsum of the back. Widespread papular crusting eruptions may also be present, along with minimal pruritus.

Top Differentials

Differentials include pediculosis and cheyletiellosis.

Diagnosis

1. Microscopy (skin scrapings, acetate tape impressions): fur mites are clasped to hairs.

Treatment and Prognosis

1. All affected cats should be treated once a week for 4 weeks.
2. Affected and all in-contact cats should be treated weekly for 4 weeks.
3. Traditional therapy is 2% to 3% lime sulfur solution every 7 days until lesions have resolved (approximately 4–8 weeks).
4. Alternative therapies that may be effective include the following:
   - Ivermectin 0.2–0.3 mg/kg PO or SC every 1 to 2 weeks for three to four treatments
   - Doramectin 0.2–0.3 mg/kg SC every 1 to 2 weeks for three to four treatments
5. Alternative treatment is ivermectin 0.3 mg/kg SQ administered twice 2 weeks apart.
6. The prognosis is good. The cat fur mite is moderately contagious to other cats and is not considered contagious to dogs, but it can cause a papular rash in humans.

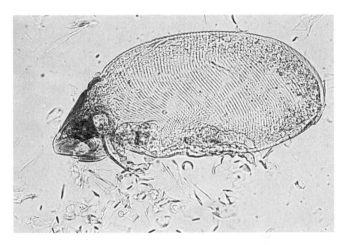

FIGURE 5-68 Cat Fur Mite. Microscopic image of a *Lynxacarus radosky* mite from a skin scraping, as seen with a 4× objective. *(Courtesy L. Messinger.)*

Fleas

Features

Fleas are small, wingless, blood-sucking insects. Although more than 2000 species and subspecies exist worldwide, *Ctenocephalides felis* is the species most commonly associated with dogs and cats. In temperate climates, problems with fleas are usually restricted to warm weather months. In warmer climates, flea problems may occur year round. Fleas are a common cause of skin disease in dogs and cats.

Dogs

Non–flea-allergic dogs may have no symptoms (asymptomatic carriers), or they may be anemic, have tapeworms, show mild skin irritation, or develop pyotraumatic dermatitis. Flea-allergic dogs have pruritic, papular, crusting eruptions with secondary seborrhea, alopecia, excoriations, pyoderma, hyperpigmentation, or lichenification. The distribution of lesions usually involves the caudodorsal lumbosacral area, the dorsal tail head, the caudomedial thighs, the abdomen, or the flanks.

Cats

Non–flea-allergic cats may have no symptoms (asymptomatic carriers), or they may be anemic, have tapeworms, or develop mild skin irritation. Flea-allergic cats often present with pruritic miliary dermatitis with variable secondary excoriations, crusting, and alopecia. Distribution of the lesions usually involves the head, neck, dorsal lumbosacral area, caudomedial thighs, or ventral abdomen. Other symptoms of fleas include symmetrical alopecia that occurs secondary to excessive grooming and eosinophilic granuloma complex lesions.

Top Differentials

Differentials include atopy, food hypersensitivity, scabies, cheyletiellosis, pyoderma, dermatophytosis, demodicosis, and *Malassezia* dermatitis.

Diagnosis

1. History and clinical findings. Response to aggressive flea control therapy.
2. Visualization of fleas or flea excreta on body (may be difficult to find in flea-allergic animals).
3. Visualization of tapeworm segments (*Dipylidium* sp.) on body or in fecal flotation.
4. Allergy testing (intradermal, serologic): positive skin test reaction to flea antigen or positive serum IgE antiflea antibody titer is highly suggestive of flea-allergic dermatitis, but false-negative results are possible.

5. Dermatohistopathology (nondiagnostic): varying degrees of superficial or deep perivascular to interstitial dermatitis, with eosinophils often predominating.
6. Response to flea treatment using every other day nitenpyram (Capstar).

Treatment and Prognosis

1. Strict flea eradication is the only effective treatment.
2. Any secondary pyoderma should be treated with appropriate long-term (minimum 3–4 weeks) systemic antibiotics that are continued at least 1 week beyond clinical resolution of the pyoderma.
3. Topical or systemic insect growth regulators (IGRs; lufenuron, piriproxyfen, methoprene) are effective alone or in combination with adulticidal therapy. IGRs are an important part of an integrated flea control program because of their ability to reduce the flea burden in the pet's environment.
4. Affected and all in-contact dogs and cats should be treated with adulticidal (orals, sprays, spot-on solutions, or dips) every 7 to 30 days, as instructed on the label. Products that contain fipronil, imidocloprid, spinosid, dinotefuran, and selamectin are especially efficacious when administered every 2 to 4 weeks. In heavily flea-infested environments, fleas may continue to be found on the animals, in spite of topical flea control.
5. In severe cases, affected animals should be administered nitenpyram, minimum dose 1 mg/kg PO, every 24 to 48 hours for 4 weeks; the environment should also be treated (see #7). Alternatively, the application of a 0.2% pyrethrin water-based spray every 1 to 2 days as a repellent may provide substantial protection for socially active dogs.

6. Flea-allergic animals should be prophylactically treated with nitenpyram, minimum dose 1 mg/kg PO, on any day that an encounter with other potentially flea-infested animals (e.g., groomer's, veterinary hospital, parks, other animal households) is planned.

7. In heavily flea-infested environments, areas where pets spend the most time should be treated. Indoor premises should be treated with an insecticide and an IGR (methoprene, piriproxyfen). Outdoor environments should be treated with insecticidal or biologic products designed for such use.

8. The prognosis is good if strict flea control is practiced. Fleas are contagious to other animals and to humans and (similar to ticks) may carry blood-borne disease.

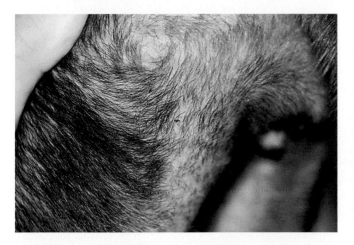

FIGURE 5-69 Fleas. Fleas on the caudal aspect of the rear leg of a dog.

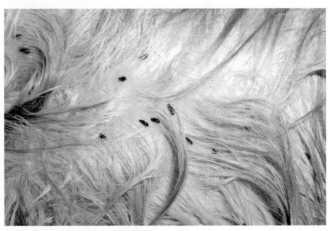

FIGURE 5-70 Fleas. Numerous fleas on the trunk of a cat.

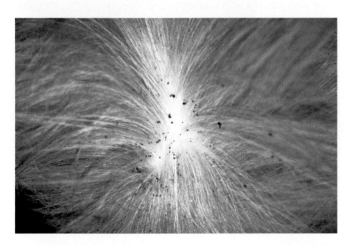

FIGURE 5-71 Fleas. Flea dirt (feces) on the skin of a cat.

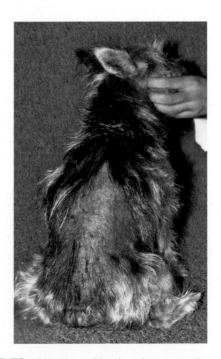

FIGURE 5-72 Fleas. Dorsal lumbar dermatitis characteristic of flea allergy dermatitis.

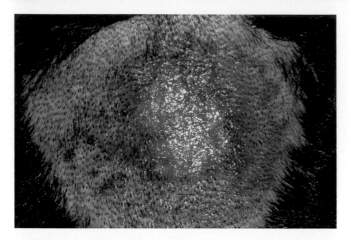

FIGURE 5-73 **Fleas.** Pyotraumatic dermatitis (hot spot) is most often associated with flea exposure. Note the expanding papular dermatitis, which suggests a superficial pyoderma.

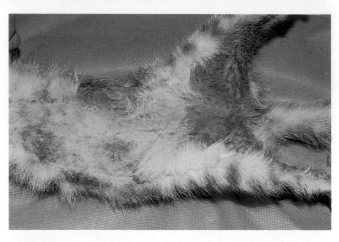

FIGURE 5-74 **Fleas.** Eosinophilic plaque on the abdomen of a flea-allergic cat. Note the similarity with food allergy and atopy.

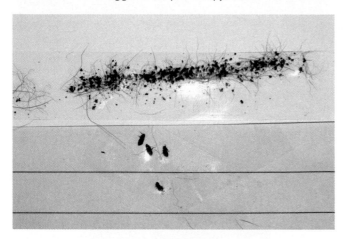

FIGURE 5-75 **Fleas.** Taping fleas or flea dirt to the discharge form may help convince owners of active flea infestations.

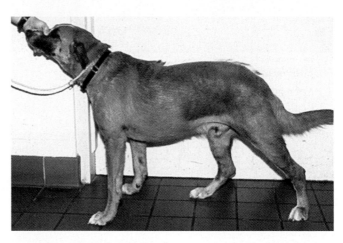

FIGURE 5-76 **Fleas.** Alopecia and hyperpigmentation in the lumbar region of a dog with flea allergy dermatitis.

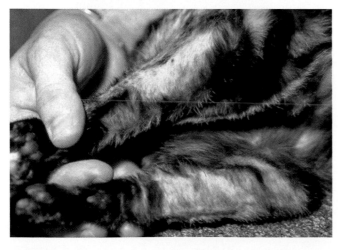

FIGURE 5-77 **Fleas.** Alopecia on the distal extremities of a flea-allergic cat.

Pediculosis (lice)

Features

Pediculosis is an infestation caused by host-specific sucking (*Linognathus setosus* [dog]) or biting (*Trichodectes canis* [dog], *Felicola subrostratus* [cat]) lice. It is uncommon in dogs and cats, with highest incidence reported in young, neglected, underfed animals.

Symptoms usually include restlessness and pruritus, with secondary seborrhea, alopecia, or excoriations. Thickly matted hairs, small papules and crusts, and, in severe infestations, anemia and debilitation may be present.

Top Differentials

Differentials include fleas, scabies, cheyletiellosis, and hypersensitivity (flea bite, food, atopy).

Diagnosis

1. Direct visualization of lice (flea combing).
2. Microscopy (acetate tape impressions, hairs): detection of lice and nits (ova).

Treatment and Prognosis

1. Affected and all in-contact same-species animals should be treated.
2. Matted hairs should be clipped away.
3. Traditional therapy is to topically treat the animal's entire body with 2% lime sulfur, pyrethrin, pyrethroid (dogs only), carbaryl, or organophosphate (dogs only) shampoo, powder, spray, or dip twice 2 weeks apart.
4. Alternative treatments include the following:
   - Ivermectin 0.2 mg/kg PO, SC twice 2 weeks apart
   - Selamectin spot-on (as per label), topically twice 2 weeks apart. Treatment administered every 2 weeks at least four times may be more effective.
   - Doramectin 0.2–0.4 mg/kg administered every week for 3 to 4 weeks
   - 0.25% fipronil pump spray 6 mL/kg, topically, twice, 2 weeks apart
   - 10% fipronil spot-on (as per label), topically, twice 2weeks apart
5. Severely anemic animals may require blood transfusions and good nursing care.
6. Bedding, grooming tools, and environment should be cleaned at least once.
7. Prophylactic use of insecticidal flea collars may protect exposed animals from infestation, but avoidance of infected animals is ideal.
8. The prognosis is good. Lice are highly contagious from dog to dog and from cat to cat, but they are not considered contagious from dogs or cats to humans.

FIGURE 5-78 Pediculosis. These white specks on the trunk of this dog were a combination of scale, lice, and nits associated with a *Trichodectes canis* infection.

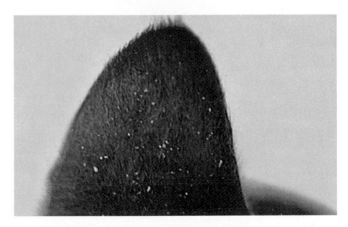

FIGURE 5-79 Pediculosis. Nits attached to the hair on the ear pinnae associated with a *Trichodectes canis* infection.

Pediculosis—*cont'd*

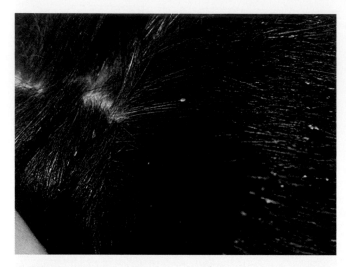

FIGURE 5-80 Pediculosis. The white nits are more clearly visible on the black fur. *(Courtesy D. Angarano.)*

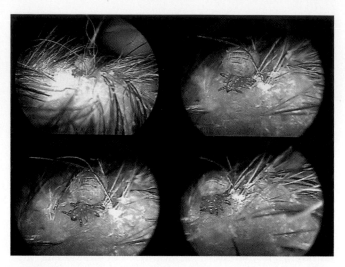

FIGURE 5-81 Pediculosis. Lice, as seen with a video otoscope.

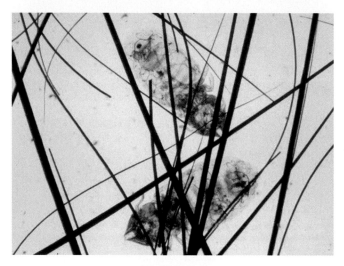

FIGURE 5-82 Pediculosis. Biting lice, as seen with a 4× objective. *(Courtesy D. Angarano.)*

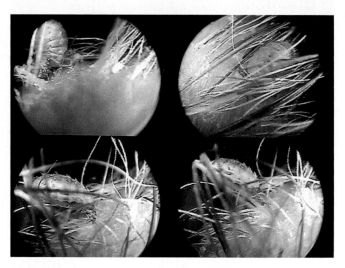

FIGURE 5-83 Pediculosis. Lice, as seen with a video otoscope.

Cuterebra

Features

Cuterebra flies lay their eggs near rabbit runs and rodent burrows. Hatched larvae crawl into the fur of a mammalian host, enter the host through a natural body opening, and migrate to a subcutaneous site. Normal hosts are rabbits, squirrels, chipmunks, and mice. *Cuterebra* are uncommon in dogs and cats, with the highest incidence of disease occurring during late summer and fall.

Infestation appears as a solitary, 1-cm-diameter, nonpainful, subcutaneous swelling that fistulates (larval breathing hole). The lesion is usually located on the head, neck, or trunk. Rarely, larvae aberrantly migrate to the central nervous system, trachea, pharynx, or nostrils, or intraocularly; they may move to other atypical sites as well.

Top Differentials

Differentials include subcutaneous abscess and dracunculiasis.

Diagnosis

1. Direct visualization of *Cuterebra* larvae within lesion: a white, cream, brown, or black larva with stout black spines covering its body.

Treatment and Prognosis

1. The breathing hole should be gently enlarged and the larvae carefully extracted with forceps.
2. Daily routine wound care should be provided.
3. If secondary bacterial infection is suspected, appropriate systemic antibiotics should be administered for 10 to 14 days.
4. The prognosis is good, but wounds tend to heal slowly. The condition is not contagious from dogs or cats to other animals or to humans.

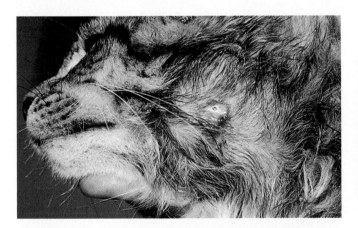

FIGURE 5-84 *Cuterebra.* Erythema and fibrosis surround the breathing hole of the *Cuterebra* on the neck of an adult cat. A purulent exudate is common.

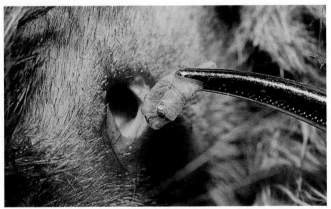

FIGURE 5-85 *Cuterebra.* Close-up of the cat in Figure 5-84. The *Cuterebra* has been removed with hemostats. The lesion consists of a fibrosed tunnel with a purulent exudate.

Cuterebra—*cont'd*

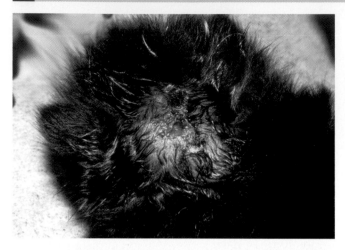

FIGURE 5-86 *Cuterebra.* This ulcerative lesion with a purulent exudate is typical of this infection.

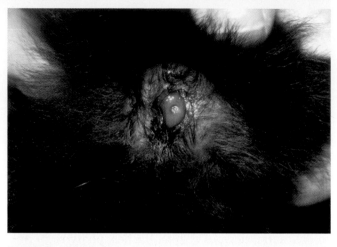

FIGURE 5-87 *Cuterebra.* Close-up of the cat in Figure 5-86. Purulent exudate can easily be expressed from the tract that contains the *Cuterebra.*

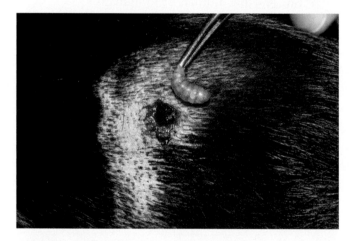

FIGURE 5-88 *Cuterebra.* The small *Cuterebra* that has been removed from its tract.

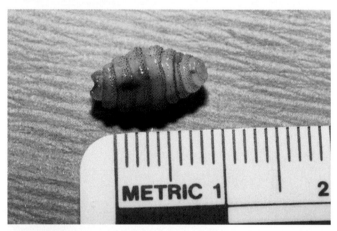

FIGURE 5-89 *Cuterebra.* The *Cuterebra* has been removed and placed on a centimeter ruler.

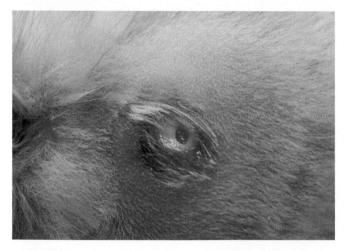

FIGURE 5-90 *Cuterebra.* Erythema and fibrosis surround the breathing hole of the *Cuterebra* on the body of a young cat.

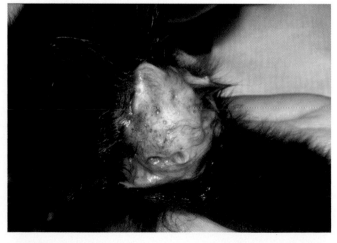

FIGURE 5-91 *Cuterebra.* Hydrogen peroxide is sometimes used (with variable efficacy) to flush the *Cuterebra* from its tract.

Fly Bite Dermatitis

Features

Lesions are caused by biting flies. Fly bite dermatitis is common in dogs housed outdoors.

Lesions include erythema and hemorrhagic crusts overlying erosions or ulcers at or near the ear tips or the most dorsal area of the ear (fold in floppy-eared dogs). Similar lesions may occasionally occur on the face. Lesions are mildly to intensely pruritic.

Top Differentials

Differentials include scabies, trauma, vasculitis, and autoimmune skin disorders.

Diagnosis

1. Usual basis: history, clinical findings, and ruling out of other differentials.

2. Response to treatment: lesions resolve with fly control.

Treatment and Prognosis

1. A topical antibiotic-steroid cream or ointment should be applied to lesions every 12 hours, and the dog should be kept indoors until lesions have healed.
2. Fly repellent, fly spray, or flea spray should be applied daily to affected skin as a preventive measure.
3. Alternatively, anecdotal reports suggest that regular use of concentrated permethrin spot-on as per label instructions may be effective in preventing fly bites.
4. The sources of flies should be identified, and these areas should be sprayed with insecticide.
5. The prognosis is good if repeated attacks by flies can be prevented.

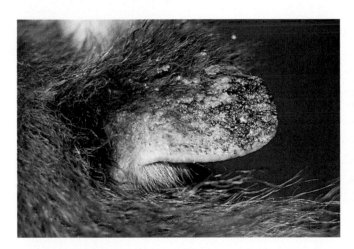

FIGURE 5-92 Fly Bite Dermatitis. Alopecia and crusting on the ear tip of a dog. Note the similarity to scabies and autoimmune skin disease.

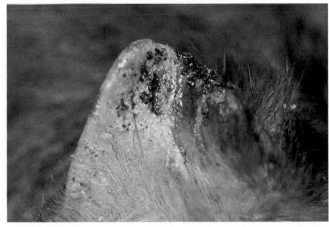

FIGURE 5-93 Fly Bite Dermatitis. Alopecia, crusting, and serosanguineous exudate on the ear tip of a dog.

Fly Bite Dermatitis—*cont'd*

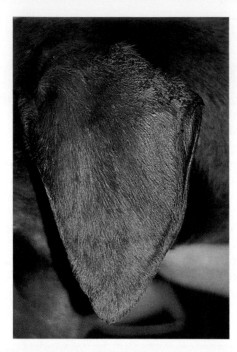

FIGURE 5-94 Fly Bite Dermatitis. Alopecia and crusting on the ear fold of a floppy-eared dog. The fly bite lesions were on the most dorsal aspect of the ear, which was located at the fold in this dog.

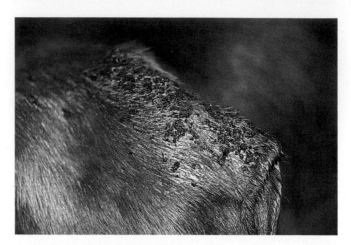

FIGURE 5-95 Fly Bite Dermatitis. Close-up of the dog in Figure 5-94. Alopecia and crusting on the dorsal ear fold.

Myiasis

Features

Myiasis is an infestation of living animals with dipteran fly larvae. Fly eggs laid on moist skin or in wounds hatch into larvae (maggots) that secrete proteolytic enzymes and digest cutaneous tissue. Myiasis is common in cats and dogs, especially in animals that are weakened, have urine-soaked skin, or are paretic.

The lesions are crateriform to irregularly shaped ulcers that are most often found around the nose, eyes, anus, genitalia, or neglected wounds. Maggots are found on skin and inside of lesions.

Diagnosis

1. Direct visualization of maggots on skin, on hair, and in lesions.

Treatment and Prognosis

1. Underlying conditions should be addressed and corrected.

2. Lesions should be clipped and cleaned to remove maggots.
3. Nitenpyram 1 mg/kg PO administered every 24 hours may be effective against maggots.
4. A pyrethrin- or pyrethroid-containing spray (dogs only) should be judiciously applied to lesions to kill remaining maggots. Too vigorous an application could kill a debilitated animal.
5. Alternatively, ivermectin 0.2–0.4 mg/kg SC once is effective against maggots.
6. If the animal's overall condition is stable, wounds should be surgically debrided, and follow-up routine daily wound care provided.
7. The animal should be housed in screened, fly-free quarters.
8. The prognosis is good to guarded, depending on predisposing factors.

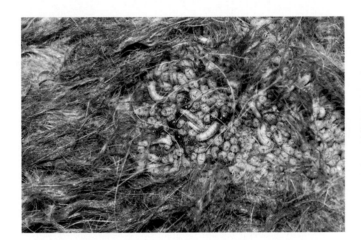

FIGURE 5-96 **Myiasis.** Numerous maggots packed into the open wound of a stray dog.

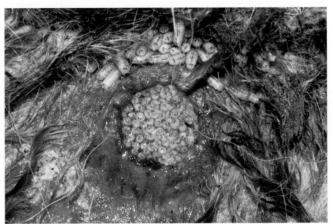

FIGURE 5-97 **Myiasis.** Same dog as in Figure 5-96. The maggots stand vertically within the ulcerated tissue to maximize occupancy. Numerous maggots can be seen crawling on the surface of the skin.

Myiasis—*cont'd*

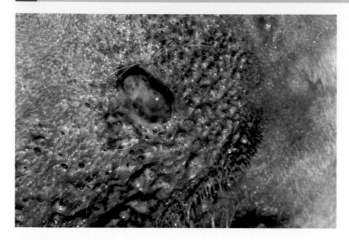

FIGURE 5-98 Myiasis. Same dog as in Figure 5-96. The maggots have been removed, leaving a deep central ulcer with numerous satellite ulcers.

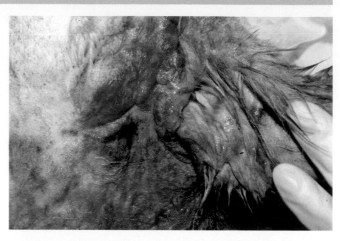

FIGURE 5-99 Myiasis. The maggots have been removed, leaving an alopecic, erythematous, papular dermatitis.

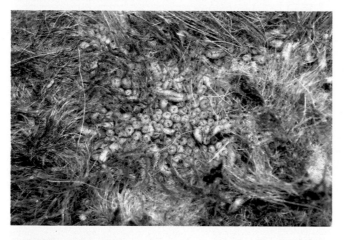

FIGURE 5-100 Myiasis. Numerous maggots on the skin of a dog.

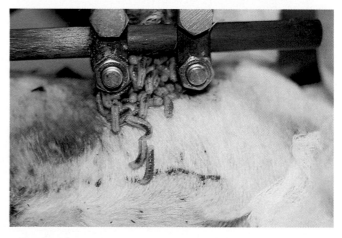

FIGURE 5-101 Myiasis. Maggots are surging out of the wound. The limb had remained bandaged for 2 weeks on this outside dog.

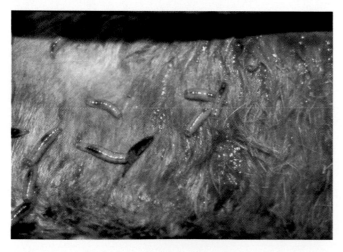

FIGURE 5-102 Myiasis. Same dog as in Figure 5-101. Maggots on the skin and hair of a dog with an external fixator. The limb had remained bandaged for 2 weeks on this outside dog.

Hookworm Dermatitis (ancylostomiasis and uncinariasis)

Features

Hookworm dermatitis is a skin reaction at sites of percutaneous larval penetration in dogs previously sensitized to hookworms. The disease is caused by *Ancylostoma* in the tropics and in warm temperate areas, and by *Uncinaria* in temperate and subarctic areas. The condition is uncommon to rare in dogs, with the highest incidence reported in dogs housed or exercised in contaminated environments, such as damp kennels with cracked and porous floors or grass and dirt runs.

Lesions are characterized by mildly to intensely pruritic, papular eruptions that appear interdigitally and on other skin areas that frequently contact the ground. Affected skin becomes uniformly erythematous, alopecic, and thickened. The feet often become swollen, hot, and painful.

Top Differentials

Differentials include bacterial pododermatitis, demodicosis, dermatophytosis, hypersensitivity (food, contact, atopy), and *Pelodera* dermatitis.

Diagnosis

1. Rule out other differentials.
2. Fecal flotation: detection of hookworm ova.
3. Dermatohistopathology (rarely diagnostic): varying degrees of perivascular dermatitis with eosinophils and neutrophils. Larvae are rarely found but, if present, are surrounded by neutrophils, eosinophils, and mononuclear cells.
4. Response to treatment: lesions resolve after anthelmintic therapy has been provided.

Treatment and Prognosis

1. Affected and all in-contact dogs should be treated with an anthelmintic such as fenbendazole, mebendazole, or pyrantel pamoate twice 3 to 4 weeks apart.
2. A system of regular anthelmintic therapy should be instituted for all dogs.
3. Environmental sanitation should be improved, with frequent removal of feces and soiled bedding. Dry, nonporous kennel floors and runs should be provided.
4. Dirt or graveled runs should be periodically treated with sodium borate 0.5 kg per square meter (10 lb/100 ft^2). Although this may be helpful, it will kill the grass.
5. The prognosis is good. A contaminated environment is a potential source of infection for other dogs and for humans.

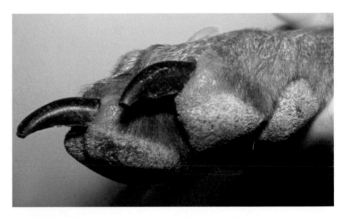

FIGURE 5-103 Hookworm Dermatitis. Alopecia, erythema, and footpad hyperkeratosis on the foot of a dog. *(Courtesy University of Florida; case material.)*

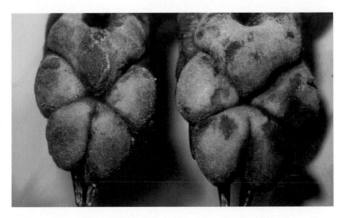

FIGURE 5-104 Hookworm Dermatitis. Close-up of the dog in Figure 5-103. Hyperkeratosis and erythema of the footpads. *(Courtesy University of Florida; case material.)*

Dracunculiasis (dracunculosis)

Features

Dracunculiasis is a skin disease that is caused by *Dracunculus*, a nematode that parasitizes subcutaneous tissues. Infection occurs when the mammalian host ingests an infected microscopic crustacean (intermediate host) while drinking contaminated water. Over the next 8 to 12 months, larvae develop into adults within the mammalian host's subcutaneous tissue. In North America, *Dracunculus insignis* primarily parasitizes raccoons, mink, and other wild mammals, with infection in dogs and cats occurring uncommonly. In Africa and Asia, *D. medinensis* (the guinea worm) infects many mammals, including dogs, horses, cattle, and humans.

Lesions are often painful or pruritic, chronic, single or multiple subcutaneous nodules on the legs, head, or abdomen that eventually fistulate (and through which female worms are stimulated to discharge their larvae when the skin contacts water).

Top Differentials

Differentials include *Cuterebra*, bacterial or fungal infection, and neoplasia.

Diagnosis

1. Cytology (fistulous exudate): eosinophils, neutrophils, macrophages, and 500-μm-long nematode larvae that have tapered tails.
2. Dermatohistopathology: subcutaneous pseudocyst that contains adult and larval nematodes surrounded by eosinophilic pyogranulomatous inflammation.

Treatment and Prognosis

1. Nodules should be surgically excised.
2. Water supplies should be decontaminated.
3. The prognosis is good. However, dracunculiasis is contagious to other animals and humans via animal-crustacean-animal transmission.

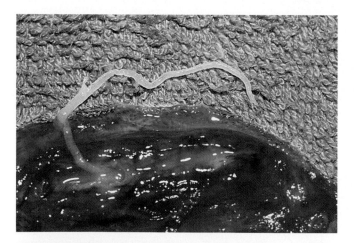

FIGURE 5-105 Dracunculiasis. The worm has been removed from the excised tissue. *(Courtesy A. Yu.)*

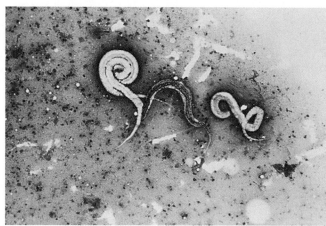

FIGURE 5-106 Dracunculiasis. Microscopic image of *Dracunculus* species. Cytology from a tissue imprint, as seen with a 10× objective. *(Courtesy A. Yu.)*

CHAPTER 6

Viral, Rickettsial, and Protozoal Skin Diseases

- Canine Distemper
- Papillomas
- Feline Rhinotracheitis Virus (feline herpesvirus-1)
- Feline Calicivirus Infection

- Feline Cowpox (catpox)
- Rocky Mountain Spotted Fever
- Canine Ehrlichiosis
- Leishmaniasis

Canine Distemper

Features

Distemper is caused by a morbillivirus that is related to the measles and rinderpest viruses. It is common in dogs, with the highest incidence reported in young, unvaccinated puppies.

Some affected dogs develop mild to severe nasal and digital hyperkeratosis (hard pad disease). More common symptoms include a pustular dermatitis that resembles impetigo, depression, anorexia, fever, bilateral serous to mucopurulent oculonasal discharge, conjunctivitis, cough, dyspnea, diarrhea, and neurologic signs.

Top Differentials

Differentials include other causes of nasodigital hyperkeratosis such as familial footpad hyperkeratosis, hereditary nasal parakeratosis of Labrador retrievers, autoimmune skin disorders, zinc-responsive dermatosis, hepatocutaneous syndrome, hypothyroidism, and idiopathic nasodigital hyperkeratosis. Additional differentials include other causes of pustular dermatitis, such as impetigo, superficial pyoderma, demodicosis, and juvenile cellulitis.

Diagnosis

1. Rule out other differentials.
2. Immunocytology or polymerase chain reaction (PCR) technique (blood, nasal or ocular discharge, saliva, conjunctival scrapings, cerebrospinal fluid [CSF]): detection of distemper antigen.
3. Dermatohistopathology (affected footpads): nonspecific changes include orthokeratotic hyperkeratosis, irregular acanthosis, thickened rete ridges, and mild mononuclear perivascular and periadnexal dermatitis. Intracytoplasmic eosinophilic viral inclusion bodies and ballooning degeneration may not be seen.
4. Immunohistochemistry (footpad, nasal planum, haired skin of the dorsal neck): detection of distemper antigen.

Treatment and Prognosis

1. No specific antiviral treatment is available.
2. Supportive care should be provided and oral or parenteral broad-spectrum antibiotics administered to prevent secondary bacterial infection.
3. The prognosis is poor for dogs with nasodigital hyperkeratosis. Canine distemper is contagious to other dogs, but not to cats or to humans.

Canine Distemper—*cont'd*

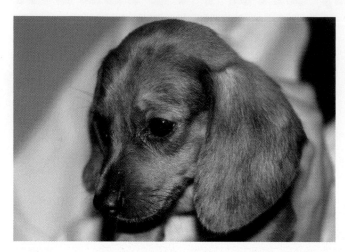

FIGURE 6-1 Canine Distemper. A puppy with mild ocular discharge.

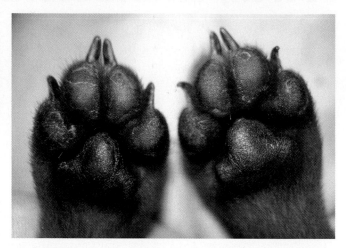

FIGURE 6-2 Canine Distemper. Same dog as in Figure 6-1. Hyperkeratosis and crusting of the footpads typical of distemper infection.

Papillomas

Features

Canine papillomavirus is characterized by benign tumors induced by infection of epithelial cells by species-specific DNA papillomaviruses. Viral oncogenes induce host epithelial cell growth and division and cause chromosomal instability and mutations. Papillomaviruses are transmitted by direct and indirect contact, with an incubation period of 1 to 2 months. Canine papillomas may persist for up to 4 to 6 months in the mouth and 6 to 12 months on the skin before regression occurs. Cellular immunity is key to papilloma regression; immunosuppressive conditions (including feline immunodeficiency virus [FIV]) and immunosuppressive medications may exacerbate and prolong infection.

At least five types of canine papillomavirus and up to eight types of feline papillomavirus have been identified; each has a distinct clinical presentation or site of infection.

Canine Oral Papillomatosis

Young dogs are most commonly affected. Canine oral papillomatosis is a usually self-limiting infection of the oral cavity and lips; it occasionally infects the nose, conjunctiva, and haired skin. Lesions begin as multiple smooth white papules and plaques and progress to verrucous cauliflower-like lesions. Lesions usually regress within 3 months.

Canine Cutaneous (Exophytic) Papillomas

These are most common in older dogs; Cocker spaniels and Kerry blue terriers may be predisposed. Lesions affect mainly the head, eyelids, and feet. Lesions are single to multiple, variably flesh-colored to pigmented, pedunculated, alopecic, smooth to fronded masses that usually measure less than 0.5 cm in diameter.

Cutaneous Inverted Papillomas These are most common in young dogs. They manifest as a self-limiting disease with lesions most commonly found on the ventral abdomen and inguinal area. Lesions are single to multiple, 1- to 2-cm-diameter, round, raised, centrally umbilicated masses.

Multiple Pigmented Plaques

These most commonly occur in young adult miniature Schnauzers and Pugs; they are possibly inherited as an autosomal dominant trait. They manifest as nonregressing lesions that occur on the ventrum and medial thighs. Lesions begin as pigmented macules and plaques that progress to scaly and hyperkeratotic flat masses. Some lesions may undergo malignant transformation into squamous cell carcinomas.

Canine Genital Papilloma

This is an infrequently reported and incompletely described venereal form of papillomavirus infection. Lesions appear as raised papillomatous plaques on the penile or vaginal mucosa.

Canine Footpad Papilloma

This is an infrequently reported disease of adult dogs that has not been consistently demonstrated to have a viral cause. (However, the author has treated two cases of canine footpad papilloma, one of which had demonstrable papillomavirus antigen on immunohistochemistry, and both of which responded to immunomodulating therapy with interferon.) Lesions are firm, hyperkeratotic masses on multiple footpads. Interdigital lesions have been described in Greyhounds. Lameness and secondary bacterial infection may occur.

Feline Oral Papilloma

Infection causes multiple raised, oval, flat-topped 4- to 8-mm masses in the oral cavity, especially the ventral tongue.

Feline Multiple Viral Papilloma

Affected cats are middle-aged or older. Lesions occur on the haired skin of the head, neck, dorsal thorax, ventral abdomen, and proximal limbs. Lesions are multiple, variably sized (3 mm–3 cm) masses that progress from pigmented macules to hyperkeratotic plaques. Disease may progress to feline multicentric squamous cell carcinoma (Bowen's disease).

Feline Solitary Cutaneous Papilloma

This is a rare lesion with no proven viral cause. Lesions occur in adult cats and have no site predilection. Clinically, they appear as small (<0.5 cm) pedunculated hyperkeratotic masses.

Diagnosis

1. Dermatohistopathology: epidermal hyperplasia and papillomatosis with ballooning degeneration of epidermal cells, variably present intranuclear inclusion bodies, and prominent keratohyaline granules.
2. Papillomavirus antigen may be detected by immunohistochemistry or PCR.

Papillomas—cont'd

Treatment and Prognosis

1. Most papillomavirus infections regress spontaneously after development of host cell–mediated immune response.
2. Surgery may be curative for persistent solitary lesions, but care should be taken with tissue handling to avoid seeding the surgical site with viral particles.
3. Cryotherapy and laser ablation are often effective, but they may need to be repeated.
4. Azithromycin, 5–10 mg/kg PO q 12–48 hours dogs and cats, has demonstrated variable success and has minimal adverse effects.
5. Interferon, 1.5–2 million units/m^2 subcutaneously three times weekly for 4 to 8 weeks (2 weeks beyond clinical cure), has been anecdotally successful in cases of oral or cutaneous viral papilloma in dogs and cats.
6. Anecdotally, 5% imiquimod cream applied topically every 24 to 48 hours until the lesion regresses has been used successfully in cases of canine cutaneous papilloma and feline Bowen's disease. An Elizabethan collar should be placed on the animal to prevent licking and medication ingestion.
7. Autogenous vaccines and immunomodulating agents (e.g., levamisole, thiabendazole) are of undocumented efficacy.
8. A new recombinant canine oral papillomavirus vaccine (COPV) produced by Georgetown University Medical Center shows promise for treatment of refractory canine oral papillomas. It consists of the major capsid protein L1 of the COPV. In the single published case report, six vaccinations were administered subcutaneously in the interscapular region. The first three boosters were administered every 2 weeks, and the last two were administered monthly. The oral papillomas regressed completely by the time the last treatment was administered, with no recurrence after 60 months.
9. Oral retinoids (i.e., acitretin 0.5–1 mg/kg PO q 24 hours) have been reported to be beneficial in one case each of canine inverted papilloma and canine pigmented plaques.
10. Antimetabolites can be used to inhibit DNA synthesis and proliferation. Topical application of 0.5% 5-fluorouracil (5-FU) solution every 24 hours for 5 days, then every 7 days for 4 to 6 weeks for cutaneous disease (dogs only). An Elizabethan collar should be placed on the dog to prevent ingestion of the medication, and the owner should wear latex gloves. Contact dermatitis or systemic toxicities are possible.
11. The prognosis is usually good, as most cases will spontaneously regress. Malignant transformation to squamous cell carcinoma is possible with canine pigmented plaque and feline multiple viral papilloma, and in rare cases of oral and corneal papilloma.

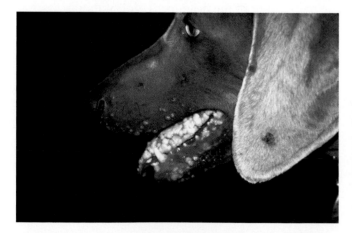

FIGURE 6-3 **Canine Papillomavirus.** Multiple oral papillomas in a 7-month-old Weimaraner.

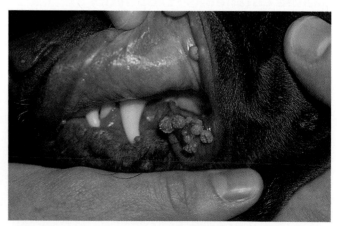

FIGURE 6-4 **Papillomavirus.** Multiple papillomas on the lips of a young dog.

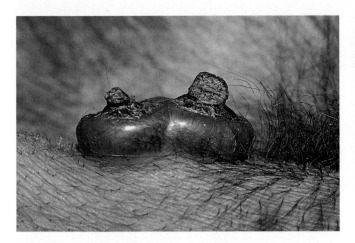

FIGURE 6-5 **Papillomavirus.** Cutaneous horns are protruding from the papillomas on the abdomen of this 6-month-old dog.

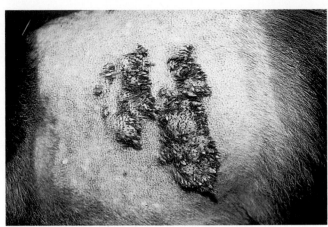

FIGURE 6-6 **Papillomavirus.** A large papillomatous plaque on the lateral thorax of an adult German shepherd.

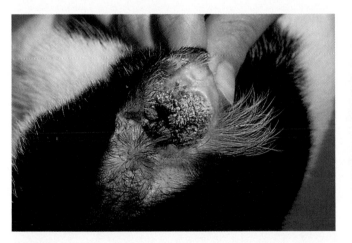

FIGURE 6-7 **Papillomavirus.** Multiple papillomas formed a plaque on the ear of this cat. *(Courtesy of A. Yu.)*

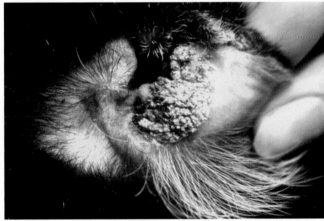

FIGURE 6-8 **Papillomavirus.** Close-up of the cat in Figure 6-7. The raised surface of the papillomatous plaque is apparent. *(Courtesy A. Yu.)*

Feline Rhinotracheitis Virus (feline herpesvirus-1)

Features

This upper respiratory disease is caused by a herpesvirus. It occurs worldwide and is common in cats, with the highest incidences reported in boarding facilities, catteries, and shelters.

Oral or superficial skin ulcers on the face, trunk, and footpads may occur but are rare. Cats usually develop a severe upper respiratory disease characterized by depression, fever, anorexia, marked sneezing, conjunctivitis, and a copious serous to mucopurulent ocular and nasal discharge, with crusting of external nares and eyelids. Ulcerative or interstitial keratitis may be seen.

Top Differentials

Differentials include other causes of upper respiratory disease such as feline calicivirus, *Bordetella*, *Chlamydia*, *Mycoplasma*, autoimmune skin diseases, and other deep infections.

Diagnosis

1. History and clinical findings.
2. Viral isolation (oropharyngeal swabs): herpesvirus.
3. Fluorescent antibody or PCR techniques (conjunctival smears): detection of rhinotracheitis viral antigen.
4. Dermatohistopathology: ulcerative and necrotic dermatitis with mixed inflammation often containing eosinophils. Epidermal cells may contain basophilic intranuclear inclusion bodies.

Treatment and Prognosis

1. No specific treatment is available.
2. Good nursing care should be provided and broad-spectrum systemic or ophthalmic antibiotics should be administered to control secondary bacterial infection.
3. For refractory ulcerative keratitis, topical antiviral eye drops may be helpful—trifluridine or idoxuridine, 1 drop q 2–6 hours.
4. For refractory herpes dermatitis, anecdotal reports suggest that antiviral medications alone or in combination may decrease clinical signs. Treatment can be attempted with one or more of the following:
   ■ Alpha-interferon 30 U PO q 12–24 hours
   ■ Lysine 200–500 mg/cat PO q 12–24 hours
5. The prognosis is usually good, with most cats recovering in 10 to 20 days. Some cats harbor latent infection, which may recrudesce with stress or immunosuppression. Feline rhinotracheitis virus is contagious to other cats, but not to dogs or to humans.

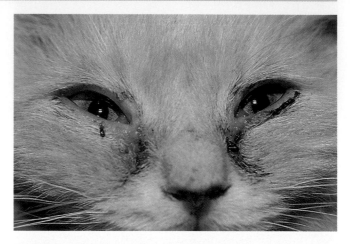

FIGURE 6-9 Feline Rhinotracheitis Virus. Ocular discharge and superficial erosions on the eyelids of a young cat.

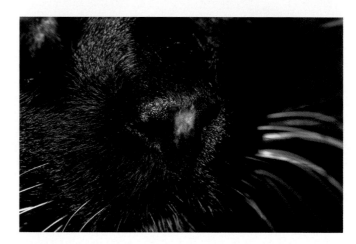

FIGURE 6-10 Feline Rhinotracheitis Virus. Focal, alopecic, erosive lesion on the nose of a cat.

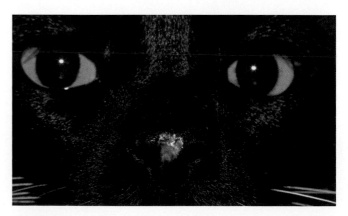

FIGURE 6-11 Feline Rhinotracheitis Virus. Same cat as in Figure 6-10. The focal erosive lesion on the nose is apparent.

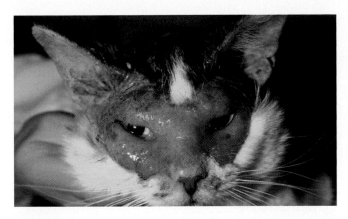

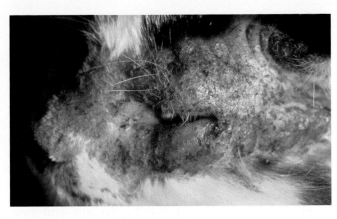

FIGURE 6-12 Feline Rhinotracheitis Virus. Severe alopecic, erythematous, erosive dermatitis in a cat with possible herpesvirus infection. *(Courtesy L. Frank.)*

FIGURE 6-13 Feline Rhinotracheitis Virus. Same cat as in Figure 6-12. The alopecic, papular crusting dermatitis affected almost the entire face. *(Courtesy L. Frank.)*

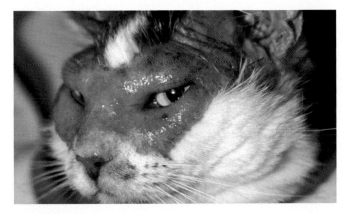

FIGURE 6-14 Feline Rhinotracheitis Virus. Same cat as in Figure 6-12. The alopecic, papular, crusting dermatitis affected almost the entire face. *(Courtesy L. Frank.)*

Feline Calicivirus Infection

Features

Feline calicivirus (FCV), a small, unenveloped RNA virus, is one of the most common viral pathogens of cats. FCV is endemic in most catteries, shelters, and large multiple-cat households, where up to one fourth of cats may be orally shedding the virus at any given time. Three forms of infection have been described: acute FCV infection, chronic FCV infection, and virulent systemic feline calicivirus disease. Although acute and chronic infections are typically caused by vaccine-sensitive FCV strains, virulent systemic FCV disease is caused by at least two different, highly virulent, vaccine-resistant FCV strains (FCV-ARI and FCV-KAOS). Acute FCV infection is common, whereas chronic FCV infection is an uncommon sequela to acute infection in cats. Virulent systemic FCV disease is rare and is characterized by acute outbreaks of rapidly spreading, often fatal infection among cats in shelter facilities, veterinary hospitals, research colonies, and multiple-cat households.

Acute FCV infection is typically a transient, self-limiting, vesiculoulcerative disease. Oral ulcers are common and may be the only clinical sign. Ulcers usually involve the tongue but can occur anywhere in the mouth (palate, gingiva), on the lips, or on the nasal philtrum. Ulcers elsewhere on the body are rare. Other symptoms may include depression, fever, mild sneezing, conjunctivitis, oculonasal discharge, arthropathy (limping), and, rarely, pneumonia. In multicat facilities, asymptomatic carrier cats are common.

Chronic FCV infection is characterized by the development of chronic, progressive, plasmacytic/lymphocytic proliferative or ulcerative gingivitis and stomatitis. Clinical signs may include halitosis, dysphagia, excessive salivation, anorexia, and weight loss.

Virulent systemic FCV infection may result in no apparent disease (asymptomatic carrier), mild to moderate disease, or severe disease and death. Affected cats usually develop symptoms acutely within 1 week of exposure and, depending on the severity of their disease, are moderately to markedly febrile. Skin lesions include oral ulcers; variable alopecia; crusting; ulcerations of the face, ear pinnae, footpads, and nares; and subcutaneous edema of the face or limbs. Other symptoms include lethargy, anorexia, nasal discharge, dyspnea, ocular discharge or conjunctivitis, limping, jaundice, pleural effusion, diarrhea, vomiting, and sudden death.

Top Differentials

Differentials include other causes of upper respiratory disease such as feline rhinotracheitis virus, *Bordetella*, *Chlamydia*, *Mycoplasma*, autoimmune skin diseases, and other deep infections.

Diagnosis

1. Often based on history and clinical findings.
2. Fluorescent antibody testing (conjunctival smears): detection of caliciviral antigen.
3. Dermatohistopathology (virulent systemic FCV): epithelial necrosis and ulceration with minimal inflammation. Superficial dermal edema or vasculitis may be present.
4. Serologic testing: seropositive for antibodies against FCV.
5. Viral culture/PCR technique (oropharyngeal swabs, tissue samples): isolation of calicivirus on viral culture with specific strain identification using PCR assays.

Treatment and Prognosis

1. No specific treatment is available.
2. Good supportive and nursing care should be provided and broad-spectrum systemic antibiotics administered to control secondary bacterial infection.
3. In virulent systemic FCV outbreaks, facilities should be temporarily closed to cats. All contaminated areas should be disinfected by thorough cleaning of rooms, cages, and instruments with a 1:32 dilution of 5% sodium hypochlorite in water.
4. The prognosis is usually good for acute FCV infection, with most cats recovering fully and uneventfully. Acute infections are rarely fatal, with mortality highest in young kittens that develop pneumonia or severe upper respiratory tract infection. Chronic FCV infection has a poor prognosis because the oral disease is progressive and extremely difficult to treat. The prognosis for virulent systemic FCV is guarded for adult cats because they are more likely than kittens to develop severe disease and die. FCV vaccines do not currently protect against virulent systemic FCV infection. Feline calicivirus is contagious to other cats, but not to dogs or to humans.

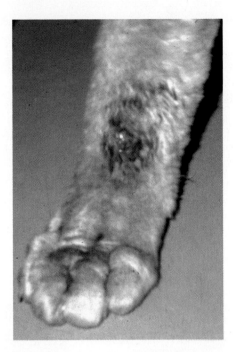

FIGURE 6-15 Feline Calicivirus. Ulcerations on the foreleg of a cat. *(Courtesy R. Malik.)*

Feline Cowpox (catpox)

Features

Feline cowpox is an orthopoxvirus infection that is primarily seen in Western Europe and Asia. It is uncommon in cats, with the highest incidence reported in rural cats that hunt wild rodents (reservoir host). Feline cowpox infections can occur any time but are most common in the autumn, when the rodent population is at its highest.

The initial lesion is a bite wound (ulcerated nodule with crust) that usually appears on the head, neck, or forelimb. It is followed 1 to 3 weeks later by the development of widespread, randomly distributed, erythematous macules and papules that enlarge into 1-cm-diameter nodules. The nodules ulcerate, scab over, and gradually dry and exfoliate 4 to 5 weeks later. The lesions may be pruritic. Some cats also have oral vesicles and ulcers. Unusual presentations may include ulcerative lesions limited to the lips and oral cavity, ulcerative stomatitis without concurrent skin lesions, widespread cutaneous edema and necrosis, and limb edema and necrosis with possible loss of digits. Except for mild pyrexia, depression, and occasionally diarrhea, affected cats usually are not systemically ill unless concurrent immunosuppressive disease is present.

Top Differentials

Differentials include bacterial and fungal infections, eosinophilic granulomas, neoplasia, and other viral infections (e.g., feline immunodeficiency virus [FIV], rhinotracheitis virus, calicivirus).

Diagnosis

1. Dermatohistopathology: epidermal hyperplasia, ballooning and reticular degeneration, microvesicles, and necrosis with keratinocytic intracytoplasmic eosinophilic inclusion bodies.
2. Serology: detection of antibodies against cowpox.
3. Immunohistochemistry (biopsy specimen): detection of cowpox antigen.
4. PCR technique (biopsy specimen): detection of cowpox antigen.
5. Viral isolation (from dry, scabbed material): feline cowpox.

Treatment and Prognosis

1. No specific treatment is available.
2. Broad-spectrum systemic antibiotics should be administered to prevent secondary bacterial infection.
3. Glucocorticosteroids are contraindicated.
4. The prognosis is good, but healed lesions may remain permanently alopecic and scarred. Infected cats are potentially contagious to other cats and to humans.

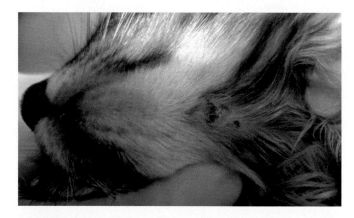

FIGURE 6-16 Feline Cowpox. Multiple crusting papular lesions on the ventral neck of a cat. *(Courtesy M. Austel.)*

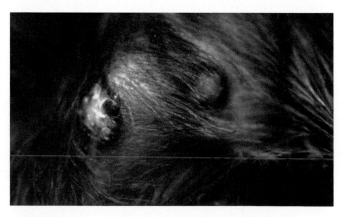

FIGURE 6-17 Feline Cowpox. Multiple papular lesions on the trunk. *(Courtesy M. Austel.)*

Rocky Mountain Spotted Fever

Features

Rocky Mountain spotted fever (RMSF) is a tick-borne zoonosis caused by *Rickettsia rickettsii*, a small, coccobacillary, gram-negative, obligate intracellular parasite. Several tick species may transmit *R. rickettsii*, but in the United States, the most important vectors are the American dog tick (*Dermacentor variabilis*) in the eastern United States and the Rocky Mountain wood tick (*D. andersoni*) in the western part of the country. Ticks acquire *R. rickettsii* when feeding on infected rodents and other small mammals. Once they infect dogs or humans, *R. rickettsii* multiply within vascular endothelium and vascular smooth muscle, inducing vasculitis and thrombosis in many organs, especially those with an abundant endarterial circulation (e.g., brain, dermis, gastrointestinal organs, heart, lung, kidneys, skeletal muscles).

The disease occurs in endemic areas of North America, Mexico, and Central and South America. In the United States, RMSF is endemic in densely populated areas of many states, but contrary to its name, it is uncommon in the Rocky Mountains. In North America, most cases are reported between March and October, when ticks are most active. It is common in dogs living in endemic areas, with the highest incidence reported in young dogs that are frequently outdoors. German shepherd dogs may be predisposed, and English Springer spaniels with suspected phosphofructokinase deficiency may have a more severe and fulminant form of the disease.

A fever usually develops 4 to 5 days after a tick bite occurs. Petechial and ecchymotic hemorrhages may appear on oral, ocular, and genital mucosae, and focal retinal hemorrhages may be seen. Discrete, clear vesicles and focal, erythematous macules may be seen on the buccal mucosae. Early on, edema, erythema, and ulceration involving the lips, ear pinna, penile sheath, scrotum, extremities, and, rarely, ventral abdomen may develop. In late-stage disease or during recovery, necrosis of the extremities can develop. Other findings may include anorexia, lethargy, peripheral lymphadenomegaly, abdominal pain, myalgia, polyarthritis, dyspnea, cough, and neurologic dysfunction (e.g., vestibular disease, seizures, coma). Occasionally, melena, epistaxis, or hematuria is seen.

Top Differentials

Differentials include other causes of vasculitis, such as other infectious agents, immune-mediated disorders, and exposure to toxins.

Diagnosis

1. Hemogram and biochemical profile: thrombocytopenia, moderate leukocytosis (minimal left shift), and hypoalbuminemia are typical.
2. Dermatohistopathology: necrotizing neutrophilic vasculitis and thrombosis.
3. Indirect immunofluorescence assay: a markedly elevated immunoglobulin (Ig)M titer in a single serum sample or a fourfold or greater increase in IgM titers to *Rickettsia* antigens from paired serum samples taken 3 weeks apart.
4. Direct immunofluorescence or immunohistochemistry (skin biopsies of early lesions): detection of *Rickettsia* antigen in vascular endothelium.
5. PCR technique (biopsy specimens): detection of *Rickettsia* DNA.

Treatment and Prognosis

1. Any attached ticks should be promptly and carefully removed with forceps or fine-tipped tweezers. The tick should not be twisted nor should its mouth parts be allowed to remain in the skin. One should not burn, puncture, squeeze, or crush the tick's body to kill it because its fluids may be infectious.
2. Appropriate supportive care should be administered if the dog is dehydrated, has kidney failure, is in shock, or has a hemorrhagic diathesis.
3. The treatment of choice is doxycycline 10–20 mg/kg PO or IV every 12 hours, or tetracycline 25–30 mg/kg PO or IV every 8 hours for 1 to 2 weeks.
4. Alternative treatments include the following:
   - Chloramphenicol (pregnant dogs or puppies <6 months old) 15–30 mg/kg PO, SC, IM, or IV q 8 hours for 1 to 2 weeks
   - Enrofloxacin (adult dogs) 5–10 mg/kg PO or SC q 12 hours for 1 to 2 weeks

Rocky Mountain Spotted Fever—*cont'd*

5. Ticks should be kept off dogs by regular treatment during the tick season with a topical insecticide labeled for use against ticks; dogs' access to tick-infested areas should be limited. In kennel situations, treatment of the premises with regular applications of an acaricide is helpful.

6. The prognosis is good if treatment is begun early in the course of the disease. Mortality from RMSF is directly related to delayed diagnosis, incorrect treat-ment, or both. In chronic cases, severe necrosis and scarred, disfigured extremities may be permanent sequelae. *Rickettsia rickettsii* are not naturally transmitted between dogs or from dogs to humans. However, dogs with RMSF may serve as sentinels for the disease in other dogs and humans. Thus, ideally, veterinarians should report cases of RMSF to their state public health authorities.

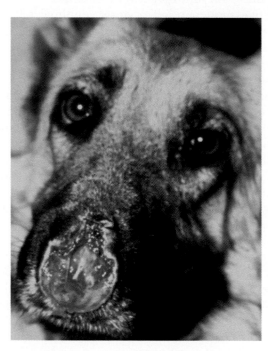

FIGURE 6-18 Rocky Mountain Spotted Fever. The severe proliferative, ulcerating lesion has almost completely destroyed this dog's nose. *(Courtesy of C. Greene.)*

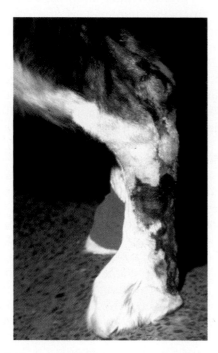

FIGURE 6-19 Rocky Mountain Spotted Fever. Ulcerated nodular lesions on the rear leg of the dog. *(Courtesy C. Greene.)*

Canine Ehrlichiosis

Features

Canine ehrlichiosis is a worldwide tick-borne disease caused by *Ehrlichia* species, which are rickettsial organisms that infect mononuclear, granulocytic, or thrombocytic cells. The most common causative agent is *Ehrlichia canis*, but other *Ehrlichia* species can also produce the disease. Clinical and subclinical infections are common in dogs.

The typical presentation is characterized by depression, lethargy, mild weight loss, and anorexia, with or without hemorrhagic tendencies. If present, bleeding usually is manifested by dermal petechiae, ecchymoses, or both. Hemorrhagic diathesis, such as epistaxis, may occur. Other symptoms may include lymphadenomegaly, splenomegaly, hepatomegaly, and, less frequently, anterior or posterior uveitis, polymyositis, polyarthritis, and central nervous system (CNS) signs (e.g., seizures, ataxia, vestibular deficits, cerebellar dysfunction).

Top Differentials

Differentials include Rocky Mountain spotted fever (RMSF) and other causes of thrombocytopenia, vasculitis, immune-mediated disorders, and cutaneous drug reactions.

Diagnosis

1. Hemogram: normochromic, normocytic nonregenerative anemia, thrombocytopenia, or leukopenia is common.
2. Indirect immunofluorescent antibody test or enzyme-linked immunosorbent assay: detection of serum anti-*Ehrlichia* antibodies. If initial test results are negative, one should consider repeating the assay 2 to 3 weeks later because false-negative results can occur in acutely ill dogs. Likewise, false-positive results (indicating exposure rather than infection) may occur, especially in healthy dogs in endemic areas.
3. PCR technique (blood, bone marrow aspirate, splenic aspirate): detection of *Ehrlichia* antigen.

Treatment and Prognosis

1. Supportive care (e.g., fluids, blood transfusions) should be provided, if needed.
2. The treatment of choice is doxycycline 10 mg/kg PO every 12 hours for 28 days.
3. Alternative treatments include the following:
   - Tetracycline 22 mg/kg PO q 8 hours for 14 to 21 days
   - Chloramphenicol (i.e., for puppies <6 months old) 15–25 mg/kg PO, SC, or IV q 8 hours for 14 to 21 days
   - Imidocarb dipropionate 5 mg/kg IM twice, 2 to 3 weeks apart
4. Clinical improvement should be seen 24 to 48 hours after treatment is initiated. Platelet counts should also begin to increase during this time, usually returning to normal within 14 days.
5. A strict tick control program should be instituted for dogs and premises.
6. In endemic areas, long-term doxycycline 3 mg/kg PO every 24 hours has been used prophylactically to prevent reinfection.
7. The prognosis is good if treatment is initiated early in the course of the disease. The prognosis is poor for dogs with chronic or severe disease. Infected dogs are not directly contagious to humans or to other dogs (except via blood transfusions), but their infection can be indirectly transmitted via tick vectors.

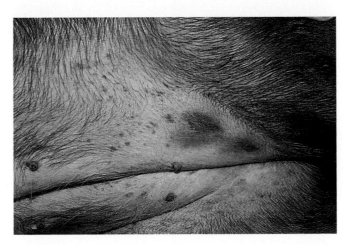

FIGURE 6-20 Canine Ehrlichiosis. Petechiae and ecchymotic hemorrhages caused by thrombocytopenia resulting from the infection.

Canine Ehrlichiosis—*cont'd*

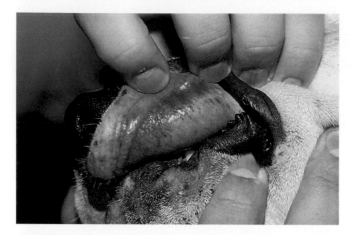

FIGURE 6-21 Canine Ehrlichiosis. Close-up of the dog in Figure 6-20. Bruising on the oral mucosa.

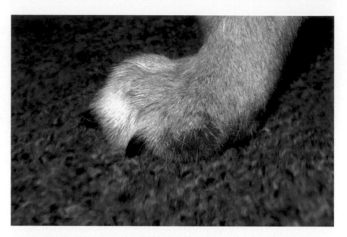

FIGURE 6-22 Canine Ehrlichiosis. A focal erythematous, alopecic lesion with superficial erosions in a dog with ehrlichiosis.

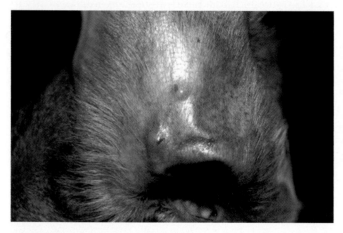

FIGURE 6-23 Canine Ehrlichiosis. Pinpoint petechiae with pustules on the ear pinna of a dog with ehrlichiosis.

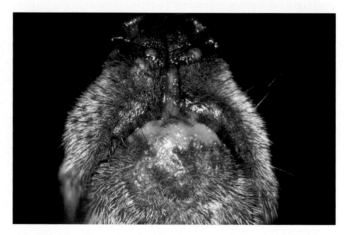

FIGURE 6-24 Canine Ehrlichiosis. Depigmentation erosive dermatitis on the chin, muzzle, and nasal planum of a dog infected with *Ehrlichia*.

Leishmaniasis

Features

Leishmaniasis is a protozoal infection transmitted by certain species of blood-sucking sandflies. The disease occurs worldwide in dogs but is most common in endemic areas where vector sandflies are found, including parts of Asia, Africa, the Middle East, southern Europe, and Latin America. Infections also occur sporadically in nonendemic regions (e.g., United States, Canada, many European countries), usually in dogs that have been imported or have visited endemic areas. However, outbreaks of visceral leishmaniasis have recently been reported in dogs from foxhound kennels in the United States that have never left the country. Cutaneous and visceral types of leishmaniasis occur rarely in cats.

Dogs

In dogs, it is seen as a visceral and cutaneous disease that develops a few months to several years after the initial infection. A progressive, symmetrical alopecia and exfoliative dermatitis with dry, silvery white scales are common. Lesions usually begin on the head, then develop on the ear pinnae and extremities and may become generalized. Some dogs develop periocular alopecia, nasal or pinnal ulcers, or nasodigital hyperkeratosis. Less common cutaneous symptoms include mucocutaneous ulcers, cutaneous or mucosal nodules, pustules, and abnormally long or brittle nails. Noncutaneous signs are variable but often include insidious, progressive mental dullness; exercise intolerance; weight loss; anorexia; muscle wasting; abnormal locomotion; conjunctivitis; signs of renal failure; and lymphadenomegaly.

Cats

In cats, it appears as single to multiple nodules that may ulcerate or crusted ulcers that develop on the ear pinnae, eyelids, lips, or nose. Rarely, visceral (disseminated) infections occur.

Top Differentials

Dogs

In dogs, leishmaniasis may mimic many other causes of seborrheic, nodular, and erosive or ulcerative skin diseases. Specific differentials depend on the clinical presentation.

Cats

Differentials in cats include bacterial or deep fungal infections and neoplasia.

Diagnosis

1. Cytology (lymph node and bone marrow aspirates): *Leishmania* organisms (amastigotes) free or in macrophages.
2. Dermatohistopathology: variable findings with orthokeratotic and parakeratotic hyperkeratosis, granulomatous perifolliculitis, superficial and deep granulomatous perivasculitis, or granulomatous interstitial dermatitis. Extracellular and intracellular (in macrophages) leishmaniae (small round to oval organisms with a round, basophilic nucleus and rodlike kinetoplast) may be difficult to find and are more easily seen with Giemsa stains.
3. Indirect immunofluorescence assay or enzyme-linked immunosorbent assay: high serum antibody titer against *Leishmania* is usually seen in dogs, but false-positive and false-negative results can occur. Serologic testing is less helpful in cats because false-negative results are common.
4. Immunohistochemistry (skin biopsies): detection of *Leishmania* antigen.
5. PCR technique (skin biopsy or bone marrow specimens): detection of *Leishmania* DNA.
6. Tissue culture: *Leishmania* spp.

Treatment and Prognosis

1. There are no reported treatments for cats.
2. Dogs traditionally are treated with meglumine antimoniate 100 mg/kg IV or SC every 24 hours for 3 to 4 weeks, or sodium stibogluconate 30–50 mg/kg IV or SC every 24 hours for 3 to 4 weeks.
3. An alternative treatment for dogs is to give long-term allopurinol PO 6–8 mg/kg every 8 hours or 15 mg/kg every 12 hours for 6 to 9 months.
4. Combination therapy with allopurinol and an antimony compound may result in a better response than is seen when either is used alone.
5. Antifungal agents (e.g., amphotericin B, ketoconazole, itraconazole) have been used with variable success. In humans, liposome-encapsulated amphotericin B has been effective in cases unresponsive to antimonials, but only a partial response to this drug has been noted in infected dogs.
6. Regardless of the treatment used, the disease is not curable. All long-term survivors require periodic retreatment when they relapse.
7. Prevention: leave dogs at home when traveling to endemic areas. In endemic areas, keep dogs indoors from 1 hour before sunset to 1 hour after dawn, use fine mesh screens on kennels and homes, and use topical repellents and insecticides on dogs.

Leishmaniasis—*cont'd*

8. The prognosis is good for dogs without renal insufficiency. After initial treatment, they have a 75% chance of surviving for longer than 4 years with a good quality of life if they are periodically retreated as needed. The prognosis is poor for dogs with renal insufficiency. Infected dogs are important reservoir hosts and are contagious to other dogs and to humans via sandfly vectors. Direct transmission from dogs to humans or between dogs is rare.

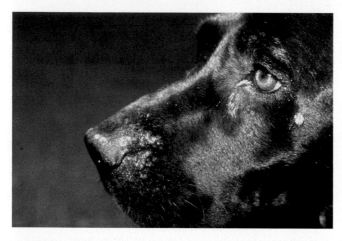

FIGURE 6-25 **Leishmaniasis.** Alopecia and crusting on the nose and periocular skin of a Labrador. Note the mild nature of the lesions.

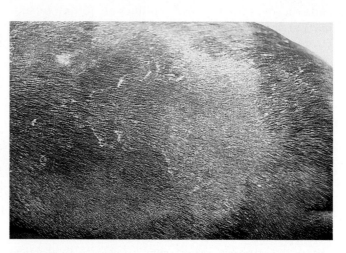

FIGURE 6-26 **Leishmaniasis.** Superficial flakes and scale (mild seborrhea) caused by the infection.

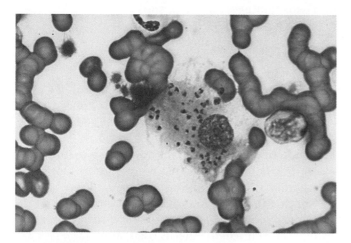

FIGURE 6-27 **Leishmaniasis.** Microscopic image of the protozoal amastigotes as viewed with a 100× (oil) objective.

CHAPTER 7

Hypersensitivity Disorders

- Canine Atopy (environmental, pollen allergies)
- Canine Food Hypersensitivity
- Acral Lick Dermatitis (lick granuloma)
- Flea Allergy Dermatitis (flea bite hypersensitivity)
- Feline Atopy
- Feline Food Hypersensitivity
- Mosquito Bite Hypersensitivity
- Feline Eosinophilic Plaque

- Feline Eosinophilic Granuloma (linear granuloma)
- Indolent Ulcer (rodent ulcer, eosinophilic ulcer)
- Feline Plasma Cell Pododermatitis
- Feline Idiopathic Ulcerative Dermatosis
- Urticaria and Angioedema (hives)
- Canine Eosinophilic Furunculosis of the Face
- Contact Dermatitis (allergic contact dermatitis)

Canine Atopy (environmental, pollen allergies)

Features

Canine atopy is a hypersensitivity reaction to inhaled (possibly a historical theory) or cutaneously absorbed environmental antigens (allergens) in genetically predisposed individuals. It is common in dogs, with age of onset ranging from 6 months to 6 years. However, in most atopic dogs, symptoms first appear at between 1 and 3 years of age.

Symptoms begin as skin erythema and pruritus (licking, chewing, scratching, rubbing), which may be seasonal or nonseasonal, depending on the offending allergen. The distribution of the pruritus usually involves the feet, flanks, groin, axillae, face, and ears. Self-trauma often results in secondary skin lesions, including salivary staining, alopecia, excoriations, scales, crusts, hyperpigmentation, and lichenification. Secondary pyoderma, *Malassezia* dermatitis, and otitis externa are common. Chronic acral lick dermatitis, recurrent pyotraumatic dermatitis, conjunctivitis, hyperhidrosis (sweating), and, rarely, allergic bronchitis or rhinitis may be seen.

Top Differentials

Differentials include food allergy, scabies, *Malassezia* dermatitis, and bacterial pyoderma, as well as other hypersensitivities (flea bite, contact), parasites (cheyletiellosis, pediculosis), and folliculitis (dermatophyte, *Demodex*).

Diagnosis

1. Seasonal foot licking is the most unique and typical symptom of atopy. If year-round allergens (house dust mites) are causing the allergy, the foot licking may be nonseasonal.
2. Allergy testing (intradermal, serologic): allergy testing can be highly variable according to the method used. Positive reactions to grass, weed, tree, mould, insect, dander, or indoor environmental allergens are seen. False-negative and false-positive reactions may occur.
3. Dermatohistopathology (nondiagnostic): superficial perivascular dermatitis that may be spongiotic or

175

Canine Atopy—cont'd

hyperplastic. Inflammatory cells are predominantly lymphocytes and histiocytes. Eosinophils are uncommon. Neutrophils or plasma cells suggest secondary infection.

Treatment and Prognosis

1. Infection prevention: any secondary pyoderma, otitis externa, and *Malassezia* dermatitis should be treated with appropriate therapies. Controlling and preventing secondary infection is an essential component of managing atopic dogs. Bathing every 3 to 7 days and treating the ears after every bath help to wash off pollens and disinfect the skin and ear canals, preventing secondary infections from recurring.
2. Symptomatic therapy (itch control):
   a. An integrated flea control program should be instituted to prevent flea bites from aggravating the pruritus.
   b. Topical therapy with antimicrobial shampoos and anti-itch conditioners, and sprays (i.e., those containing oatmeal, pramoxine, antihistamines, or glucocorticoids) applied every 2 to 7 days or as needed may help reduce clinical symptoms.
   c. Systemic antihistamine therapy reduces clinical symptoms in many cases (Table 7-1). Antihistamines can be used alone or in combination with glucocorticoids or essential fatty acids for a synergistic effect. One- to 2-week-long therapeutic trials with different antihistamines may be required to determine which is most effective.

   d. Oral essential fatty acid supplements (180 mg ecosopentanoic acid [EPA]/10 lb) help control pruritus in 20% to 50% of cases, but 8 to 12 weeks of therapy may be needed before beneficial effects are seen. Also, a synergistic effect is often noted when essential fatty acid supplements are administered in combination with glucocorticoids or antihistamines.
   e. Dextromethorphan, an opioid antagonist, may be a useful adjunct in managing the licking, chewing, and biting behaviors associated with allergic dermatitis in dogs. Dextromethorphan 2 mg/kg PO should be administered every 12 hours. A beneficial effect should be seen within 2 weeks.
   f. Systemic glucocorticoid therapy is often effective (75%) in controlling pruritus but almost always results in adverse effects ranging from mild (polyuria [PU]/polydipsia [PD]) to severe (immune dysfunction, demodicosis, and calcinosis cutis). It is a therapeutic option if the allergy season is very short but may result in unacceptable adverse effects, especially if used over the long term.
      ■ Potent, long-acting injectable steroids are contraindicated for the treatment of allergies because of their comparatively short anti-inflammatory benefits (3 weeks) relative to their prolonged metabolic and immunodepressive effects (6–10 weeks).
      ■ Injectable short-acting steroids (dexamethasone sodium phosphate 0.5–1 mg/kg or prednisolone acetate 0.1–1 mg/kg) are effective at providing relief and may last 2 to 3 weeks if no concurrent secondary infection occurs. This treatment option allows the clinician to more closely control and monitor the patient's use of steroids compared with oral treatments administered by the owner.
      ■ Temaril-P (trimeprazine and prednisolone combination) is a unique drug that provides significant antipruritic effects at a relatively lower dose of the prednisolone. One tablet per 10 to 20 kg should be administered every 24 to 48 hours. The dosage should be tapered to the lowest possible dose and frequency.
      ■ Prednisone 0.25–1 mg/kg (or methylprednisolone 0.2–0.8 mg/kg) PO should be administered every 24 to 48 hours for 3 to 7 days. The dosage should be tapered to the lowest possible dose and frequency.
      ■ All dogs treated with long-term steroids (>3 months) should be frequently monitored for liver disease and urinary tract infection (UTI).
3. Allergy treatment (immune modulation)
   a. Exposure to offending allergens should be reduced, if possible, by their removal from the

TABLE 7-1 Antihistamine Therapy in Dogs*

Antihistamine	Dose
Chlorpheniramine	0.2–3 mg/kg PO q 8–12 hours
Diphenhydramine	1–4 mg/kg PO q 8 hours
Hydroxyzine	3–7 mg/kg PO q 8 hours
Amitriptyline	1–2 mg/kg PO q 12 hours
Cyproheptadine	0.1–2 mg/kg PO q 8–12 hours
Trimeprazine	0.5–5 mg/kg PO q 8–12 hours
Brompheniramine	0.5–2 mg/kg PO q 12 hours
Clemastine	0.05–1.5 mg/kg PO q 12 hours
Terfenadine	0.25–1.5 mg/kg PO q 12–24 hours
Astemizole	1 mg/kg PO q 12–24 hours
Promethazine	1–2.5 mg/kg PO q 12 hours
Loratadine	0.5 mg/kg PO q 24 hours
Cetirizine	0.5–1 mg/kg PO q 24 hours
Doxepin	0.5–1 mg/kg PO q 8–12 hours
Dimenhydrinate	8 mg/kg PO q 8 hours
Tripelennamine	1 mg/kg PO q 12 hours
Clomipramine	1–3 mg/kg PO q 24 hours

Antihistamines in bold are preferred by the author.

environment. High-efficiency particulate air (HEPA) and charcoal filters should be used to reduce pollens, molds, and dust in the home. For house dust mite–sensitive dogs, household treatments for carpets, mattresses, and upholstery with the acaricide benzyl benzoate once a month for approximately 3 months, then every 3 months thereafter, may effectively eliminate house dust mites from the environment. Old dog beds should be discarded as these accumulate house dust mite antigens. Dehumidifying the house to below 40% relative humidity decreases house dust mite, mould, and flea antigen loads. To achieve this, high-efficiency dehumidifiers that are capable of pulling several liters of water from the air per day are required.

b. Cyclosporine (Atopica) helps control pruritus in 75% of atopic dogs. A dose of 5 mg/kg PO should be administered every 24 hours until beneficial effects are seen (approximately 4–6 weeks). Then, dosage frequency should be tapered down to every 48 to 72 hours. For long-term control, approximately 25% of dogs require daily dosing, 50% can be controlled with every-other-day dosing, and approximately 25% can be controlled with twice-weekly dosing. Glucocorticoids can be used initially to speed response. As of this writing, no statistically significant increases in tumor risk or severe infection resulting from the immune effects of cyclosporine have been noted.

c. Immunotherapy (allergy vaccine): 60% to 75% of atopic dogs show good (some medical therapy still needed) to excellent (no other therapy needed) response. Clinical improvement is usually noted within 3 to 5 months of initiation of immunotherapy, but it can take up to 1 year in some dogs.

4. The prognosis is good, although lifelong therapy for control is needed in most dogs. Relapses (pruritic flare-ups with/without secondary infections) are common, so individualized treatment adjustments to meet patient needs may be required periodically. In dogs that become poorly controlled, one should rule out secondary infection (e.g., that caused by bacteria or *Malassezia*); sarcoptic mange; demodicosis; and concurrent food, flea bite, and recently acquired hypersensitivity to additional environmental allergens. Because a strong genetic component is present, the breeding of any male or female dog with clinical signs of atopic dermatitis should be discouraged.

Author's Note

Our profession has excelled at reducing the use of steroids for arthritis; however, we have failed to make similar achievements for allergic disease, including atopy. Because the two diseases have many similarities, including chronicity and multimodal therapeutic options, our goal should be to minimize the use of steroids for allergic disease through the use of alternative, safer treatment options. To achieve best medicine, the frequency of steroid use should be similar for patients with arthritis and those with allergy.

The use of long-acting, injectable steroids should be stopped because of their profound impact on the metabolic and immune systems, as well as growing concern of legal liability for the practitioner.

Author's Note

The only real, long-term options for treating the allergic immune response to environmental allergens are avoidance, allergy vaccine, and cyclosporine (Atopica). Based on typical general practice demographics, every full-time small animal veterinarian should have approximately 20 to 30 patients that are no longer controlled with symptomatic therapy and need more aggressive treatment (allergy vaccine or cyclosporine).

Text continued on page 183.

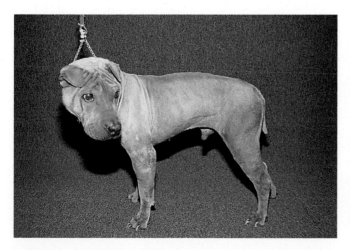

FIGURE 7-1 Canine Atopy. Subtle symptoms, including alopecia, erythema, and excoriations on the face, extremities, and flank of an adult Shar pei.

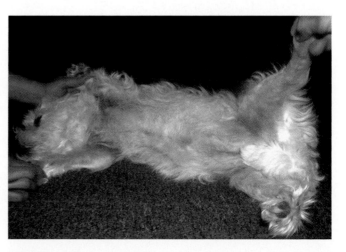

FIGURE 7-2 Canine Atopy. Alopecia with erythema and hyperpigmentation on the ventrum of an atopic dog, demonstrating typical lesion distribution for atopy. Note the similarity in distribution with *Malassezia* dermatitis.

Canine Atopy—*cont'd*

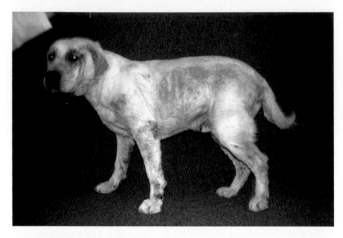

FIGURE 7-3 Canine Atopy. Generalized alopecia and hyperpigmentation in a severely pruritic Labrador. The lesions are especially noticeable on the face, axilla, and flank.

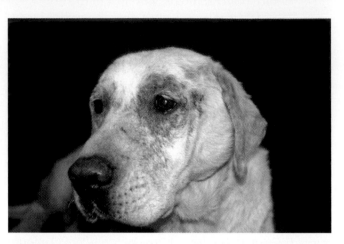

FIGURE 7-4 Canine Atopy. Close-up of the dog in Figure 7-3. The periocular alopecia and hyperpigmentation caused by facial pruritus are typical of allergic disease.

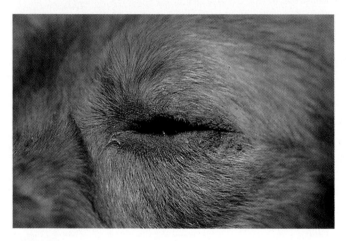

FIGURE 7-5 Canine Atopy. Periocular alopecia, erythema, hyperpigmentation, and lichenification caused by pruritus.

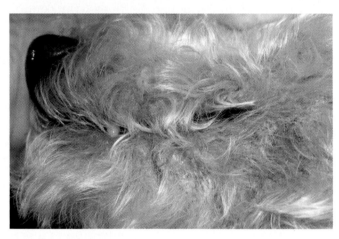

FIGURE 7-6 Canine Atopy. Perioral dermatitis with alopecia, erythema, and crusting caused by a secondary bacterial and yeast infection associated with underlying allergic disease.

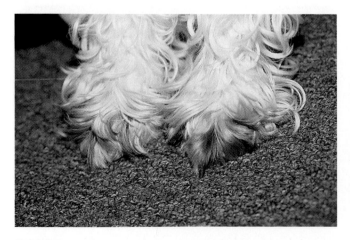

FIGURE 7-7 Canine Atopy. Pododermatitis demonstrating the salivary staining caused by chronic licking.

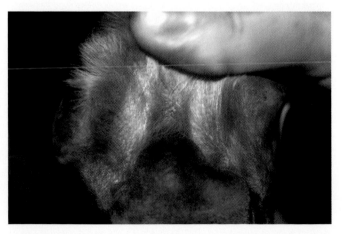

FIGURE 7-8 Canine Atopy. Pododermatitis with alopecia and erythema affecting the interdigital tissue between the central pad and digits. Pododermatitis and foot pruritus are some of the most consistent findings of atopy.

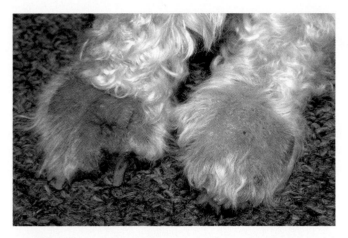

FIGURE 7-9 Canine Atopy. Pododermatitis demonstrating alopecia, erythema, hyperpigmentation, and lichenification caused by a secondary yeast infection associated with underlying allergic disease.

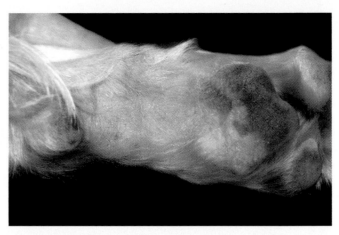

FIGURE 7-10 Canine Atopy. Alopecia and erythema on the caudal aspect of the distal extremities just proximal to the central footpad is a common finding in allergic dogs.

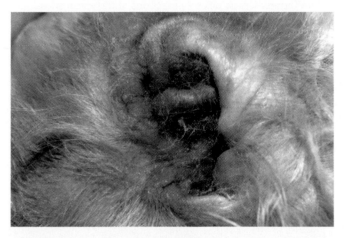

FIGURE 7-11 Canine Atopy. Erythema and lichenification of the ear canal associated with secondary yeast otitis. Otitis (sterile or infectious) is a common finding in allergic dogs.

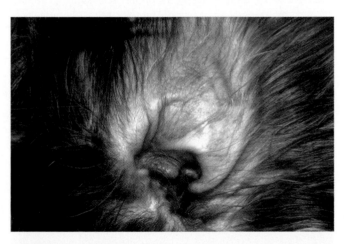

FIGURE 7-12 Canine Atopy. Sterile otitis caused by allergy often presents with erythema of the ear pinna and external canal.

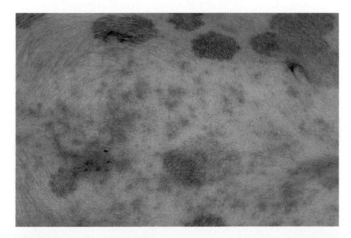

FIGURE 7-13 Canine Atopy. Secondary bacterial pyoderma is one of the most common findings in allergic dogs. The erythematous papular rash on the abdomen of this dog was caused by a secondary pyoderma associated with underlying atopy.

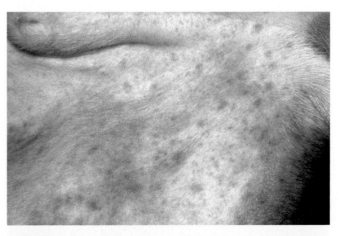

FIGURE 7-14 Canine Atopy. Secondary bacterial pyoderma (erythematous papular rash) on the inguinal area of an allergic dog.

Canine Atopy—cont'd

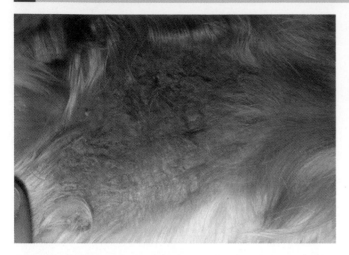

FIGURE 7-15 Canine Atopy. Secondary *Malassezia* dermatitis caused by underlying allergy. The alopecic, erythematous, lichenified lesion on the ventral neck of this allergic dog is typical of *Malassezia* dermatitis.

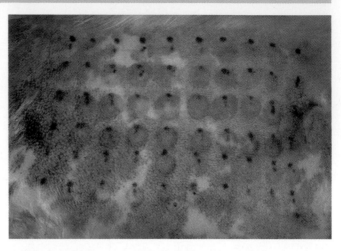

FIGURE 7-16 Canine Atopy. An intradermal allergy test demonstrating numerous positive reactions with typical wheal and flare reactions.

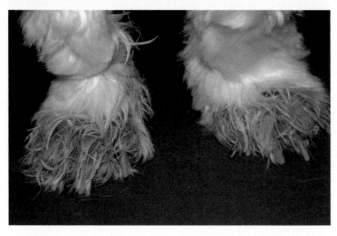

FIGURE 7-17 Canine Atopy. Severe erythema of the feet caused by intense pruritus and by the patient self-mutilating his feet.

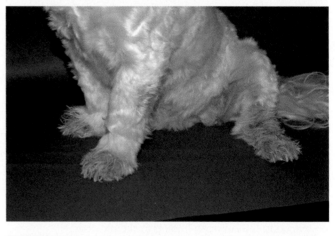

FIGURE 7-18 Canine Atopy. Same dog as in Figure 7-17 demonstrating the severe pododermatitis typical of atopy. Note the erythema on the abdomen, which is common with allergies.

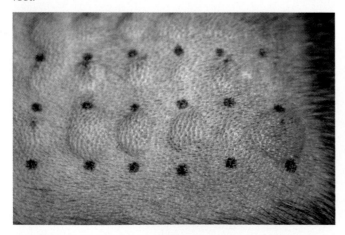

FIGURE 7-19 Canine Atopy. This intradermal allergy test (IDAT) demonstrates positive reactions with classic erythematous, well-demarcated, raised reactions.

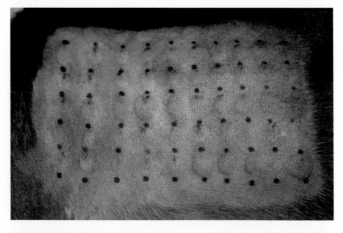

FIGURE 7-20 Canine Atopy. Same patient as in Figure 7-19. This intradermal allergy test (IDAT) demonstrates positive reactions with classic erythematous, well-demarcated, raised reactions. Note the difference between negative and positive reactions.

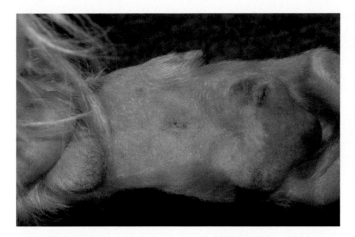

FIGURE 7-21 Canine Atopy. Erythema on the proximal carpus or tarsus is a classic symptom of atopy and usually occurs with podopruritus.

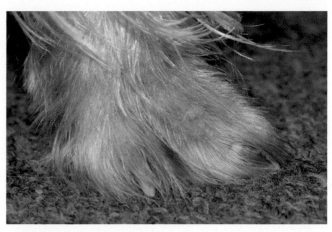

FIGURE 7-22 Canine Atopy. Erythema on the feet caused by a combination of the underlying allergic reaction and the patient licking.

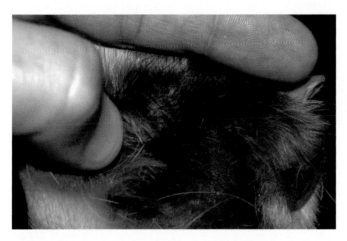

FIGURE 7-23 Canine Atopy. Dermatitis (erythema and lichenification) of the interdigital space is an extremely common symptom of atopy. Often a secondary bacterial or yeast infection is present.

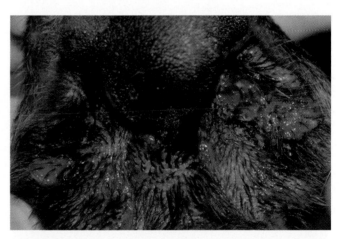

FIGURE 7-24 Canine Atopy. Severe interdigital dermatitis with ulceration caused by secondary bacterial and yeast infections.

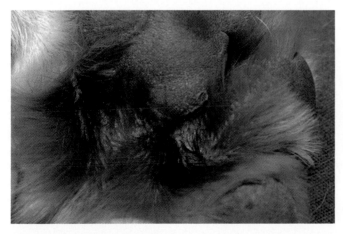

FIGURE 7-25 Canine Atopy. Uninfected interdigital dermatitis typical of atopy alone.

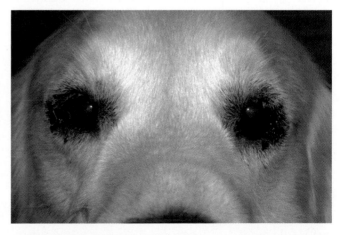

FIGURE 7-26 Canine Atopy. Periocular alopecia, lichenification, and mild crusting in an atopic dog. Periocular inflammation with resulting dermatitis is a common feature of atopy.

Canine Atopy—*cont'd*

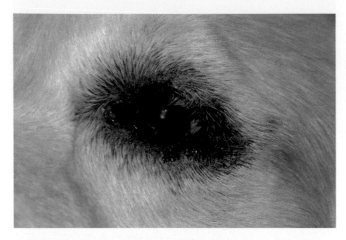

FIGURE 7-27 Canine Atopy. Same dog as in Figure 7-26. Periocular dermatitis caused by the allergic reaction is obvious.

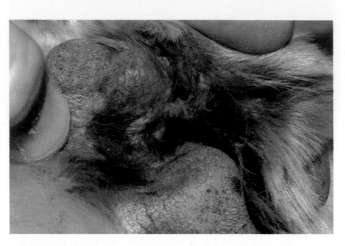

FIGURE 7-28 Canine Atopy. Interdigital dermatitis with salivary staining is extremely common in atopic patients.

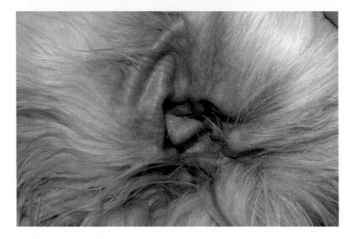

FIGURE 7-29 Canine Atopy. Sterile, allergic otitis in a dog with atopy. Note the generalized erythema without obvious otic exudate.

Canine Food Hypersensitivity

Features

Canine food hypersensitivity is an adverse reaction to a food or food additive. It can occur at any age, from recently weaned puppies to elderly dogs that have been eating the same dog food for years. Approximately 30% of dogs diagnosed with food allergy are younger than 1 year of age. Food allergy is common in dogs.

Canine food hypersensitivity is characterized by nonseasonal pruritus that may or may not respond to steroid therapy. The pruritus may be regional or generalized and usually involves the ears, feet, inguinal or axillary areas, face, neck, and perineum. Affected skin is often erythematous, and a papular rash may be present. Self–trauma-induced lesions include alopecia, excoriations, scales, crusts, hyperpigmentation, and lichenification. Secondary superficial pyoderma, *Malassezia* dermatitis, and otitis externa are common. Other symptoms that may be seen are acral lick dermatitis, chronic seborrhea, and recurring pyotraumatic dermatitis. Some dogs are minimally pruritic, with the only symptom being recurrent infection with pyoderma, *Malassezia* dermatitis, or otitis. In these cases, the pruritus is present only when secondary infections are left untreated. Occasionally, urticaria or angioedema may occur. Concurrent gastrointestinal signs (e.g., frequent bowel movements, vomiting, diarrhea, flatulence) are reported in 20% to 30% of cases.

Top Differentials

Differentials include atopy, scabies, *Malassezia* dermatitis, and bacterial pyoderma, as well as other hypersensitivities (flea bite, contact), parasites (cheyletiellosis, pediculosis), and folliculitis (dermatophyte, *Demodex*).

Diagnosis

1. Perianal dermatitis with or without recurrent otitis is the most common and unique feature of food allergy. However, food allergy can manifest in many patterns and should be suspected for atypical pruritic patients, including those with recurrent infections without pruritus.
2. Dermatohistopathology (nondiagnostic): varying degrees of superficial perivascular dermatitis. Mononuclear cells or neutrophils may predominate. Eosinophils may be more numerous than in atopy.
3. Food allergy testing (intradermal, serologic) (nondiagnostic): not recommended because test results are unreliable. Some dogs will have positive reactions to storage mite antigens, which may be clinically relevant, or that may be caused by cross-reactivity with other insects. Storage mites are ubiquitous, and their clinical significance is currently unknown.
4. Response to hypoallergenic diet trial: symptoms improve within 10 to 12 weeks of initiation of a strict home-cooked or commercially prepared restricted diet (one protein and one carbohydrate source). The hypoallergenic diet should not contain food ingredients previously administered in dog food, treats, or table scraps, nor should flavored heartworm preventive, flavored medications, nutritional supplements, or chewable treats (i.e., pig ears, cow hooves, rawhide, dog biscuits, table food such as cheese) be administered during the hypoallergenic diet trial. Beef and dairy are the most common food allergens in dogs, and avoiding these alone may result in clinical improvement. Other common food allergies include chicken, eggs, soy, corn, and wheat.
5. Provocative challenge: recurrence of symptoms within hours to days of reintroduction of suspect allergen into the diet.

Treatment and Prognosis

1. Infection prevention: any secondary pyoderma, otitis externa, and *Malassezia* dermatitis should be treated with appropriate therapies. Controlling and preventing secondary infection is an essential component of managing atopic dogs. Bathing every 3 to 7 days and treating the ears after every bath helps wash off pollens and disinfect the skin and ear canals, preventing secondary infections from recurring.
2. Symptomatic therapy (itch control) is variably effective for food allergy:
   a. An integrated flea control program should be instituted to prevent flea bites from aggravating the pruritus.
   b. Topical therapy with antimicrobial shampoos and anti-itch conditioners, and sprays (i.e., those containing oatmeal, pramoxine, antihistamines, or glucocorticoids) applied every 2 to 7 days or as needed may help reduce clinical symptoms.
   c. Systemic antihistamine therapy reduces clinical symptoms in many cases (see Table 7-1). One- to 2-week-long therapeutic trials with different antihistamines may be required to determine which is most effective.
   d. Oral essential fatty acid supplements (180 mg ecosopentanoic acid [EPA]/10 lb) help control pruritus in 20% to 50% of cases, but 8 to 12 weeks of therapy may be needed before beneficial effects are seen. Also, a synergistic effect is often

Canine Food Hypersensitivity—*cont'd*

noted when essential fatty acid supplements are administered in combination with glucocorticoids or antihistamines.

e. Dextromethorphan, an opioid antagonist, may be a useful adjunct in managing the licking, chewing, and biting behaviors associated with allergic dermatitis in dogs. Dextromethorphan 2 mg/kg PO should be administered every 12 hours. A beneficial effect should be seen within 2 weeks.

f. Systemic glucocorticoid therapy is only variably effective (unpredictable minimal to good response) in controlling pruritus caused by food allergy but almost always results in adverse effects ranging from mild (PU/PD) to severe (immune dysfunction, demodicosis, and calcinosis cutis) (see "Atopy" section).

■ Potent, long-acting injectable steroids are contraindicated for the treatment of allergies because of their comparatively short anti-inflammatory benefits (3 weeks) relative to their prolonged metabolic and immunodepressive effects (6–10 weeks).

■ Injectable short-acting steroids (dexamethasone sodium phosphate 0.5–1 mg/kg or prednisolone acetate 0.1–1 mg/kg) are effective at providing relief and may last 2 to 3 weeks if no concurrent secondary infection occurs. This treatment option allows the clinician to more closely control and monitor the patient's use of steroids compared with oral treatments administered by the owner.

■ All dogs treated with long-term steroids (>3 months) should be frequently monitored for liver disease and UTI.

3. Food allergy treatment

a. Offending dietary allergen(s) should be avoided. A balanced home-cooked diet or a commercial hypoallergenic diet should be provided.

b. To identify offending substances to be avoided (challenge phase after food allergy has been confirmed with the dietary trial), one new food item should be added to the hypoallergenic diet every 2 to 4 weeks. If the item is allergenic, clinical symptoms will recur within 7 to 10 days. *Note*: Some dogs (approximately 20%) should be fed home-cooked diets to remain symptom-free. For these dogs, commercial hypoallergenic diets are ineffective, presumably because their hypersensitivity relates to a food preservative or dye.

c. Anecdotal reports suggest that higher doses (10 mg/kg) of cyclosporine (Atopica) may be beneficial in reducing the allergic immune response and symptoms of food allergy.

4. The prognosis is good. In dogs that are poorly controlled, owner noncompliance should be ruled out, along with development of hypersensitivity to an ingredient in the hypoallergenic diet, secondary infection (caused by bacteria, *Malassezia*, dermatophyte), scabies, demodicosis, atopy, flea allergy dermatitis, and contact hypersensitivity.

Author's Note

Recent food industry changes have caused an explosion of products available by prescription or over the counter, and the listing is beyond the scope of this text.

Many of the over-the-counter diets are sufficiently restricted and of high enough quality to produce clinical benefit when a food-allergic patient is restricted to one of the nonbeef and nondairy products.

Food allergy is responsible for most of the very unusual clinical symptom patterns in dogs with recurrent infection (with or without pruritus).

Poor owner compliance should be expected, making the long-term management of food-allergic patients difficult and frustrating; repeated lapses in diet result in flare-ups of pruritus and secondary infection.

Author's Note

The use of long-acting, injectable steroids should be stopped because of their profound impact on the metabolic and immune systems, as well as growing concern for the legal liability of the practitioner.

Text continued on page 189.

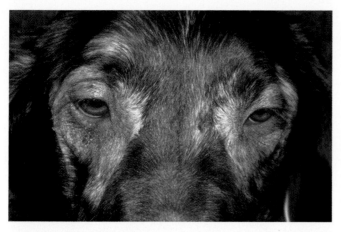

FIGURE 7-30 Canine Food Hypersensitivity. Severe periocular dermatitis (alopecia, erythema, and hyperpigmentation) is a common finding in allergic dogs.

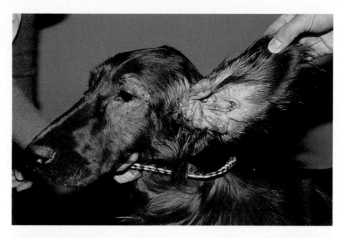

FIGURE 7-31 Canine Food Hypersensitivity. Alopecia, erythema, and excoriations around the eye and ear. The crusting papular rash is due to a secondary superficial pyoderma associated with the allergic disease.

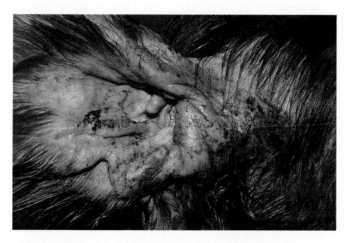

FIGURE 7-32 Canine Food Hypersensitivity. Close-up of the dog in Figure 7-31. Erythema, alopecia, and papular rash involving the ear pinnae. No infectious otitis is present—only external lesions associated with the underlying allergy.

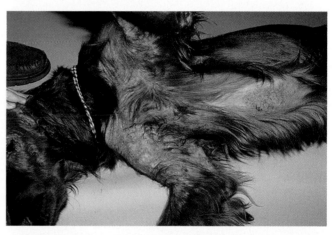

FIGURE 7-33 Canine Food Hypersensitivity. Close-up of the dog in Figure 7-31. Alopecia and erythema in the axillary area. Mild hyperpigmentation and lichenification are caused by a secondary yeast dermatitis. Note the similarity to lesions seen with atopy.

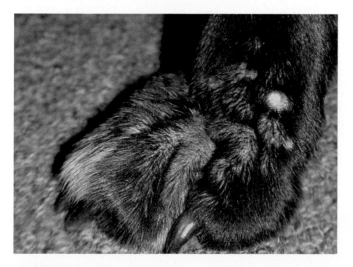

FIGURE 7-34 Canine Food Hypersensitivity. Pododermatitis is a common symptom of allergic dermatitis in dogs. Alopecia and hyperpigmentation on the dorsal foot are apparent.

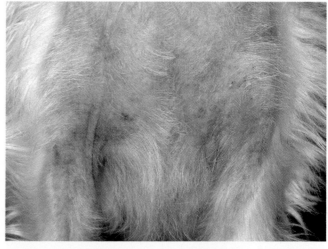

FIGURE 7-35 Canine Food Hypersensitivity. Alopecia and erythema with papules and early lichenification on the ventral neck and axillary area, caused by a secondary yeast dermatitis associated with underlying allergic disease.

Canine Food Hypersensitivity—cont'd

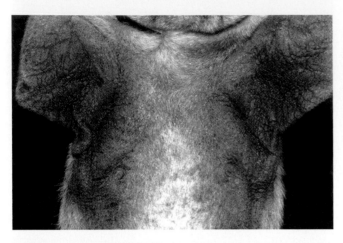

FIGURE 7-36 **Canine Food Hypersensitivity.** Secondary *Malassezia* dermatitis caused by underlying allergy, demonstrating the classic alopecic, hyperpigmented, lichenified "elephant skin" dermatitis and axillary area of an allergic dog.

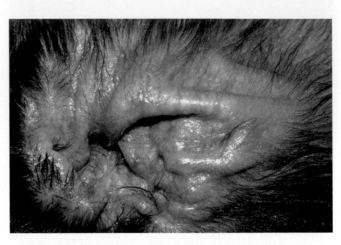

FIGURE 7-37 **Canine Food Hypersensitivity.** Otitis is an extremely common finding in allergic dogs. The erythematous pinna and external canal without secondary infection were caused by primary allergic disease in this patient.

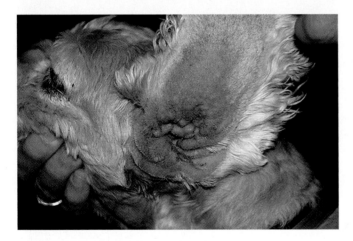

FIGURE 7-38 **Canine Food Hypersensitivity.** Chronic otitis in a food-allergic Cocker spaniel. Severe swelling and stenosis of the external ear canal and lichenification of the pinna with erythema and hyperpigmentation are chronic changes.

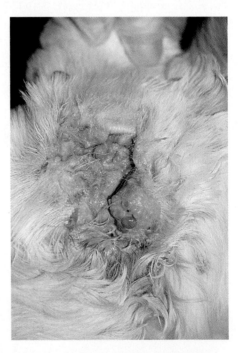

FIGURE 7-39 **Canine Food Hypersensitivity.** Severe allergic otitis with secondary bacterial infection in a Cocker spaniel. Lateral ear canal resection without dietary therapy failed to resolve the underlying cause of the chronic otitis.

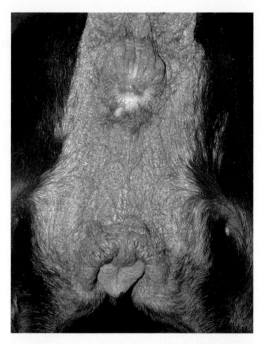

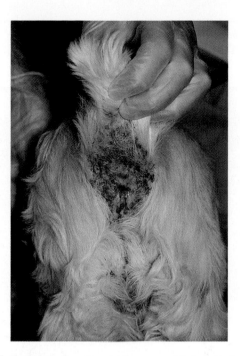

FIGURE 7-40 **Canine Food Hypersensitivity.** Perianal dermatitis is a common finding in food-allergic dogs. Alopecic, hyperpigmented, lichenified perianal skin is caused by chronic inflammation and pruritus.

FIGURE 7-41 **Canine Food Hypersensitivity.** Perianal dermatitis in a food-allergic Cocker spaniel.

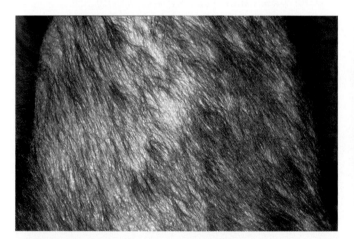

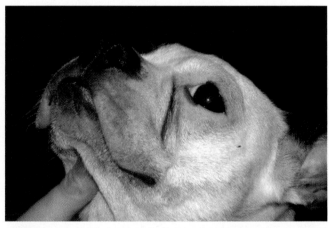

FIGURE 7-42 **Canine Food Hypersensitivity.** Secondary bacterial pyoderma is common in allergic dogs. The moth-eaten hair coat with underlying erythematous skin was caused by secondary bacterial infection associated with the underlying allergy.

FIGURE 7-43 **Canine Food Hypersensitivity.** Facial dermatitis (alopecia, erythema, and pruritus) is a common finding in allergic dogs.

Canine Food Hypersensitivity—*cont'd*

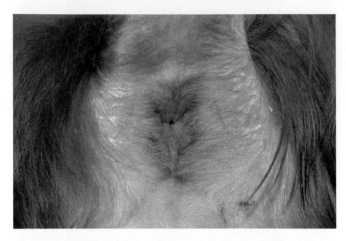

FIGURE 7-44 **Canine Food Hypersensitivity.** Perianal dermatitis is one of the most consistent and unique features of food allergy.

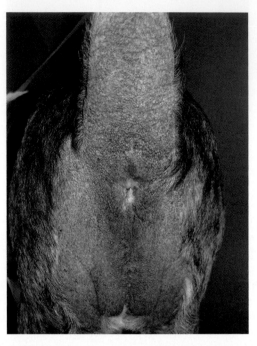

FIGURE 7-45 **Canine Food Hypersensitivity.** Severe lichenification, hyperpigmentation, and alopecia affecting the perianal area of this food-allergic dog.

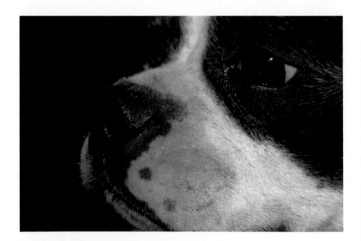

FIGURE 7-46 **Canine Food Hypersensitivity.** Facial dermatitis with pruritus is not a unique feature of food allergy and is indistinguishable from the facial dermatitis caused by atopy.

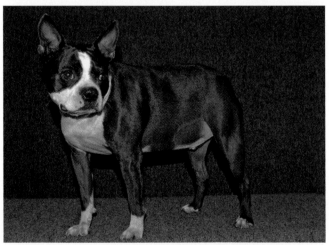

FIGURE 7-47 **Canine Food Hypersensitivity.** From a distance, this food-allergic dog appears to have minimal lesions; however, multiple areas of alopecia and erythema affecting the face, abdomen, and feet are apparent. Note the identical pattern to atopy.

Acral Lick Dermatitis (lick granuloma)

Features

Acral lick dermatitis is first noted as excessive, compulsive licking at a focal area on a limb, resulting in a firm, proliferative, ulcerative, alopecic lesion. Causes of the licking are multifactorial, and, although environmental stress (e.g., boredom, confinement, loneliness, separation anxiety) may be a contributor, other factors are usually more important (Box 7-1). This dermatitis is common in dogs, with the highest incidence in middle-aged to older, large-breed dogs, especially Doberman pinschers, Great Danes, Golden retrievers, Labrador retrievers, German shepherds, and Boxers.

The lesion usually begins as a small area of dermatitis that slowly enlarges because of persistent licking. The affected area becomes alopecic, firm, raised, thickened, and plaquelike to nodular, and it may be eroded or ulcerated. With chronicity, extensive fibrosis, hyperpigmentation, and secondary bacterial infection are common. Lesions are usually single but may be multiple, and they most often are found on the dorsal aspect of the carpus, metacarpus, tarsus, or metatarsus.

Top Differentials

Differentials include demodicosis, dermatophyte kerion, fungal or bacterial granuloma, and neoplasia.

Diagnosis

1. Usually based on history, clinical findings, and ruling out other differentials.
2. Dermatohistopathology: ulcerative and hyperplastic epidermis, mild neutrophilic and mononuclear perivascular dermatitis, and varying degrees of dermal fibrosis.

BOX 7-1 Underlying Causes of Acral Lick Dermatitis

- Hypersensitivity (atopy, food)
- Fleas
- Trauma (cut, bruise)
- Foreign body reaction
- Infection (bacterial, fungal)
- Demodicosis
- Hypothyroidism
- Neuropathy
- Osteopathy
- Arthritis

3. Bacterial culture (exudates, biopsy specimen): *Staphylococcus* is often isolated. Mixed gram-positive and gram-negative infections are common.

Treatment and Prognosis

1. The underlying causes should be identified and corrected (see Box 7-1).
2. One should treat for secondary bacterial infection with long-term systemic antibiotics (minimum 6–8 weeks, and as long as 4–6 months in some dogs). Antibiotic therapy should be continued at least 3 to 4 weeks beyond regression of the lesion. The antibiotic should be selected according to bacterial culture and sensitivity results.
3. Anecdotal reports suggest good efficacy with combined antibiotic, amitriptyline (2 mg/kg q 12 hours), and hydrocodone (0.25 mg/kg q 8–12 hours) administered until lesions resolve. Then, one drug should be discontinued every 2 weeks until it can be determined which drug (if any) may be required for maintenance therapy.
4. Topical application of analgesic, steroidal, or bad-tasting medications every 8 to 12 hours may help stop the licking, but response is unpredictable and often disappointing.
5. When no underlying cause can be found, treatment with behavior-modifying drugs may be beneficial in some dogs (Table 7-2). Trial treatment periods of up

TABLE 7-2 Drugs for Psychogenic Dermatoses in Dogs

Drug	Dose
Anxiolytics	
Phenobarbital	2–6 mg/kg PO q 12 hours
Diazepam	0.2 mg/kg PO q 12 hours
Hydroxyzine	2.2 mg/kg PO q 8 hours
Tricyclic Antidepressants	
Fluoxetine	1 mg/kg PO q 24 hours
Amitriptyline	1–3 mg/kg PO q 12 hours
Imipramine	2–4 mg/kg PO q 24 hours
Clomipramine	1–3 mg/kg PO q 24 hours
Endorphin Blocker	
Naltrexone	2 mg/kg PO q 24 hours
Endorphin Substitute	
Hydrocodone	0.25 mg/kg PO q 8 hours
Topical Products	
Fluocinolone acetonide + Flunixin meglumine	
Deep Heet + Bitter Apple	

Acral Lick Dermatitis—*cont'd*

to 5 weeks should be used until the most effective drug is identified. Lifelong treatment is often necessary.

6. Alternative medical treatments such as cold laser therapy or acupuncture have been beneficial in some patients.

7. Mechanical barriers such as wire muzzles and bandaging, Elizabethan collars, and side braces may be helpful.

8. Surgical excision or laser ablation is not recommended because postoperative complications, especially wound dehiscence, are common. Laser ablation may help sterilize the lesion and deaden nerve endings; however, response is highly variable.

9. The prognosis is variable. Chronic lesions that are unresponsive or extensively fibrotic and those for which no underlying cause can be found have a poor prognosis for resolution. Although this disease is rarely life threatening, its course may be intractable.

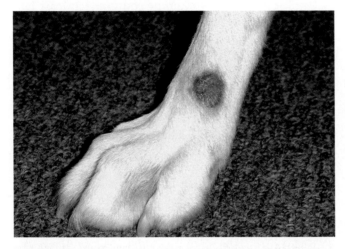

FIGURE 7-48 Acral Lick Dermatitis. This focal alopecic erosive lesion on the medial aspect of the distal leg is typical of this disease.

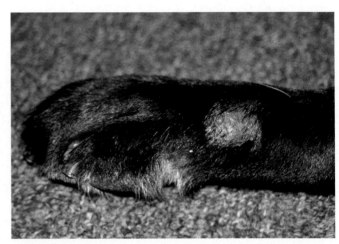

FIGURE 7-50 Acral Lick Dermatitis. A focal area of alopecia and thickening on the distal extremity.

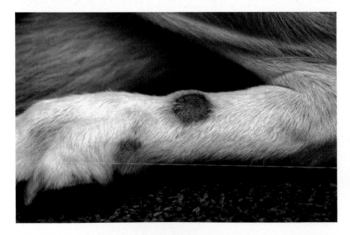

FIGURE 7-49 Acral Lick Dermatitis. A focal alopecic erosive lesion demonstrating the raised infiltrative nature typical of this disease.

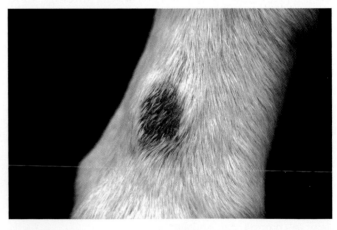

FIGURE 7-51 Acral Lick Dermatitis. A focal area of alopecia with tissue thickening and minimal erosion.

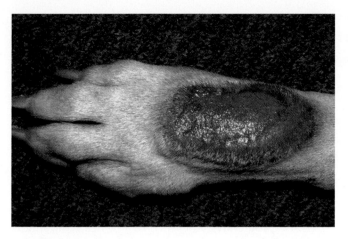

FIGURE 7-52 A large alopecic lesion demonstrating severe swelling and tissue erosion. Alopecia and erosions are the result of persistent licking.

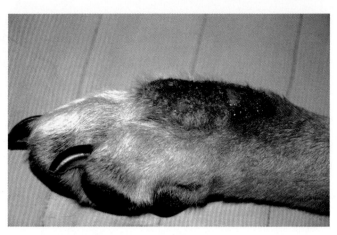

FIGURE 7-53 Acral Lick Dermatitis. Same dog as in Figure 7-52. The swollen infiltrative nature of the lesion causes it to protrude from the surrounding, more normal skin.

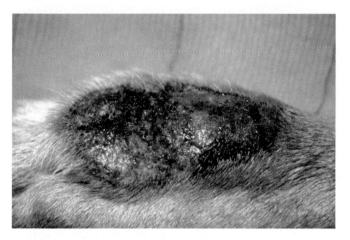

FIGURE 7-54 Acral Lick Dermatitis. Close-up of the lesion in Figure 7-53. Alopecia and the erosive surface of the swollen lesion are apparent.

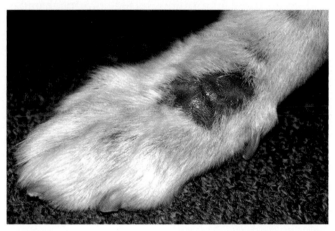

FIGURE 7-55 Acral Lick Dermatitis. A focal area of alopecia with hyperpigmentation and erosion on the foot.

Flea Allergy Dermatitis (flea bite hypersensitivity)

Features

Flea allergy dermatitis is a common skin disease in dogs and cats sensitized to flea saliva proteins through repeated and intermittent flea bites. Symptoms are usually seasonal (warm weather months and in the fall) in temperate zones and are often nonseasonal in subtropical and tropical areas. Fall is often the most severe season according to when the first cold snap occurs.

Dogs

Distribution typically involves the caudodorsal lumbosacral area, dorsal tail head, caudomedial thighs, abdomen, and flanks. Lesions include pruritic, papular, crusting eruptions with secondary erythema, seborrhea, alopecia, excoriations, pyoderma, hyperpigmentation, and lichenification.

Cats

Cats do not have a pattern unique to flea allergy dermatitis. Patients commonly present with pruritic miliary dermatitis with secondary excoriations, crusting, and alopecia of the neck, dorsal lumbosacral area, caudomedial thighs, and ventral abdomen. Other symptoms include symmetrical alopecia secondary to excessive grooming and eosinophilic granuloma complex lesions.

Top Differentials

Differentials include atopy, food hypersensitivity, other ectoparasites (scabies, cheyletiellosis, pediculosis, demodicosis), superficial pyoderma, dermatophytosis, demodicosis, and *Malassezia* dermatitis.

Diagnosis

1. Lumbar dermatitis in the dog is the most consistent and unique feature of flea allergy dermatitis. Flea allergy should be highly suspected in any cat with skin disease.
2. Visualization of fleas or flea excreta on the body: may be difficult with flea-allergic animals as flea-allergic animals are very effective at removing fleas through grooming.
3. Allergy testing (intradermal, serologic): positive skin test reaction to flea antigen or positive serum immunoglobulin (Ig)E antiflea antibody titer is highly suggestive, but false-negative results are possible.
4. Dermatohistopathology (nondiagnostic): varying degrees of superficial or deep perivascular to interstitial dermatitis, with eosinophils often predominating.
5. Response to aggressive flea control (nitenpyram administered every other day for 1 month): symptoms resolve.

Treatment and Prognosis

1. Integrated flea management program (insect growth regulator combined with an adulticide combined with environmental treatments) is essential because of the progressive tolerance of the flea to available adulticides. Over time, specific active ingredients typically lose efficacy as the result of chronic exposure and genetic drift of the flea.
2. Topical or systemic insect growth regulators (lufenuron, piriproxyfen, methoprene) may be effective alone or used in combination with adulticidal therapy.
3. Affected and all in-contact dogs and cats should be treated with adulticidal flea sprays, spot-on solutions, orals, or dips every 7 to 30 days, as instructed on the label. Products that contain Spinosad, imidocloprid, dinoteferon, selamectin, or fipronil are especially effective when administered every 2 to 4 weeks. In heavily flea-infested environments, fleas may continue to be found on animals for several months in spite of topical flea control. In these cases, affected animals should also be administered nitenpyram at a minimum dose of 1 mg/kg PO every 24 to 48 hours for 2 to 4 weeks, or until fleas are no longer seen. The environment should be treated (see number 5 below). Alternatively, the application of a 0.2% pyrethrin water-based spray every 1 to 2 days as a repellent may provide substantial protection for socially active dogs.
4. Flea-allergic animals should be treated prophylactically with nitenpyram, minimum dose 1 mg/kg PO, on any day that an encounter is planned with other potentially flea-infested animals (e.g., a visit to the groomer, veterinary hospital, park, another household with animals). No more than one treatment with nitenpyram should be administered per day.
5. In heavily flea-infested environments, areas where pets spend the most time should be treated. Indoor premises should be treated with an insecticide and an insect growth regulator (e.g., methoprene, piriproxyfen). The outdoor environment should be treated with insecticidal or biologic products designed for such use.
6. Flea control therapy should be continued from spring until first snowfall in temperate areas and year-round in warm climates. Year-round flea infestations can be perpetuated indoors and on wildlife despite extreme cold outdoors.

7. Symptomatic therapy (itch control):
   a. Topical therapy with antimicrobial shampoos and anti-itch conditioners, and sprays (i.e., those containing oatmeal, pramoxine, antihistamines, or glucocorticoids) applied every 2 to 7 days or as needed may help reduce clinical symptoms.
   b. Systemic antihistamine therapy reduces clinical symptoms in many cases (see Table 7-1).
   c. Systemic glucocorticoid therapy is often effective (75%) in controlling pruritus but almost always results in adverse effects ranging from mild (PU/PD) to severe (immune dysfunction, demodicosis, and calcinosis cutis). It is a therapeutic option if the allergy season is very short but may result in unacceptable adverse effects, especially if used over the long term.
      - Potent, long-acting injectable steroids are contraindicated for the treatment of allergies because of their comparatively short anti-inflammatory benefits (3 weeks) relative to their prolonged metabolic and immunodepressive effects (6–10 weeks).
      - Injectable short-acting steroids (dexamethasone sodium phosphate 0.5–1 mg/kg or prednisolone acetate 0.1–1 mg/kg) are effective at providing relief and may last 2 to 3 weeks if no concurrent secondary infection occurs. This treatment option allows the clinician to more closely control and monitor the patient's use of steroids compared with oral treatments administered by the owner.
      - Temaril-P (trimeprazine and prednisolone combination) is a unique drug that provides significant antipruritic effects at a relatively lower dose of the prednisolone. One tablet per 10 to 20 kg should be administered every 24 to 48 hours. The dosage should be tapered to the lowest possible dose and frequency.
      - Prednisone 0.25–1 mg/kg (or methylprednisolone 0.2–0.8 mg/kg) PO should be administered every 24 to 48 hours for 3 to 7 days. The dosage should be tapered to the lowest possible dose and frequency.
      - All dogs treated with long-term steroids (>3 months) should be frequently monitored for liver disease and UTI.
8. The prognosis is good if strict flea control is practiced. Fleas may infest other in-contact animals and humans. They may carry blood-borne diseases in a manner similar to ticks.

Author's Note

The use of long-acting, injectable steroids should be stopped because of their profound impact on the metabolic and immune systems, as well as growing concern for the legal liability of the practitioner.

Any dog with lumbar dermatitis or any cat with skin disease should be highly suspected of having flea allergy dermatitis, even if the patient has been treated with seemingly good flea control therapies.

A nitenpyram trial (every other day for 1 month) is the most efficient and cost-effective way to convince the owner and yourself of the role of flea allergy in a pruritic patient.

Text continued on page 198.

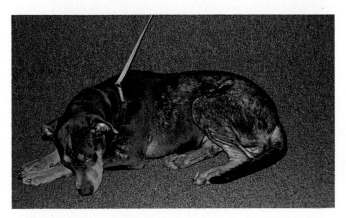

FIGURE 7-56 Flea Allergy Dermatitis. Moth-eaten alopecia on the lumbar and caudal flank area is typical of flea allergy dermatitis in dogs.

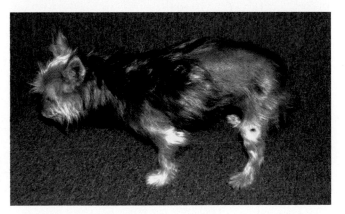

FIGURE 7-57 Flea Allergy Dermatitis. Lumbar dermatitis caused by a flea allergy. Most lesions in flea-allergic patients are caudal to the rib cage.

Flea Allergy Dermatitis—*cont'd*

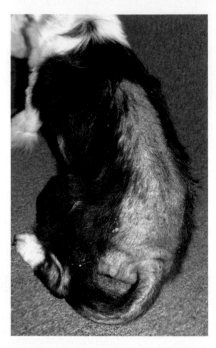

FIGURE 7-58 Flea Allergy Dermatitis. Severe lumbar and tail head dermatitis in a flea-allergic dog.

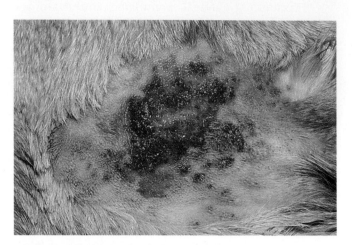

FIGURE 7-59 Flea Allergy Dermatitis. Hot spots (pyotraumatic dermatitis) are usually caused by exposure to fleas. Severe, erythematous, moist, erosive dermatitis with expanding papular rash is typical of pyotraumatic dermatitis.

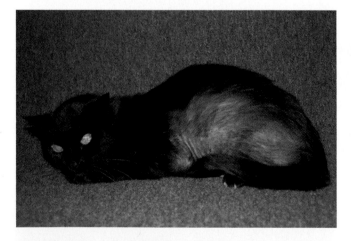

FIGURE 7-60 Flea Allergy Dermatitis. Allergic alopecia on the caudal flanks of a flea-allergic cat.

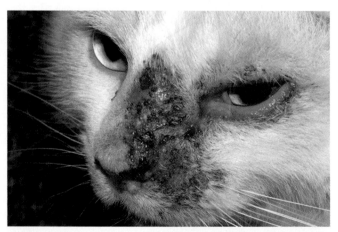

FIGURE 7-61 Flea Allergy Dermatitis. Eosinophilic plaque on the face of a flea-allergic cat. Severe, erythematous, erosive dermatitis with crust formation developed acutely after flea exposure.

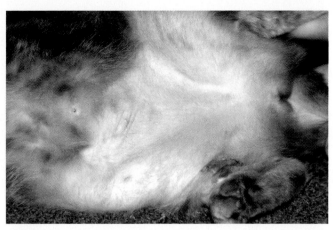

FIGURE 7-62 Flea Allergy Dermatitis. Preauricular dermatitis with a focal eosinophilic plaque in a flea allergic cat.

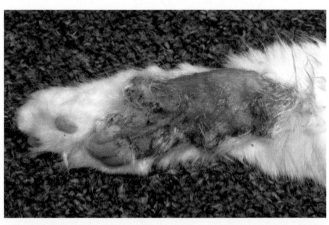

FIGURE 7-63 Flea Allergy Dermatitis. Allergic alopecia on the abdomen of a flea allergic cat. Lack of apparent cutaneous inflammation often leads to the misdiagnosis of psychogenic alopecia. Note the small eosinophilic plaque on the proximal region of the right inner thigh.

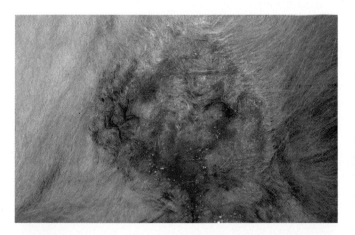

FIGURE 7-64 Flea Allergy Dermatitis. An eosinophilic plaque caused by flea allergy dermatitis in a cat. Alopecic, moist, erosive dermatitis is apparent.

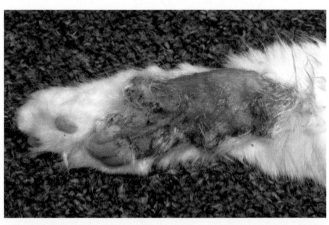

FIGURE 7-65 Flea Allergy Dermatitis. An eosinophilic plaque caused by flea allergy dermatitis on the distal limb of the cat.

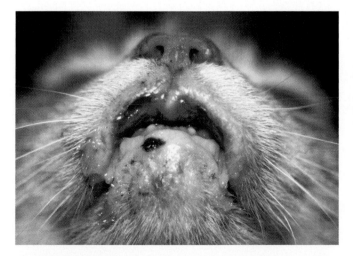

FIGURE 7-66 Flea Allergy Dermatitis. Eosinophilic granulomas affecting the chin and upper lips of this cat were caused by an underlying flea allergy. The skin is alopecic, erythematous, and swollen, as is typical of an eosinophilic granuloma.

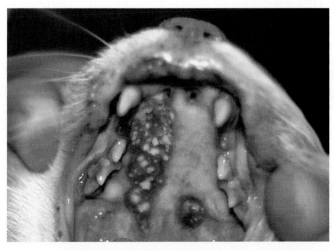

FIGURE 7-67 Flea Allergy Dermatitis. An oral eosinophilic granuloma in a flea allergic cat. Feline oral eosinophilic granulomas are often a manifestation of flea allergy.

Flea Allergy Dermatitis—*cont'd*

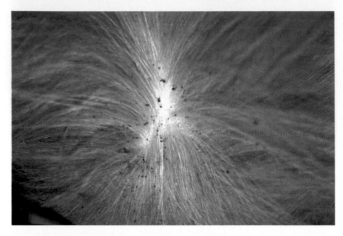

FIGURE 7-68 **Flea Allergy Dermatitis.** Same cat as in Figure 7-67. Digested blood passed as feces forms a dark coagulate typical of "flea dirt."

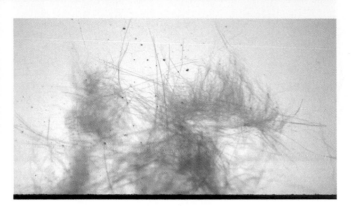

FIGURE 7-69 **Flea Allergy Dermatitis.** Hairs and flea dirt collected with a flea comb and placed on paper.

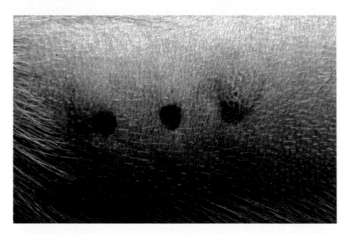

FIGURE 7-70 **Flea Allergy Dermatitis.** An intradermal allergy test using flea antigen *(right)* was positive in this flea allergic dog. Histamine *(left)* and saline *(middle)* were used as positive and negative controls.

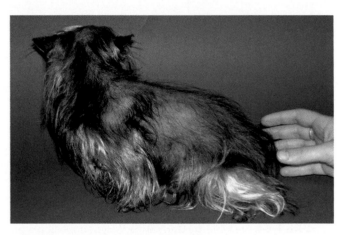

FIGURE 7-71 **Flea Allergy Dermatitis.** Characteristic lumbar dermatitis is demonstrated by visible alopecia covering the back half of this dog's body.

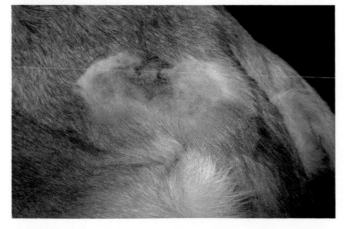

FIGURE 7-72 A focal lesion on the lumbar region of a dog. Note the similarity to a hot spot (pyotraumatic dermatitis) but without the moist exudate.

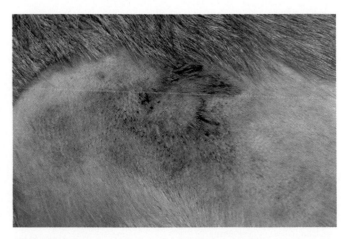

FIGURE 7-73 **Flea Allergy Dermatitis.** Close-up of the dog in Figure 7-72. The focal lesion clearly demonstrates erythema and mild crusting.

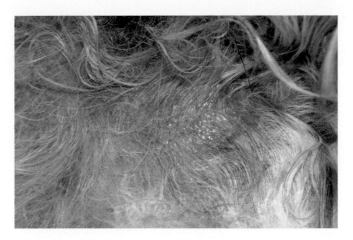

FIGURE 7-74 Flea Allergy Dermatitis. Severe erythema with a moist exudate starting to form, which likely will lead to the formation of a hot spot (pyotraumatic dermatitis).

Feline Atopy

Features

Feline atopy is a type 1 hypersensitivity reaction to environmental antigens (allergens), a genetic or heritable predisposition is suspected. It is uncommon in cats and is less common than flea hypersensitivity and food allergy.

Cats do not have a pattern unique to atopy. The primary symptom is pruritus (chewing, scratching, excessive grooming), which may be seasonal or non-seasonal, depending on the offending allergens. This pruritus may concentrate around the head, neck, and ears, or it may involve other areas such as the ventral abdomen, caudal thighs, forelegs, or lateral thorax. Self-trauma usually results in alopecia that can be bilaterally symmetrical. Remaining hairs are broken off and do not epilate easily. The alopecic skin may appear otherwise normal or may be secondarily excoriated. Miliary dermatitis, ceruminous otitis externa, and eosinophilic granuloma complex lesions are common. With chronicity, secondary pyoderma or peripheral lymphadenomegaly may develop. Atopy may be linked with chronic bronchitis or asthma in some cats.

Top Differentials

Differentials include flea allergy dermatitis, other hypersensitivities (food, mosquito bite), dermatophytosis, ectoparasites (cheyletiellosis, ear mites, feline scabies, demodicosis), psychogenic alopecia, pemphigus, and cutaneous lymphoma.

Diagnosis

1. Rule out other differentials, especially flea allergy dermatitis, dermatophytosis, mites, and food allergy.
2. Allergy testing (intradermal, serologic): allergy testing can be highly variable according to the method used. Positive reactions to grass, tree, mould, weed, insect, dander, feathers, or indoor environmental allergens are seen. False-negative reactions are common. False-positive reactions can occur. Systemic fluorescein administration may improve the diagnostic accuracy of intradermal skin testing in cats.
3. Dermatohistopathology (nondiagnostic): variably mild to marked perivascular or diffuse inflammation with lymphocytes, mast cell hyperplasia, and eosinophils. Epidermal hyperplasia, spongiosis, erosions, ulcers, and serocellular crusts may be present.

Treatment and Prognosis

1. Infection prevention: any secondary pyoderma or otitis should be treated with appropriate therapies for 2 to 4 weeks.
2. Symptomatic therapy (itch control): pruritus can be controlled with antihistamines, essential fatty acid supplements, and glucocorticoids.
   a. An integrated flea control program should be instituted to prevent flea bites from aggravating the pruritus.
   b. Systemic antihistamines may reduce clinical symptoms in 40% to 70% of atopic cats. A beneficial effect should occur within 1 to 2 weeks of initiation of therapy (Table 7-3).
   c. Oral essential fatty acid supplements may help control pruritus in 20% to 50% of cats. A beneficial effect should occur within 8 to 12 weeks of initiation of therapy. A synergistic effect may be seen when essential fatty acid supplements are administered in combination with other therapies.
   d. Systemic glucocorticoids control pruritus but almost always result in adverse effects ranging from mild to severe. Effective therapies include the following:
      ■ Prednisolone 2 mg/kg PO q 24 hours until pruritus and lesions resolve (approximately 2–8 weeks), then 2 mg/kg PO q 48 hours for 2–4 weeks, tapered down to the lowest possible alternate-day dosage if long-term maintenance therapy is needed
      ■ Dexamethasone 2 mg PO q 1–3 days to reduce pruritus, then tapered to the lowest possible frequency required
3. Allergy treatment (immune modulation)
   a. The caregiver can reduce exposure to offending allergens by removing them from the environment, if possible. HEPA air and charcoal filters can be used to reduce pollens, molds, and dust in the home. For house dust mite–sensitive cats, household treatments of carpets, mattresses, and

TABLE 7-3 Antihistamine Therapy for Cats*

Antihistamine	Dose
Chlorpheniramine	2–4 mg/cat PO q 12–24 hours
Amitriptyline	5–10 mg/cat PO q 12–24 hours
Clemastine	0.68 mg/cat PO q 12 hours
Cyproheptadine	2 mg/cat PO q 12 hours
Hydroxyzine	5–10 mg/cat PO q 8–12 hours
Diphenhydramine	2–4 mg/cat PO q 12 hours

Antihistamines in bold are preferred by authors.

upholstery with the acaricide benzyl benzoate once a month for approximately 3 months, then every 3 months thereafter, may effectively eliminate house dust mites from the environment. Old cat beds should be discarded, as these may accumulate house dust mite antigens. Dehumidifying the house to below 40% relative humidity decreases house dust mite, mould, and flea antigen loads. To achieve this, high-efficiency dehumidifiers that are capable of pulling several liters of water per day from the air are required.

b. Cyclosporine (Atopica) 7.5 mg/kg PO can be administered every 24 hours until beneficial effects are seen (approximately 4–6 weeks). Then, try to taper down dosage frequency to every 48 to 72 hours. Many cats can be maintained on every 72-hour dosing, making this therapy extremely cost effective. Cats should be feline leukemia virus (FeLV) and feline immunodeficiency virus (FIV) negative. The risk of toxoplasmosis infection is a matter of concern; however, this risk seems to be very low as of this writing.

c. Immunotherapy (allergy vaccine) is indicated if medical therapy is ineffective or unacceptable to the owner, or if it results in undesirable adverse effects. Overall, 50% to 70% of atopic cats show favorable responses to immunotherapy. Clinical improvement is usually noted within 3 to 8 months but can take up to 1 year in some cats.

4. The prognosis is good for most cats, but successful management usually requires lifelong therapy.

Author's Note

Although extremely common, long-acting injectable steroids should be used only as a last resort because life-threatening cardiac effects have been identified in up to 11% of cats, as have other better known medical risks, including diabetes and urinary tract infection.

Cyclosporine (Atopica) is extremely well tolerated in cats and has very few adverse effects. It is interesting to note that cyclosporine seems to be able to control most of the immunologic causes of feline dermatitis with the exception of flea allergy, dermatophytosis, and mites.

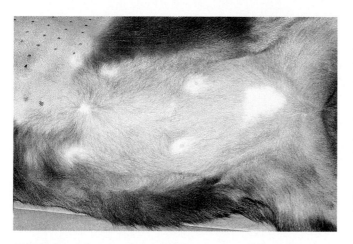

FIGURE 7-75 Feline Atopy. Allergic alopecia on the abdomen of a cat. Similar alopecic lesions with excessive grooming can be caused by flea allergy, food allergy, and mite infestations.

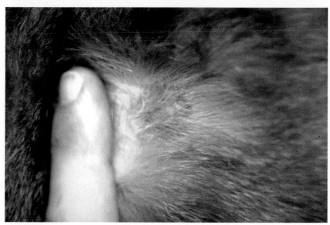

FIGURE 7-77 Feline Atopy. Focal erythema with slight alopecia on the flank of an atopic cat. This lesion was a mild eosinophilic plaque.

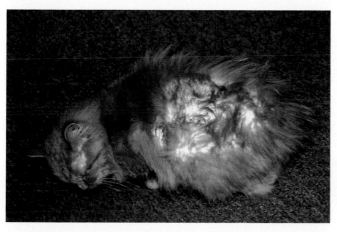

FIGURE 7-76 Feline Atopy. Multifocal alopecia on the flank and lumbar area of a cat with atopy.

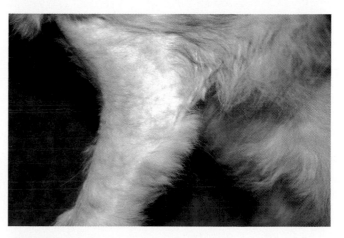

FIGURE 7-78 Feline Atopy. Allergic alopecia affecting almost the entire front limb of an atopic cat. Note the general absence of dermatitis (apparent inflammation), which often leads to the misdiagnosis of psychogenic alopecia.

Feline Atopy—*cont'd*

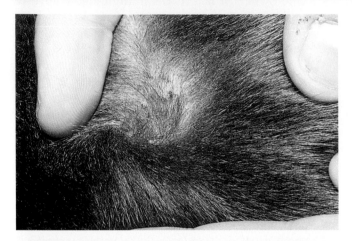

FIGURE 7-79 Feline Atopy. Small focal crusts typical of miliary dermatitis in an atopic cat.

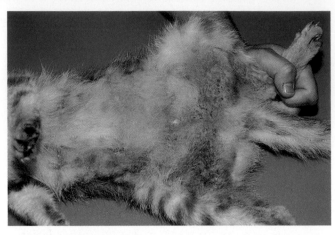

FIGURE 7-80 Feline Atopy. Alopecia and early eosinophilic plaques on the abdomen of an allergic cat.

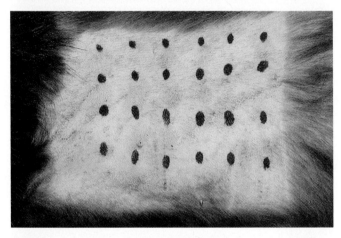

FIGURE 7-81 Feline Atopy. This intradermal allergy test demonstrates several positive reactions. Note the subtlety of the reactions, which is typical of allergy tests in cats.

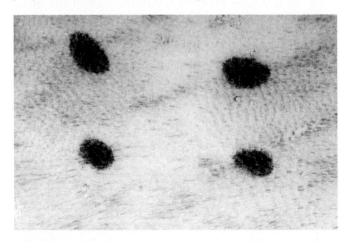

FIGURE 7-82 Feline Atopy. Close-up of the intradermal allergy test in Figure 7-81. Positive reactions appear as erythematous macules.

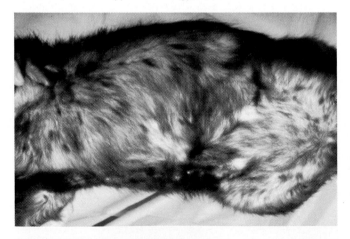

FIGURE 7-83 Feline Atopy. Generalized moth-eaten alopecia on the trunk of an atopic cat.

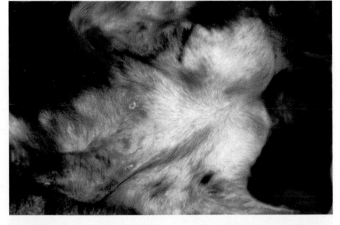

FIGURE 7-84 Feline Atopy. Allergic alopecia on the abdomen of an atopic cat. Cutaneous inflammation can be mild and easily overlooked.

Feline Food Hypersensitivity

Features

Feline food hypersensitivity is an adverse reaction to a food or food additive. It can occur at any age. It is uncommon in cats—less common than flea hypersensitivity—but may be more common than feline atopy.

Cats do not have a unique pattern of food allergy. Feline food hypersensitivity is characterized by nonseasonal pruritus that may or may not respond to glucocorticoid therapy. Distribution of the pruritus may be localized to the head and neck, or it may be generalized and involve the trunk, ventrum, and limbs. Skin lesions are variable and may include alopecia, erythema, miliary dermatitis, eosinophilic granuloma complex lesions, excoriations, crusts, and scales. *Malassezia* or ceruminous otitis externa may be seen. Concurrent gastrointestinal symptoms (e.g., diarrhea, vomiting) may be reported.

Top Differentials

Differentials include flea allergy dermatitis, atopy, mosquito bite hypersensitivity, dermatophytosis, ectoparasites (cheyletiellosis, ear mites, feline scabies, demodicosis), psychogenic alopecia and pemphigus, and cutaneous lymphoma.

Diagnosis

1. Rule out other differentials, especially flea allergy dermatitis, dermatophytosis, mites, and atopy.
2. Dermatohistopathology (nondiagnostic): varying degrees of superficial or deep perivascular dermatitis in which eosinophils or mast cells often predominate.
3. Food allergy testing (intradermal or serologic) (nondiagnostic): not recommended because test results are unreliable.
4. Response to hypoallergenic diet trial: symptoms improve within 10 to 12 weeks of initiation of a strict home-cooked or commercially prepared restricted diet (one protein and one carbohydrate source). The diet should not contain food ingredients previously included in cat food, treats, or table scraps provided.
5. Provocative challenge: symptoms recur within hours to days of reintroduction of suspect allergen into the diet.

Treatment and Prognosis

1. Infection prevention: any secondary pyoderma or otitis should be treated with appropriate therapies for 2 to 4 weeks.

2. Symptomatic therapy (itch control): pruritus can be controlled with antihistamines, essential fatty acid supplements, and glucocorticoids.
   a. An integrated flea control program should be instituted to prevent flea bites from aggravating the pruritus.
   b. Systemic antihistamines may reduce clinical symptoms in 40% to 70% of atopic cats. A beneficial effect should occur within 1 to 2 weeks of initiation of therapy (see Table 7-3).
   c. Oral essential fatty acid supplements may help control pruritus in 20% to 50% of cats. A beneficial effect should occur within 8 to 12 weeks of initiation of therapy. A synergistic effect may be seen when essential fatty acid supplements are administered in combination with other therapies.
   d. Systemic glucocorticoids control pruritus but almost always result in adverse effects ranging from mild to severe. Effective therapies include the following:
      - Prednisolone 2 mg/kg PO q 24 hours until pruritus and lesions resolve (approximately 2–8 weeks), then 2 mg/kg PO q 48 hours for 2–4 weeks, tapered down to the lowest possible alternate-day dosage if long-term maintenance therapy is needed
      - Dexamethasone, 2 mg PO q 1–3 days to reduce the pruritus, then tapered to the lowest possible frequency required
3. Allergy treatment
   a. Offending dietary allergen(s) should be avoided. A balanced home-cooked diet or a commercially prepared hypoallergenic diet should be provided.
   b. Cyclosporine (Atopica) 7.5 mg/kg PO can be administered every 24 hours until beneficial effects are seen (approximately 4–6 weeks). Then, try to taper down dosage frequency to every 48 to 72 hours. Many cats can be maintained on every 72 hour dosing, making this therapy extremely cost effective. Cats should be FeLV and FIV negative. The risk of toxoplasmosis infection is a matter of concern; however, this risk seems to be very low as of this writing.
4. The prognosis is good if the cat accepts the hypoallergenic diet. If the cat relapses, owner noncompliance should be ruled out, along with the development of food hypersensitivity to the new diet, dermatophytosis, ectoparasites, concurrent atopy, and flea allergy dermatitis.

Feline Food Hypersensitivity—*cont'd*

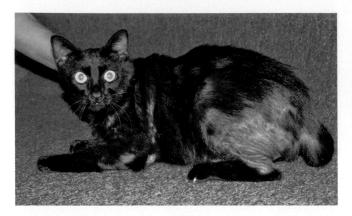

FIGURE 7-85 **Feline Food Hypersensitivity.** Allergic alopecia on the lumbar and caudal thigh regions of a food-allergic cat.

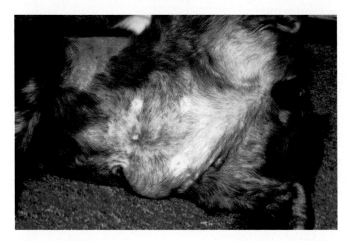

FIGURE 7-86 **Feline Food Hypersensitivity.** Close-up of the cat in Figure 7-85. Alopecia is often the predominant lesion in allergic cats. Note that the skin is in good condition with little apparent inflammation.

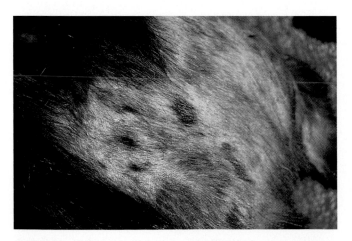

FIGURE 7-87 **Feline Food Hypersensitivity.** Close-up of the cat in Figure 7-86. Allergic alopecia on the abdomen is apparent.

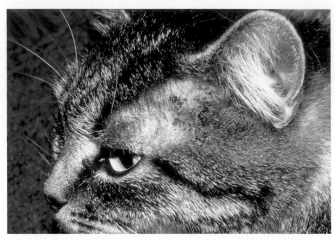

FIGURE 7-88 **Feline Food Hypersensitivity.** Preauricular dermatitis consisting of alopecia and a crusting papular rash typical of miliary dermatitis.

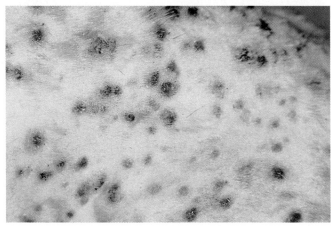

FIGURE 7-89 **Feline Food Hypersensitivity.** Severe eosinophilic papular dermatitis on the trunk of a cat. A papular rash covered most of the cat's body.

Author's Note

Although extremely common, long-acting injectable steroids should be used only as a last resort because life-threatening cardiac effects have been identified in up to 11% of cats, as have other better known medical risks, including diabetes and urinary tract infection.

Cyclosporine (Atopica) is extremely well tolerated in cats and has very few adverse effects. It is interesting to note that cyclosporine seems to be able to control most of the immunologic causes of feline dermatitis with the exception of flea allergy, dermatophytosis, and mites.

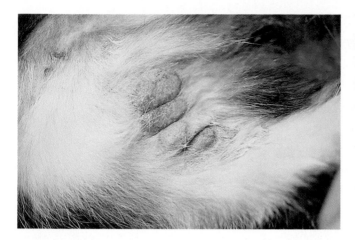

FIGURE 7-90 **Feline Food Hypersensitivity.** An eosinophilic plaque on the abdomen of a food-allergic cat.

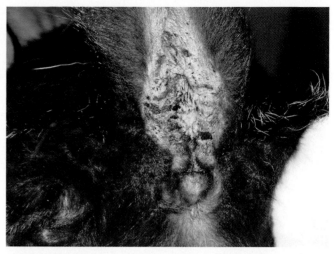

FIGURE 7-91 **Feline Food Hypersensitivity.** Perianal dermatitis in a food-allergic cat. Perianal dermatitis is a common finding in food-allergic animals.

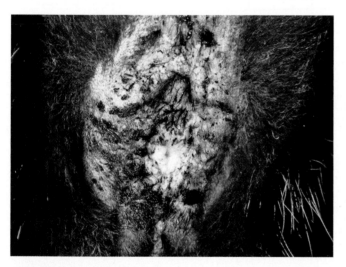

FIGURE 7-92 **Feline Food Hypersensitivity.** Perianal dermatitis in a food-allergic cat.

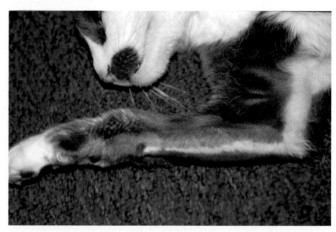

FIGURE 7-93 **Feline Food Hypersensitivity.** Allergic alopecia covering almost the entire front limb of this allergic cat.

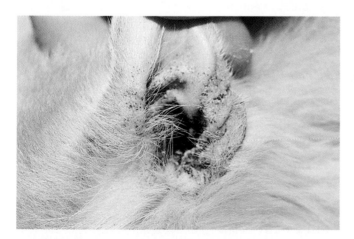

FIGURE 7-94 **Feline Food Hypersensitivity.** Otitis externa caused by a secondary bacterial and yeast infection associated with allergy. The otitis resolved after secondary infections were treated and a dietary food trial was provided.

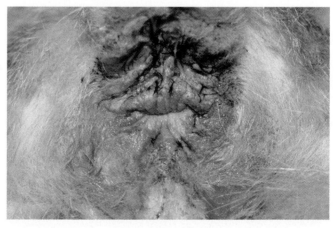

FIGURE 7-95 **Feline Food Hypersensitivity.** Severe erythema and alopecia affecting the perianal area of a food-allergic cat.

Feline Food Hypersensitivity—*cont'd*

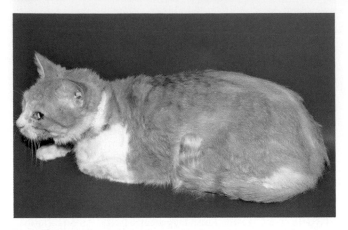

FIGURE 7-96 Feline Food Hypersensitivity. At a distance, this food-allergic cat has only mild lesions affecting the face and dorsal lumbar region.

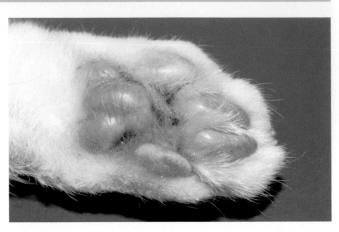

FIGURE 7-97 Feline Food Hypersensitivity. Same cat as in Figure 7-96. The feet look healthy until the interdigital space is more closely examined.

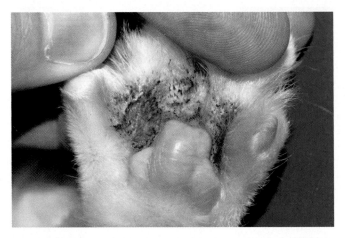

FIGURE 7-98 Feline Food Hypersensitivity. Same cat as in Figure 7-96. The interdigital dermatitis had a secondary bacterial infection caused by the allergy.

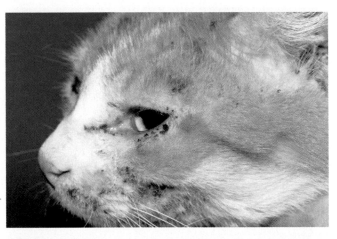

FIGURE 7-99 Feline Food Hypersensitivity. Facial dermatitis, alopecia, and erythema with crust formation demonstrating the pruritic nature of this disease.

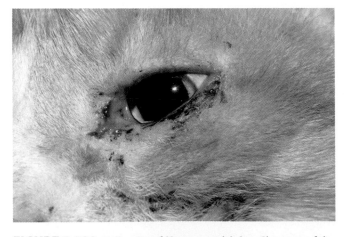

FIGURE 7-100 Feline Food Hypersensitivity. Close-up of the same cat as in Figure 7-99. Crusting, erythematous lesions are apparent.

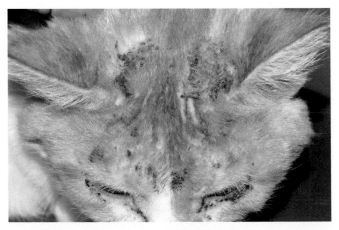

FIGURE 7-101 Feline Food Hypersensitivity. Same cat as in Figure 7-100. Alopecia with erythema and crust formation is apparent.

Mosquito Bite Hypersensitivity

Features

Mosquito bite hypersensitivity is an uncommon seasonal disease in cats sensitized to mosquito bites.

It appears as mildly to severely pruritic papules, pustules, erosions, and crusts on the bridge of the nose and on the outer ear pinnae. Lesions may be hypopigmented or hyperpigmented and symmetrical. The bridge of the nose is often swollen. The footpads, especially on the outer margins, may be hyperkeratotic, hyperpigmented or hypopigmented, fissured, painful, swollen, or ulcerated. Peripheral lymphadenomegaly may be present.

Top Differentials

Differentials include flea allergy dermatitis, food allergy, atopy, dermatophytosis, ear mites, demodicosis, plasma cell pododermatitis, and autoimmune skin disorders.

Diagnosis

1. Seasonal history, clinical findings, and response to confinement to a mosquito-free environment. Lesions improve within 4 to 7 days.
2. Dermatohistopathology (nondiagnostic): hyperplastic, superficial perivascular to diffuse eosinophilic dermatitis.

Treatment and Prognosis

1. The cat should be confined indoors, especially at dawn and dusk, when mosquitoes are most active.
2. To repel mosquitoes, the caregiver should apply a water-based dilute pyrethrin spray topically to affected areas every 24 hours. Caution should be used when cats are treated with pyrethroid products. Topical mosquito repellents marketed for human use (e.g., DEET) may be toxic to cats.
3. If mosquito exposure cannot be avoided, therapies used to control atopy may be beneficial.
4. The prognosis is good, but permanent scarring is a potential sequela in severely affected cats.

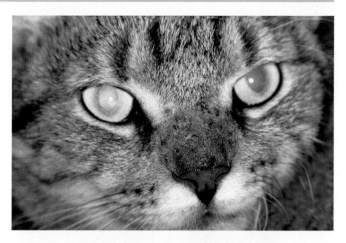

FIGURE 7-102 Mosquito Bite Hypersensitivity. Alopecia and crusts on the bridge of the nose caused by biting mosquitoes.

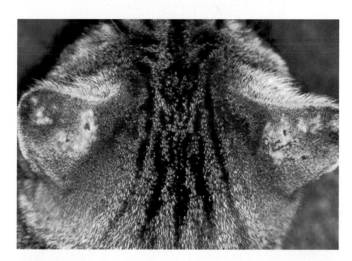

FIGURE 7-103 Mosquito Bite Hypersensitivity. Close-up of the cat in Figure 7-102. Alopecia and crusts on the ear pinnae caused by hypersensitivity to mosquito bites. Note the similarity to autoimmune skin disease.

Mosquito Bite Hypersensitivity—*cont'd*

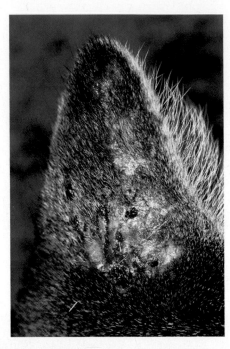

FIGURE 7-104 **Mosquito Bite Hypersensitivity.** Close-up of the cat in Figure 7-102. Alopecia and crusts on the ear pinna.

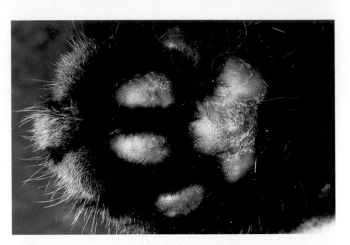

FIGURE 7-105 **Mosquito Bite Hypersensitivity.** Close-up of the cat in Figure 7-102. Hyperkeratosis and crusting of the footpads. Note the similarity to plasma cell pododermatitis and autoimmune skin disease.

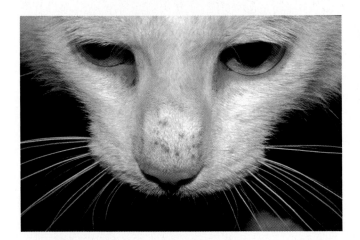

FIGURE 7-106 **Mosquito Bite Hypersensitivity.** Multifocal alopecia and crusting on the nose of a cat.

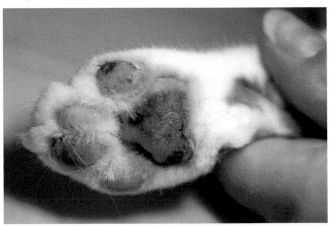

FIGURE 7-107 **Mosquito Bite Hypersensitivity.** Hyperkeratosis and crusting of the footpads. Note the similarity to autoimmune skin disease and plasma cell pododermatitis.

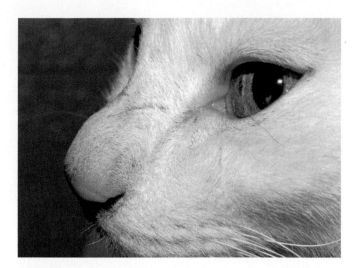

FIGURE 7-108 **Mosquito Bite Hypersensitivity.** Nasal swelling in an allergic cat. The skin is in good condition. Notice the similarity to early *Cryptococcus* infection in cats.

Feline Eosinophilic Plaque

Features

Feline eosinophilic plaque is an inflammatory skin disease that is usually associated with an underlying hypersensitivity, most often flea allergy but possibly food allergy or atopy. It is common in cats, with the highest incidence in young adult to middle-aged cats.

Feline eosinophilic plaque manifests as single to multiple well-circumscribed, raised, erythematous, eroded or ulcerated plaques. Lesions are usually intensely pruritic and may appear anywhere on the body, but they are most commonly found on the ventral abdomen and medial thighs. Regional lymphadenomegaly may be present.

Top Differentials

Differentials include bacterial or fungal granulomas and neoplasia.

Diagnosis

1. Usually based on history, clinical findings, and ruling out other differentials.
2. Cytology (impression smear): eosinophils are usually seen, but neutrophils and bacteria may predominate if the lesion is secondarily infected.
3. Dermatohistopathology: hyperplastic, superficial, and deep perivascular to diffuse eosinophilic dermatitis. Eosinophilic microabscesses may be seen.
4. Hemogram: peripheral eosinophilia is common.

Treatment and Prognosis

1. Any secondary pyoderma with appropriate therapies for 2 to 4 weeks.
2. Any underlying allergies should be identified and managed, especially flea allergy dermatitis treatments. A month-long nitenpyram trial (every other day) may be the only study to prove a link to flea allergy in some patients.
3. Systemic antihistamines may reduce clinical symptoms in 40% to 70% of atopic cats. A beneficial effect should occur within 2 weeks of initiation of therapy (see Table 7-3).
4. Cyclosporine (Atopica) 7.5 mg/kg PO can be administered every 24 hours until beneficial effects are seen (approximately 4–6 weeks). Then, try to taper down dosage frequency to every 48 to 72 hours. Many cats can be maintained on every 72 hour dosing, making this therapy extremely cost effective. Cats should be FeLV and FIV negative. The risk of toxoplasmosis infection is a matter of concern; however this risk seems to be very low as of this writing.

5. Systemic glucocorticoids may produce rapid reductions in lesion severity and pruritus but almost always result in adverse effects ranging from mild to severe. Effective therapies include the following:
   - To induce remission, prednisolone 2 mg/kg PO every 12 hours should be administered until lesions resolve (approximately 2–8 weeks). Significant improvement should be seen within 2 to 4 weeks. Once lesions have resolved, oral prednisolone therapy should be gradually tapered to the lowest possible alternate-day dose.
   - Dexamethasone 2 mg PO q 1–3 days to reduce pruritus, then tapered to the lowest possible frequency required
   - Triamcinolone (induction dose) 0.8 mg/kg PO q 24 hours
6. Alternative medical therapies that may be effective include the following:
   - Trimethoprim sulfa 125 mg q 12 hours
   - Doxycycline 5–10 mg/kg q 12 hours
   - Oral essential fatty acid supplements may help control pruritus in 20% to 50% of cats. A beneficial effect should occur within 8 to 12 weeks of initiation of therapy. A synergistic effect may be seen when essential fatty acid supplements are administered in combination with other therapies.
7. Other treatments that may be effective in some cats include surgical excision, laser therapy, and radiation therapy; however, adverse effects and wound complications are common.
8. The prognosis is variable. Cats with underlying allergies that are successfully managed have a good prognosis. Cats with recurring lesions for which no underlying cause can be found usually require long-term therapy to keep lesions in remission. These cats have a poorer prognosis as they may become refractory to or may develop unacceptable adverse effects as the result of medical therapy.

Author's Note

Although extremely common, long-acting injectable steroids should be used only as a last resort because life-threatening cardiac effects have been identified in up to 11% of cats, as have other better known medical risks, including diabetes and urinary tract infection.

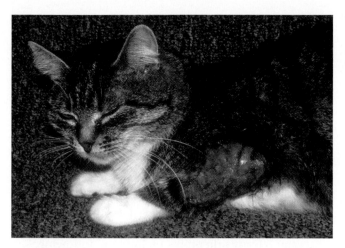

FIGURE 7-109 **Feline Eosinophilic Plaque.** A large alopecic, erythematous, eroded lesion with a moist exudate typical of this disease. Note that the location is atypical.

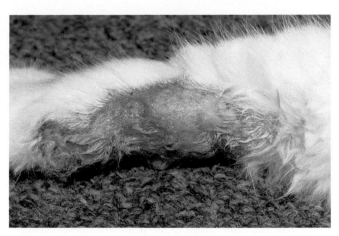

FIGURE 7-110 **Feline Eosinophilic Plaque.** An alopecic, erythematous lesion with a moist exudate on the distal front leg of the cat. This eosinophilic plaque was caused by flea allergy dermatitis.

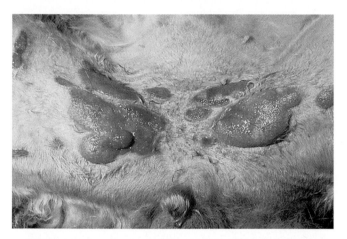

FIGURE 7-111 **Feline Eosinophilic Plaque.** These multifocal erosive plaques on the abdomen were intensely pruritic. Note the intense erythema and moist exudate typical of this syndrome.

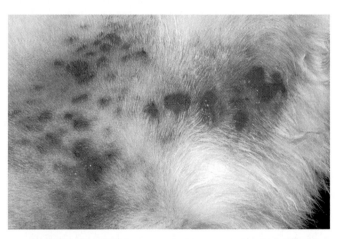

FIGURE 7-112 **Feline Eosinophilic Plaque.** Multiple small alopecic, erythematous plaques on the abdomen of a flea-allergic cat.

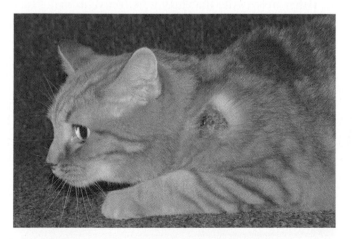

FIGURE 7-113 **Feline Eosinophilic Plaque.** A large eosinophilic plaque on the shoulder of a flea-allergic cat.

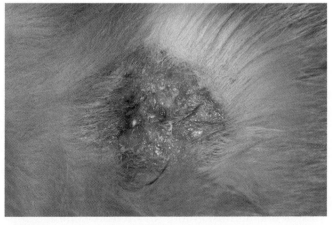

FIGURE 7-114 **Feline Eosinophilic Plaque.** Close-up of the lesion in Figure 7-113. The alopecic, erythematous, erosive lesion and the moist exudate are typical of this disease.

Feline Eosinophilic Granuloma (linear granuloma)

Features

Feline eosinophilic granuloma is an inflammatory cutaneous or oral mucosal disease that is usually associated with an underlying hypersensitivity, most often flea allergy but also food allergy and atopy. It is common in cats.

Cutaneous lesions usually occur singly and may be raised, firm, linear plaques or papular to nodular, edematous, or firm swellings. The lesions may be mildly erythematous, alopecic, eroded, or ulcerated, but they usually are neither painful nor pruritic. Lesions can occur anywhere on the body but are most common on the caudal aspect of the thigh (linear granuloma) and chin or lip (swelling). A regional lymphadenomegaly may be present. Oral lesions are characterized by papules, nodules, or well-circumscribed plaques and are found on the tongue or palate. Cats with oral lesions may be dysphagic.

Top Differentials

Differentials include bacterial or fungal granuloma and neoplasia.

Diagnosis

1. Usually based on history, clinical findings, and ruling out other differentials.
2. Cytology (impression smear): many eosinophils are seen, but neutrophils and bacteria may predominate if the lesion is secondarily infected.
3. Dermatohistopathology: nodular to diffuse granuloma composed of eosinophils, histiocytes, and multinucleated giant cells with foci of collagen degeneration.
4. Hemogram: peripheral eosinophilia may be present.

Treatment and Prognosis

1. Any secondary pyoderma with appropriate therapies for 2 to 4 weeks.
2. Any underlying allergies should be identified and managed, especially flea allergy dermatitis treatments. A month-long nitenpyram trial (every other day) may be the only study to prove a link to flea allergy in some patients.
3. Systemic antihistamines may reduce clinical symptoms in 40% to 70% of atopic cats. A beneficial effect should occur within 2 weeks of initiation of therapy (see Table 7-3).
4. Cyclosporine (Atopica) 7.5 mg/kg PO can be administered every 24 hours until beneficial effects are seen (approximately 4–6 weeks). Then, try to taper down dosage frequency to every 48 to 72 hours. Many cats can be maintained on every 72 hour dosing, making this therapy extremely cost effective. Cats should be FeLV and FIV negative. The risk of toxoplasmosis infection is a matter of concern; however; this risk seems to be very low as of this writing.
5. Systemic glucocorticoids may produce rapid reductions in lesion severity and pruritus but almost always result in adverse effects ranging from mild to severe. Effective therapies include the following:
   - To induce remission, prednisolone 2 mg/kg PO every 12 hours should be administered until lesions resolve (approximately 2–8 weeks). Significant improvement should be seen within 2 to 4 weeks. Once lesions have resolved, oral prednisolone therapy should be gradually tapered to the lowest possible alternate-day dose.
   - Dexamethasone 2 mg PO q 1–3 days to reduce pruritus, then tapered to the lowest possible frequency required
   - Triamcinolone (induction dose) 0.8 mg/kg PO q 24 hours
6. Alternative medical therapies that may be effective include the following:
   - Trimethoprim sulfa 125 mg q 12 hours
   - Doxycycline 5–10 mg/kg q 12 hours

   Oral essential fatty acid supplements may help control pruritus in 20% to 50% of cats. A beneficial effect should occur within 8 to 12 weeks of initiation of therapy. A synergistic effect may be seen when essential fatty acid supplements are administered in combination with other therapies.
7. Other treatments that may be effective in some cats include surgical excision, laser therapy, and radiation therapy; however, adverse effects and wound complications are common.
8. The prognosis is variable. Cats with underlying allergies that are managed successfully have an excellent prognosis. Cats with recurring lesions for which no underlying cause can be found usually require long-term therapy to keep lesions in remission. These cats have a poorer prognosis as they may become refractory to or may develop unacceptable adverse effects as the result of medical therapy.

Author's Note

Although extremely common, long-acting injectable steroids should be used only as a last resort because life-threatening cardiac effects have been identified in up to 11% of cats, as have other better known medical risks, including diabetes and urinary tract infection.

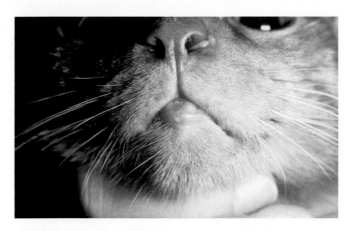

FIGURE 7-115 **Feline Eosinophilic Granuloma.** Tissue swelling and erythema on the lower lip of a cat. Note the similarity to an indolent ulcer, which usually occurs on the upper lip. *(Courtesy D. Angarano.)*

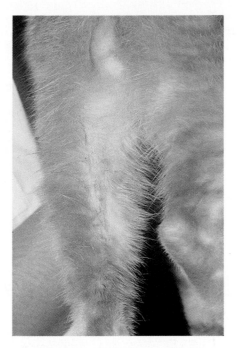

FIGURE 7-116 **Feline Eosinophilic Granuloma.** A thickened linear region of alopecia and erythema on the caudal rear leg. The inflammation associated with linear eosinophilic granulomas creates a distinctive palpable lesion. *(Courtesy D. Angarano.)*

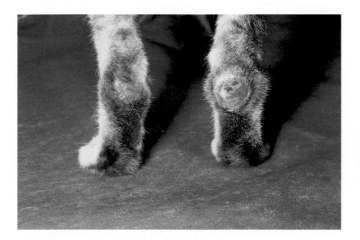

FIGURE 7-117 **Feline Eosinophilic Granuloma.** A circular eosinophilic granuloma on the rear leg.

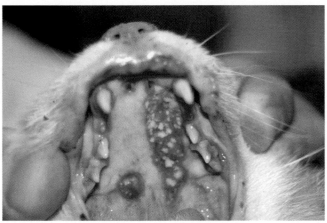

FIGURE 7-118 **Feline Eosinophilic Granuloma.** Multiple coalescing granulomas on the hard palate of a flea-allergic cat.

Feline Eosinophilic Granuloma—*cont'd*

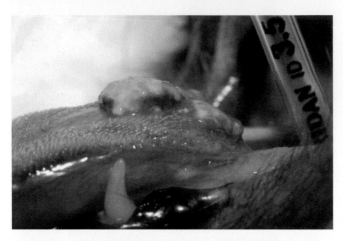

FIGURE 7-119 **Feline Eosinophilic Granuloma.** These large, coalescing granulomas developed over several weeks. The cat was having difficulty swallowing, necessitating aggressive medical intervention.

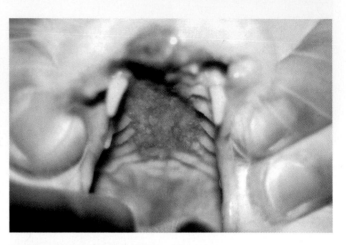

FIGURE 7-120 **Feline Eosinophilic Granuloma.** Eosinophilic granuloma on the hard palate of an adult cat.

Indolent Ulcer (rodent ulcer, eosinophilic ulcer)

Features

Indolent ulcer is an ulcerative skin disease that is usually associated with an underlying hypersensitivity, most often flea allergy but also food allergy and atopy. It is common in cats.

The lesion begins as a small, crater-like ulcer with raised margins that most commonly affects the upper lip. It usually is unilateral but can be bilateral. The ulcer may enlarge progressively and become disfiguring, but it is not painful or pruritic. Regional lymphadenomegaly may be present.

Top Differentials

Differentials include neoplasia and infection (bacterial, fungal, viral).

Diagnosis

1. Usually based on history and clinical findings.
2. Dermatohistopathology: hyperplastic, ulcerative, superficial perivascular to interstitial dermatitis and fibrosis. Inflammatory cells are primarily neutrophils and mononuclear cells; eosinophils are not typically found.

Treatment and Prognosis

1. Any secondary pyoderma with appropriate therapies for 2 to 4 weeks.
2. Any underlying allergies should be identified and managed, especially flea allergy dermatitis treatments. A month-long nitenpyram trial (every other day) may be the only study to prove a link to flea allergy in some patients.
3. Systemic antihistamines may reduce clinical symptoms in 40% to 70% of atopic cats. A beneficial effect should occur within 2 weeks of initiation of therapy (see Table 7-3).
4. Cyclosporine (Atopica) 7.5 mg/kg PO can be administered every 24 hours until beneficial effects are seen (approximately 4–6 weeks). Then, try to taper down dosage frequency to every 48 to 72 hours. Many cats can be maintained on every 72 hour dosing, making this therapy extremely cost effective. Cats should be FeLV and FIV negative. The risk of toxoplasmosis infection is a matter of concern; however, this risk seems to be very low as of this writing.
5. Systemic glucocorticoids may produce rapid reductions in lesion severity and pruritus but almost always result in adverse effects ranging from mild to severe. Effective therapies include the following:
   - To induce remission, prednisolone 2 mg/kg PO every 12 hours should be administered until lesions resolve (approximately 2–8 weeks). Significant improvement should be seen within 2 to 4 weeks. Once lesions have resolved, oral prednisolone therapy should be gradually tapered to the lowest possible alternate-day dose.
   - Dexamethasone 2 mg PO q 1–3 days to reduce pruritus, then tapered to the lowest possible frequency required
   - Triamcinolone (induction dose) 0.8 mg/kg PO q 24 hours
6. Alternative medical therapies that may be effective include the following:
   - Trimethoprim sulfa 125 mg q 12 hours
   - Doxycycline 5–10 mg/kg q 12 hours

   Oral essential fatty acid supplements may help control pruritus in 20% to 50% of cats. A beneficial effect should occur within 8 to 12 weeks of initiation of therapy. A synergistic effect may be seen when essential fatty acid supplements are administered in combination with other therapies.
7. Other treatments that may be effective in some cats include surgical excision, laser therapy, and radiation therapy; however, adverse effects and wound complications are common.
8. The prognosis is variable, depending on the underlying cause. Cats with underlying allergies that are managed successfully have an excellent prognosis. Cats with recurring lesions for which no underlying cause can be found usually require long-term therapy to keep lesions in remission. These cats have a poorer prognosis as they may become refractory to or may develop unacceptable adverse effects as the result of medical therapy.

Author's Note

Although extremely common, long-acting injectable steroids should be used only as a last resort because life-threatening cardiac effects have been identified in up to 11% of cats, as have other better known medical risks, including diabetes and urinary tract infection.

Indolent Ulcer—*cont'd*

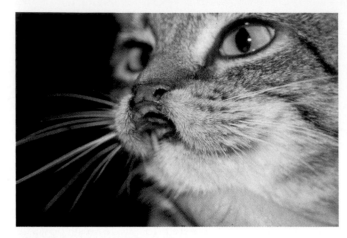

FIGURE 7-121 Indolent Ulcer. Severe tissue destruction of the upper lip caused by a severe ulcerative lesion in a flea-allergic cat.

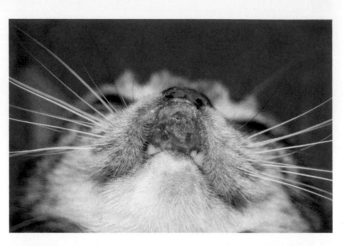

FIGURE 7-122 Indolent Ulcer. Close-up of the cat in Figure 7-121. Severe tissue destruction and ulceration of the upper lip are apparent. The entire upper lip extending to the nasal planum has been destroyed.

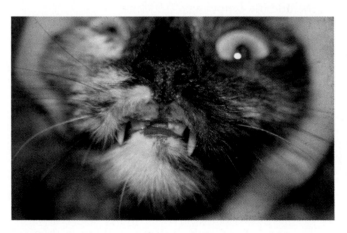

FIGURE 7-123 Indolent Ulcer. Alopecia and ulceration of the upper lip in a cat.

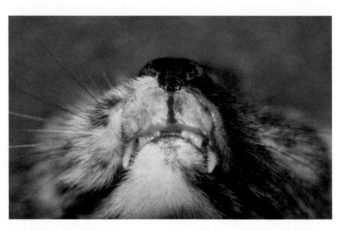

FIGURE 7-124 Indolent Ulcer. Close-up of the cat in Figure 7-123. Tissue destruction and ulceration of the upper lip are apparent.

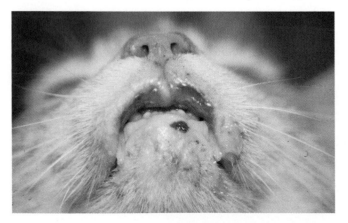

FIGURE 7-125 Indolent Ulcer. The alopecic erythematous lesion with severe tissue swelling and ulceration of the upper lip is characteristic of this disease. The lesions on the chin are atypical of this syndrome and may be more representative of an eosinophilic granuloma.

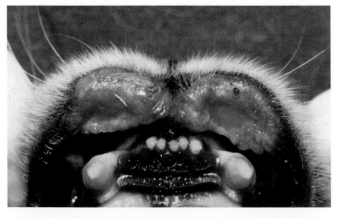

FIGURE 7-126 Indolent Ulcer. Tissue swelling and ulceration of the upper lip are characteristic of indolent ulcers.

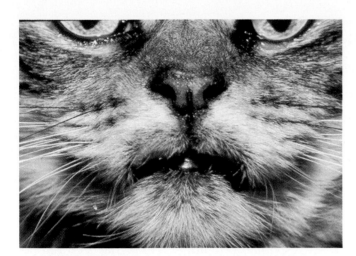

FIGURE 7-127 **Indolent Ulcer.** Same cat as in Figure 7-126. The lesion appears mild with slight alopecia and swelling.

Feline Plasma Cell Pododermatitis

Features

Feline plasma cell pododermatitis is a plasmacytic inflammatory disease of the footpads. Although the exact pathogenesis is unknown, persistent hypergammaglobulinemia, marked plasma cell tissue infiltration, and a beneficial response to glucocorticoid therapy suggest an immune-mediated cause. It is rare in cats.

Feline plasma cell pododermatitis is characterized by asymptomatic swelling of multiple footpads, which become soft and spongy. The metacarpal and metatarsal pads are most commonly affected, but digital pads also may be involved. Swollen footpads may ulcerate and bleed easily, resulting in pain and lameness. Regional lymphadenomegaly may be seen. Occasionally, concurrent plasmacytic dermatitis causes swelling on the bridge of the nose, plasmacytic stomatitis, immune-mediated glomerulonephritis, or renal amyloidosis.

Top Differentials

Differentials include eosinophilic granulomas, bacterial or fungal granulomas, neoplasia, autoimmune disorders, and mosquito bite hypersensitivity.

Diagnosis

1. Rule out other differentials.
2. Cytology (aspirate): numerous plasma cells. Smaller numbers of lymphocytes and neutrophils may be seen.
3. Dermatohistopathology: perivascular to diffuse dermal infiltration with plasma cells and Mott cells (plasma cells containing immunoglobulin that stain bright pink). Variable numbers of neutrophils and lymphocytes may be present.

Treatment and Prognosis

1. Asymptomatic lesions may regress spontaneously without treatment.
2. Any underlying allergies should be identified and managed, especially flea allergy dermatitis treatments. A month-long nitenpyram trial (every other day) may be the only study to prove a link to flea allergy in some patients.
3. Any secondary pyoderma with appropriate therapies for 2 to 4 weeks.
4. For painful or ulcerated lesions, treatment with systemic glucocorticoids is usually effective, although bleeding ulcers may require surgical intervention. Prednisolone 4 mg/kg PO should be administered every 24 hours until lesions resolve, then gradually tapered off. Improvement should be noted within 2 to 3 weeks, and resolution by 10 to 14 weeks. Alternative steroids include the following:
   - Dexamethasone 2 mg PO q 1–3 days to reduce pruritus, then tapered to the lowest possible frequency required
   - Triamcinolone (induction dose) 0.8 mg/kg PO q 24 hours
5. Cyclosporine (Atopica) 5–10 mg/kg PO can be administered every 24 hours until beneficial effects are seen (approximately 4–6 weeks). Then, try to taper down dosage frequency to every 48 to 72 hours. Many cats can be maintained on every 72 hour dosing, making this therapy extremely cost effective. Cats should be FeLV and FIV negative. The risk of toxoplasmosis infection is a matter of concern; however, this risk seems to be very low as of this writing.
6. Doxycycline 5–10 mg/kg PO every 12 hours may be effective. Improvement should be seen within 1 to 2 months. Treatment is continued until the footpads have completely healed. In some cats, doxycycline therapy may have to be continued indefinitely to maintain remission.
7. Bleeding ulcers may require surgical intervention. Wide surgical excision of affected footpads may be curative without concurrent use of medical therapy.
8. The prognosis is good for most cats unless concurrent stomatitis or renal disease is present.

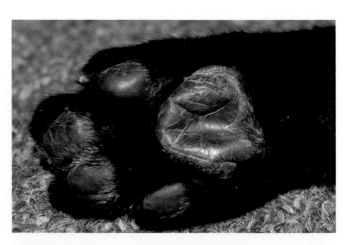

FIGURE 7-128 Plasma Cell Pododermatitis. The central footpad is swollen with a doughy texture when palpated. Mild hyperkeratosis is also present.

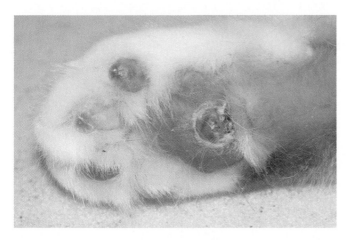

FIGURE 7-129 Plasma Cell Pododermatitis. A focal area of ulceration and crusting caused by the abnormal structure of the central pad is associated with abnormal cellular infiltrate.

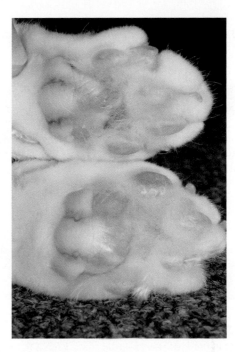

FIGURE 7-130 Plasma Cell Pododermatitis. The footpads of this white cat appear bruised or discolored. The footpads also had a doughy texture when palpated.

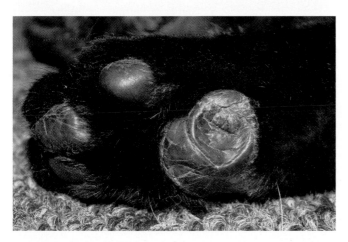

FIGURE 7-131 Plasma Cell Pododermatitis. Hyperkeratosis and swelling of the central footpad. Notice the indentations caused by the abnormal tissue architecture associated with the cellular infiltrate.

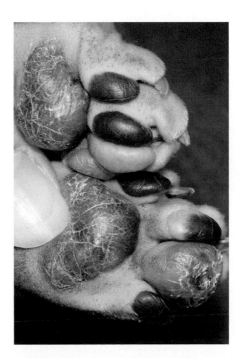

FIGURE 7-132 Plasma Cell Pododermatitis. Severe swelling and hyperkeratosis of the footpads. The severely affected digital footpad is an atypical presentation for this syndrome.

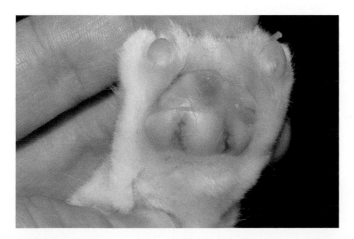

FIGURE 7-133 Plasma Cell Pododermatitis. Soft, mushy footpads are characteristic of this syndrome. Note the bruising of the deep tissue and the more severely affected central pad.

Feline Plasma Cell Pododermatitis—*cont'd*

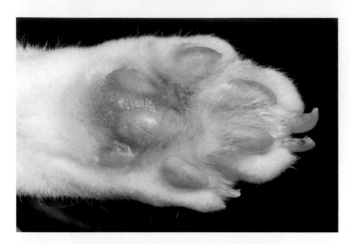

FIGURE 7-134 Plasma Cell Pododermatitis. The central footpad is usually more severely affected.

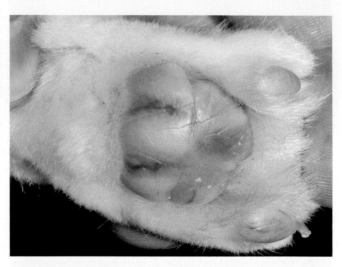

FIGURE 7-135 Plasma Cell Pododermatitis. Deep bruising of the footpads caused by the cellular infiltrate. As the disease progresses, the footpad will become soft and spongy with possible ulceration.

Feline Idiopathic Ulcerative Dermatosis

Features

Feline idiopathic ulcerative dermatosis is an ulcerative skin disease of unknown origin. It is rare in cats.

The lesion is a heavily crusted, nonhealing ulcer that is surrounded by a border of thickened skin. It may be painful and occurs most commonly on the dorsal midline of the caudal neck or between the shoulder blades. A peripheral lymphadenomegaly may be present. No signs of systemic illness are seen.

Top Differentials

Differentials include injection reaction; foreign body reaction; trauma; burn; bacterial, fungal, or viral infection; *Demodex gatoi*; hypersensitivity (flea, food, atopy); and neoplasia.

Diagnosis

1. Rule out other differentials.
2. Dermatohistopathology: extensive epidermal ulceration and superficial dermal necrosis with minimal to mild dermal inflammation. Chronic lesions may also have a subepidermal band of dermal fibrosis extending peripherally from the ulcer.

Treatment and Prognosis

1. Find and treat any underlying diseases (flea hypersensitivity, food allergy, ectoparasitism). A lime sulfur trial should be considered because some mites (*D gatoi*) are difficult to find.
2. For painful or ulcerated lesions, treatment with systemic glucocorticoids may be effective. Prednisolone 4 mg/kg PO should be administered every 24 hours until lesions resolve, then gradually tapered off. Improvement should be noted within 2 to 3 weeks, and resolution by 10 to 14 weeks. Alternative steroids include the following:
   - Dexamethasone 2 mg PO q 1–3 days to reduce pruritus, then tapered to the lowest possible frequency required
   - Triamcinolone (induction dose) 0.8 mg/kg PO q 24 hours
3. For severe, refractory lesions that fail to respond and have no identifiable underlying disease, wide surgical excision should be attempted but may be unsuccessful.
4. A restraint device may be needed to prevent the cat from mutilating the affected area.
5. The prognosis is guarded to poor because lesions often are refractory to medical therapy and too extensive to be surgically excised.

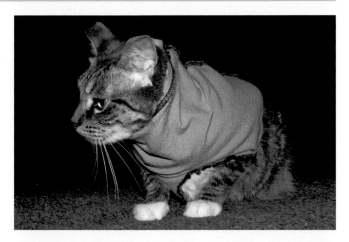

FIGURE 7-136 Feline Idiopathic Ulcerative Dermatosis. This cat required a bandage to prevent aggressive self-mutilation of the dorsal cervical area.

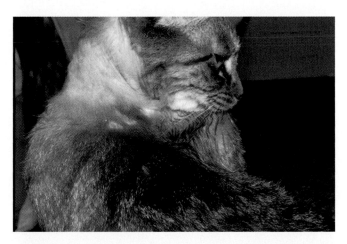

FIGURE 7-137 Feline Idiopathic Ulcerative Dermatosis. Same cat as in Figure 7-136. As soon as the bandage was removed, the cat began tearing at the cervical skin.

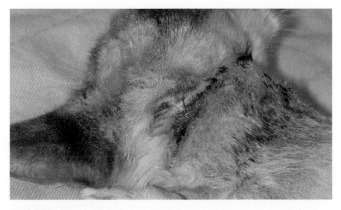

FIGURE 7-138 Feline Idiopathic Ulcerative Dermatosis. Severe dermatitis on the dorsal cervical region. The linear ulcer persisted because of the cat's self-mutilation.

Feline Idiopathic Ulcerative Dermatosis—*cont'd*

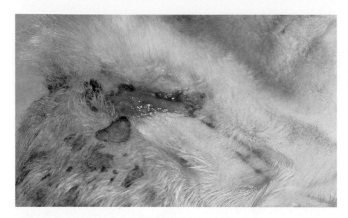

FIGURE 7-139 Feline Idiopathic Ulcerative Dermatosis. Same cat as in Figure 7-138. The ulcerative lesion and linear excoriations are apparent.

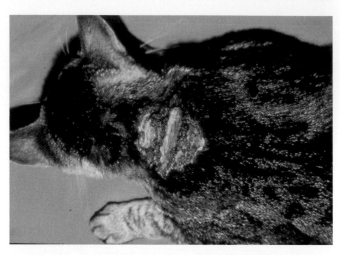

FIGURE 7-140 Feline Idiopathic Ulcerative Dermatosis. A large ulcer on the dorsal cervical region of an adult cat. *(Courtesy D. Angarano.)*

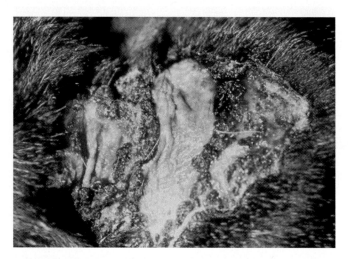

FIGURE 7-141 Feline Idiopathic Ulcerative Dermatosis. Close-up of the cat in Figure 7-140. Deep ulceration. *(Courtesy D. Angarano.)*

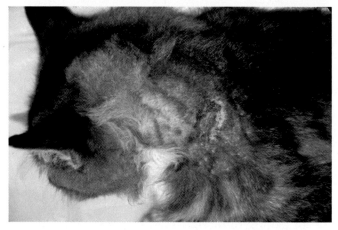

FIGURE 7-142 Feline Idiopathic Ulcerative Dermatosis. A focal area of ulcerative dermatitis caused by the cat's self-mutilation behavior. This lesion was thought to be associated with an underlying feline immunodeficiency virus (FIV) infection.

Urticaria and Angioedema (hives)

Features

Urticaria and angioedema manifests as a cutaneous hypersensitivity reaction to immunologic and nonimmunologic stimuli such as drugs, vaccines, bacterins, food or food additives, stinging or biting insects, and plants. It is uncommon in dogs and rare in cats.

It begins as an acute onset of variably pruritic wheals (urticaria) or large, edematous swellings (angioedema). Urticarial lesions may resolve and appear elsewhere on the body. Angioedema is usually localized, especially to the head, whereas urticaria may be localized or generalized. Affected skin is often erythematous, but hair loss does not occur. Dyspnea from pharyngeal, nasal, or laryngeal angioedema may be present. Rarely, anaphylactic shock with hypotension, collapse, gastrointestinal signs, or death may result.

Top Differentials

Urticaria

Differentials include folliculitis (caused by bacteria, dermatophyte, *Demodex*), vasculitis, erythema multiforme, and neoplasia (lymphoreticular, mast cell).

Angioedema

Differentials include juvenile cellulitis, bacterial or fungal cellulitis, neoplasia, and snake bite.

Diagnosis

1. History and clinical findings.
2. Diascopy: a glass slide is pressed onto the erythematous lesion. If the lesion blanches (turns white), the lesion is caused by vasodilatation (urticaria). If the lesion remains red, the lesion is the result of petechiae or ecchymosis (vasculitis, tick-borne disease).
3. Dermatohistopathology: vascular dilatation and edema in superficial and middle dermis, or superficial perivascular to interstitial dermatitis with varying numbers of mononuclear cells, neutrophils, mast cells, and, rarely, eosinophils.

Treatment and Prognosis

1. A single treatment with prednisone or prednisolone 2 mg/kg PO, IM, or IV is usually effective. Alternatively, dexamethasone sodium phosphate 0.5–1 mg/kg IM.
2. Concurrent administration of diphenhydramine 2–4 mg/kg PO or IM every 8 hours for 2 to 3 days may also be helpful.
3. If angioedema is severe enough to interfere with breathing, a rapid-acting steroid such as dexamethasone sodium phosphate (1–2 mg/kg IV) or prednisolone sodium succinate (100–500 mg/dog IV) should be administered once. For life-threatening anaphylaxis, one should administer 1:10,000 epinephrine 0.5 to 1.0 mL IV once (if reaction is severe), or 0.2 to 0.5 mL SC once (if reaction is mild to moderate).
4. The suspected cause should be identified and future exposure avoided. Insects, drugs (especially vaccines), and food allergens are most likely to cause recurrent urticaria.
5. Long-term antihistamine therapy may help prevent or control chronic urticaria of unknown cause.
6. The prognosis is good for animals that do not develop anaphylactic shock.

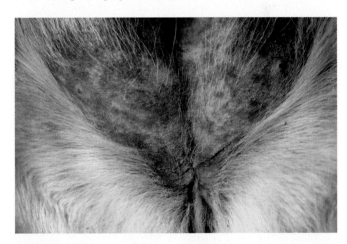

FIGURE 7-143 Urticaria and Angioedema. These intensely erythematous macules were caused by an acute urticarial reaction likely associated with food allergy.

Urticaria and Angioedema—*cont'd*

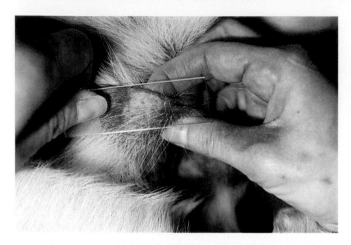

FIGURE 7-144 Urticaria and Angioedema. Diascopy being performed on the dog in Figure 7-143. Blanching indicates vasodilatation (urticaria) rather than ecchymotic hemorrhage (vasculitis).

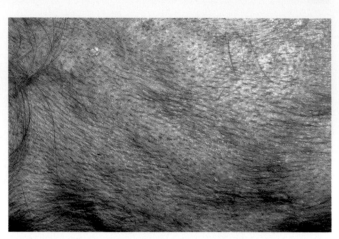

FIGURE 7-145 Urticaria and Angioedema. This erythematous lesion was caused by a large area of urticaria that coalesced to form an edematous plaque. Note that the erythematous raised lesions are well demarcated from adjacent normal skin.

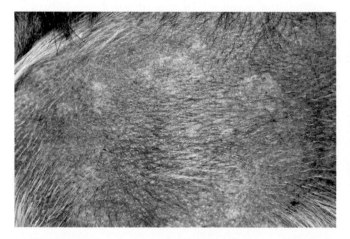

FIGURE 7-146 Urticaria and Angioedema. Intense erythema associated with an acute allergic reaction.

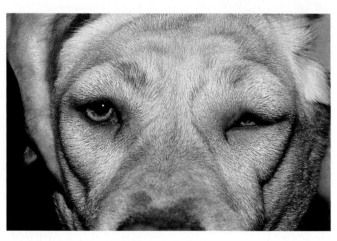

FIGURE 7-147 Urticaria and Angioedema. Severe swelling of the face and periocular tissue developed after a venomous insect sting.

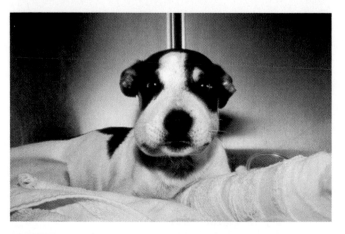

FIGURE 7-148 Urticaria and Angioedema. Swelling on the muzzle resembling angioedema caused by a snakebite.

Author's Note

Recurrent cases should be evaluated for allergic disease and maintained on a hypoallergenic diet and therapy used for allergic disease.

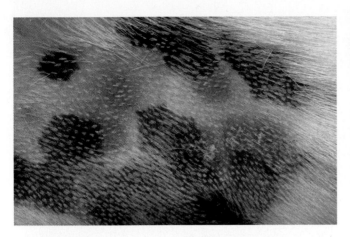

FIGURE 7-149 Urticaria and Angioedema. Focal erythematous lesions typical of urticaria on the abdomen of a dog.

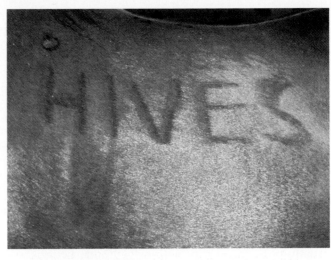

FIGURE 7-150 Urticaria and Angioedema. Dermatographism in a horse (too cool to resist). *(Courtesy of S. Sargent).*

Canine Eosinophilic Furunculosis of the Face

Features

Canine eosinophilic furunculosis of the face is an acute, usually self-limiting disease of the face. Although its exact pathogenesis is not known, a hypersensitivity reaction to insect stings or spider bites is suspected. It is uncommon to rare in dogs, with the highest incidence in inquisitive, young adult, medium-sized and large dogs with ready access to the outdoors.

Blisters, erythematous papules and nodules, ulceration, crusts, and hemorrhage may develop acutely and usually peak in severity within 24 hours. Lesions are minimally pruritic to nonpruritic but may be painful and typically involve the muzzle, bridge of the nose, and periocular areas. Occasionally, the ventral abdomen, chest, or ear pinnae may be involved.

Top Differentials

Differentials include nasal pyoderma, dermatophytosis, demodicosis, and autoimmune skin diseases.

Diagnosis

1. History, clinical findings, and rule out other differentials.
2. Cytology (blister, pustule, exudates): numerous eosinophils are seen. Neutrophils and bacteria also may be seen if lesions are secondarily infected.
3. Dermatohistopathology: eosinophilic perifolliculitis, folliculitis, and furunculosis. Infiltration with neutrophils, lymphocytes, and macrophages, along with areas of dermal hemorrhage and collagen degeneration, is common.

Treatment and Prognosis

1. Any secondary pyoderma should be treated with appropriate systemic antibiotics for 3 to 4 weeks.
2. Prednisone 1–2 mg/kg PO should be administered every 24 hours, until lesions are markedly improved (approximately 7–10 days); then, 1–2 mg/kg PO should be administered every 48 hours for 10 more days.
3. Hot packs and hydrotherapy may speed clinical improvement.
4. The prognosis is good. Without glucocorticoid treatment, spontaneous recovery usually occurs within 3 weeks, but systemic prednisone hastens resolution of the lesions.

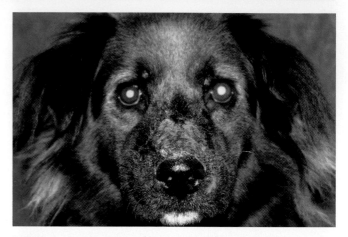

FIGURE 7-151 Canine Eosinophilic Furunculosis of the Face. Alopecic, erythematous, erosive dermatitis with a moist exudate is typical of eosinophilic furunculosis.

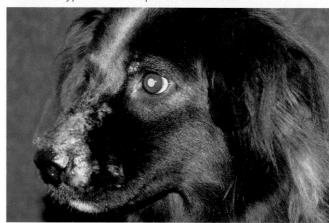

FIGURE 7-152 Canine Eosinophilic Furunculosis of the Face. Same dog as in Figure 7-151. Moist, erosive dermatitis on the muzzle is apparent. Note that the nasal planum is usually spared, thereby differentiating this disease from autoimmune skin disease.

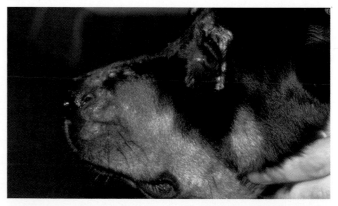

FIGURE 7-153 Canine Eosinophilic Furunculosis of the Face. Alopecia, erythema, and papules on the muzzle and around the eye caused by venomous insect stings.

Contact Dermatitis (allergic contact dermatitis)

Features

Contact dermatitis is a reaction that usually requires prolonged contact with the offending allergen. Contact hypersensitivity to plants, carpet deodorizers, detergents, floor waxes, fabric cleaners, fertilizers, mulch, concrete, plastic dishes, rubber chew toys, leather/rawhide, and wool or synthetic carpets and rugs may develop. It is uncommon to rare in dogs and cats.

Mildly to intensely pruritic skin lesions include erythema, macules, papules, alopecia, plaques, vesicles, excoriations, hyperpigmentation, lichenification, and crusts. Secondary pyoderma and *Malassezia* dermatitis may be present. Thinly haired skin that frequently contacts the ground (interdigital areas, axillae, groin, scrotum, pressure points, perineum, chin, ear flaps) is usually affected, but haired skin can be involved if the offending allergen is a liquid. The lips and muzzle are typically affected if the offending allergen is rawhide, a rubber chew toy, or a plastic dish.

Top Differentials

Differentials include parasites (canine scabies, demodicosis, *Pelodera*, hookworm dermatitis), atopy, food hypersensitivity, pyoderma, dermatophytosis, and *Malassezia* dermatitis.

Diagnosis

1. Rule out other differentials.
2. Dermatohistopathology (nondiagnostic): varying degrees of superficial perivascular dermatitis. Mononuclear cells or neutrophils may predominate. Evidence of pyoderma or seborrhea may also be present.

3. Patch testing: patch testing is very difficult and extremely variable in veterinary species. A skin reaction (erythema, swelling, macules, or papules) develops 48 to 72 hours after the suspect allergen is applied to a shaved skin site. False-negative and false-positive reactions can occur.
4. Avoidance/provocative exposure: removing the animal from its environment and hospitalizing it in a stainless steel cage for 3 to 5 days results in significant clinical improvement. Symptoms recur shortly after reintroduction into the regular environment.

Treatment and Prognosis

1. The animal should be bathed with a hypoallergenic shampoo to remove surface contact allergens.
2. Any secondary pyoderma or *Malassezia* dermatitis should be treated with appropriate therapies.
3. The offending allergen should be identified, and contact with it should be avoided.
4. If the allergen cannot be identified or avoided, the use of mechanical barriers such as socks or a T-shirt may be effective.
5. For short-term control of pruritus, a glucocorticoid-containing topical preparation should be applied to

Author's Note

Contact dermatitis is very rare and is overdiagnosed. Dogs and cats have fur coats that protect the skin from contact reactions much better than is possible in humans; however, many owners are aware of the concept of contact allergens and may jump to this diagnosis prematurely.

Most patients diagnosed with contact dermatitis actually have atopy, food allergy, or scabies with secondary infection, including pyoderma and Malassezia dermatitis.

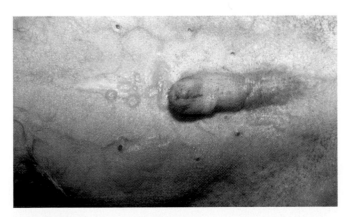

FIGURE 7-154 Contact Dermatitis. Acute urticarial reaction on the abdomen of a Dachshund after application of an iodine surgical scrub.

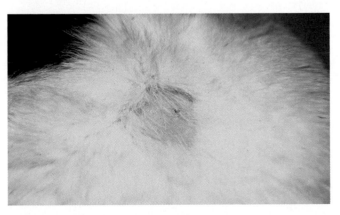

FIGURE 7-155 Contact Dermatitis. Focal area of alopecia caused by application of a spot-on flea control product.

Contact Dermatitis—*cont'd*

affected areas every 12 hours, or prednisone 1 mg/kg (dogs) or 2 mg/kg (cats) PO should be administered every 24 hours for 5 to 10 days.

6. For long-term control (if allergen cannot be identified or avoided), therapy as described for canine and feline atopy may be beneficial.

7. Alternatively, long-term treatment with pentoxifylline (dogs) 10–25 mg/kg PO every 12 hours may be effective in controlling pruritus.

8. The prognosis is good if the offending allergen is identified and avoided. The prognosis is poor if the allergen cannot be identified or avoided.

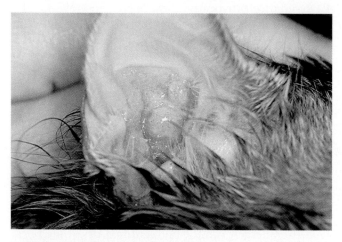

FIGURE 7-156 Contact Dermatitis. Focal erythema and edema caused by topical otic medication.

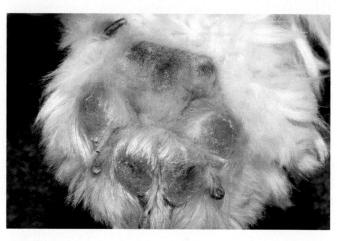

FIGURE 7-158 Contact Dermatitis. Hyperkeratosis, depigmentation, and swelling of the footpad caused by contact with a caustic substance.

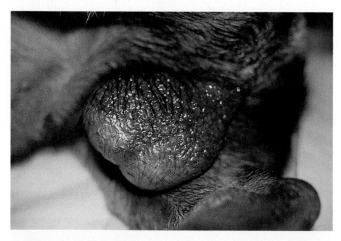

FIGURE 7-157 Contact Dermatitis. Severe erosive dermatitis on the scrotum of a dog.

CHAPTER 8

Autoimmune and Immune-Mediated Skin Disorders

- Pemphigus Foliaceus
- Pemphigus Erythematosus
- Pemphigus Vulgaris
- Bullous Pemphigoid
- Discoid Lupus Erythematosus (DLE)
- Systemic Lupus Erythematosus (SLE)
- Canine Subcorneal Pustular Dermatosis
- Sterile Eosinophilic Pustulosis
- Sterile Nodular Panniculitis

- Idiopathic Sterile Granuloma and Pyogranuloma
- Canine Eosinophilic Granuloma
- Cutaneous Vasculitis
- Erythema Multiforme (EM) and Toxic Epidermal Necrolysis (TEN)
- Cutaneous Drug Reaction (drug eruption)
- Injection Reaction and Post–Rabies Vaccination Alopecias

Pemphigus Foliaceus

Features

Pemphigus foliaceus is an autoimmune skin disease that is characterized by the production of autoantibodies against a component of the adhesion molecules on keratinocytes. The deposition of antibody in intercellular spaces causes the cells to detach from each other within the uppermost epidermal layers (acantholysis). Pemphigus foliaceus is probably the most common autoimmune skin disease in dogs and cats. Any age, sex, or breed can be affected, but among dogs, Akitas and Chow Chows may be predisposed. Pemphigus foliaceus is usually idiopathic, but some cases may be drug induced, or it may occur as a sequela to a chronic inflammatory skin disease.

The primary lesions are superficial pustules. However, intact pustules are often difficult to find because they are obscured by the hair coat, are fragile, and rupture easily. Secondary lesions include superficial erosions, crusts, scales, epidermal collarettes, and alopecia. Lesions on the nasal planum, ear pinnae, and footpads are unique and characteristic of autoimmune skin disease. The disease often begins on the bridge of the nose, around the eyes, and on the ear pinnae, before it becomes generalized. Nasal depigmentation frequently accompanies facial lesions. Skin lesions are variably pruritic and may wax and wane. Footpad hyperkeratosis

Author's Note

The most efficient way to confirm an autoimmune skin disease is through biopsy; however, using a dermatopathologist will greatly increase the usefulness of reported results. Unfortunately, there is a paucity of dermatohistopathologists; currently vin.com and itchnot.com provide the most current listings.

Historically, steroid therapy has been the mainstay of treatment for these diseases. We are beginning to realize the usefulness of nonsteroid alternatives (Table 8-1) in many cases, with mild cases often not requiring any steroid therapy.

The goal of therapy is to control 90% of the symptoms 90% of the time while minimizing the adverse effects of treatments. Normally, flare-ups will occur, and it is important to differentiate infection (especially pyoderma and demodicosis) from an actual disease flare.

Pemphigus Foliaceus—*cont'd*

is common and may be the only symptom in some dogs and cats. Oral lesions are rare. Mucocutaneous involvement is usually minimal in dogs. In cats, lesions around the nail beds and nipples are a unique and common feature of pemphigus. With generalized skin disease, concurrent lymphadenomegaly, limb edema, fever, anorexia, and depression may be present.

Top Differentials

Differentials include demodicosis, superficial pyoderma, dermatophytosis, other autoimmune skin diseases, subcorneal pustular dermatosis, eosinophilic pustulosis, drug eruption, dermatomyositis, zinc-responsive dermatosis, cutaneous epitheliotropic lym-

TABLE 8-1 Immunosuppressive Therapies for Autoimmune and Immune-Mediated Skin Disease

Drug—Species	Induction Dosage	Maintenance Dosage
Topical Therapy		
Steroids (hydrocortisone, dexamethasone, triamcinolone, fluocinolone, betamethasone, mometasone, etc.)	Applied every 12 hours	Taper to lowest effective dose
Tacrolimus	Applied every 12 hours	Taper to lowest effective dose
Conservative Oral Treatments With Very Few Adverse Effects		
Essential fatty acids—dogs and cats		180 mg EPA/10 lb PO daily
Vitamin E		400 IU PO daily
Tetracycline and niacinamide—dogs	Dogs >10 kg—500 mg of each drug PO q 8 hours Dogs <10 kg—250 mg of each drug PO q 8 hours	Dogs >10 kg—500 mg of each drug PO q 12–24 hours Dogs >10 kg—250 mg of each drug PO q 12–24 hours
Doxycycline may be substituted for tetracycline	5–10 mg/kg q 12 hours	Then, taper to lowest effective dose
Cyclosporine (Atopica)—dogs and cats	5–12.5 mg/kg PO q 12–24 hours	After remission is achieved, taper slowly to lowest effective dose
Reliably Effective Treatments But Adverse Effects Are Common and May Be Severe		
Prednisone—dogs	1–3 mg/kg PO q 12–24 hours	0.5–2 mg/kg PO q 48 hours
Prednisolone—cats	2–2.5 mg/kg PO q 12–24 hours	2.5–5 mg/kg PO q 2–7 days
Methylprednisolone—dogs	0.8–1.4 mg/kg PO q 12–24 hours	0.4–0.8 mg/kg PO q 48 hours
Triamcinolone—dogs	0.1–0.3 mg/kg PO q 12–24 hours	0.1–0.2 mg/kg PO q 48–72 hours
Triamcinolone—cats	0.3–1 mg/kg PO q 12–24 hours	0.6–1 mg/kg PO q 2–7 days
Dexamethasone—dogs and cats	0.1–0.2 mg/kg PO q 12–24 hours	0.05–0.1 mg/kg PO q 48–72 hours
Azathioprine—dogs	1.5–2.5 mg/kg PO q 24–48 hours	1.5–2.5 mg/kg PO q 48–72 hours
Chlorambucil—dogs and cats	0.1–0.2 mg/kg PO q 24 hours	0.1–0.2 mg/kg PO q 48 hours
Dapsone—dogs only	1 mg/kg PO q 8 hours	Taper to lowest effective dose
Aggressive Treatments With Few Studies Documenting Efficacy and Safety		
Methylprednisolone sodium succinate (pulse therapy)—dogs and cats	1 mg/kg IV over a 3- to 4-hour period q 24 hours for 2–3 consecutive days	Alternate-day oral glucocorticosteroid
Dexamethasone (pulse therapy)—dogs and cats	1 mg/kg IV once or twice 24 hours apart	Alternate-day oral glucocorticosteroid
Cyclophosphamide—dogs and cats	50 mg/m^2 (or 1.5 mg/kg) PO q 48 hours	25–50 mg/m^2 (or 0.75–1.5 mg/kg) PO q 48 hours
Mycophenolate mofetil	10–20 mg/kg q 8–12 hours	Then, taper to lowest effective dose
Leflunomide	2 mg/kg q 12 hours	Then, taper to lowest effective dose

phoma, hepatocutaneous syndrome, and mosquito bite hypersensitivity (cats).

Diagnosis

1. Rule out other differentials.
2. Cytology (pustule): neutrophils and acantholytic cells are seen. Eosinophils may also be present.
3. Antinuclear antibodies (ANA): negative, but false-positives are common.
4. Dermatohistopathology: subcorneal pustules containing neutrophils and acantholytic cells, with variable numbers of eosinophils.
5. Immunofluorescence or immunohistochemistry (skin biopsy specimens): detection of intercellular antibody deposition is suggestive, but false-positive and false-negative results are common. Positive results should be confirmed histologically.
6. Bacterial culture (pustule): usually sterile, but occasionally bacteria are isolated if secondary infections are present.

Treatment and Prognosis

1. Symptomatic shampoo therapy to remove crusts may be helpful.
2. To treat or prevent secondary pyoderma in dogs, appropriate long-term systemic antibiotics should be administered (minimum 4 weeks). Dogs treated with antibiotics during the induction phase of immunosuppressive therapy have significantly higher survival rates than do dogs treated with immunosuppressive drugs alone. Antibiotics should be continued until concurrent immunosuppressive therapy has the pemphigus under control.
3. The goal of treatment is to control the disease and its symptoms with the safest treatments used at the lowest possible doses. Typically, combinations of therapies (see Table 8-1) will have to be used to provide a multimodal treatment plan, minimizing the adverse effects of any one therapy. Depending on the severity of the disease, more or less aggressive treatments will have to be selected. To push the disease into remission, higher doses are used initially and then are tapered over 2 to 3 months to the lowest effective dose.
   a. **Topical therapy** applied every 12 hours with steroid-containing products or tacrolimus will help reduce focal inflammation and will lower the doses of systemic treatments required to control the symptoms. Once in remission, the frequency of application should be minimized to reduce local adverse effects.
   b. **Conservative systemic treatments** (see Table 8-1) include drugs that help reduce the inflammation with few to no adverse effects. These treatments help reduce the need for more aggressive therapy such as steroids or chemotherapeutics.
   c. **Steroid therapy** is one of the most reliably predictable treatments for autoimmune skin disease; however, adverse effects associated with the high doses needed to control symptoms may be severe. Although glucocorticoid therapy alone may be effective in maintaining remission, the dosages needed may result in undesirable adverse effects, especially in dogs. **For this reason, the use of nonsteroidal immunosuppressive drugs, alone or in combination with glucocorticoids, is usually recommended for long-term maintenance.**
      - Immunosuppressive doses of oral prednisone or methylprednisolone should be administered daily (see Table 8-1). After lesions resolve (after approximately 2–8 weeks), the dosage should be gradually tapered over a period of several (8–10) weeks until the lowest possible alternate-day dosage that maintains remission is being administered. If no significant improvement is seen within 2 to 4 weeks of initiation of therapy, a concurrent skin infection should be ruled out, then alternative or additional immunosuppressive medications considered.
      - Alternative steroids for prednisone- and methylprednisolone-refractory cases include triamcinolone and dexamethasone (see Table 8-1).
      - In cats, treatment with immunosuppressive doses of triamcinolone or dexamethasone is often more effective than therapy with prednisolone or methylprednisolone. Oral triamcinolone or dexamethasone should be administered daily until remission is achieved (approximately 2–8 weeks), then the dosage should be gradually tapered until the lowest possible and least frequent dosage that maintains remission is being administered (see Table 8-1).
      - If unacceptable adverse effects develop, or if no significant improvement is seen within 2 to 4 weeks of initiation of therapy, consider using an alternate glucocorticosteroid or a nonsteroidal immunosuppressive drug (see Table 8-1).
   d. **Nonsteroidal immunosuppressive drugs** that may be effective include cyclosporine (Atopica), azathioprine (dogs only), chlorambucil, cyclophosphamide, mycophenolate mofetil, and leflunomide (see Table 8-1). A beneficial response occurs within 8 to 12 weeks of initiation of therapy. Once remission is achieved, gradually attempt to taper the dosage and frequency of the nonsteroidal immunosuppressive drug for long-term maintenance.

Pemphigus Foliaceus—cont'd

4. The prognosis is fair to good. Although some animals remain in remission after immunosuppressive therapy is tapered and discontinued, most animals require lifelong therapy to maintain remission. Regular monitoring of clinical signs, hemograms, and serum biochemistry panels with treatment adjustments as needed is essential. Potential complications of immunosuppressive therapy include unacceptable drug adverse effects and immunosuppression-induced bacterial infection, dermatophytosis, or demodicosis.

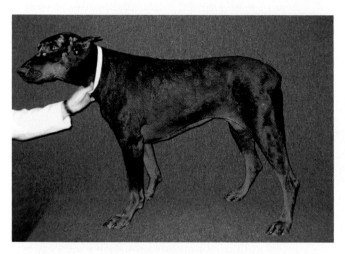

FIGURE 8-1 **Pemphigus Foliaceus.** An adult Doberman with pemphigus foliaceus. Note the diffuse pattern of lesions.

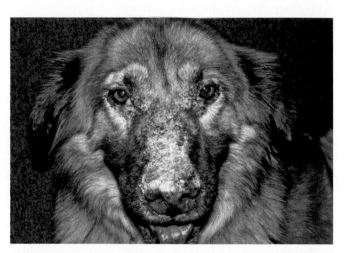

FIGURE 8-3 **Pemphigus Foliaceus.** Alopecic, crusting, papular dermatitis on the face. Lesions on the nasal planum and ear pinnae are characteristic of autoimmune skin disease.

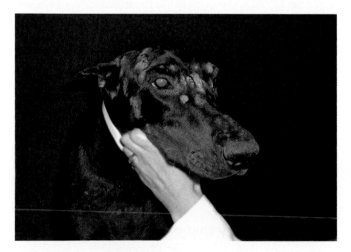

FIGURE 8-2 **Pemphigus Foliaceus.** Same dog as in Figure 8-1. Alopecic, crusting, papular lesions on the face are apparent. Note the similarity of lesions to folliculitis; however, the pattern of distribution is unique.

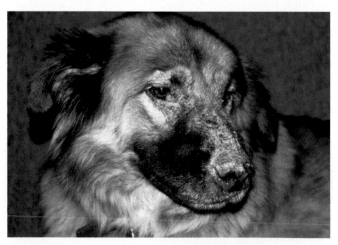

FIGURE 8-4 **Pemphigus Foliaceus.** Same dog as in Figure 8-3. Alopecic, crusting, papular dermatitis on the face and nasal planum is characteristic of autoimmune skin disease. Note the similarity to folliculitis lesions; however, no follicles are present on the nasal planum, making these lesions a unique feature.

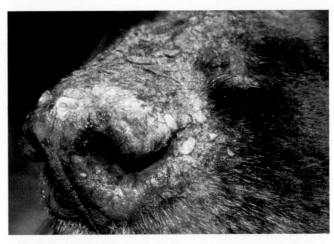

FIGURE 8-5 Pemphigus Foliaceus. Crusting erosive dermatitis on the nasal planum with depigmentation and loss of the normal cobblestone texture is a unique feature of autoimmune skin disease.

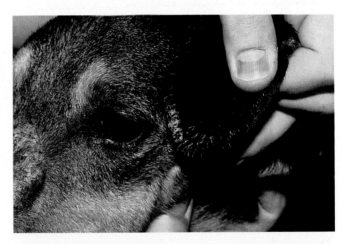

FIGURE 8-6 Pemphigus Foliaceus. Same dog as in Figure 8-5. Lesions on the nasal planum are characteristic of autoimmune skin disease.

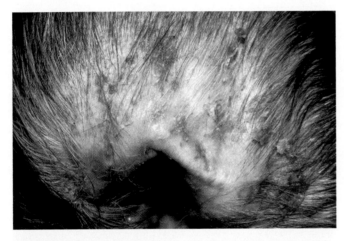

FIGURE 8-7 Pemphigus Foliaceus. Crusting papular dermatitis on the ear pinna of a dog with pemphigus foliaceus. Lesions on the nasal planum, ear pinnae, and footpads are characteristic of autoimmune skin disease.

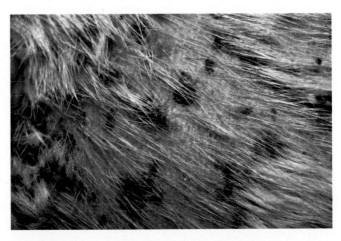

FIGURE 8-8 Pemphigus Foliaceus. Alopecic, crusting dermatitis on the ear margin of a Doberman with pemphigus foliaceus. Note the similarity to scabies; however, this dog was not intensely pruritic.

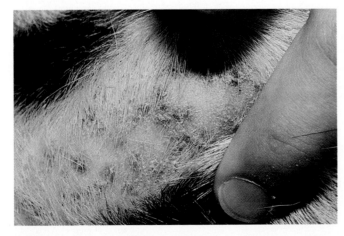

FIGURE 8-9 Pemphigus Foliaceus. Alopecic, crusting, papular, dermatitis that covered the entire cutaneous surface area of this Dalmatian. Note the similarity to folliculitis.

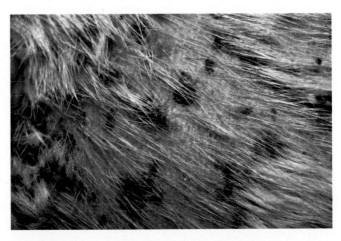

FIGURE 8-10 Pemphigus Foliaceus. Alopecia with a crusting papular rash on the trunk.

Pemphigus Foliaceus—*cont'd*

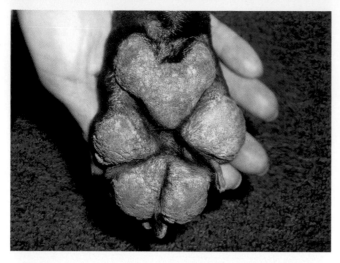

FIGURE 8-11 Pemphigus Foliaceus. Hyperkeratosis and crusting of the footpads are characteristic of autoimmune skin disease. Note that the lesions are on the actual pad rather than on the interdigital surface, which would be typical of allergic dermatitis or bacterial or yeast pododermatitis.

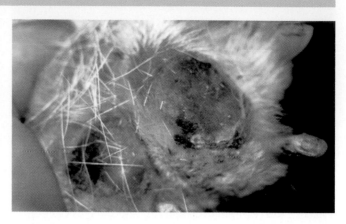

FIGURE 8-12 Pemphigus Foliaceus. Hyperkeratosis and crusting of the footpads.

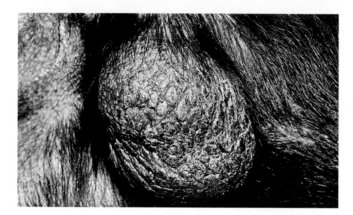

FIGURE 8-13 Pemphigus Foliaceus. Hyperkeratosis and crusting of the scrotum of a dog with pemphigus foliaceus.

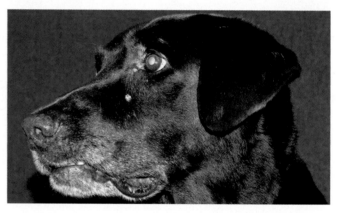

FIGURE 8-14 Pemphigus Foliaceus. Depigmentation of the nasal planum with loss of the normal cobblestone texture is an early change associated with autoimmune skin disease.

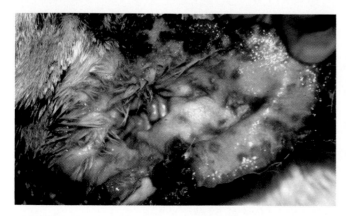

FIGURE 8-15 Pemphigus Foliaceus. Severe moist dermatitis is a rare feature of pemphigus foliaceus.

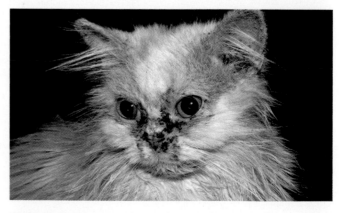

FIGURE 8-16 Pemphigus Foliaceus. Facial dermatitis (alopecic, crusting, papular rash) in a cat. Note the similarity to facial dermatitis of Persian cats.

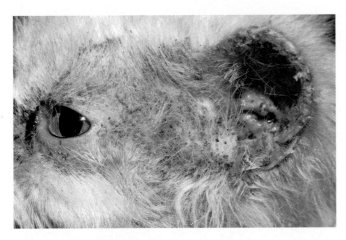

FIGURE 8-17 **Pemphigus Foliaceus.** Close-up of the cat in Figure 8-16. The alopecic, crusting, papular dermatitis on the face and ear pinna is characteristic of autoimmune skin disease.

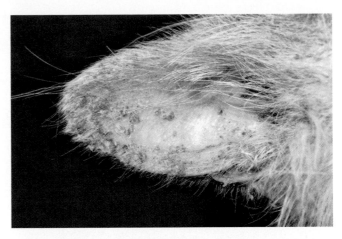

FIGURE 8-18 **Pemphigus Foliaceus.** Same cat as in Figure 8-16. The crusting papular rash on the ear pinna is a unique feature of autoimmune skin disease.

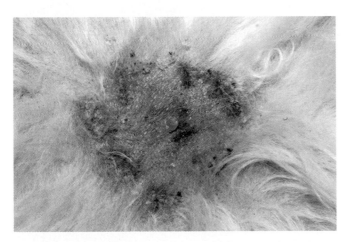

FIGURE 8-19 **Pemphigus Foliaceus.** Same cat as in Figure 8-16. Alopecic, crusting, erosive dermatitis around the nipples is a common and unique feature of pemphigus foliaceus in cats.

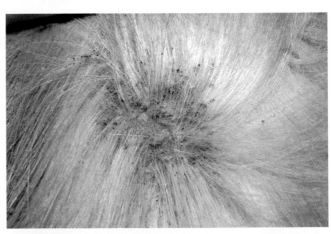

FIGURE 8-20 **Pemphigus Foliaceus.** Papular crusting dermatitis. Note the similarity with dermatophytosis, ectoparasitism, and other allergic causes.

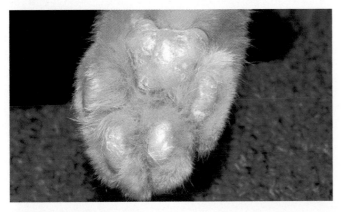

FIGURE 8-21 **Pemphigus Foliaceus.** Hyperkeratosis and crusting on the footpads are common features of autoimmune skin disease.

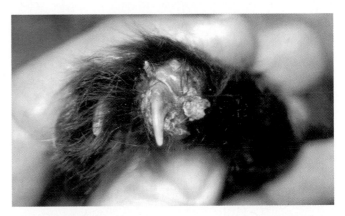

FIGURE 8-22 **Pemphigus Foliaceus.** Crusting dermatitis of the nail beds (paronychia) is a common and unique feature of pemphigus foliaceus in cats.

Pemphigus Foliaceus—*cont'd*

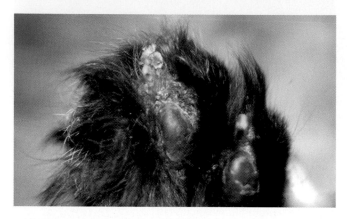

FIGURE 8-23 **Pemphigus Foliaceus.** Paronychia and hyper-keratosis of the footpads in a cat with pemphigus foliaceus.

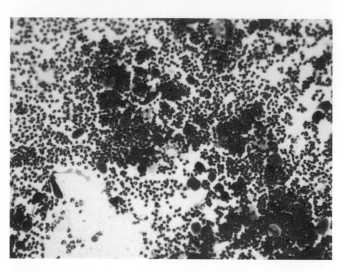

FIGURE 8-24 **Pemphigus Foliaceus.** Microscopic image of acantholytic cells and numerous neutrophils as viewed with a 10× objective.

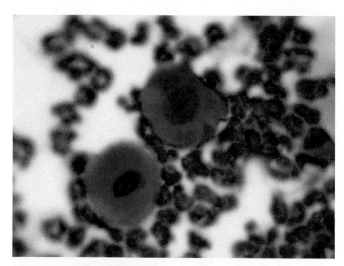

FIGURE 8-25 **Pemphigus Foliaceus.** Microscopic image of acantholytic cells as viewed with a 100× (oil) objective.

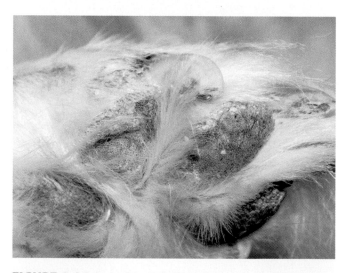

FIGURE 8-26 **Pemphigus Foliaceus.** Severe crusting on the footpads of an affected dog.

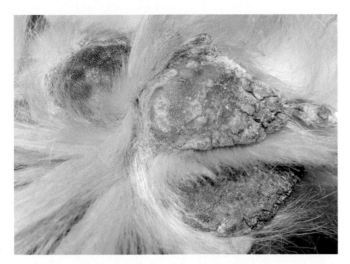

FIGURE 8-27 Pemphigus Foliaceus. Severe crusting of the footpads developed over several weeks in a middle-aged dog.

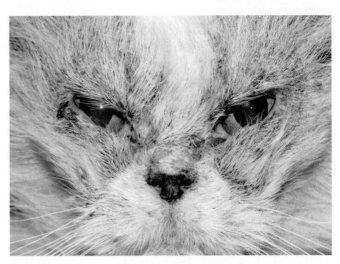

FIGURE 8-28 Pemphigus Foliaceus. Severe facial crusting with alopecia in a cat. The nasal planum is affected but not to the extent that a dog's nasal planum typically is affected.

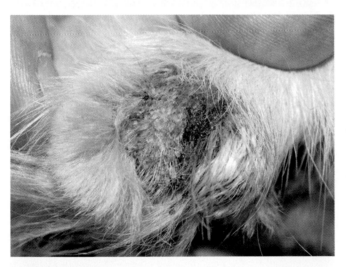

FIGURE 8-29 Pemphigus Foliaceus. Severe paronychia, exudative dermatitis with crusting, is a common feature of pemphigus in cats.

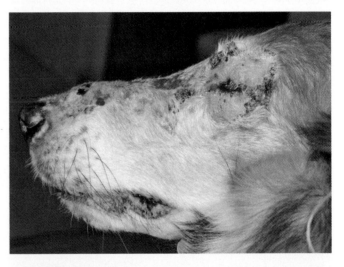

FIGURE 8-30 Pemphigus Foliaceus. Severe erosive dermatitis with crusting alopecia on the face of an affected dog. The lesions on the nasal planum, around the eyes, and on the lips are typical of pemphigus.

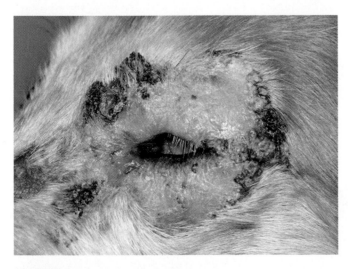

FIGURE 8-31 Pemphigus Foliaceus. Close-up of the dog as in Figure 8-30. Alopecia with crusting around the eye is apparent.

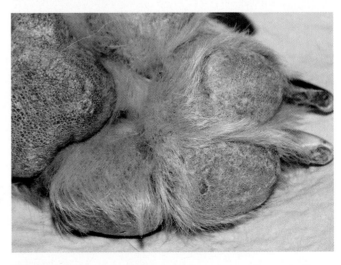

FIGURE 8-32 Pemphigus Foliaceus. Same dog as in Figure 8-30. Crusting of the footpads is a characteristic feature of most autoimmune skin diseases.

Pemphigus Foliaceus—*cont'd*

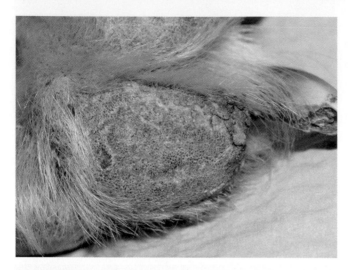

FIGURE 8-33 **Pemphigus Foliaceus.** Close-up of the footpad demonstrating the thickened keratin and crusting of the pad, especially at the margin.

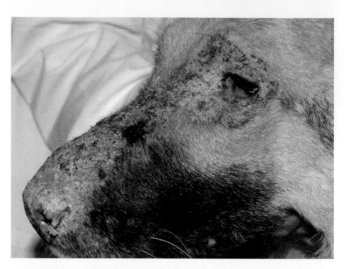

FIGURE 8-34 **Pemphigus Foliaceus.** Severe erosive, crusting, alopecic dermatitis on the face of a dog with pemphigus. Depigmentation, loss of normal cobblestone texture, erosion, and crusting on the nasal planum are characteristic of autoimmune skin disease.

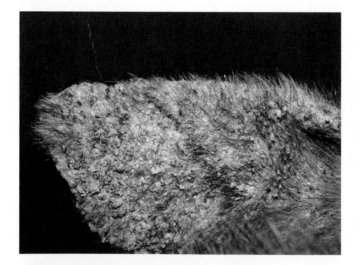

FIGURE 8-35 **Pemphigus Foliaceus.** Severe crusting on the ear pinna of a dog with pemphigus. Crusted ear pinnae (with or without otitis externa) is a common characteristic of autoimmune skin disease.

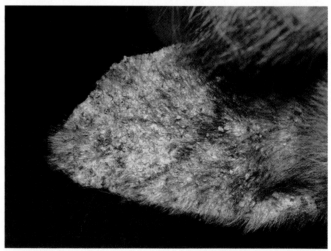

FIGURE 8-36 **Pemphigus Foliaceus.** Severe alopecic, crusting dermatitis on the ear pinna is typical of pemphigus and other autoimmune skin diseases.

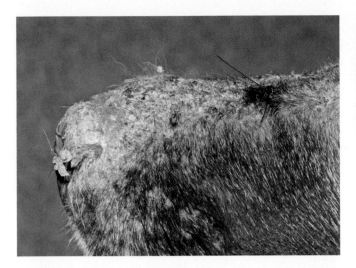

FIGURE 8-37 Pemphigus Foliaceus. Severe erosive, depigmenting, crusting dermatitis of the nasal planum is a classic characteristic of autoimmune skin disease.

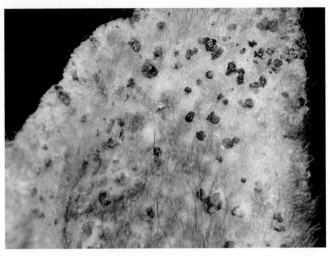

FIGURE 8-38 Pemphigus Foliaceus. Severe alopecia with punctate, crusted erosions on the ear pinna of a dog with pemphigus.

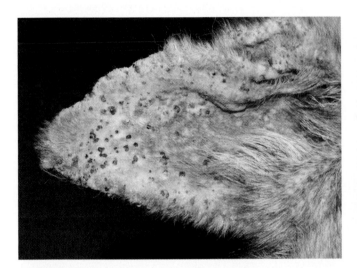

FIGURE 8-39 Pemphigus Foliaceus. Severe crusting dermatitis on the ear pinna typical of autoimmune skin disease. Note that the ear canal appears to be normal; otitis externa may or may not be present in patients with autoimmune skin disease.

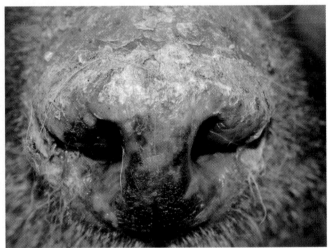

FIGURE 8-40 Pemphigus Foliaceus. Severe crusting, erosive dermatitis on the nasal planum of a dog with pemphigus. Loss of normal cobblestone texture and depigmentation usually occur first, followed by erosive, crusting lesions as the disease progresses.

Pemphigus Foliaceus—*cont'd*

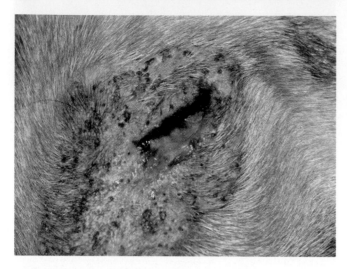

FIGURE 8-41 Pemphigus Foliaceus. Alopecic, crusting dermatitis around the eye of a dog with pemphigus.

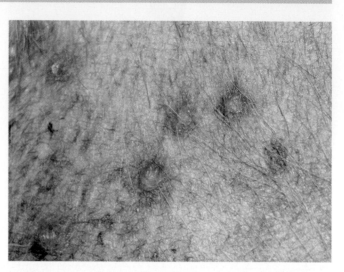

FIGURE 8-42 Pemphigus Foliaceus. Pustules on the skin of a dog with pemphigus. Pustules are the primary lesions caused by pemphigus; however, they usually are destroyed very quickly by the dog's normal activity.

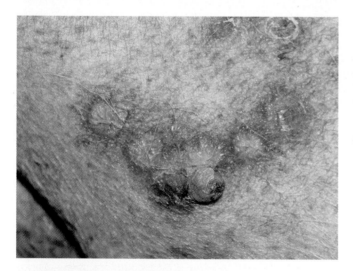

FIGURE 8-43 Pemphigus Foliaceus. Pustular dermatitis on the skin of a dog with pemphigus.

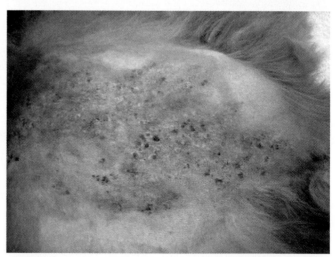

FIGURE 8-44 Pemphigus Foliaceus. Severe crusting dermatitis caused by a drug-induced pemphigus after the dog was treated with Promeris. Pemphigus-induced Promeris drug reactions have been well documented. *(Courtesy S. Sargent.)*

Pemphigus Erythematosus

Features

This disease may be a benign form of pemphigus foliaceus or a crossover between pemphigus and lupus erythematosus. It is uncommon in cats and common in dogs, with an increased incidence in German shepherds, collies, and Shetland Sheep dogs.

The disease is usually limited to the face (bridge of the nose and around the eyes) and ear pinnae. Superficial erosions, scales, and crusts are typical. Pustules may be present but are usually difficult to find. Skin lesions may be minimally to mildly pruritic. Concurrent nasal depigmentation is common. The oral cavity is not involved.

Top Differentials

Differentials include demodicosis, nasal pyoderma, dermatophytosis, discoid lupus erythematosus, pemphigus foliaceus, dermatomyositis, nasal solar dermatitis, mosquito bite hypersensitivity (cats), uveodermatologic syndrome, and zinc-responsive dermatosis.

Diagnosis

1. Rule out other differentials.
2. Cytology (pustule): neutrophils and acantholytic cells are seen. Eosinophils may also be present.
3. Antinuclear antibody (ANA) test: may be positive; however, a positive result is only supportive and is not pathognomonic for pemphigus erythematosus because positive titers can be associated with many other chronic diseases.
4. Dermatohistopathology: subcorneal pustules that contain neutrophils and acantholytic cells with or without eosinophils. Lichenoid infiltration with mononuclear cells, plasma cells, neutrophils, or eosinophils may also be present.
5. Immunofluorescence or immunohistochemistry (skin biopsy specimen): detection of intercellular antibody deposition. Antibody deposition along the dermal-epidermal junction may also be present. False-positive and false-negative results are common. Positive results should be confirmed histologically.
6. Bacterial culture (pustule): usually sterile, but occasionally bacteria are isolated if secondary infection is present.

Treatment and Prognosis

1. Sunlight exposure should be avoided and topical sunscreens used to prevent ultraviolet light from exacerbating nasal lesions. Products containing titanium dioxide are especially effective.
2. Symptomatic shampoo therapy may be helpful for removing crusts.
3. To treat or prevent secondary pyoderma in dogs, appropriate long-term systemic antibiotics should be administered (minimum 4 weeks). Dogs treated with antibiotics during the induction phase of immunosuppressive therapy have significantly higher survival rates than dogs treated with immunosuppressive drugs alone. Antibiotics should be continued until concurrent immunosuppressive therapy has the pemphigus under control.
4. The goal of treatment is to control the disease and its symptoms with the safest treatments used at the lowest possible doses. Typically, combinations of therapies (see Table 8-1) will have to be used to provide a multimodal treatment plan, minimizing the adverse effects of any one therapy. Depending on the severity of the disease, more or less aggressive treatments will have to be selected. To push the disease into remission, higher doses are used initially and then are tapered over 2 to 3 months to the lowest effective dose.
   a. **Topical therapy** applied every 12 hours with steroid-containing products or tacrolimus will help reduce focal inflammation and will lower the doses of systemic treatments required to control the symptoms. Once in remission, the frequency of application should be minimized to reduce local adverse effects.
   b. **Conservative systemic treatments** (see Table 8-1) include drugs that help reduce the inflammation with few to no adverse effects. These treatments help reduce the need for more aggressive therapy such as steroids or chemotherapeutics.
   c. **Steroid therapy** is one of the most reliably predictable treatments for autoimmune skin disease; however, adverse effects associated with the high doses needed to control symptoms may be severe. Although glucocorticoid therapy alone may be effective in maintaining remission, the dosages needed may result in undesirable adverse effects, especially in dogs. **For this reason, the use of nonsteroidal immunosuppressive drugs, alone or in combination with glucocorticoids, is usually recommended for long-term maintenance.**
      - Immunosuppressive doses of oral prednisone or methylprednisolone should be administered daily (see Table 8-1). After lesions resolve (after approximately 2–8 weeks), the dosage should be gradually tapered over a period of several (8–10) weeks until the lowest possible

Pemphigus Erythematosus—*cont'd*

alternate-day dosage that maintains remission is being administered. If no significant improvement is seen within 2 to 4 weeks of initiation of therapy, concurrent skin infection should be ruled out, then alternative or additional immunosuppressive medications considered.

■ Alternative steroids for prednisone- and methylprednisolone-refractory cases include triamcinolone and dexamethasone (see Table 8-1).

■ In cats, treatment with immunosuppressive doses of triamcinolone or dexamethasone often is more effective than therapy with prednisolone or methylprednisolone. Oral triamcinolone or dexamethasone should be administered daily until remission is achieved (approximately 2–8 weeks), then the dosage should be gradually tapered until the lowest possible and least frequent dosage that maintains remission is being administered (see Table 8-1).

■ If unacceptable adverse effects develop, or if no significant improvement is seen within 2 to 4 weeks of initiation of therapy, consider using an alternate glucocorticosteroid or a nonsteroidal immunosuppressive drug (see Table 8-1).

d. **Nonsteroidal immunosuppressive drugs** that may be effective include cyclosporine (Atopica), azathioprine (dogs only), chlorambucil, cyclophosphamide, mycophenolate mofetil, and leflunomide (see Table 8-1). A beneficial response occurs within 8 to 12 weeks of initiation of therapy. Once remission is achieved, gradually attempt to taper the dosage and frequency of the nonsteroidal immunosuppressive drug for long-term maintenance.

5. The prognosis is good because even without treatment, this disease usually remains benign and localized. If systemic immunosuppressive drugs are used, regular monitoring of clinical signs, hemograms, and serum biochemistry panels, with treatment adjustments as needed, is essential. Potential complications of systemic immunosuppressive therapy include unacceptable drug adverse effects and immunosuppression-induced secondary bacterial infection, dermatophytosis, or demodicosis.

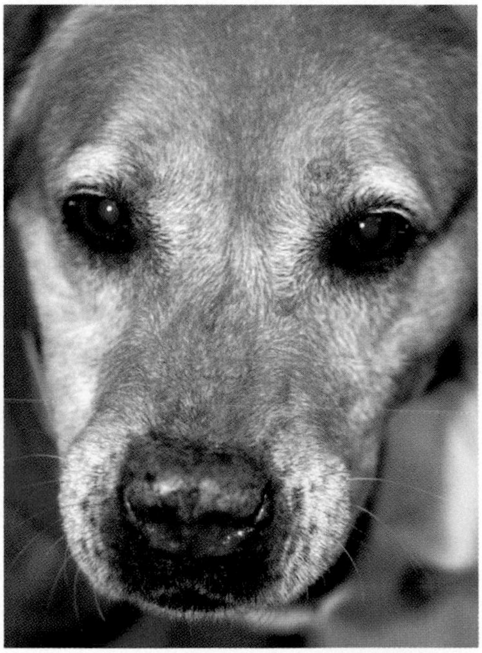

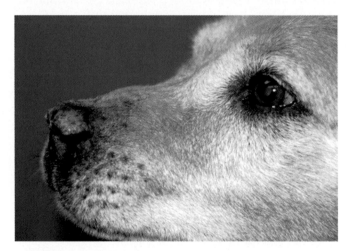

FIGURE 8-46 Pemphigus Erythematosus. Same dog as in Figure 8-45. Depigmenting erosive lesions on the nasal planum.

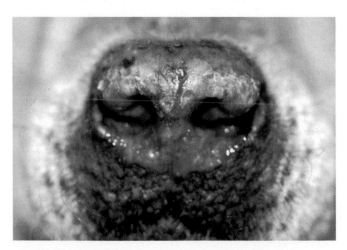

FIGURE 8-47 Pemphigus Erythematosus. Depigmentation and erosions on the nasal planum.

FIGURE 8-45 Pemphigus Erythematosus. Depigmentation and erosive dermatitis on the nasal planum. Lesions on the nasal planum are a common and unique feature of autoimmune skin disease.

Pemphigus Vulgaris

Features

Pemphigus vulgaris is an autoimmune skin disease characterized by the production of autoantibodies against antigens in or near the epidermal-dermal junction. The deposition of antibody in intercellular spaces causes cell detachment within the deeper epidermal layers (acantholysis). It is the most severe form of pemphigus and is rare among dogs and cats.

Erosions, ulcers, and, rarely, vesicles and bullae occur on the skin (especially on the axillae and groin), mucocutaneous junctions (nail beds, lips, nares, eyelids), and mucous membranes (oral cavity, anus, vulva, prepuce, conjunctiva). Concurrent fever, depression, and anorexia are common. Marked salivation and halitosis may accompany oral lesions. Lesions on the nasal planum, ear pinnae, and footpads are unique and characteristic of autoimmune skin disease.

Top Differentials

Differentials include bullous pemphigoid, systemic lupus erythematosus, erythema multiforme/toxic epidermal necrolysis, drug reaction, infection (bacterial, fungal), vasculitis, and cutaneous epitheliotropic lymphoma.

Diagnosis

1. Rule out other differentials.
2. Dermatohistopathology: suprabasilar clefts and vesicles with varying degrees of perivascular, interstitial, or lichenoid inflammation; acantholysis and acantholytic cells.
3. Immunofluorescence or immunohistochemistry (skin biopsy specimens): detection of intercellular antibody deposition. False-positive and false-negative results are common. Positive results should be confirmed histologically.
4. Bacterial culture (vesicle, bulla): usually sterile, but occasionally bacteria are isolated if secondary infection is present.

Treatment and Prognosis

1. Symptomatic shampoo therapy may be helpful for removing crusts.
2. To treat or prevent secondary pyoderma in dogs, appropriate long-term systemic antibiotics should be administered (minimum 4 weeks). Dogs treated with antibiotics during the induction phase of immunosuppressive therapy have significantly higher survival rates than dogs treated with immunosuppressive drugs alone. Antibiotics should be continued until concurrent immunosuppressive therapy has the pemphigus under control.
3. The goal of treatment is to control the disease and its symptoms with the safest treatments used at the lowest possible doses. Typically, combinations of therapies (see Table 8-1) will have to be used to provide a multimodal treatment plan, minimizing the adverse effects of any one therapy. Depending on the severity of the disease, more or less aggressive treatments will have to be selected. To push the disease into remission, higher doses are used initially and then are tapered over 2 to 3 months to the lowest effective dose.

Because Pemphigus vulgaris is usually severe, aggressive therapy is usually required.

Although glucocorticoid therapy alone may be effective in maintaining remission, the dosages needed may result in undesirable adverse effects, especially in dogs. **For this reason, the use of nonsteroidal immunosuppressive drugs, alone or in combination with glucocorticoids, is usually recommended for long-term maintenance.**

a. Immunosuppressive doses of oral prednisone or methylprednisolone should be administered daily (see Table 8-1). After lesions resolve (after approximately 2–8 weeks), the dosage should be gradually tapered over a period of several (8–10) weeks until the lowest possible alternate-day dosage that maintains remission is being administered. If no significant improvement is seen within 2 to 4 weeks of initiation of therapy, concurrent skin infection should be ruled out, then alternative or additional immunosuppressive medications considered.

b. Alternative steroids for prednisone- and methylprednisolone-refractory cases include triamcinolone and dexamethasone (see Table 8-1).

c. In cats, treatment with immunosuppressive doses of triamcinolone or dexamethasone is often more effective than therapy with prednisolone or methylprednisolone. Oral triamcinolone or dexamethasone should be administered daily until remission is achieved (approximately 2–8 weeks), then the dosage should be gradually tapered until the lowest possible and least frequent dosage that maintains remission is being administered (see Table 8-1).

d. If unacceptable adverse effects develop, or if no significant improvement is seen within 2 to 4 weeks of initiation of therapy, consider using an alternate glucocorticosteroid or a nonsteroidal immunosuppressive drug (see Table 8-1).

Pemphigus Vulgaris—*cont'd*

4. Nonsteroidal immunosuppressive drugs are usually needed in addition to steroidal therapy to control severe lesions and minimize the side effects of steroids. Treatments that may be effective include cyclosporine (Atopica), azathioprine (dogs only), chlorambucil, cyclophosphamide, mycophenolate mofetil, and leflunomide (see Table 8-1). A beneficial response occurs within 8 to 12 weeks of initiation of therapy. Once remission is achieved, gradually attempt to taper the dosage and frequency of the nonsteroidal immunosuppressive drug for long-term maintenance.

5. The prognosis is fair to poor, and lifelong therapy is usually required to maintain remission. Regular monitoring of clinical signs, hemograms, and serum biochemistry panels, with treatment adjustments as needed, is essential. Potential complications of immunosuppressive therapy include unacceptable drug adverse effects and immunosuppression-induced bacterial infection, dermatophytosis, or demodicosis.

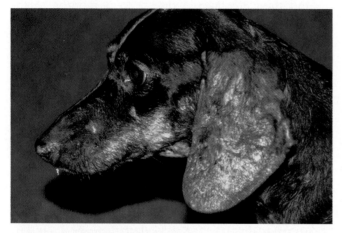

FIGURE 8-48 Pemphigus Vulgaris. Severe alopecic, crusting, erosive dermatitis on the nasal planum, face, and ear pinna of an adult dog with pemphigus vulgaris. The nasal planum, ear pinnae, and footpads are unique features of autoimmune skin disease.

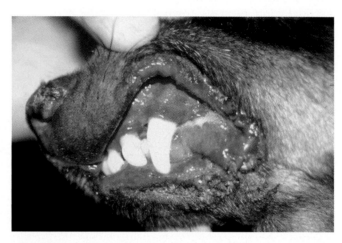

FIGURE 8-50 Pemphigus Vulgaris. Erosive dermatitis on the lips and gingiva. Lesions on the oral mucosa can be seen with pemphigus vulgaris, bullous pemphigoid, systemic lupus erythematosus (SLE), and vasculitis.

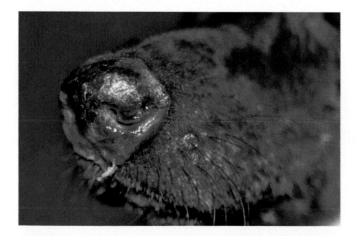

FIGURE 8-49 Pemphigus Vulgaris. Swelling, depigmentation, and erosions on the nasal planum.

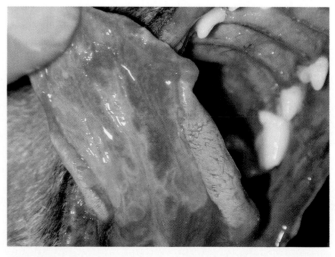

FIGURE 8-51 Pemphigus Vulgaris. Erosive lesions on the tongue.

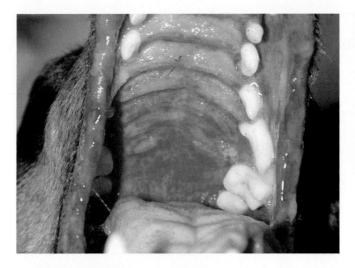

FIGURE 8-52 Pemphigus Vulgaris. Erosive lesions on the palate of a dog with pemphigus vulgaris.

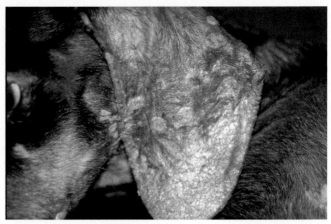

FIGURE 8-53 Pemphigus Vulgaris. Alopecic, erosive dermatitis on the ear pinna of a dog. Note the erosive nature of pemphigus vulgaris compared with the typical crusting seen in pemphigus foliaceus.

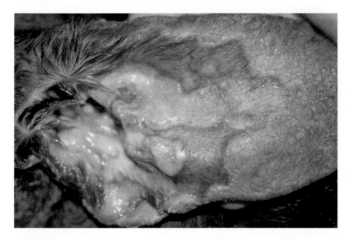

FIGURE 8-54 Pemphigus Vulgaris. Alopecic, erosive dermatitis on the ear pinna.

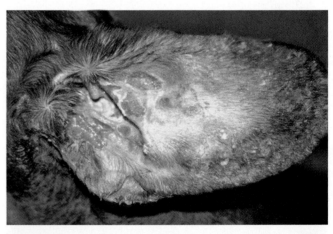

FIGURE 8-55 Pemphigus Vulgaris. Alopecic, crusting, erosive dermatitis on the ear pinna.

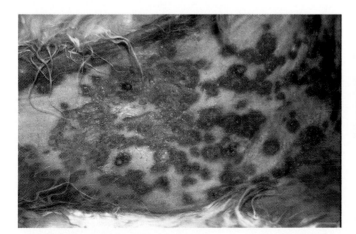

FIGURE 8-56 Pemphigus Vulgaris. Alopecic, erosive dermatitis on the abdomen. Note the punctate nature of the lesions, which can coalesce to form large erosive plaques. These lesions are similar to erythema multiforme and cutaneous drug reactions.

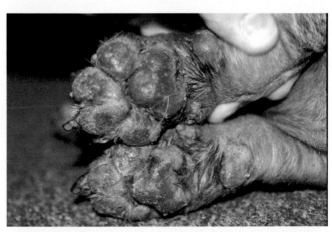

FIGURE 8-57 Pemphigus Vulgaris. Erosive dermatitis on the footpads. Footpad lesions are a common feature of autoimmune skin disease. Note the erosive nature of pemphigus vulgaris compared with the crusting typically seen in pemphigus foliaceus.

Pemphigus Vulgaris—*cont'd*

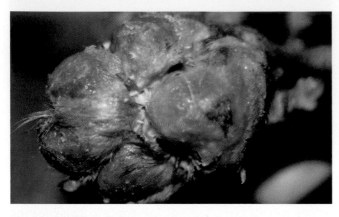

FIGURE 8-58 Pemphigus Vulgaris. Complete erosion of the footpads in a dog with pemphigus vulgaris.

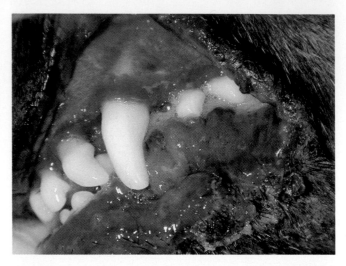

FIGURE 8-59 Pemphigus Vulgaris. Erosive lesions on the gingiva. Lesions on the oral mucosa can be seen with pemphigus vulgaris, bullous pemphigoid, systemic lupus erythematosus (SLE), and vasculitis.

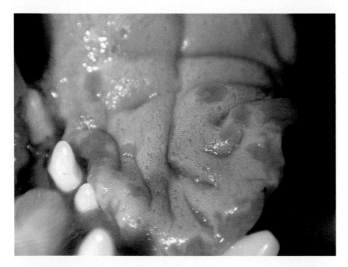

FIGURE 8-60 Pemphigus Vulgaris. Erosive lesions on the tongue of a dog with pemphigus vulgaris.

Bullous Pemphigoid

Features

Bullous pemphigoid is an autoimmune skin disease characterized by the production of autoantibodies against basement membrane zone (lamina lucida) antigens that cause the epidermis to separate from the underlying dermis. Fragile vesicles and bullae form and rupture, leaving ulcerated lesions. The condition is rare in dogs.

Bullous pemphigoid manifests as an ulcerative disease of the skin (especially on the head, neck, axillae, and ventral abdomen), mucocutaneous junctions (nares, eyelids, lips), mucous membranes (oral cavity, anus, vulva, prepuce, conjunctiva), and footpads. Vesicles and bullae are rare. Severely affected dogs may be anorectic, depressed, and febrile. Lesions on the nasal planum, ear pinnae, and footpads are unique and characteristic of autoimmune skin disease.

Top Differentials

Differentials include pemphigus vulgaris, systemic lupus erythematosus, erythema multiforme/toxic epidermal necrolysis, drug eruption, vasculitis, cutaneous epitheliotropic lymphoma, and infection (bacterial, fungal).

Diagnosis

1. Rule out other differentials.
2. Dermatohistopathology: subepidermal clefts and vesicles with a mild perivascular to marked lichenoid mononuclear and neutrophilic inflammation. Eosinophils may also be present.
3. Immunofluorescence or immunohistochemistry (skin biopsy specimens): deposition of immunoglobulin along the dermal-epidermal junction. False-positive and false-negative results are common. Positive results should be confirmed histologically.
4. Bacterial culture (vesicle, bulla): usually sterile, but occasionally, bacteria are isolated if secondary infection is present.

Treatment and Prognosis

1. Symptomatic shampoo therapy may be helpful for removing crusts.
2. To treat or prevent secondary pyoderma in dogs, appropriate long-term systemic antibiotics should be administered (minimum 4 weeks). Dogs treated with antibiotics during the induction phase of immunosuppressive therapy have significantly higher survival rates than dogs treated with immunosuppressive drugs alone. Antibiotics should be continued until concurrent immunosuppressive therapy has the autoimmune disease under control.
3. The goal of treatment is to control the diseases and its symptoms with the safest treatments used at the lowest possible doses. Typically, combinations of therapies (see Table 8-1) will have to be used to provide a multimodal treatment plan, minimizing the adverse effects of any one therapy. Depending on the severity of the disease, more or less aggressive treatments will have to be selected. To push the disease into remission, higher doses are used initially and then are tapered over 2 to 3 months to the lowest effective dose.

Because bullous pemphigoid is usually severe, aggressive therapy is usually required.

Although glucocorticoid therapy alone may be effective in maintaining remission, the dosages needed may result in undesirable adverse effects, especially in dogs. **For this reason, the use of nonsteroidal immunosuppressive drugs, alone or in combination with glucocorticoids, is usually recommended for long-term maintenance.**

a. Immunosuppressive doses of oral prednisone or methylprednisolone should be administered daily (see Table 8-1). After lesions resolve (after approximately 2–8 weeks), the dosage should be gradually tapered over a period of several (8–10) weeks until the lowest possible alternate-day dosage that maintains remission is being administered. If no significant improvement is seen within 2 to 4 weeks of initiation of therapy, a concurrent skin infection should be ruled out, then alternative or additional immunosuppressive medications considered.

b. Alternative steroids for prednisone- and methylprednisolone-refractory cases include triamcinolone and dexamethasone (see Table 8-1).

c. In cats, treatment with immunosuppressive doses of triamcinolone or dexamethasone is often more effective than therapy with prednisolone or methylprednisolone. Oral triamcinolone or dexamethasone should be administered daily until remission is achieved (approximately 2–8 weeks), then the dosage should be gradually tapered until the lowest possible and least frequent dosage that maintains remission is being administered (see Table 8-1).

d. If unacceptable adverse effects develop, or if no significant improvement is seen within 2 to 4 weeks of initiation of therapy, consider using an

Bullous Pemphigoid—*cont'd*

alternate glucocorticosteroid or a nonsteroidal immunosuppressive drug (see Table 8-1).

4. Nonsteroidal immunosuppressive drugs are usually needed in addition to steroidal therapy to control severe lesions and minimize the side effects of steroids. Treatments that may be effective include cyclosporine (Atopica), azathioprine (dogs only), chlorambucil, cyclophosphamide, mycophenolate mofetil, and leflunomide (see Table 8-1). A beneficial response occurs within 8 to 12 weeks of initiation of therapy. Once remission is achieved, gradually attempt to taper the dosage and frequency of the nonsteroidal immunosuppressive drug for long-term maintenance

5. The prognosis is fair to poor. Lifelong therapy is usually required to maintain remission. Regular monitoring of clinical signs, hemograms, and serum biochemistry panels, with treatment adjustments as needed, is essential. Potential complications of immunosuppressive therapy include unacceptable drug adverse effects and immunosuppression-induced bacterial infection, dermatophytosis, or demodicosis.

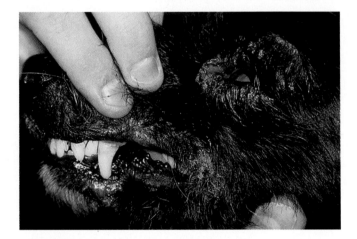

FIGURE 8-61 Bullous Pemphigoid. Alopecia, ulcers, and crusts around the mouth of an adult Scottie.

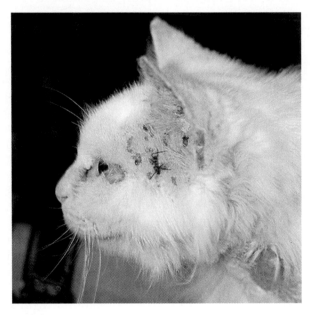

FIGURE 8-62 Bullous Pemphigoid. Alopecia and ulcers on the face of an adult cat.

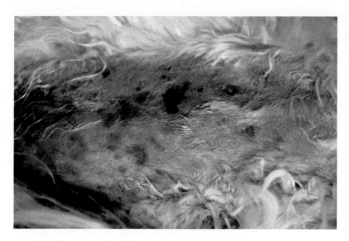

FIGURE 8-63 Bullous Pemphigoid. Close-up of the cat in Figure 8-62. Numerous ulcers on the trunk.

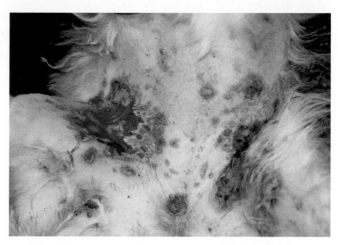

FIGURE 8-64 Bullous Pemphigoid. Severe ulcerative dermatitis on the abdomen. The punctate lesions coalesced to form large ulcerative lesions. Note the similarity to erythema multiforme, cutaneous drug reactions, and vasculitis.

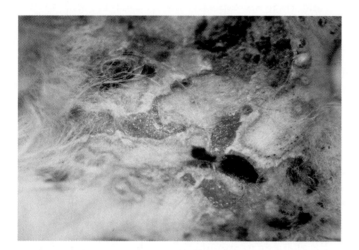

FIGURE 8-65 Bullous Pemphigoid. Same dog as in Figure 8-64. Coalescing ulcerative lesions with a serpentine, well-demarcated margin. Note the similarity to cutaneous drug reactions and vasculitis.

Discoid Lupus Erythematosus (DLE)

Features

This disease is considered by many to be a benign variant of systemic lupus erythematosus. It is common in dogs and rare in cats.

Dogs

Nasal depigmentation, erythema, scaling, erosions, ulcerations, and crusting are characteristic. Similar lesions may involve the lips, bridge of the nose, periocular skin, ear pinnae, and, less commonly, distal limbs or genitalia. Hyperkeratotic footpads and oral ulcers are rarely present.

Cats

In cats, the disease appears as erythema, alopecia, and crusting on the face and ear pinnae. Nasal lesions are uncommon.

Top Differentials

Differentials include nasal pyoderma, demodicosis, dermatophytosis, pemphigus erythematosus or foliaceus, dermatomyositis, uveodermatologic syndrome, nasal solar dermatitis, nasal depigmentation, and mosquito bite hypersensitivity (cats).

Diagnosis

1. Rule out other differentials.
2. Dermatohistopathology: findings may include hydropic or lichenoid interface dermatitis, focal thickening of the basement membrane zone, pigmentary incontinence, apoptotic keratinocytes, and perivascular and periadnexal accumulations of mononuclear and plasma cells.
3. Immunofluorescence or immunohistochemistry (skin biopsy specimens): patchy deposition of immunoglobulin or complement at the basement membrane zone. Not diagnostic in itself because false-positive results are possible and false-negative results are common.

Treatment and Prognosis

1. Sunlight exposure should be avoided and topical sunscreens used to prevent ultraviolet light from exacerbating nasal lesions. Products containing titanium dioxide are especially helpful.
2. Symptomatic shampoo therapy may be helpful for removing crusts.
3. To treat or prevent secondary pyoderma in dogs, appropriate long-term systemic antibiotics should be administered (minimum 4 weeks). Dogs treated with antibiotics during the induction phase of immunosuppressive therapy have significantly higher survival rates than dogs treated with immunosuppressive drugs alone. Antibiotics should be continued until concurrent immunosuppressive therapy has the autoimmune disease under control.
4. The goal of treatment is to control the disease and its symptoms with the safest treatments used at the lowest possible doses. Typically, combinations of therapies (see Table 8-1) will have to be used to provide a multimodal treatment plan, minimizing the adverse effects of any one therapy. Depending on the severity of the disease, more or less aggressive treatments will have to be selected. To push the disease into remission, higher doses are used initially and then are tapered over 2 to 3 months to the lowest effective dose.
    a. Topical therapy applied every 12 hours with steroid-containing products or tacrolimus will help reduce focal inflammation and will lower the doses of systemic treatments required to control symptoms. Once in remission, the frequency of application should be minimized to reduce local adverse effects.
    b. Conservative systemic treatments (see Table 8-1) include drugs that help reduce inflammation with few to no adverse effects. These treatments help reduce the need for more aggressive therapies such as steroids or chemotherapeutics.
    c. Steroid therapy is one of the most reliably predictable treatments for autoimmune skin disease; however, adverse effects associated with the high doses needed to control symptoms may be severe. Although glucocorticoid therapy alone may be effective in maintaining remission, the dosages needed may result in undesirable adverse effects, especially in dogs. **For this reason, the use of nonsteroidal immunosuppressive drugs, alone or in combination with glucocorticoids, is usually recommended for long-term maintenance.**
       ■ Immunosuppressive doses of oral prednisone or methylprednisolone should be administered daily (see Table 8-1). After lesions resolve (after approximately 2–8 weeks), the dosage should be gradually tapered over a period of several (8–10) weeks until the lowest possible alternate-day dosage that maintains remission is being administered. If no significant improvement is seen within 2 to 4 weeks of initiation of therapy, concurrent skin infection should be

ruled out, then alternative or additional immunosuppressive medications considered.

- Alternative steroids for prednisone- and methylprednisolone-refractory cases include triamcinolone and dexamethasone (see Table 8-1).
- If unacceptable adverse effects develop, or if no significant improvement is seen within 2 to 4 weeks of initiation of therapy, consider using an alternate glucocorticosteroid or a nonsteroidal immunosuppressive drug (see Table 8-1).

d. Nonsteroidal immunosuppressive drugs that may be effective include cyclosporine (Atopica), azathioprine (dogs only), chlorambucil, cyclophosphamide, mycophenolate mofetil, and leflunomide (see Table 8-1). A beneficial response occurs within 8 to 12 weeks of initiation of therapy. Once remission is achieved, gradually attempt to taper the dosage and frequency of the nonsteroidal immunosuppressive drug for long-term maintenance.

5. The prognosis is good, but lifelong treatment is usually necessary. Permanent scarring or leukoderma (depigmentation) and, rarely, squamous cell carcinoma are possible sequelae.

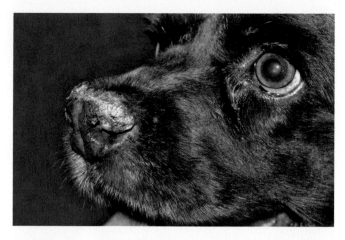

FIGURE 8-67 Discoid Lupus Erythematosus. Depigmentation, crusting, erosive dermatitis on the nasal planum of a dog.

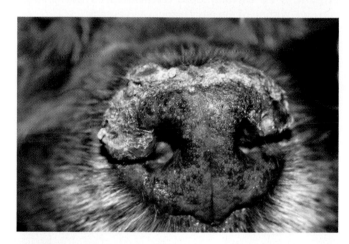

FIGURE 8-68 Discoid Lupus Erythematosus. Depigmentation, crusts, and erosions on the nasal planum typical of autoimmune skin disease.

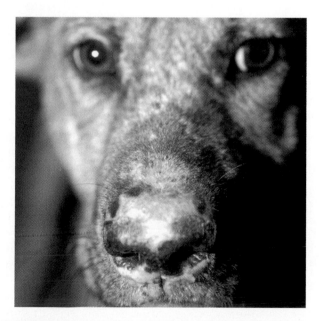

FIGURE 8-66 Discoid Lupus Erythematosus. Focal alopecia and depigmentation on the nasal planum and bridge of the nose. Lesions on the nasal planum are unique features of autoimmune skin disease.

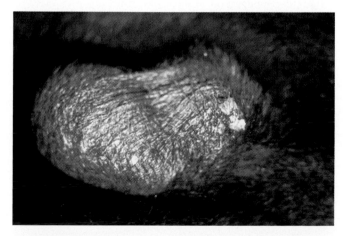

FIGURE 8-69 Discoid Lupus Erythematosus. Hyperkeratosis and crusting on the scrotum.

Discoid Lupus Erythematosus (DLE)—cont'd

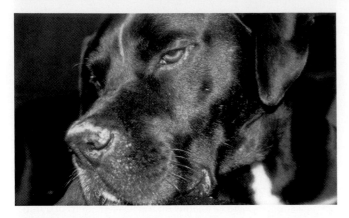

FIGURE 8-70 Discoid Lupus Erythematosus. Depigmentation and crusting of the nasal planum and eyelids.

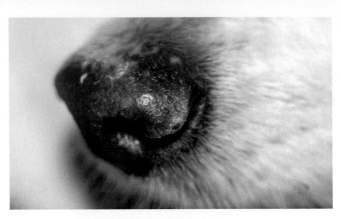

FIGURE 8-71 Discoid Lupus Erythematosus. Erythema and depigmentation of the nasal planum. The normal cobblestone texture has been destroyed, leaving a smooth appearance.

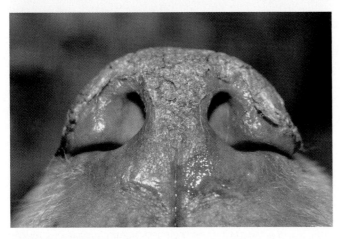

FIGURE 8-72 Discoid Lupus Erythematosus. Close-up of the nasal planum demonstrating loss of the normal cobblestone surface, depigmentation, erosion, and crusts.

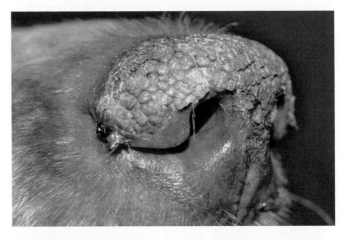

FIGURE 8-73 Discoid Lupus Erythematosus. Severe crust accumulation on the nasal planum that also has multifocal erosion and depigmentation.

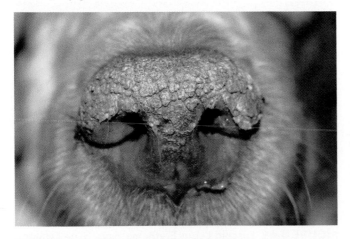

FIGURE 8-74 Discoid Lupus Erythematosus. Severe crusting can be caused by noninflammatory nasal hyperkeratosis; however, depigmentation and ulceration are classic features of autoimmune skin disease.

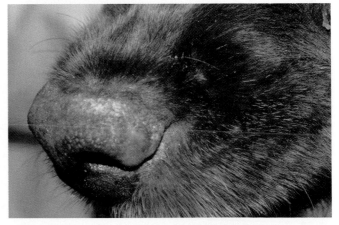

FIGURE 8-75 Discoid Lupus Erythematosus. Early and mild disease often will first present with depigmentation and ulceration on the margins of the nasal planum. Note that the normal cobblestone surface structure is still present, indicating mild and early lesions.

Systemic Lupus Erythematosus (SLE)

Features

Systemic lupus erythematosus is a multisystemic immune-mediated disease characterized by the production of a variety of autoantibodies (e.g., ANA, rheumatoid factor, anti-RBC antibodies) that form circulating immune complexes. It is rare in cats and uncommon in dogs, with collies, Shetland Sheep dogs, and German shepherds possibly predisposed.

Dogs

Symptoms are often nonspecific and may wax and wane. Cutaneous signs are common and variable and often mimic those seen in many other skin disorders. Mucocutaneous or mucosal erosions and ulcers may be present. Skin lesions may include erosions, ulcers, scales, erythema, alopecia, crusting, and scarring. Lesions may be multifocal or diffuse. They can occur anywhere on the body, but the face, ears, and distal extremities are most commonly affected. Peripheral lymphadenomegaly is often present. Other symptoms may include fluctuating fever, polyarthritis, polymyositis, renal failure, blood dyscrasias, pleuritis, pneumonitis, pericarditis or myocarditis, central or peripheral neuropathy, and lymphedema. Lesions on the nasal planum, ear pinnae, and footpads are unique and characteristic of autoimmune skin disease.

Vesicular cutaneous lupus erythematosus, formerly known as ulcerative dermatosis of Shetland Sheep dogs and rough collie dogs (UDSSC), is thought to be a vesicular variant of cutaneous lupus erythematosus. It is uncommon in Shetland Sheep dogs, rough collie dogs, and their crosses. It typically occurs in adulthood, with lesions usually first appearing in the summer months. Some dogs may go into remission during winter, then relapse in early summer. The primary lesions are vesicles and bullae. However, these lesions are often difficult to find because they are fragile and rupture easily. Secondary lesions include annular, polycyclic, and serpiginous ulcerations. These ulcerations typically involve sparsely haired skin (e.g., groin, axillae, ventral abdomen, medial thighs) and may progress to involve the mucocutaneous junctions, concave aspects of the ear pinnae, oral cavity, and footpads. Affected dogs may become debilitated and develop sepsis from secondary bacterial skin infection.

Cats

Cutaneous lesions are variable and may include an erythematous, alopecic, scaling, crusting, and scarring dermatosis; an exfoliative erythroderma; and excessive scaling (seborrhea). Lesions can appear anywhere on the body, but the face, ear pinnae, and paws are most often affected. Oral ulcers may be present. Other symptoms may include fever, polyarthritis, renal failure, neurologic or behavioral abnormalities, hematologic abnormalities, and myopathy.

Top Differentials

Differentials include other causes of polysystemic disease such as drug reaction, rickettsial infection, other infections (viral, bacterial, fungal), neoplasia, and other autoimmune and immune-mediated disorders.

Diagnosis

1. A definitive diagnosis is often difficult to make. All other differentials should be ruled out. The following findings are supportive, and, when several are present together (clusters of symptoms), are highly suggestive of systemic lupus erythematosus:
   - Hemogram: anemia (that may or may not be Coombs-positive), thrombocytopenia, leukopenia, or leukocytosis
   - Urinalysis: proteinuria
   - Arthrocentesis (polyarthritis): sterile purulent inflammation (may or may not be rheumatoid factor–positive)
   - ANA test: a good screening test because most patients with systemic lupus erythematosus have positive ANA titers. However, a positive result is only supportive and is not pathognomonic for systemic lupus erythematosus because positive titers can be associated with many other chronic or infectious diseases such as bartonellosis, ehrlichiosis, and leishmaniasis. False-negatives can occur (10%).
   - Lupus erythematosus (LE) cell test: a positive result is highly suggestive, but this test is not a good screening test because false-negative results are common.
2. Titers for rickettsial infection should be performed to rule out tick-borne disease.
3. Dermatohistopathology: focal thickening of the basement membrane zone, subepidermal vacuolation, hydropic or lichenoid interface dermatitis, or leukocytoclastic vasculitis is characteristic. However, these changes are not always seen, and findings may be nonspecific.
4. Immunofluorescence or immunohistochemistry (skin biopsy specimens): patchy deposition of immunoglobulin or complement at the basement membrane zone. Not diagnostic in itself because

Systemic Lupus Erythematosus (SLE)—*cont'd*

false-positive results are possible and false-negative results are common.

Treatment and Prognosis

1. Symptomatic shampoo therapy may be helpful for removing crusts.
2. To treat or prevent secondary pyoderma in dogs, appropriate long-term systemic antibiotics should be administered (minimum 4 weeks). Dogs treated with antibiotics during the induction phase of immunosuppressive therapy have significantly higher survival rates than dogs treated with immunosuppressive drugs alone. Antibiotics should be continued until concurrent immunosuppressive therapy has the autoimmune disease under control.
3. The goal of treatment is to control the disease and its symptoms with the safest treatments used at the lowest possible doses. Typically, combinations of therapies (see Table 8-1) will have to be used to provide a multimodal treatment plan, minimizing the adverse effects of any one therapy. Depending on the severity of the disease, more or less aggressive treatments will have to be selected. To push the disease into remission, higher doses are used initially and then are tapered over 2 to 3 months to the lowest effective dose.
   a. Topical therapy applied every 12 hours with steroid-containing products or tacrolimus will help reduce focal inflammation and will lower the doses of systemic treatments required to control symptoms. Once in remission, frequency of application should be minimized to reduce local adverse effects.
   b. Conservative systemic treatments (see Table 8-1) include drugs that help reduce inflammation with few to no adverse effects. These treatments help reduce the need for more aggressive therapies such as steroids or chemotherapeutics.
   c. Steroid therapy is one of the most reliably predictable treatments for autoimmune skin disease; however, adverse effects associated with the high doses needed to control symptoms may be severe. Although glucocorticoid therapy alone may be effective in maintaining remission, the dosages needed may result in undesirable adverse effects, especially in dogs. **For this reason, the use of nonsteroidal immunosuppressive drugs, alone or in combination with glucocorticoids, is usually recommended for long-term maintenance.**
      ■ Immunosuppressive doses of oral prednisone or methylprednisolone should be adminis-

tered daily (see Table 8-1). After lesions resolve (after approximately 2–8 weeks), the dosage should be gradually tapered over a period of several (8–10) weeks until the lowest possible alternate-day dosage that maintains remission is being administered. If no significant improvement is seen within 2 to 4 weeks of initiation of therapy, a concurrent skin infection should be ruled out, then alternative or additional immunosuppressive medications considered.
      ■ Alternative steroids for prednisone- and methylprednisolone-refractory cases include triamcinolone and dexamethasone (see Table 8-1).
      ■ In cats, treatment with immunosuppressive doses of triamcinolone or dexamethasone often is more effective than therapy with prednisolone or methylprednisolone. Oral triamcinolone or dexamethasone should be administered daily until remission is achieved (approximately 2–8 weeks), then the dosage should be gradually tapered until the lowest possible and least frequent dosage that maintains remission is being administered (see Table 8-1).
      ■ If unacceptable adverse effects develop, or if no significant improvement is seen within 2 to 4 weeks of initiation of therapy, consider using an alternate glucocorticosteroid or a nonsteroidal immunosuppressive drug (see Table 8-1).
   d. Nonsteroidal immunosuppressive drugs that may be effective include cyclosporine (Atopica), azathioprine (dogs only), chlorambucil, cyclophosphamide, mycophenolate mofetil, and leflunomide (see Table 8-1). A beneficial response occurs within 8 to 12 weeks of initiation of therapy. Once remission is achieved, gradually attempt to taper the dosage and frequency of the nonsteroidal immunosuppressive drug for long-term maintenance.
4. The prognosis is guarded if hemolytic anemia, thrombocytopenia, or glomerulonephritis is present. In up to 40% of cases, death occurs during the first year of treatment as the result of renal failure, poor response to therapy, drug complications, or secondary systemic infection (pneumonia, sepsis). The prognosis is more favorable for animals that respond to glucocorticoid therapy alone, with approximately 50% having long-term survival times. Regular monitoring of clinical signs, hemograms, and serum biochemistry panels, with treatment adjustments as needed, is essential.

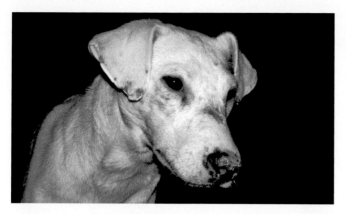

FIGURE 8-76 Systemic Lupus Erythematosus. Alopecic, erythematous, erosive dermatitis on the face, nasal planum, and ear pinnae of an adult Jack Russell terrier. Lesions on the nasal planum and ear pinnae are unique features of autoimmune skin disease.

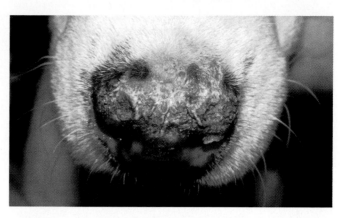

FIGURE 8-77 Systemic Lupus Erythematosus. Same dog as in Figure 8-76. Depigmentation and crusting erosions on the nasal planum.

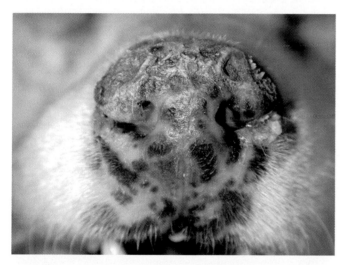

FIGURE 8-78 Systemic Lupus Erythematosus. Severe crusting, erosive dermatitis with depigmentation on the nasal planum.

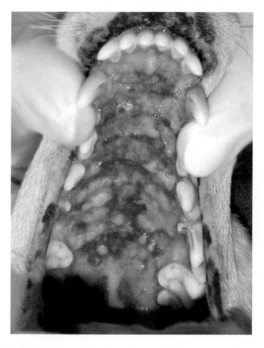

FIGURE 8-80 Systemic Lupus Erythematosus. Erosions on the palate of a dog.

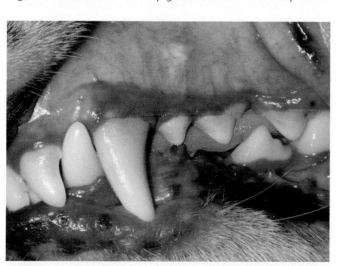

FIGURE 8-79 Systemic Lupus Erythematosus. Erosive dermatitis on the gingiva. Lesions on the oral mucosa can be seen with pemphigus vulgaris, bullous pemphigoid, systemic lupus erythematosus (SLE), and vasculitis.

Systemic Lupus Erythematosus (SLE)—cont'd

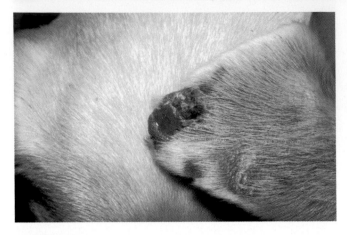

FIGURE 8-81 Systemic Lupus Erythematosus. Alopecic, crusting lesions on the ear pinna. The notch defect is indicative of an underlying vasculitis associated with systemic lupus erythematosus (SLE).

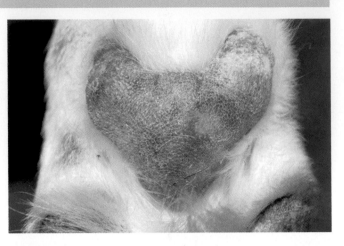

FIGURE 8-82 Systemic Lupus Erythematosus. Hyperkeratosis and crusting on the footpad. Lesions on the footpad are characteristic features of autoimmune skin disease.

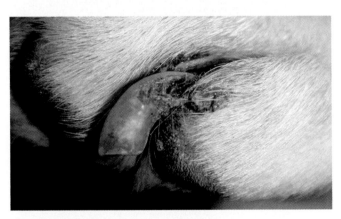

FIGURE 8-83 Systemic Lupus Erythematosus. Inflammation of the nail bed with dystrophic nail formation suggests an underlying vasculitis associated with systemic lupus erythematosus (SLE).

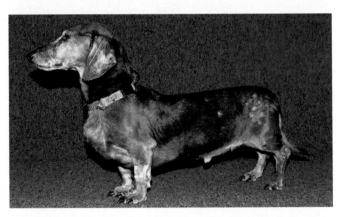

FIGURE 8-84 Systemic Lupus Erythematosus. An adult Dachshund with systemic lupus erythematosus (SLE) demonstrating the generalized pattern of lesions.

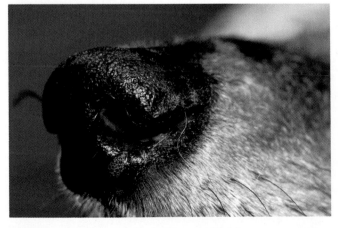

FIGURE 8-85 Systemic Lupus Erythematosus. Crusting erosive dermatitis on the nasal planum. Note the subtle depigmentation on the medial surface of the nostril.

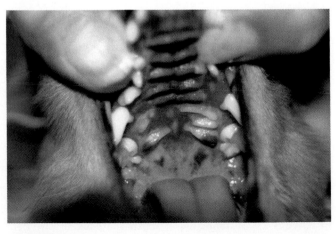

FIGURE 8-86 Systemic Lupus Erythematosus. Erosive dermatitis on the palate of a dog.

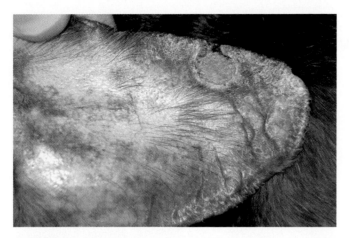

FIGURE 8-87 Systemic Lupus Erythematosus. Crusting dermatitis with hyperpigmentation on the ear margin. The large circular crust is caused by an underlying vasculitis.

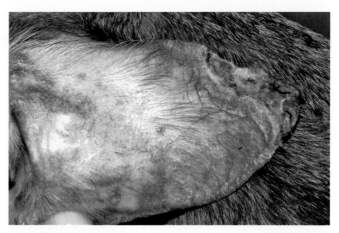

FIGURE 8-88 Systemic Lupus Erythematosus. Same dog as in Figure 8-87. The underlying vasculitis has caused necrosis of the distal ear pinna. Crusting and hyperpigmentation of the remaining ear margin can be noted.

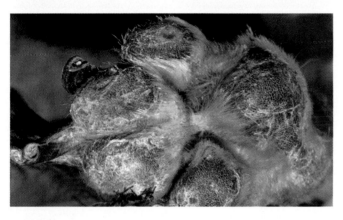

FIGURE 8-89 Systemic Lupus Erythematosus. Hyperkeratosis and crusting on the footpads. The crusting lesion on the center of the footpad is characteristic of vasculitis.

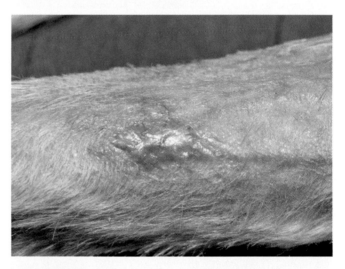

FIGURE 8-90 Systemic Lupus Erythematosus. A focal lesion caused by vasculitis on the distal limb of a dog. Note that the alopecia is a result of chronic inflammation.

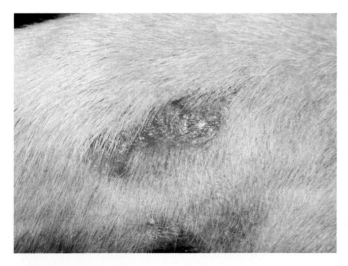

FIGURE 8-91 Systemic Lupus Erythematosus. Same dog as in Figure 8-90 demonstrating a more mild lesion.

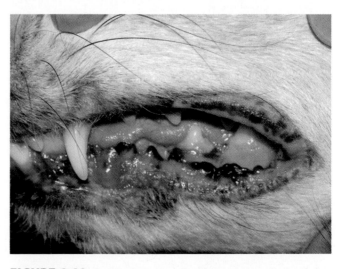

FIGURE 8-92 Systemic Lupus Erythematosus. Perioral dermatitis in a dog. Note the similarity to allergy and mucocutaneous pyoderma.

Systemic Lupus Erythematosus (SLE)—*cont'd*

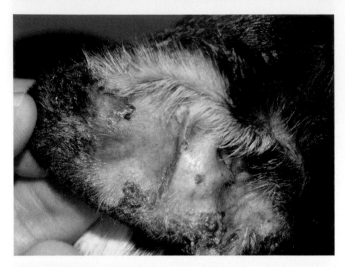

FIGURE 8-93 Systemic Lupus Erythematosus. Severe ulcerative, crusting dermatitis on the ear pinna of a dog with systemic lupus erythematosus (SLE).

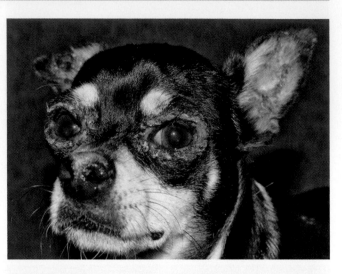

FIGURE 8-94 Systemic Lupus Erythematosus. Severe ulcerative, crusting dermatitis surrounding the eyes and ear pinnae of an affected dog. Notice that the nasal planum is less severely affected, which seems to be common in systemic lupus erythematosus (SLE).

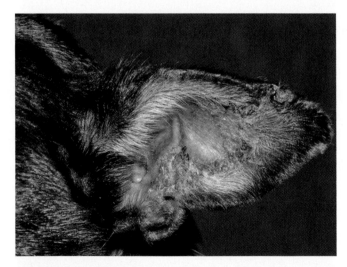

FIGURE 8-95 Systemic Lupus Erythematosus. Severe ulcerative, crusting dermatitis on the ear pinna of a dog with systemic lupus erythematosus (SLE).

Canine Subcorneal Pustular Dermatosis

Features

Canine subcorneal pustular dermatosis appears as a sterile, superficial, pustular skin disease of unknown cause but may be a variant of pemphigus foliaceus. It is rare in dogs, with miniature Schnauzers possibly predisposed.

Multifocal to generalized pustules with secondary crusts, circumscribed areas of alopecia, epidermal collarettes, and scaling are noted. Lesions usually involve the head and trunk. Footpads may be scaly. Lesions may wax and wane, and pruritus varies from none to intense. Peripheral lymphadenomegaly may be present. Concurrent systemic signs of illness (e.g., fever, anorexia, depression) are rare.

Top Differentials

Differentials include demodicosis, dermatophytosis, superficial pyoderma, pemphigus foliaceus, systemic lupus erythematosus, and drug eruption. If lesions are pruritic, differentials should include scabies, hypersensitivity (flea bite, food, atopy), and sterile eosinophilic pustulosis.

Diagnosis

1. Rule out other differentials.
2. Cytology (pustule): numerous neutrophils are seen. An occasional acantholytic keratinocyte may also be present, but no bacteria are found.
3. Dermatohistopathology: subcorneal pustules containing nondegenerative neutrophils. Acantholytic keratinocytes may also be seen.
4. Bacterial culture (pustule): no growth unless secondary infection is present.

Treatment and Prognosis

1. Treat as for pemphigus foliaceus (see Table 8-1).
2. Dapsone 1 mg/kg PO should be administered every 8 hours until lesions resolve (approximately 2–4 weeks). The dosage should gradually be tapered down to 1 mg/kg PO every 24 to 72 hours, or as infrequently as possible to maintain remission.
3. The prognosis is good if response to dapsone is seen. In some dogs, dapsone therapy can eventually be discontinued, whereas others require lifelong therapy for control.

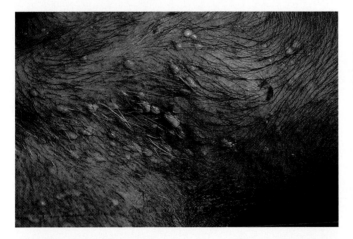

FIGURE 8-96 Canine Subcorneal Pustular Dermatosis. These large nonfollicular pustules are characteristic of this disease. *(Courtesy D. Angarano.)*

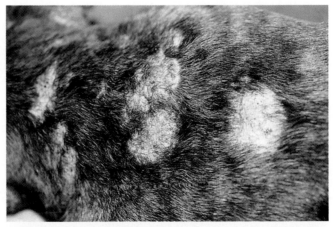

FIGURE 8-97 Canine Subcorneal Pustular Dermatosis. These alopecic, crusting plaques developed after the initial pustular lesions had formed. These generalized lesions will resolve when treated with dapsone.

Sterile Eosinophilic Pustulosis

Features

Sterile eosinophilic pustulosis manifests as a sterile, superficial, pustular skin disease of unknown cause. It is rare in dogs.

Usually, an acute eruption of multifocal to generalized erythematous papules and pustules appears over the trunk, with secondary erosions, circumscribed areas of alopecia, and hyperpigmentation, epidermal collarettes, and scaling. Lesions are pruritic. Concurrent peripheral lymphadenomegaly, depression, anorexia, or fever occasionally may be present.

Top Differentials

Differentials include superficial pyoderma, dermatophytosis, demodicosis, pemphigus foliaceus, systemic lupus erythematosus, drug eruption, and subcorneal pustular dermatosis.

Diagnosis

1. Rule out other differentials.
2. Cytology (pustule): numerous eosinophils are seen. Neutrophils and occasional acantholytic keratinocytes also may be present, but no bacteria are found.
3. Dermatohistopathology: eosinophilic intraepidermal pustules, folliculitis, and furunculosis.

4. Hemogram: peripheral eosinophilia is common.
5. Bacterial culture (pustule): no growth unless secondarily infected.

Treatment and Prognosis

1. Treat as for pemphigus foliaceus (see Table 8-1).
2. Alternatively, treatment with dapsone (as described for subcorneal pustular dermatosis in this chapter) or with a combination antihistamine and fatty acid supplement, may be effective in some dogs.
3. The prognosis for cure is poor, but most dogs can be kept in remission with maintenance medical therapy.

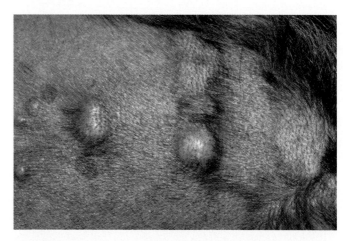

FIGURE 8-99 Sterile Eosinophilic Pustulosis. These large pustules are filled with eosinophils.

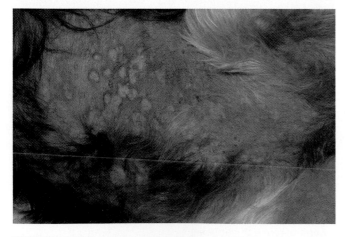

FIGURE 8-98 Sterile Eosinophilic Pustulosis. These large eosinophilic pustules developed over the entire body. Note that the surrounding skin is intensely erythematous.

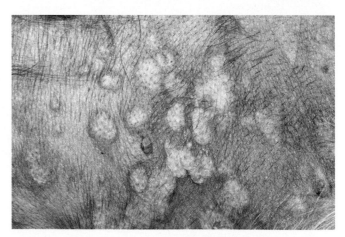

FIGURE 8-100 Sterile Eosinophilic Pustulosis. Numerous large pustules are coalescing on the trunk. Note that the pustules are not centered over hair follicles, which would be suggestive of folliculitis.

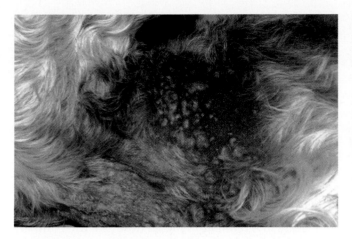

FIGURE 8-101 **Sterile Eosinophilic Pustulosis.** Large fluctuant pustules on the abdomen of a Schnauzer. Note that the purulent exudate is composed almost entirely of eosinophils when examined cytologically.

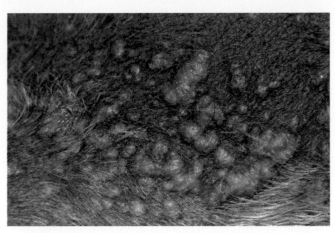

FIGURE 8-102 **Sterile Eosinophilic Pustulosis.** Close-up of the large fluctuant pustules in Figure 8-101, which contain eosinophils almost exclusively.

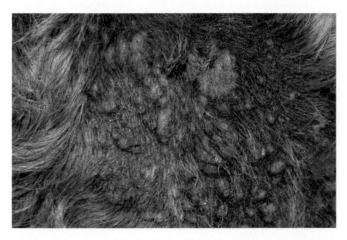

FIGURE 8-103 **Sterile Eosinophilic Pustulosis.** Close-up of the large fluctuant pustules in Figure 8-101, which contain eosinophils almost exclusively.

Sterile Nodular Panniculitis

Features

Sterile nodular panniculitis is an idiopathic inflammatory disease of subcutaneous fat. It is rare in dogs and cats.

Lesions are characterized by one or more deep-seated subcutaneous nodules that may be a few millimeters to a few centimeters in diameter. These nodules may be painful and fluctuant to firm; they may ulcerate and drain a yellowish, oily exudate. Lesions can occur anywhere on the body and in some dogs may wax and wane. Concurrent fever, anorexia, and depression may be present.

Top Differentials

Differentials include infection (bacterial, mycobacteria, fungal), foreign body reaction, drug reaction, postinjection reaction, systemic lupus erythematosus, neoplasia, and vitamin E deficiency (steatitis in cats).

Diagnosis

1. Rule out other differentials.
2. Cytology (aspirate): neutrophils and foamy (lipid-containing) macrophages. No microorganisms are seen.
3. Dermatohistopathology (excisional biopsy): suppurative, pyogranulomatous, granulomatous, eosinophilic, necrotizing, or fibrosing septal or diffuse panniculitis. Special stains do not reveal infectious agents.
4. Microbial cultures (tissue): negative for anaerobic and aerobic bacteria, mycobacteria, and fungi.

Treatment and Prognosis

1. If the lesion is solitary, complete surgical excision is usually curative.
2. To treat or prevent secondary pyoderma in dogs, appropriate long-term systemic antibiotics should be administered (minimum 4 weeks). Dogs treated with antibiotics during the induction phase of immunosuppressive therapy have significantly higher survival rates than dogs treated with immunosuppressive drugs alone. Antibiotics should be continued until concurrent immunosuppressive therapy has the autoimmune disease under control.
3. The goal of treatment is to control the disease and its symptoms with the safest treatments used at the lowest possible doses. Typically, combinations of therapies (see Table 8-1) will have to be used to provide a multimodal treatment plan, minimizing the adverse effects of any one therapy. Depending on the severity of the disease, more or less aggressive treatments will have to be selected. To push the disease into remission, higher doses are used initially and then are tapered over 2 to 3 months to the lowest effective dose.
   a. Conservative systemic treatments (see Table 8-1) include drugs that help reduce inflammation with few to no adverse effects. These treatments help reduce the need for more aggressive therapies such as steroids or chemotherapeutics.
   b. Steroid therapy is one of the most reliably predictable treatments for autoimmune skin disease; however, adverse effects associated with the high doses needed to control symptoms may be severe. Although glucocorticoid therapy alone may be effective in maintaining remission, the dosages needed may result in undesirable adverse effects, especially in dogs. **For this reason, the use of nonsteroidal immunosuppressive drugs, either alone or in combination with glucocorticoids, is usually recommended for long-term maintenance.**
      ■ Immunosuppressive doses of oral prednisone or methylprednisolone should be administered daily (see Table 8-1). After lesions resolve (after approximately 2–8 weeks), the dosage should be gradually tapered over a period of several (8–10) weeks until the lowest possible alternate-day dosage that maintains remission is being administered. If no significant improvement is seen within 2 to 4 weeks of initiation of therapy, concurrent skin infection should be ruled out, then alternative or additional immunosuppressive medications considered.
      ■ Alternative steroids for prednisone- and methylprednisolone-refractory cases include triamcinolone and dexamethasone (see Table 8-1).
      ■ In cats, treatment with immunosuppressive doses of triamcinolone or dexamethasone is often more effective than therapy with prednisolone or methylprednisolone. Oral triamcinolone or dexamethasone should be administered daily until remission is achieved (approximately 2–8 weeks), then the dosage should be gradually tapered until the lowest

possible and least frequent dosage that maintains remission is being administered (see Table 8-1).

- If unacceptable adverse effects develop, or if no significant improvement is seen within 2 to 4 weeks of initiation of therapy, consider using an alternate glucocorticosteroid or a nonsteroidal immunosuppressive drug (see Table 8-1).

4. The prognosis after treatment is good, although healed lesions may leave scars.

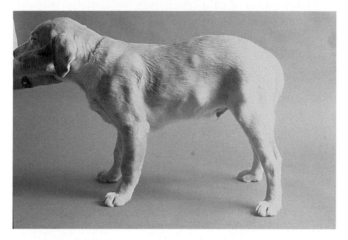

FIGURE 8-104 **Sterile Nodular Panniculitis.** Multiple nodules on the trunk of this young Labrador slowly enlarged and eventually drained. *(Courtesy J. A. MacDonald.)*

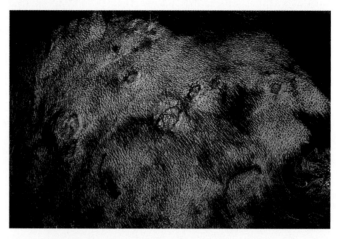

FIGURE 8-106 **Sterile Nodular Panniculitis.** Multiple nodules and draining tracts on the dorsum.

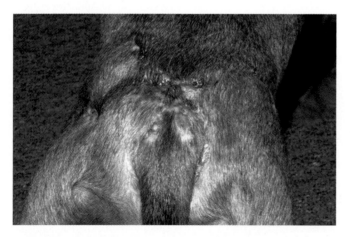

FIGURE 8-105 **Sterile Nodular Panniculitis.** Alopecic nodules with drainage on the lumbar area of an adult Dachshund.

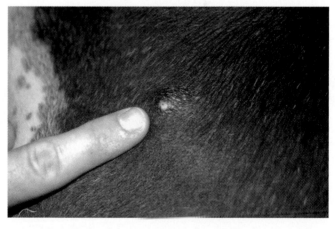

FIGURE 8-107 **Sterile Nodular Panniculitis.** An alopecic nodule on the flank of a dog just before its rupture and drainage.

Sterile Nodular Panniculitis—*cont'd*

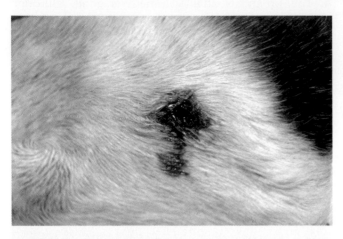

FIGURE 8-108 Sterile Nodular Panniculitis. A ruptured nodule draining a serosanguineous fluid that forms a crust.

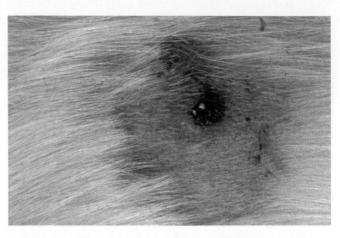

FIGURE 8-109 Sterile Nodular Panniculitis. Nodular lesions often drain a clear oily fluid. *(Courtesy J. A. MacDonald.)*

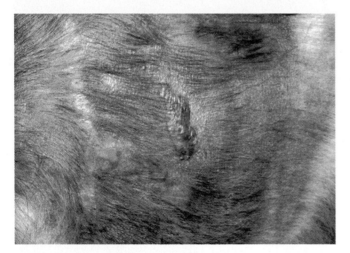

FIGURE 8-110 Sterile Nodular Panniculitis. Alopecic nodules on the trunk. *(Courtesy A. Yu.)*

Idiopathic Sterile Granuloma and Pyogranuloma

Features

Idiopathic sterile granuloma and pyogranuloma is a skin disease that is thought to be immune-mediated, although its exact pathogenesis is unknown. It is uncommon in dogs, with the highest incidences in collies, Golden retrievers, Boxers, and large, short-coated breeds.

It manifests as nonpainful and nonpruritic, firm dermal papules and nodules that may become alopecic or ulcerated. Lesions can appear anywhere on the body but are found most commonly on the bridge of the nose or muzzle, around the eyes, and on the ear pinnae and feet.

Top Differentials

Differentials include infection (bacteria, mycobacteria, fungus), parasites (leishmania, Dirofilaria, tick bites), foreign body reaction, and neoplasia.

Diagnosis

1. Rule out other differentials.
2. Cytology (aspirate): (pyo)granulomatous inflammation with no microorganisms.
3. Dermatohistopathology: nodular to diffuse (pyo) granulomatous dermatitis. Special stains do not reveal infectious agents.
4. Microbial cultures (tissue): negative for anaerobic and aerobic bacteria, mycobacteria, and fungi

Treatment and Prognosis

1. Solitary lesions should be surgically excised, if possible.
2. For nonsurgical or multiple lesions, treat as for pemphigus foliaceus (see Table 8-1).
3. The prognosis is good for most dogs, although life-long therapy may be needed for some dogs.

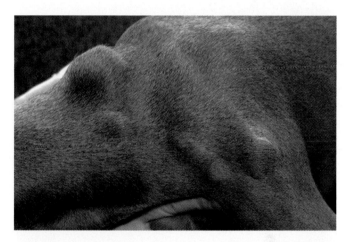

FIGURE 8-112 Idiopathic Sterile Granuloma and Pyogranuloma. Same dog as in Figure 8-111. Large granulomas on the neck and shoulder progressively enlarged over previous weeks.

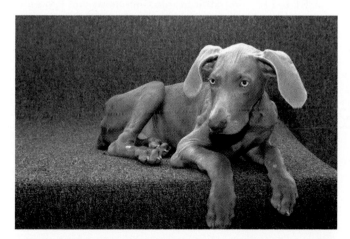

FIGURE 8-111 Idiopathic Sterile Granuloma and Pyogranuloma. Multiple large granulomas in a young Weimaraner puppy.

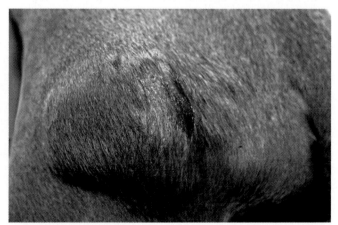

FIGURE 8-113 Idiopathic Sterile Granuloma and Pyogranuloma. Same dog as in Figure 8-111. Numerous large granulomas covered the puppy's entire body.

Idiopathic Sterile Granuloma and Pyogranuloma—*cont'd*

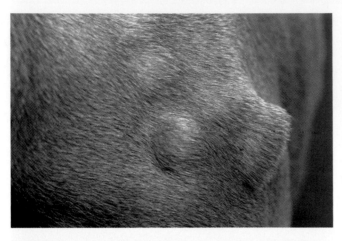

FIGURE 8-114 **Idiopathic Sterile Granuloma and Pyogranuloma.** Same dog as in Figure 8-111. Large granulomas over the shoulder.

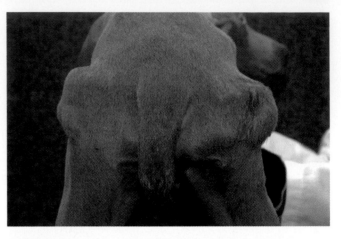

FIGURE 8-115 **Idiopathic Sterile Granuloma and Pyogranuloma.** Same dog as in Figure 8-111. Two large granulomas over the pelvis were bilaterally symmetrical.

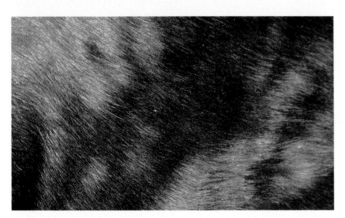

FIGURE 8-116 **Idiopathic Sterile Granuloma and Pyogranuloma.** Numerous small granulomas on the trunk of a dog. The hair coat appears wavy or undulating, but the granulomas are easily palpated.

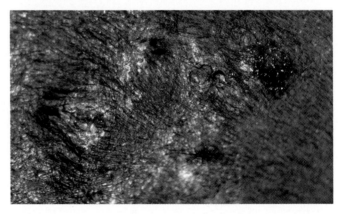

FIGURE 8-117 **Idiopathic Sterile Granuloma and Pyogranuloma.** Multiple granulomas that have ruptured and drained a serosanguineous fluid, which formed crusts.

Canine Eosinophilic Granuloma

Features

Canine eosinophilic granuloma is an eosinophilic disease characterized by nodules and plaques in the mouth or tonsils, or on the skin. The exact cause is unknown, but skin lesions may represent a hypersensitivity reaction to arthropod bites or stings. It is rare in dogs, with the highest incidences reported in young Siberian huskies and Cavalier King Charles spaniels.

Oral lesions are characterized by plaques or proliferative masses. These are most commonly found on the palate and the lateral or ventral aspect of the tongue. Oral lesions may be painful. Halitosis is usually the presenting complaint.

Cutaneous lesions are papules, plaques, and nodules. These are neither painful nor pruritic and most commonly occur on the ventral abdomen and flanks.

Top Differentials

Differentials include bacterial and fungal granulomas and neoplasia.

Diagnosis

1. Rule out other differentials.
2. Dermatohistopathology: eosinophilic and histiocytic granulomas with foci of collagen degeneration.
3. Microbial cultures (biopsy specimens): negative for anaerobic and aerobic bacteria, mycobacteria, and fungi.

Treatment and Prognosis

1. Solitary lesions may regress spontaneously without therapy.
2. Symptomatic therapy as for atopy (antihistamines to reduce and control eosinophilic reactions, essential fatty acids, cyclosporine) may be helpful (see Chapter 7).
3. Systemic glucocorticoid therapy is usually curative. Prednisone 0.5–2.0 mg/kg PO should be administered every 24 hours until lesions resolve (approximately 2–3 weeks), then should be tapered off.
4. The prognosis is good.

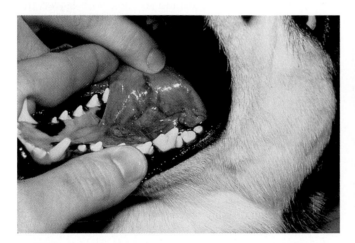

FIGURE 8-118 Canine Eosinophilic Granuloma. An eosinophilic plaque on the tongue of a Siberian husky. *(Courtesy J. Noxon.)*

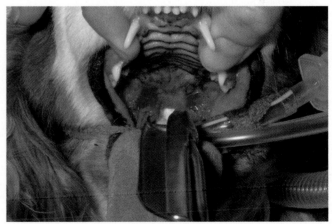

FIGURE 8-119 Canine Eosinophilic Granuloma. Eosinophilic granulomatous inflammation of the tonsils in a Cavalier King Charles spaniel.

Cutaneous Vasculitis

Features

Cutaneous vasculitis is an inflammatory disease of blood vessels that is usually secondary to immune complex deposition within the vessel walls. Vasculitis may be associated with underlying infection (bacterial, rickettsial, viral, fungal), malignancy, food hypersensitivity, drug reaction, rabies vaccination, metabolic disease (diabetes mellitus, uremia), systemic lupus erythematosus, or exposure to cold (cold agglutinin disease), or it may be idiopathic. It is uncommon in dogs and rare in cats.

In most cases, clinical signs are characterized by purpura, necrosis, and punctate ulcers, especially on the ear pinnae, lips, oral mucosa, footpads, tail, and scrotum. Acrocyanosis may be seen. Urticarial vasculitis (acute onset of intense erythroderma with coalescing erythematous wheals that do not blanche) has been described in dogs with underlying food hypersensitivity. In some dogs with rabies vaccine–induced alopecia, the focal area of alopecia that develops at the site of vaccination is followed 1 to 5 months later by the appearance of multifocal cutaneous lesions caused by generalized ischemic dermatopathy. These lesions are characterized by variable alopecia, crusting, hyperpigmentation, erosions, and ulcers on the pinnal margins, periocular areas, skin overlying bony prominences, tip of the tail, and footpads. Lingual erosions and ulcers also may be seen. Animals with cutaneous vasculitis may have concurrent anorexia, depression, fever, arthropathy, myopathy, and pitting edema of the extremities.

Top Differentials

Differentials include systemic lupus erythematosus, erythema multiforme/toxic epidermal necrolysis, bullous pemphigoid, pemphigus vulgaris, frostbite, and cutaneous drug reaction. For dogs with ear pinnal lesions only, the differentials should also include ear margin dermatosis.

Diagnosis

1. Rule out other differentials.
2. Titers for rickettsial infection should be performed to rule out tick-borne disease.
3. Dermatohistopathology: neutrophilic, eosinophilic, or lymphocytic vasculitis. In rabies vaccine–induced ischemic dermatopathy, cases of moderate to severe follicular atrophy, hyalinization of collagen, cell-poor interface dermatitis, and mural folliculitis may occur.

Treatment and Prognosis

1. Any underlying cause should be identified and corrected.
2. To treat or prevent secondary pyoderma in dogs, appropriate long-term systemic antibiotics should be administered (minimum 4 weeks). Dogs treated with antibiotics during the induction phase of immunosuppressive therapy have significantly higher survival rates than dogs treated with immunosuppressive drugs alone. Antibiotics should be continued until concurrent immunosuppressive therapy has the autoimmune disease under control.
3. The goal of treatment is to control the disease and its symptoms with the safest treatments used at the lowest possible doses. Typically, combinations of therapies (see Table 8-1) will have to be used to provide a multimodal treatment plan, minimizing the adverse effects of any one therapy. Depending on the severity of the disease, more or less aggressive treatments will have to be selected. To push the disease into remission, higher doses are used initially and then are tapered over 2 to 3 months to the lowest effective dose.
   a. Topical therapy applied every 12 hours with steroid-containing products or tacrolimus will help reduce focal inflammation and will lower the doses of systemic treatments required to control symptoms. Once in remission, the frequency of application should be minimized to reduce local adverse effects.
   b. Conservative systemic treatments (see Table 8-1) include drugs that help reduce inflammation with few to no adverse effects. These treatments help reduce the need for more aggressive therapy such as steroids or chemotherapeutics.
   c. Steroid therapy is one of the most reliably predictable treatments for autoimmune skin disease; however, adverse effects associated with the high doses needed to control symptoms may be severe. Although glucocorticoid therapy alone may be effective in maintaining remission, the dosages needed may result in undesirable adverse effects, especially in dogs. **For this reason, the use of nonsteroidal immunosuppressive drugs, alone or in combination with glucocorticoids, is usually recommended for long-term maintenance.**
      ■ Immunosuppressive doses of oral prednisone or methylprednisolone should be administered daily (see Table 8-1). After lesions resolve (after approximately 2–8 weeks), the dosage

should be gradually tapered over a period of several (8–10) weeks until the lowest possible alternate-day dosage that maintains remission is being administered. If no significant improvement is seen within 2 to 4 weeks of initiation of therapy, concurrent skin infection should be ruled out, then alternative or additional immunosuppressive medications considered.

- Alternative steroids for prednisone- and methylprednisolone-refractory cases include triamcinolone and dexamethasone (see Table 8-1).
- In cats, treatment with immunosuppressive doses of triamcinolone or dexamethasone often is more effective than therapy with prednisolone or methylprednisolone. Oral triamcinolone or dexamethasone should be administered daily until remission is achieved (approximately 2–8 weeks), then the dosage should be gradually tapered until the lowest possible and least frequent dosage that maintains remission is being administered (see Table 8-1).
- If unacceptable adverse effects develop, or if no significant improvement is seen within 2 to 4 weeks of initiation of therapy, consider using an alternate glucocorticosteroid or a nonsteroidal immunosuppressive drug (see Table 8-1).

d. Alternative therapies that may be effective include the following:

- Dapsone (dogs only) 1 mg/kg PO q 8 hours until lesions resolve (approximately 2–3 weeks). Once remission is achieved, the dosage is slowly tapered by giving 1 mg/kg PO q 12 hours for 2 weeks, then 1 mg/kg q 24 hours for 2 weeks, followed by 1 mg/kg q 48 hours.
- Sulfasalazine 10–20 mg/kg (maximum 3 g/day) PO q 8 hours until lesions resolve (approximately 2–4 weeks). Once remission is achieved, the dosage is tapered by giving 10 mg/kg q 12 hours for 3 weeks, followed by 10 mg/kg PO q 24 hours.

e. Nonsteroidal immunosuppressive drugs that may be effective include cyclosporine (Atopica), azathioprine (dogs only), chlorambucil, cyclophosphamide, mycophenolate mofetil, and leflunomide (see Table 8-1). A beneficial response occurs within 8 to 12 weeks of initiation of therapy. Once remission is achieved, gradually attempt to taper the dosage and frequency of the nonsteroidal immunosuppressive drug for long-term maintenance.

4. Regardless of the drug used, in some patients, therapy eventually can be discontinued after 4 to 6 months; in others, long-term maintenance therapy is needed to maintain remission.

5. The prognosis is variable, depending on the underlying cause, the extent of cutaneous lesions, and the degree of involvement of other organs.

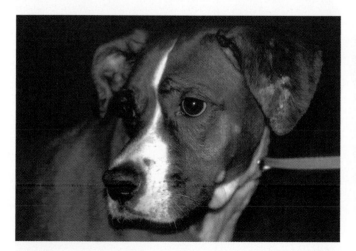

FIGURE 8-120 Cutaneous Vasculitis. Alopecic, crusting lesions on the ear pinnae. The nasal planum is unaffected. Note the similarity to scabies; however, this dog was minimally pruritic.

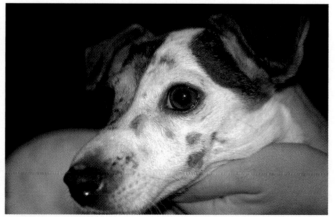

FIGURE 8-121 Cutaneous Vasculitis. Alopecic, erythematous lesions on the face of an adult Jack Russell terrier.

Cutaneous Vasculitis—*cont'd*

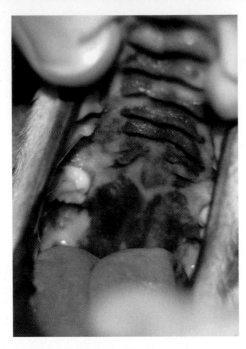

FIGURE 8-122 **Cutaneous Vasculitis.** Same dog as in Figure 8-121. Erosive lesions on the palate are typical of vasculitis. Lesions on the oral mucosa are commonly seen with vasculitis, pemphigus vulgaris, bullous pemphigoid, and systemic lupus erythematosus (SLE).

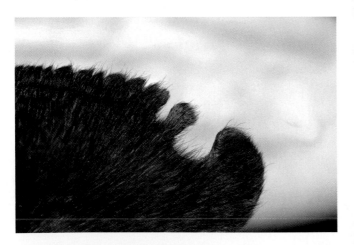

FIGURE 8-124 **Cutaneous Vasculitis.** Multiple notch defects on the ear margin of an adult Dachshund. No inflammation is evident to indicate active vasculitis.

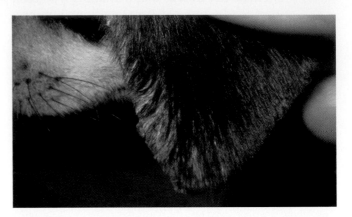

FIGURE 8-123 **Cutaneous Vasculitis.** Alopecic, crusting lesions on the ear margin are typical of vasculitis. Note the similarity to scabies; however, this dog is not intensely pruritic.

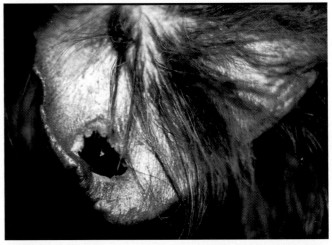

FIGURE 8-125 **Cutaneous Vasculitis.** A large notch defect caused by chronic vasculitis on the ear pinna.

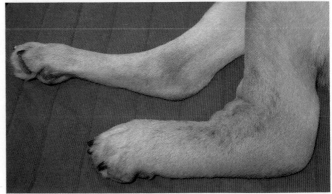

FIGURE 8-126 **Cutaneous Vasculitis.** Peripheral edema caused by vascular leakage associated with vasculitis.

...ema Multiforme (EM) and Toxic Epidermal Necrolysis (TEN)

...ures

...pathogenesis of these two diseases is unknown, ...may represent a host-specific cell-mediated ...nsitivity reaction induced by various antigens ...hemicals, drugs, infectious agents [bacteria, ...], malignancies) that alter keratinocytes, making ...targets of an aberrant immune response. Some ...igators believe that EM and TEN are two distinct ...ses; others believe that TEN is a more severe clini-...form of EM. These diseases are uncommon in dogs ...rare in cats.

...Lesions often develop over the dorsum and resemble ...thermal (heating pad) or chemical burn. Lesions ...sually occur acutely and are multifocal to diffuse. The ...skin, mucocutaneous junctions, and oral cavity may be ...involved. Erythema multiforme is characterized by ery-...thematous macules to slightly raised papules or plaques ...that spread peripherally and clear centrally to produce ...annular or serpiginous "target" or "bulls-eye" lesions. ...Rarely, generalized scaling, crusting, erythema, and alo-...pecia may occur. Toxic epidermal necrolysis is character-...ized by painful vesicles, bullae, ulcers, and epidermal ...necrosis. Concurrent depression, anorexia, and fever ...may be present, especially with TEN.

Top Differentials

Differentials include thermal or chemical burn, urti-caria, deep infection (bacterial, fungal), bullous pemphigoid, pemphigus vulgaris, systemic lupus ery-thematosus, vesicular cutaneous lupus erythematosus, vasculitis, epitheliotropic lymphoma, and cutaneous drug reaction.

Diagnosis

1. Rule out other differentials.
2. Dermatohistopathology: damage is limited to the epidermis with individual keratinocyte necrosis (apoptosis) to full-thickness necrosis of the epider-mis. The epithelial cells of outer root sheaths of hair follicles may be similarly affected. Biopsy should be performed early to differentiate from a burn (damage in the deep dermal tissues).

Treatment and Prognosis

1. Discontinue the use of all suspect drugs adminis-tered within 2 to 4 weeks before lesion development, and do not use any related drugs or drugs with a similar chemical structure. In cases with no known drug or chemical exposure, one should thoroughly

search for an underlying infectious disease or neoplasia.
2. Appropriate symptomatic and supportive care (e.g., whirlpool baths, fluids, electrolytes, parenteral nutri-tion) should be provided as needed. To prevent sec-ondary bacterial skin infection, systemic antibiotics that are unrelated to any suspect drugs should be administered.
3. Mild cases of EM may resolve spontaneously within 2 to 4 weeks.
4. Treat as for pemphigus foliaceus (see Table 8-1).
5. In more severe cases, treatment with prednisone 2 mg/kg (dogs) or 4 mg/kg (cats) PO every 24 hours may be helpful. Significant improvement may be seen within 1 to 2 weeks. After lesions resolve (approximately 2–8 weeks), the dosage should be gradually tapered over a period of 4 to 6 weeks. In most cases, steroid therapy can be discontinued.
6. For refractory cases, treatment with human intrave-nous immunoglobulin (IVIG) may be effective. A 5% to 6% solution of human IVIG is prepared with the use of saline (0.9% NaCl), according to the man-ufacturer's recommendations. Then, 0.5 to 1 g/kg is infused IV over a 4- to 6-hour period, once or twice, 24 hours apart.
7. The prognosis is fair to good for EM and poor to guarded for TEN, especially if an underlying cause cannot be found.

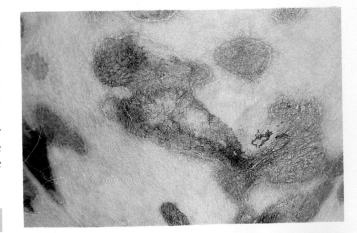

FIGURE 8-141 Erythema Multiforme and Toxic Epidermal Necrolysis. Well-demarcated areas of erythema, erosion, and hyperpigmentation. Note the distinct, well-demarcated serpen-tine borders, which are typical of vasculitis, cutaneous drug reac-tions, or autoimmune skin disease.

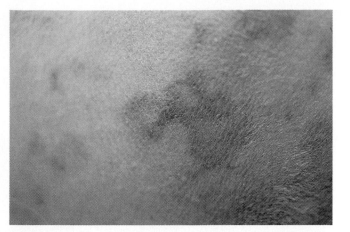

FIGURE 8-127 Cutaneous Vasculitis. This erythematous lesion with a well-demarcated serpentine border is characteristic of vasculitis, cutaneous drug reactions (erythema multiforme), or autoimmune skin disease.

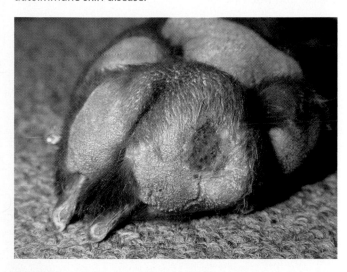

FIGURE 8-129 Cutaneous Vasculitis. A focal ulcerative lesion on the center of the footpad is a unique feature of vascular disease.

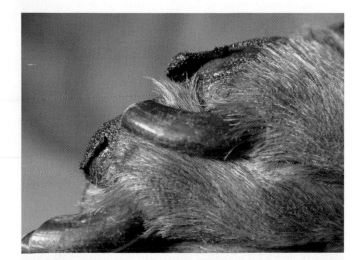

FIGURE 8-131 Cutaneous Vasculitis. Sloughing of the foot-pads in a dog with vasculitis. Footpad lesions can also be seen with autoimmune skin disease.

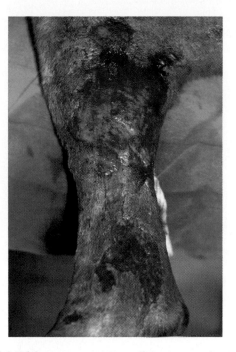

FIGURE 8-128 Cutaneous Vasculitis. Severe ulcerative der-matitis on the leg of an adult Greyhound. Note the well-demar-cated serpentine border, which is characteristic of vasculitis, cutaneous drug reactions (erythema multiforme), or autoim-mune skin disease.

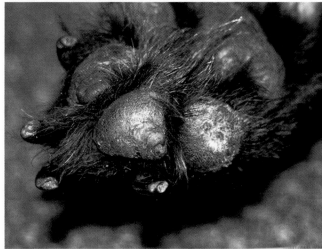

FIGURE 8-130 Cutaneous Vasculitis. Crusting lesions on the footpad (especially central pad lesions) are unique features of vasculitis.

Cutaneous Vasculitis—cont'd

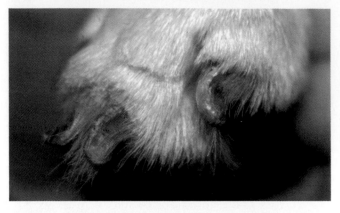

FIGURE 8-132 **Cutaneous Vasculitis.** Sloughing and dystrophic formation of the nails are common features of vasculitis. Note the similarity to autoimmune skin disease or lupoid onychodystrophy.

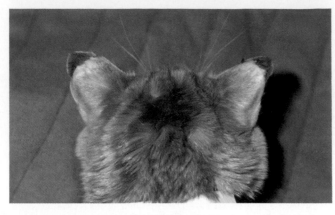

FIGURE 8-133 **Cutaneous Vasculitis.** Necrosis of the ear tips in a cat with vasculitis.

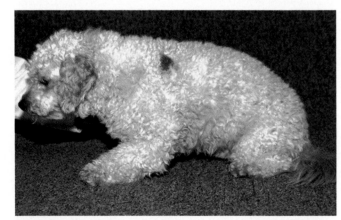

FIGURE 8-134 **Cutaneous Vasculitis.** A focal alopecic, hyperpigmented lesion at the site of previous rabies vaccine administration. Vaccine reactions are often associated with vasculitis.

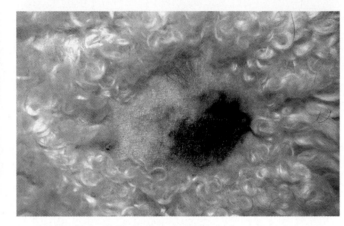

FIGURE 8-135 **Cutaneous Vasculitis.** Close-up of the dog in Figure 8-134. The focal area of alopecia with hyperpigmentation is typical of rabies vaccine reactions. A focal vasculitis lesion or generalized vasculitis can develop weeks to months after vaccine administration.

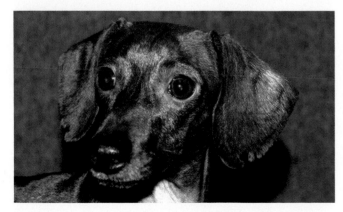

FIGURE 8-136 **Cutaneous Vasculitis.** An adult Dachshund with bilateral notched ears typical of vasculitis.

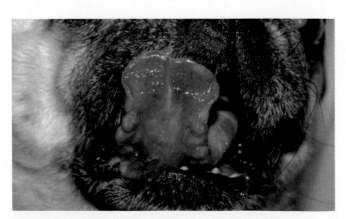

FIGURE 8-137 **Cutaneous Vasculitis.** Lingual erosions and ulcerations caused by cutaneous vasculitis. Oral lesions are less common than ear-margin and footpad crusting, ulcerated lesions.

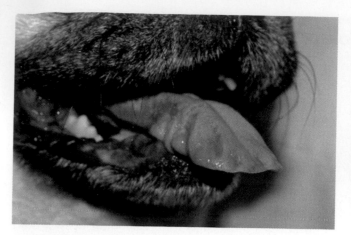

FIGURE 8-138 **Cutaneous Vasculitis.** Same dog as in Figure 8-137. Multifocal erosions on the lateral margin of the tongue are apparent.

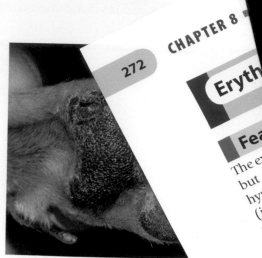

FIGURE 8-139 Cutaneous Vascul on the footpads of a dog with vascu center of the affected footpad is a n presentation.

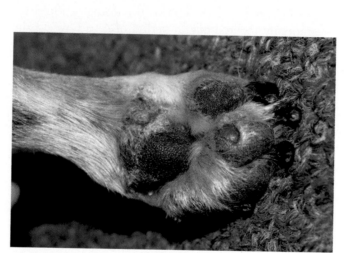

FIGURE 8-140 **Cutaneous Vasculitis.** Ulcerations on the footpads of a dog with vasculitis.

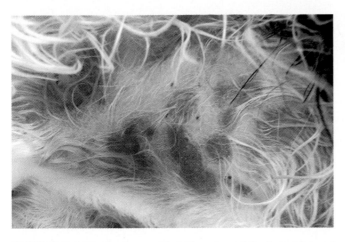

FIGURE 8-142 Erythema Multiforme and Toxic Epidermal Necrolysis. Focal areas of erosive dermatitis on the inguinal surface. Note the well-demarcated borders, which are characteristic.

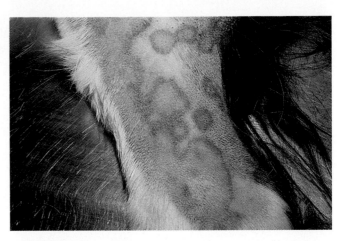

FIGURE 8-143 Erythema Multiforme and Toxic Epidermal Necrolysis. Erythematous lesions on the distal limb of an adult dog. The well-demarcated serpentine margins are apparent.

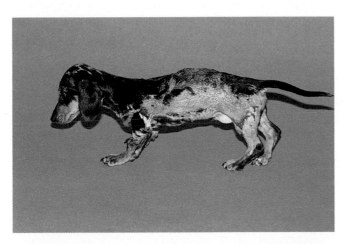

FIGURE 8-144 Erythema Multiforme and Toxic Epidermal Necrolysis. Alopecia, crusting, ulceration, and granulation tissue on the dorsum of a 6-month-old Dachshund. Epidermal necrosis developed over several weeks after routine vaccination.

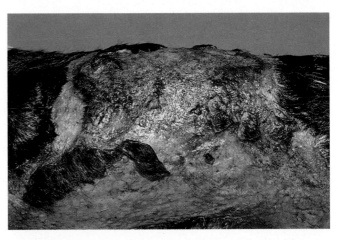

FIGURE 8-145 Erythema Multiforme and Toxic Epidermal Necrolysis. Close-up of the dog in Figure 8-144. The lesion was beginning to form granulation tissue. The remaining skin was necrotic and will eventually slough.

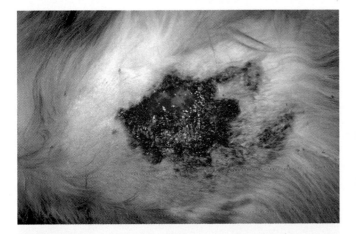

FIGURE 8-146 Erythema Multiforme and Toxic Epidermal Necrolysis. A focal area of full-thickness necrosis. Note the well-demarcated serpentine margin, which is characteristic.

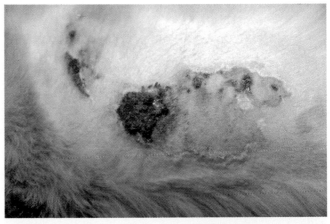

FIGURE 8-147 Erythema Multiforme and Toxic Epidermal Necrolysis. Well-demarcated erythema, with crusts covering areas of full-thickness necrosis. Note the progression of lesions from well-demarcated serpentine erythema to crusting lesions that conceal the epidermal necrosis. Over time, the entire area will likely necrose and slough.

Erythema Multiforme (EM) and Toxic Epidermal Necrolysis (TEN)—cont'd

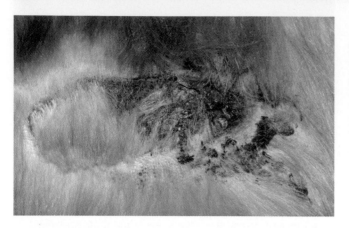

FIGURE 8-148 Erythema Multiforme and Toxic Epidermal Necrolysis. Focal area of cutaneous necrosis with ulceration and crusting. Note the well-demarcated margins, which are typical of a cutaneous drug reaction.

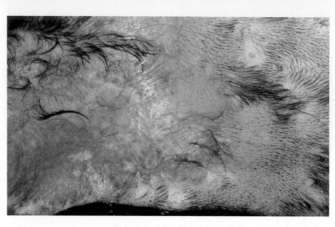

FIGURE 8-149 Erythema Multiforme and Toxic Epidermal Necrolysis. Well-demarcated alopecic erosions are very characteristic of a cutaneous drug reaction, including erythema multiforme. Note the classic serpentine margins.

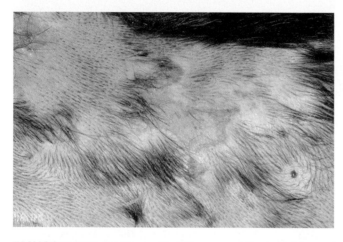

FIGURE 8-150 Erythema Multiforme and Toxic Epidermal Necrolysis. Multiple focal areas of alopecia and erosion in the characteristic well-demarcated serpentine pattern.

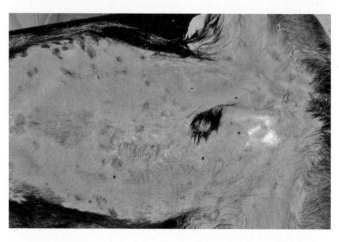

FIGURE 8-151 Erythema Multiforme and Toxic Epidermal Necrolysis. Generalized lesion on the abdomen of an affected dog. Note the widespread well-demarcated erosive lesions.

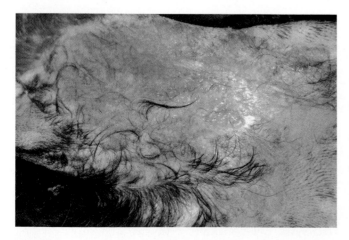

FIGURE 8-152 Erythema Multiforme and Toxic Epidermal Necrolysis. Close-up of a severely erosive lesion demonstrating the characteristic demarcation typical of this disease.

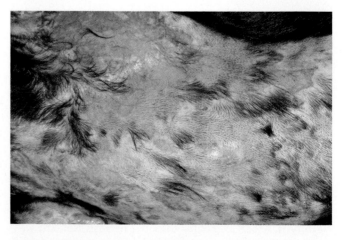

FIGURE 8-153 Erythema Multiforme and Toxic Epidermal Necrolysis. Generalized erosive dermatitis on the abdomen of an affected dog.

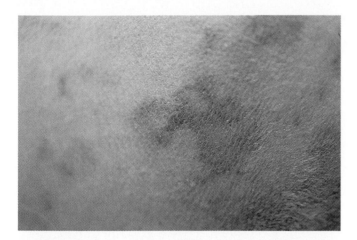

FIGURE 8-127 Cutaneous Vasculitis. This erythematous lesion with a well-demarcated serpentine border is characteristic of vasculitis, cutaneous drug reactions (erythema multiforme), or autoimmune skin disease.

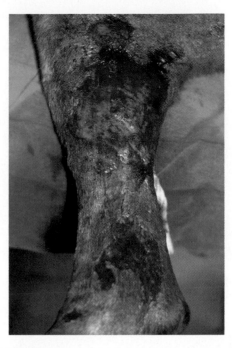

FIGURE 8-128 Cutaneous Vasculitis. Severe ulcerative dermatitis on the leg of an adult Greyhound. Note the well-demarcated serpentine border, which is characteristic of vasculitis, cutaneous drug reactions (erythema multiforme), or autoimmune skin disease.

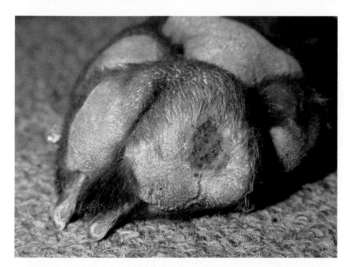

FIGURE 8-129 Cutaneous Vasculitis. A focal ulcerative lesion on the center of the footpad is a unique feature of vascular disease.

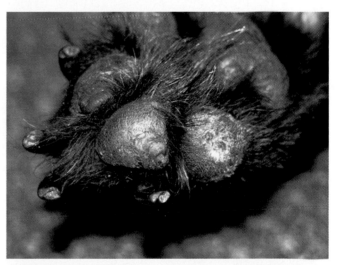

FIGURE 8-130 Cutaneous Vasculitis. Crusting lesions on the footpad (especially central pad lesions) are unique features of vasculitis.

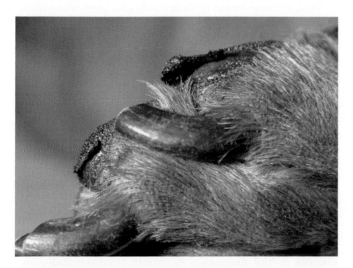

FIGURE 8-131 Cutaneous Vasculitis. Sloughing of the footpads in a dog with vasculitis. Footpad lesions can also be seen with autoimmune skin disease.

Cutaneous Vasculitis—*cont'd*

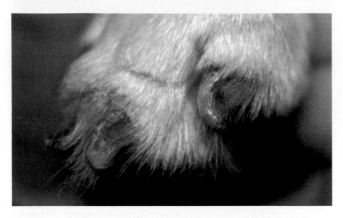

FIGURE 8-132 Cutaneous Vasculitis. Sloughing and dystrophic formation of the nails are common features of vasculitis. Note the similarity to autoimmune skin disease or lupoid onychodystrophy.

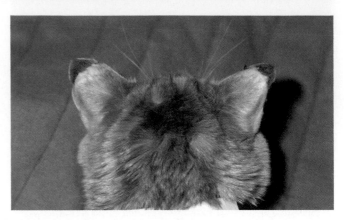

FIGURE 8-133 Cutaneous Vasculitis. Necrosis of the ear tips in a cat with vasculitis.

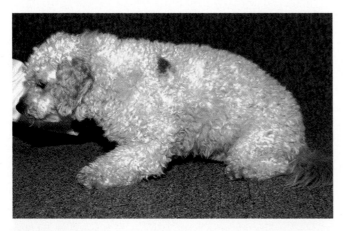

FIGURE 8-134 Cutaneous Vasculitis. A focal alopecic, hyperpigmented lesion at the site of previous rabies vaccine administration. Vaccine reactions are often associated with vasculitis.

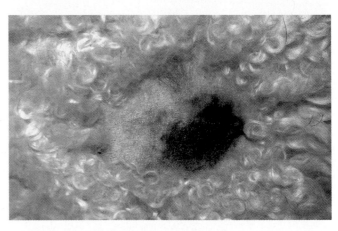

FIGURE 8-135 Cutaneous Vasculitis. Close-up of the dog in Figure 8-134. The focal area of alopecia with hyperpigmentation is typical of rabies vaccine reactions. A focal vasculitis lesion or generalized vasculitis can develop weeks to months after vaccine administration.

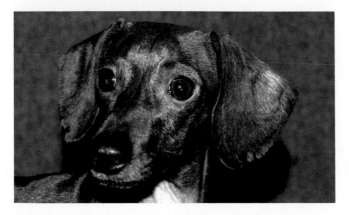

FIGURE 8-136 Cutaneous Vasculitis. An adult Dachshund with bilateral notched ears typical of vasculitis.

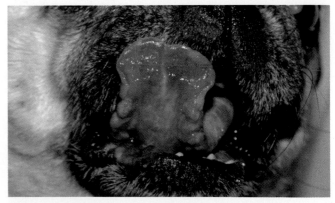

FIGURE 8-137 Cutaneous Vasculitis. Lingual erosions and ulcerations caused by cutaneous vasculitis. Oral lesions are less common than ear-margin and footpad crusting, ulcerated lesions.

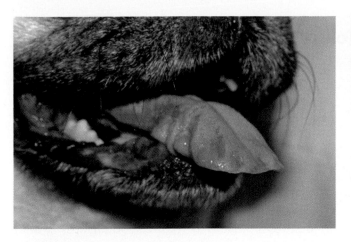

FIGURE 8-138 Cutaneous Vasculitis. Same dog as in Figure 8-137. Multifocal erosions on the lateral margin of the tongue are apparent.

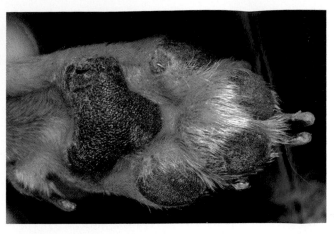

FIGURE 8-139 Cutaneous Vasculitis. Multifocal ulcerations on the footpads of a dog with vasculitis. Focal lesion at the center of the affected footpad is a more common clinical presentation.

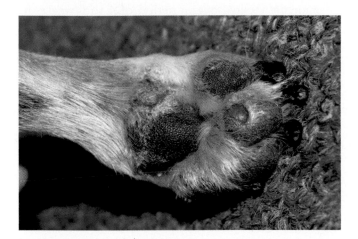

FIGURE 8-140 Cutaneous Vasculitis. Ulcerations on the footpads of a dog with vasculitis.

Erythema Multiforme (EM) and Toxic Epidermal Necrolysis (TEN)

Features

The exact pathogenesis of these two diseases is unknown, but they may represent a host-specific cell-mediated hypersensitivity reaction induced by various antigens (i.e., chemicals, drugs, infectious agents [bacteria, viruses], malignancies) that alter keratinocytes, making them targets of an aberrant immune response. Some investigators believe that EM and TEN are two distinct diseases; others believe that TEN is a more severe clinical form of EM. These diseases are uncommon in dogs and rare in cats.

Lesions often develop over the dorsum and resemble a thermal (heating pad) or chemical burn. Lesions usually occur acutely and are multifocal to diffuse. The skin, mucocutaneous junctions, and oral cavity may be involved. Erythema multiforme is characterized by erythematous macules to slightly raised papules or plaques that spread peripherally and clear centrally to produce annular or serpiginous "target" or "bulls-eye" lesions. Rarely, generalized scaling, crusting, erythema, and alopecia may occur. Toxic epidermal necrolysis is characterized by painful vesicles, bullae, ulcers, and epidermal necrosis. Concurrent depression, anorexia, and fever may be present, especially with TEN.

Top Differentials

Differentials include thermal or chemical burn, urticaria, deep infection (bacterial, fungal), bullous pemphigoid, pemphigus vulgaris, systemic lupus erythematosus, vesicular cutaneous lupus erythematosus, vasculitis, epitheliotropic lymphoma, and cutaneous drug reaction.

Diagnosis

1. Rule out other differentials.
2. Dermatohistopathology: damage is limited to the epidermis with individual keratinocyte necrosis (apoptosis) to full-thickness necrosis of the epidermis. The epithelial cells of outer root sheaths of hair follicles may be similarly affected. Biopsy should be performed early to differentiate from a burn (damage in the deep dermal tissues).

Treatment and Prognosis

1. Discontinue the use of all suspect drugs administered within 2 to 4 weeks before lesion development, and do not use any related drugs or drugs with a similar chemical structure. In cases with no known drug or chemical exposure, one should thoroughly search for an underlying infectious disease or neoplasia.
2. Appropriate symptomatic and supportive care (e.g., whirlpool baths, fluids, electrolytes, parenteral nutrition) should be provided as needed. To prevent secondary bacterial skin infection, systemic antibiotics that are unrelated to any suspect drugs should be administered.
3. Mild cases of EM may resolve spontaneously within 2 to 4 weeks.
4. Treat as for pemphigus foliaceus (see Table 8-1).
5. In more severe cases, treatment with prednisone 2 mg/kg (dogs) or 4 mg/kg (cats) PO every 24 hours may be helpful. Significant improvement may be seen within 1 to 2 weeks. After lesions resolve (approximately 2–8 weeks), the dosage should be gradually tapered over a period of 4 to 6 weeks. In most cases, steroid therapy can be discontinued.
6. For refractory cases, treatment with human intravenous immunoglobulin (IVIG) may be effective. A 5% to 6% solution of human IVIG is prepared with the use of saline (0.9% NaCl), according to the manufacturer's recommendations. Then, 0.5 to 1 g/kg is infused IV over a 4- to 6-hour period, once or twice, 24 hours apart.
7. The prognosis is fair to good for EM and poor to guarded for TEN, especially if an underlying cause cannot be found.

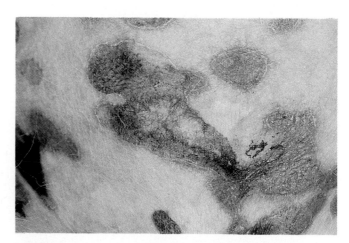

FIGURE 8-141 Erythema Multiforme and Toxic Epidermal Necrolysis. Well-demarcated areas of erythema, erosion, and hyperpigmentation. Note the distinct, well-demarcated serpentine borders, which are typical of vasculitis, cutaneous drug reactions, or autoimmune skin disease.

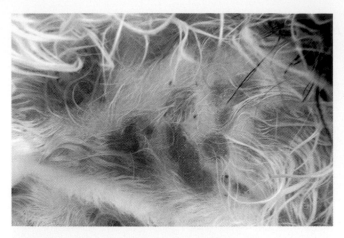

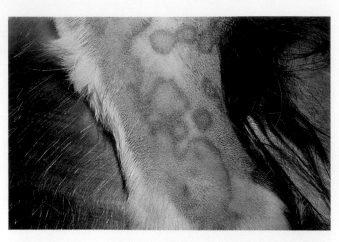

FIGURE 8-142 Erythema Multiforme and Toxic Epidermal Necrolysis. Focal areas of erosive dermatitis on the inguinal surface. Note the well-demarcated borders, which are characteristic.

FIGURE 8-143 Erythema Multiforme and Toxic Epidermal Necrolysis. Erythematous lesions on the distal limb of an adult dog. The well-demarcated serpentine margins are apparent.

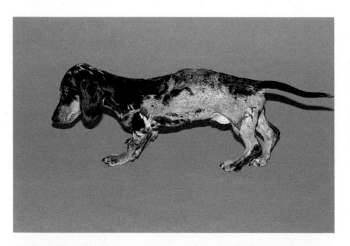

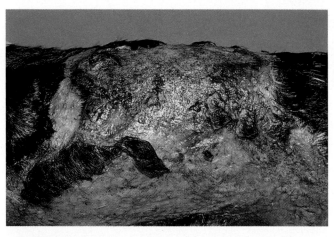

FIGURE 8-144 Erythema Multiforme and Toxic Epidermal Necrolysis. Alopecia, crusting, ulceration, and granulation tissue on the dorsum of a 6-month-old Dachshund. Epidermal necrosis developed over several weeks after routine vaccination.

FIGURE 8-145 Erythema Multiforme and Toxic Epidermal Necrolysis. Close-up of the dog in Figure 8-144. The lesion was beginning to form granulation tissue. The remaining skin was necrotic and will eventually slough.

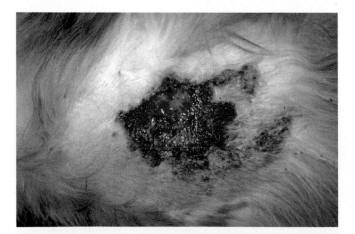

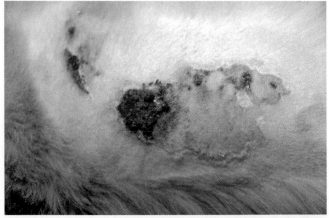

FIGURE 8-146 Erythema Multiforme and Toxic Epidermal Necrolysis. A focal area of full-thickness necrosis. Note the well-demarcated serpentine margin, which is characteristic.

FIGURE 8-147 Erythema Multiforme and Toxic Epidermal Necrolysis. Well-demarcated erythema, with crusts covering areas of full-thickness necrosis. Note the progression of lesions from well-demarcated serpentine erythema to crusting lesions that conceal the epidermal necrosis. Over time, the entire area will likely necrose and slough.

Erythema Multiforme (EM) and Toxic Epidermal Necrolysis (TEN)—*cont'd*

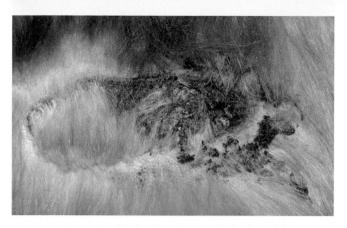

FIGURE 8-148 **Erythema Multiforme and Toxic Epidermal Necrolysis.** Focal area of cutaneous necrosis with ulceration and crusting. Note the well-demarcated margins, which are typical of a cutaneous drug reaction.

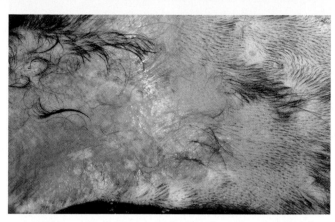

FIGURE 8-149 **Erythema Multiforme and Toxic Epidermal Necrolysis.** Well-demarcated alopecic erosions are very characteristic of a cutaneous drug reaction, including erythema multiforme. Note the classic serpentine margins.

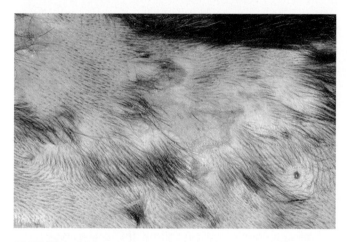

FIGURE 8-150 **Erythema Multiforme and Toxic Epidermal Necrolysis.** Multiple focal areas of alopecia and erosion in the characteristic well-demarcated serpentine pattern.

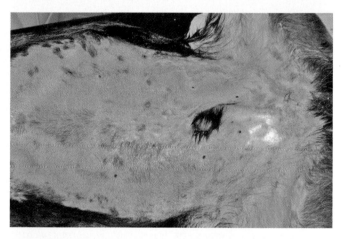

FIGURE 8-151 **Erythema Multiforme and Toxic Epidermal Necrolysis.** Generalized lesion on the abdomen of an affected dog. Note the widespread well-demarcated erosive lesions.

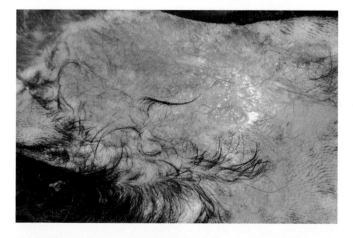

FIGURE 8-152 **Erythema Multiforme and Toxic Epidermal Necrolysis.** Close-up of a severely erosive lesion demonstrating the characteristic demarcation typical of this disease.

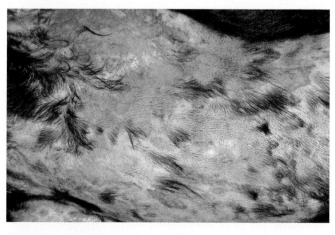

FIGURE 8-153 **Erythema Multiforme and Toxic Epidermal Necrolysis.** Generalized erosive dermatitis on the abdomen of an affected dog.

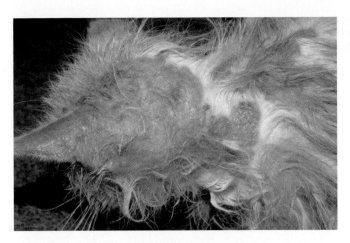

FIGURE 8-154 **Erythema Multiforme and Toxic Epidermal Necrolysis.** Characteristic, well-demarcated lesions in a cat typical of cutaneous drug reaction and vasculitis.

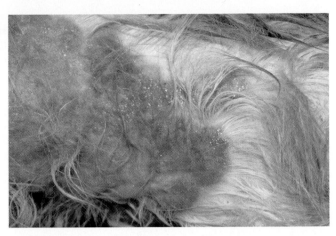

FIGURE 8-155 **Erythema Multiforme and Toxic Epidermal Necrolysis.** Well-demarcated erythematous dermatitis on the neck of a cat.

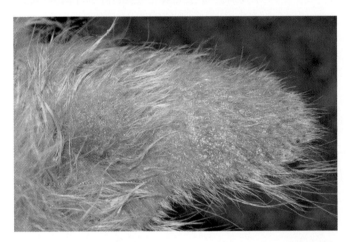

FIGURE 8-156 **Erythema Multiforme and Toxic Epidermal Necrolysis.** Severe erythema with alopecia and scale formation on the ear pinna of a cat.

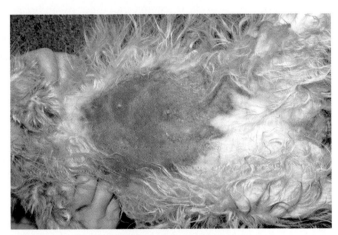

FIGURE 8-157 **Erythema Multiforme and Toxic Epidermal Necrolysis.** Severe erythema and alopecia in a focal well-demarcated lesion on a cat.

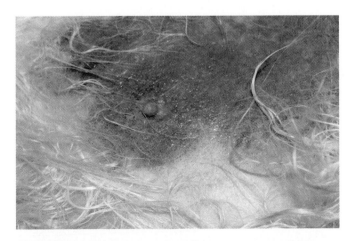

FIGURE 8-158 **Erythema Multiforme and Toxic Epidermal Necrolysis.** Close-up of focal erythema and erosive dermatitis on the abdomen of a cat.

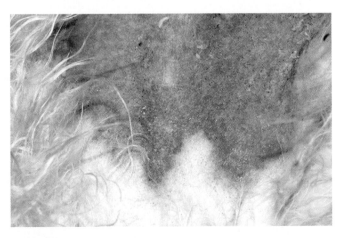

FIGURE 8-159 **Erythema Multiforme and Toxic Epidermal Necrolysis.** Close-up of a characteristic erythema multiforme lesion. Note the sharp, well-demarcated margin.

Erythema Multiforme (EM) and Toxic Epidermal Necrolysis (TEN)—*cont'd*

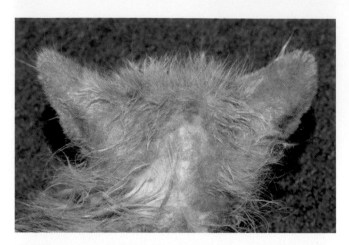

FIGURE 8-160 **Erythema Multiforme and Toxic Epidermal Necrolysis.** Severe alopecia, erythema with erosions, and scale formation on the head of a cat with erythema multiforme.

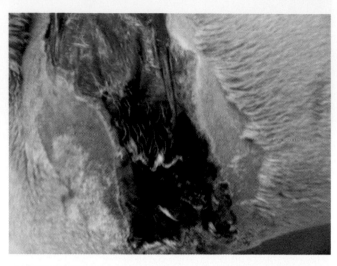

FIGURE 8-161 **Erythema Multiforme and Toxic Epidermal Necrolysis.** Toxic epidermal necrolysis. This well-demarcated area of dead skin was caused by a cutaneous drug reaction.

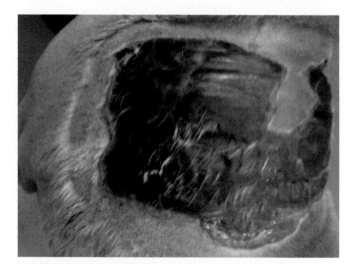

FIGURE 8-162 **Erythema Multiforme and Toxic Epidermal Necrolysis.** This well-demarcated area of dead skin was caused by a cutaneous drug reaction. The entire area of dead skin will slough, requiring aggressive wound management.

Cutaneous Drug Reaction (drug eruption)

Features

A cutaneous drug reaction is a cutaneous or mucocutaneous reaction to a topical, oral, or injectable drug. An adverse drug reaction can occur after one treatment, after several treatments, or after years of treatment. It is uncommon in dogs and cats.

Clinical signs are extremely variable and may include papules, plaques, pustules, vesicles, bullae, purpura, erythema, urticaria, angioedema, alopecia, erythema multiforme or toxic epidermal necrolysis lesions, scaling or exfoliation, erosions, ulcerations, and otitis externa. Lesions may be localized, multifocal or diffuse, and painful or pruritic. Concurrent fever, depression, or lameness may be present.

Top Differentials

Cutaneous drug reactions mimic many other skin disorders, especially other immune-mediated and autoimmune diseases. Specific differentials depend on the clinical presentation.

Diagnosis

1. History of recent drug administration and rule out other differentials.
2. Hemogram: anemia, thrombocytopenia, leukopenia, or leukocytosis may be present.
3. Serum biochemistry panel: variable abnormalities reflecting damage to other organs may be present.
4. Dermatohistopathology (nondiagnostic): findings are variable and reflect the gross appearance of the lesions.

Treatment and Prognosis

1. Discontinue the use of all suspect drugs administered within 2 to 4 weeks before lesion development, and do not use any related drugs or drugs with a similar chemical structure. In cases with no known drug or chemical exposure, one should thoroughly search for an underlying infectious disease or neoplasia.

2. Appropriate symptomatic and supportive care (e.g., whirlpool baths, fluids, electrolytes, parenteral nutrition) should be provided as needed. To prevent secondary bacterial skin infection, systemic antibiotics that are unrelated to any suspect drugs should be administered.

3. Treat as for pemphigus foliaceus (see Table 8-1).

4. In more severe cases, treatment with prednisone 2 mg/kg (dogs) or 4 mg/kg (cats) PO every 24 hours may be helpful. Significant improvement may be seen within 1 to 2 weeks. After lesions resolve (approximately 2–8 weeks), the dosage should be gradually tapered over a period of 4 to 6 weeks. In most cases, steroid therapy can be discontinued.

5. For refractory cases, treatment with human intravenous immunoglobulin (IVIG) may be effective. A 5% to 6% solution of human IVIG is prepared with the use of saline (0.9% NaCl), according to the manufacturer's recommendations. Then, 0.5 to 1 g/kg is infused IV over a 4- to 6-hour period, once or twice, 24 hours apart.

6. Future use of the offending drug, any related drug, or drugs with similar chemical structures should be avoided.

7. The prognosis is good except with multiorgan involvement or extensive epidermal necrosis.

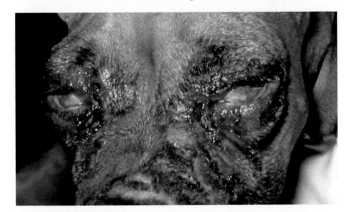

FIGURE 8-163 Cutaneous Drug Reaction. Severe crusting erosive dermatitis on the face of an adult Boxer. This dog also had a secondary methicillin-resistant *Staphylococcus aureus* infection, likely obtained from the owner, who worked in the human health care industry.

Cutaneous Drug Reaction—*cont'd*

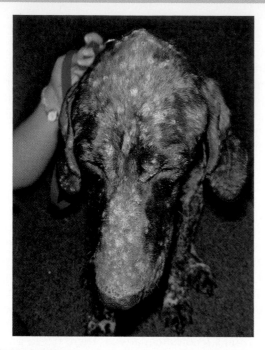

FIGURE 8-164 Cutaneous Drug Reaction. Multiple alopecic, crusting nodules covering the entire head. This nodular dermatitis was thought to be caused by systemic antibiotic administration.

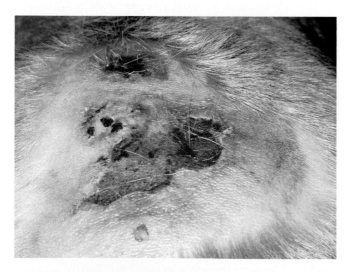

FIGURE 8-166 Cutaneous Drug Reaction. Erosive dermatitis with focal areas of crust formation. Note the well-demarcated serpentine border, which is characteristic of vasculitis, cutaneous drug reactions, or autoimmune skin disease.

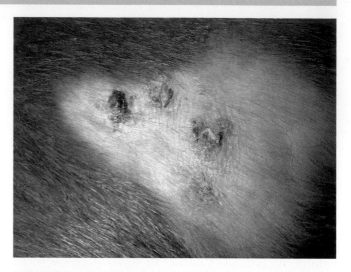

FIGURE 8-165 Cutaneous Drug Reaction. Multiple foci of crusting nodules on the trunk.

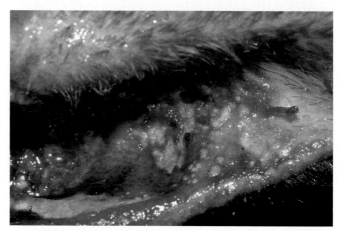

FIGURE 8-167 Cutaneous Drug Reaction. Ulcerative dermatitis on the ear pinna. The islands of epidermal regrowth are originating from the hair follicles.

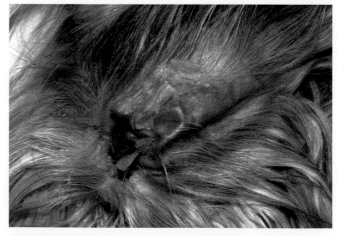

FIGURE 8-168 Cutaneous Drug Reaction. Erythematous dermatitis on the ear pinna with large adherent flakes of epidermis. The dermatitis was caused by a topical otic treatment.

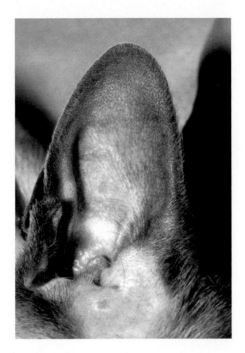

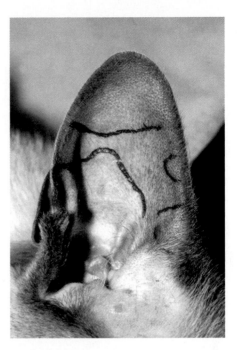

FIGURE 8-169 Cutaneous Drug Reaction. Erythematous plaques with a well-demarcated serpentine border on the ear pinna of a cat. This subtle dermatitis was caused by a systemic antibiotic.

FIGURE 8-170 Cutaneous Drug Reaction. Same cat as in Figure 8-169. The serpentine borders of the lesion have been traced to make them more apparent.

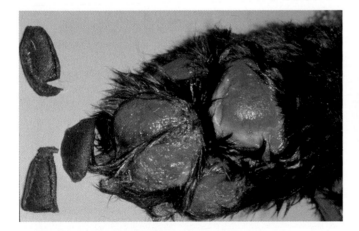

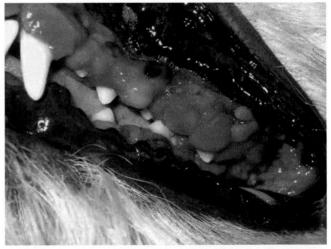

FIGURE 8-171 Cutaneous Drug Reaction. Sloughing of the footpads, leaving an ulcerative lesion. *(Courtesy P. White.)*

FIGURE 8-172 Cutaneous Drug Reaction. Gingival hyperplasia is an uncommon adverse reaction to cyclosporine. Hyperplasia often resolves after discontinuation of the drug. *(Courtesy S. Sargent.)*

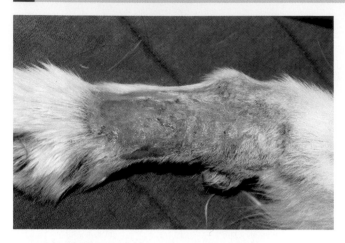

FIGURE 8-173 Cutaneous Drug Reaction. Focal radiation therapy reaction on the carpus of a dog.

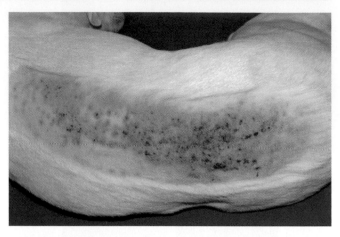

FIGURE 8-174 Cutaneous Drug Reaction. Deep, multifocal, punctate lesions limited to the dorsum and developing within hours to days after bathing are a unique feature of postbathing folliculitis and furunculosis.

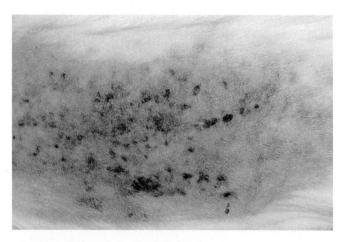

FIGURE 8-175 Cutaneous Drug Reaction. Same dog as in Figure 8-174. Multifocal, punctate lesions on the dorsum are a typical feature of postbathing folliculitis and furunculosis.

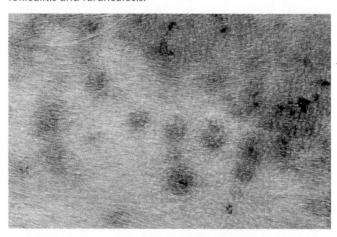

FIGURE 8-176 Cutaneous Drug Reaction. Same dog as in Figure 8-174. Close-up image of the focal, punctate lesion.

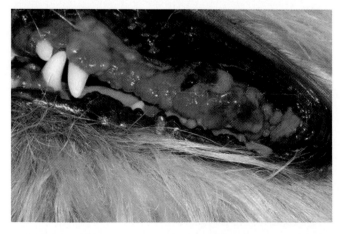

FIGURE 8-177 Cutaneous Drug Reaction. Gingival hyperplasia developed during cyclosporine therapy. *(Courtesy S. Sargent.)*

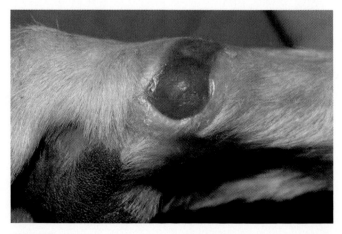

FIGURE 8-178 Cutaneous Drug Reaction. Focal lesion caused by radiation therapy.

Injection Reaction and Post–Rabies Vaccination Alopecias

Features

With this condition, a focal area of alopecia occurs at the site where a subcutaneous injection of rabies vaccine, praziquantel, glucocorticoids, or progestational compounds has been administered. It is uncommon in dogs and cats.

A focal, circumscribed to ovoid area of alopecia develops at the injection site (over the shoulder, back, posterolateral thigh) 2 to 4 months post injection. In dogs, affected skin is usually thin, atrophic, and hypopigmented if the lesion is glucocorticoid- or progesterone-induced. With the canine rabies vaccine, the injection site lesion is characterized by a 2- to 5-cm, slowly enlarging, flat to slightly indurated patch of alopecia with variable erythema that may become mildly scaly, shiny, and centrally hyperpigmented. Rarely, this focal area of rabies vaccine–induced alopecia is followed 1 to 5 months later by the development of multifocal cutaneous lesions from vasculitis. In cats, both pruritic, ulcerative, plaquelike to nodular lesions and lesions similar to those seen in dogs from rabies vaccination have been associated with injection reactions.

Top Differentials

Dogs

In dogs, differentials include localized demodicosis, dermatophytosis, superficial pyoderma, alopecia areata, and topical steroid reaction.

Cats

In cats, differentials include localized demodicosis, dermatophytosis, idiopathic ulcerative dermatosis, and neoplasia.

Diagnosis

1. Based on history, clinical findings, and rule out other differentials.
2. Dermatohistopathology: with rabies vaccine reactions, nodular perivascular accumulations of lymphocytes, plasma cells, and histiocytes in the deep dermis and panniculus are usually present. Vasculitis and follicular atrophy may also be seen. With glucocorticoid or progesterone injection reactions, varying degrees of dermal and pilosebaceous atrophy are usually seen.

Treatment and Prognosis

1. For dogs, no treatment is usually needed. Spontaneous hair regrowth is typical but can take as long as a year to occur.
2. Pentoxifylline 25 mg/kg PO administered every 12 hours for approximately 3 to 4 months.
3. Tetracycline and niacinamide or doxycycline (see Table 8-1) may be effective.
4. Essential fatty acids (180 mg EPA/10 lb) may reduce inflammation.
5. For dogs with rabies vaccine–induced lesions that continue to enlarge, treatment with prednisone may be effective. Give prednisone, initially 0.5 mg/kg PO every 12 hours and tapered over time to 0.5 mg/kg PO every 48 hours. The lesion should stop expanding, but hair regrowth may not be complete.
6. Topical treatment with steroids or tacrolimus may be effective (apply every 12–72 hours to control inflammation).
7. For dogs whose lesions remain permanently alopecic, surgical excision is curative.
8. Cats with pruritic lesions may be difficult to manage medically. Systemic antibiotics for secondary pyoderma may be indicated.
9. For cats with chronic lesions, surgical excision should be considered.
10. The prognosis is usually good, but hair regrowth may not be complete or may have altered pigmentation.

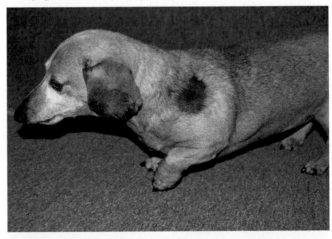

FIGURE 8-179 Injection Reaction. Focal area of alopecia and hyperpigmentation at the site of vaccine administration in an adult Dachshund.

Injection Reaction and Post–Rabies Vaccination Alopecias—cont'd

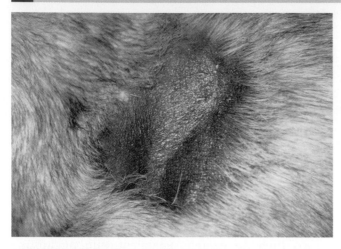

FIGURE 8-180 Injection Reaction. Same dog as in Figure 8-179. The focal area of alopecia and hyperpigmentation is apparent. No evidence of ulcerative vasculitis or secondary infection can be seen.

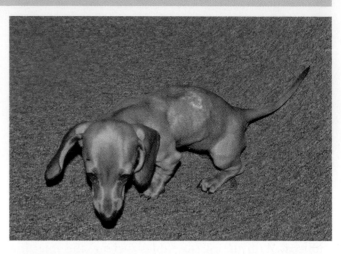

FIGURE 8-181 Injection Reaction. A Dachshund puppy with a focal area of alopecia on the dorsum caused by vaccine administration.

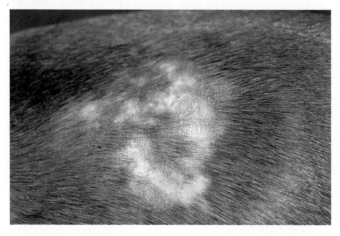

FIGURE 8-182 Injection Reaction. Close-up of the dog in Figure 8-181. Focal area of alopecia and hyperpigmentation on the dorsum. No evidence of ulcerative vasculitis or secondary infection can be seen.

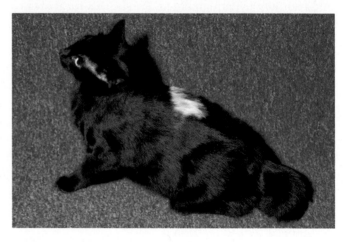

FIGURE 8-183 Injection Reaction. Focal area of white hair (leukotrichia) develops shortly after a steroid injection.

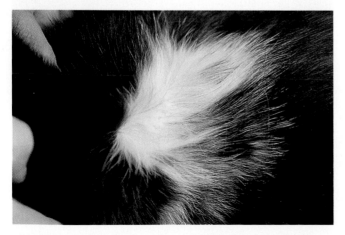

FIGURE 8-184 Injection Reaction. Close-up of the cat in Figure 8-183. Focal leukotrichia at the site of injection is apparent.

CHAPTER 9

Hereditary, Congenital, and Acquired Alopecias

- Excessive Shedding
- Alopecic Breeds
- Canine Hypothyroidism
- Canine Hyperadrenocorticism (Cushing's disease)
- Postclipping Alopecia
- Alopecia X (adrenal sex hormone imbalance, congenital adrenal hyperplasia, castration-responsive dermatosis, adult-onset hyposomatotropism, growth hormone–responsive dermatosis, pseudo-Cushing's disease, follicular arrest of plush-coated breeds, hair cycle arrest)
- Feline Paraneoplastic Alopecia/Dermatitis
- Feline Hyperadrenocorticism
- Sex Hormone Dermatosis—Intact Male Dogs
- Sex Hormone Dermatosis—Intact Female Dogs
- Congenital Hypotrichosis
- Color Dilution Alopecia (color mutant alopecia)
- Black Hair Follicular Dysplasia
- Canine Pattern Baldness
- Idiopathic Bald Thigh Syndrome of Greyhounds
- Canine Recurrent Flank Alopecia (seasonal flank alopecia, cyclic flank alopecia, cyclic follicular dysplasia)
- Miscellaneous Canine Follicular Dysplasias
- Feline Preauricular and Pinnal Alopecias
- Anagen and Telogen Defluxion
- Traction Alopecia
- Alopecia Areata
- Feline Psychogenic Alopecia (neurodermatitis)

Excessive Shedding

Features

Shedding is a normal phenomenon in dogs and cats, but some animals shed more than others—a common owner complaint. Some animals shed more in spring and fall, and others shed excessively year round. In spite of continual hair loss, no alopecia or skin abnormalities are associated. Although hairs may epilate easily, focal areas of alopecia cannot be created.

Top Differentials

Differentials include superficial pyoderma, dermatophytosis, demodicosis, anagen or telogen defluxion, and causes of endocrine alopecia.

Diagnosis

1. Based on history, clinical findings, and rule out other differentials.

Treatment and Prognosis

1. The animal should be groomed every day to remove shed hairs before they fall off.
2. The diet should be balanced.
3. Daily fatty acid supplementation may be helpful.
4. Sometimes outdoor animals improve when brought indoors and vice versa.
5. The prognosis is good. Although excessive shedding is annoying to owners, affected animals are otherwise healthy.

Excessive Shedding—*cont'd*

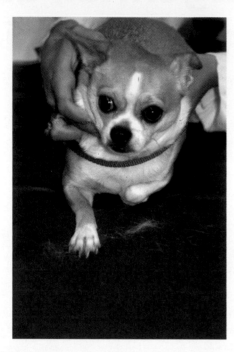

FIGURE 9-1 **Excessive Shedding.** This adult Chihuahua presented with excessive shedding. No cutaneous or systemic abnormalities were observed.

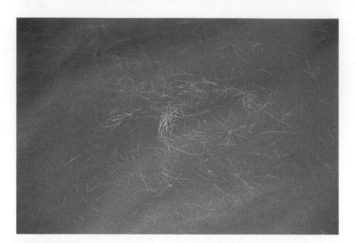

FIGURE 9-2 **Excessive Shedding.** A large amount of hair was shed in just a few minutes from the dog in Figure 9-1.

Alopecic Breeds

Features

These dogs and cats are bred deliberately to produce hairless offspring. Alopecic breeds include the Mexican Hairless dog, Chinese Crested dog, Inca Hairless dog, American Hairless terrier, and Sphinx cat.

Generalized truncal alopecia at birth is typical. Mild secondary pyodermas or seborrhea may develop in dogs. Sphinx cats, because of reluctance to groom, often become greasy, seborrheic, and malodorous. Comedones and milia are common.

Diagnosis

1. Based on signalment, history, and clinical findings.
2. Dermatohistopathology: atrophic, decreased numbers or complete absence of hair follicles.

Adnexa are often similarly affected. Follicular dilatation and hyperkeratosis are common.

Treatment and Prognosis

1. Antiseborrheic follicular flushing (comedolytic) antibacterial shampoo baths and conditioners should be used as needed for secondary seborrhea and pyoderma.
2. The prognosis is good. These animals are meant to be hairless.

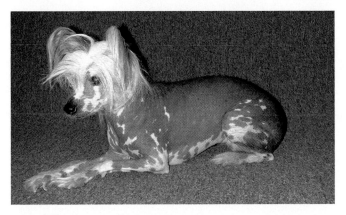

FIGURE 9-3 Alopecic Breeds. This Chinese Crested demonstrates the characteristic pattern of alopecia typical of this breed.

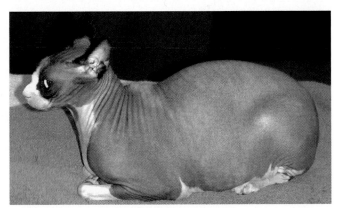

FIGURE 9-5 Alopecic Breeds. A Sphinx cat, demonstrating the almost total alopecia typical of this breed.

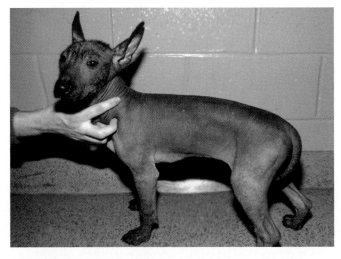

FIGURE 9-4 Alopecic Breeds. A Mexican Hairless dog with generalized alopecia.

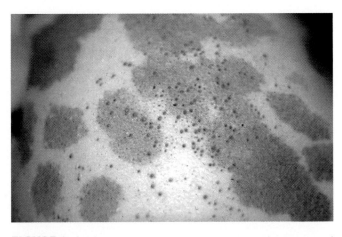

FIGURE 9-6 Alopecic Breeds. Numerous comedones caused by occlusion of dystrophic hair follicles. As these breeds age, comedones and milia are common.

Alopecic Breeds—*cont'd*

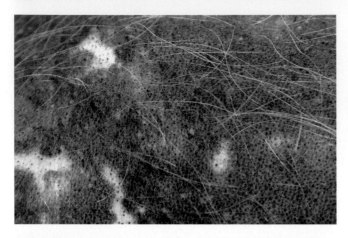

FIGURE 9-7 **Alopecic Breeds.** Numerous comedones on the trunk of an adult Chinese Crested.

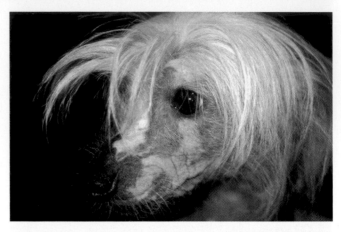

FIGURE 9-8 **Alopecic Breeds.** The Chinese Crested with facial alopecia typical of the breed.

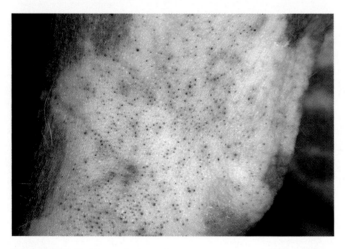

FIGURE 9-9 **Alopecic Breeds.** Numerous comedones on the inner thigh of a Chinese Crested.

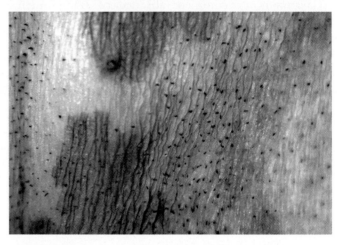

FIGURE 9-10 **Alopecic Breeds.** Numerous comedones on the abdomen.

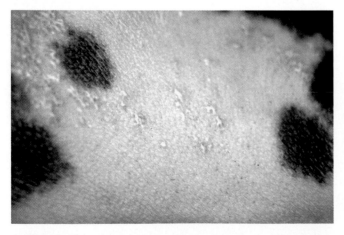

FIGURE 9-11 **Alopecic Breeds.** Over time, the occluded follicles form milia, which appear as white, papular lesions.

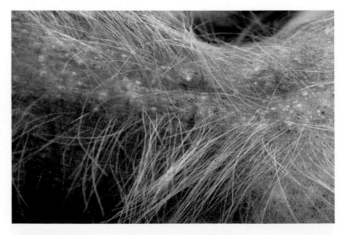

FIGURE 9-12 **Alopecic Breeds.** Numerous comedones and milia on the neck of an older Chinese Crested.

Canine Hypothyroidism

Features

This endocrinopathy is most often associated with primary thyroid dysfunction caused by lymphocytic thyroiditis or idiopathic thyroid atrophy. It is common in dogs, with highest incidence in middle-aged to older dogs. Young adult large and giant-breed dogs also are occasionally affected. Congenital hypothyroidism is extremely rare.

A variety of cutaneous symptoms can be seen. Alopecia on the bridge of the nose occurs in some dogs as an early symptom. The hair coat may be dull, dry, and brittle. Bilaterally symmetrical alopecia that spares the extremities may occur, with easily epilated hairs. Alopecic skin may be hyperpigmented, thickened, or cool to the touch. Thickened and droopy facial skin from dermal mucinosis, chronic seborrhea sicca or oleosa, or ceruminous otitis externa may be present. Seborrheic skin and ears may be secondarily infected with yeast or bacteria. In some dogs, the only symptom is recurrent pyoderma or adult-onset generalized demodicosis. Pruritus is not a primary feature of hypothyroidism and, if present, reflects secondary pyoderma, *Malassezia* infection, or demodicosis. Noncutaneous symptoms of hypothyroidism are variable and may include aggression, lethargy or mental dullness, exercise intolerance, weight gain or obesity, thermophilia (cold intolerance), bradycardia, vague neuromyopathic or gastrointestinal signs, central nervous system involvement (e.g., head tilt, nystagmus, hemiparesis, cranial nerve dysfunction, hypermetria), and reproductive problems (e.g., decreased libido, prolonged anestrus, infertility). Puppies with congenital hypothyroidism are disproportionate dwarfs with short limbs and neck relative to their body length.

Top Differentials

Differentials include other causes of endocrine alopecia, superficial pyoderma, *Malassezia* dermatitis, and demodicosis.

Diagnosis

1. Rule out other differentials.
2. Hemogram and serum biochemistry panel: nonspecific findings may include a mild, nonregenerative anemia, hypercholesterolemia, or elevated creatine kinase.
3. Dermatohistopathology: usually, nonspecific endocrine changes or findings consistent with pyoderma, *Malassezia* dermatitis, or seborrhea are seen. If present, dermal mucinosis is highly suggestive of hypothyroidism, but this can be a normal finding in some breeds (e.g., Shar pei).
4. Serum total thyroxine (TT_4), free thyroxine (FT_4) by equilibrium dialysis, and endogenous thyroid-stimulating hormone (TSH) assays: low TT_4, low FT_4, and high TSH are highly suggestive of hypothyroidism, but false-positive and false-negative results can occur, especially with TT_4 and TSH. For example, although TT_4 is a good screening test, it should not be used alone to make a diagnosis because its serum level can be artificially increased or decreased by several factors, such as nonthyroidal illness, autoantibodies, and drug therapy (Box 9-1).

BOX 9-1 Factors and Drugs That May Affect Total Thyroxine (TT_4) Serum Levels in Dogs

Reduced TT_4 Values
- Normal hourly fluctuations
- Nonthyroidal illness
- Prolonged fasting
- Age >7 years
- Breed = Greyhounds
- Autoantibodies
- Phenobarbital
- Furosemide
- Glucocorticoids
- Sulfonamides
- Nonsteroidal antiinflammatories (e.g., Rimadyl, Etogesic)
- Salicylates
- Tricyclic antidepressants
- Phenylbutazone
- Mitotane
- General anesthesia

Increased TT_4 Values
- Normal hourly fluctuations
- Recovery phase of illness
- Age <3 months
- Obesity
- Autoantibodies
- Diestrus, pregnancy
- Estrogen
- Progesterone
- Insulin
- Narcotic analgesics

Canine Hypothyroidism—*cont'd*

Treatment and Prognosis

1. Any secondary seborrhea, pyoderma, *Malassezia* dermatitis, or demodicosis should be treated with appropriate topical and systemic therapies.

2. Levothyroxine 0.02 mg/kg PO should be administered every 12 hours until symptoms resolve (approximately 8–16 weeks). Some dogs then can be maintained with 0.02 mg/kg PO every 24 hours; others require lifelong twice-daily dosing to maintain remission.

3. Dogs with concurrent heart disease should be started on levothyroxine more gradually. Treatment should begin with 0.005 mg/kg PO every 12 hours; dosage should be increased by 0.005 mg/kg every 2 weeks until 0.02 mg/kg every 12 hours is being administered.

4. After 2 to 4 months of therapy, serum TT_4 level should be measured 4 to 6 hours after medication administration and should be in the high normal to supranormal range. If the level is low or within the normal range, and if minimal clinical improvement has been seen, the dosage of levothyroxine should be increased and the serum TT_4 level checked 2 to 4 weeks later.

5. If signs of thyrotoxicosis from oversupplementation (e.g., anxiety, panting, polydipsia, polyuria) occur, the serum TT_4 level should be evaluated. If the level is markedly elevated, medication should be temporarily stopped until adverse effects abate; it then should be reinstituted at a lower dose or a less frequent dosage schedule.

6. The prognosis is good with lifelong replacement thyroxine therapy, although hypothyroidism-induced neuromuscular abnormalities may not completely resolve.

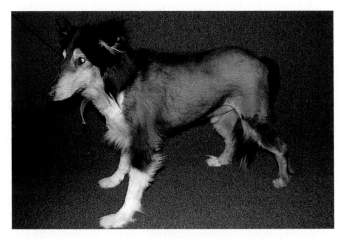

FIGURE 9-14 Canine Hypothyroidism. Generalized truncal alopecia in an adult collie.

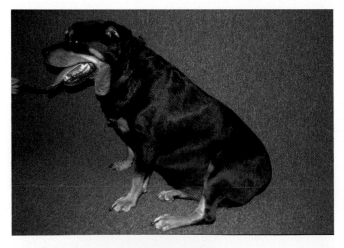

FIGURE 9-13 Canine Hypothyroidism. An obese Rottweiler with hypothyroidism. Note that the hair coat lacks the bilaterally symmetrical alopecia that is considered characteristic of this disease.

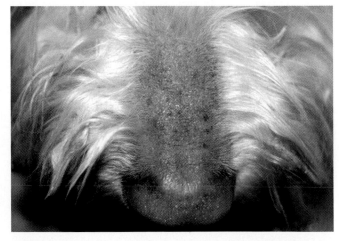

FIGURE 9-15 Canine Hypothyroidism. Mild alopecia on the bridge of the nose may be an early lesion of hypothyroidism.

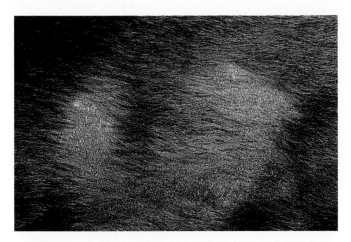

FIGURE 9-16 Canine Hypothyroidism. Alopecia and hyperpigmentation with no evidence of secondary superficial pyoderma on the trunk.

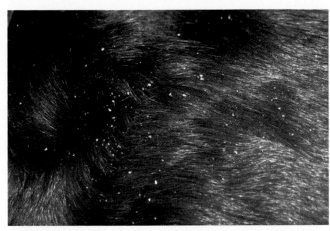

FIGURE 9-17 Canine Hypothyroidism. Generalized seborrhea sicca can be caused by numerous underlying conditions, including hypothyroidism.

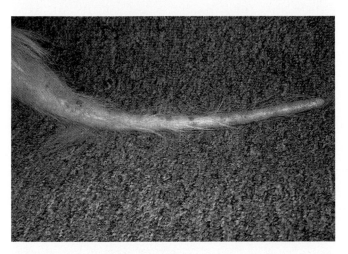

FIGURE 9-18 Canine Hypothyroidism. General alopecia of the tail caused by hypothyroidism.

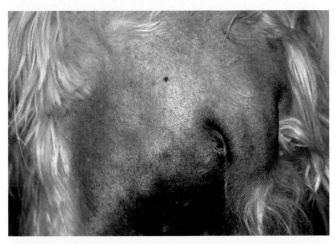

FIGURE 9-19 Canine Hypothyroidism. Alopecia on the lumbar area and tail head. Note the similarity to flea allergy dermatitis and postclipping alopecia.

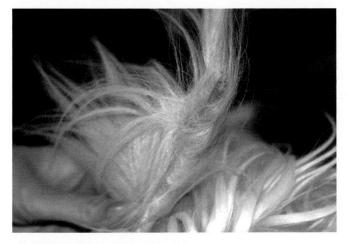

FIGURE 9-20 Canine Hypothyroidism. Alopecia of the tail tip.

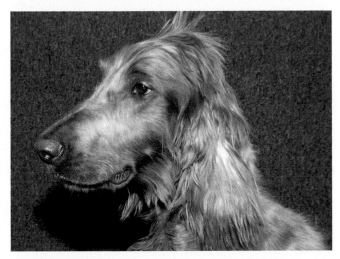

FIGURE 9-21 Canine Hypothyroidism. The hair of this affected Irish Setter became faded over time as a result of the follicular arrest that occurs with hypothyroidism.

Canine Hypothyroidism—*cont'd*

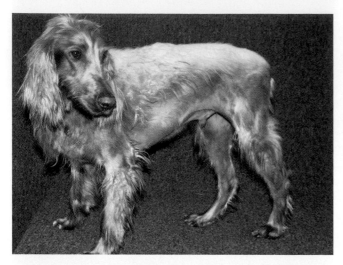

FIGURE 9-22 Canine Hypothyroidism. Severe fading of the hair coat with partial alopecia in a hypothyroid Irish Setter.

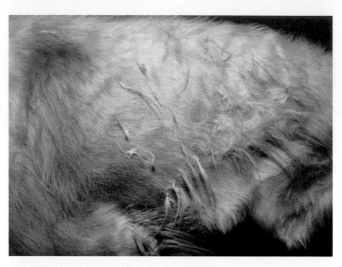

FIGURE 9-23 Canine Hypothyroidism. Same dog as in Figure 9-22. The extremely faded hair coat also demonstrates partial alopecia (the matting is not typical of this disease).

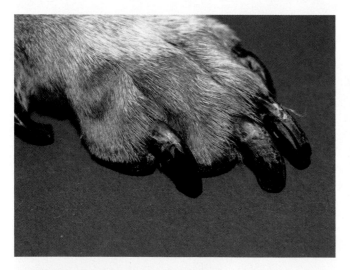

FIGURE 9-24 Canine Hypothyroidism. Same dog as in Figure 9-22. Faded hair is apparent on the dorsal surface of the foot. Note the abnormal nails, which developed as a result of the metabolic effects of hypothyroidism.

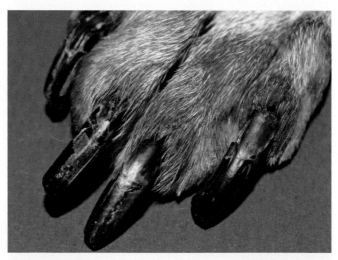

FIGURE 9-25 Canine Hypothyroidism. Same dog as in Figure 9-22. Abnormal nails developed as a result of the abnormal metabolism caused by the disease.

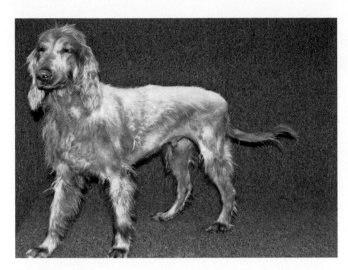

FIGURE 9-26 Canine Hypothyroidism. Generalized fading caused by the lack of normal follicular cycling and hair renewal.

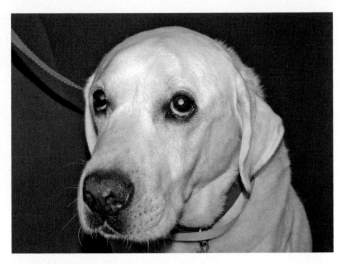

FIGURE 9-27 Canine Hypothyroidism. A tragic facial expression is characteristic of this disease.

Canine Hyperadrenocorticism (Cushing's disease)

Features

Spontaneously occurring hyperadrenocorticism is associated with excessive production of endogenous steroid hormones (principally glucocorticoids, but sometimes mineralocorticoids or sex hormones) by the adrenal cortex. The disease is caused by a hyperfunctioning adrenal tumor (15%–20% of cases) or pituitary tumor (80%–85% of cases). Pituitary-dependent hyperadrenocorticism (PDH) is caused by excessive production of adrenocorticotropic hormone (ACTH), usually from a pituitary microadenoma or macroadenoma. Iatrogenically induced disease occurs secondary to excessive administration of exogenous glucocorticoids. Iatrogenic hyperadrenocorticism can occur at any age and is common, especially in chronically pruritic dogs and dogs with immune-mediated disorders that are controlled with long-term glucocorticoids. Spontaneously occurring hyperadrenocorticism is also common and tends to occur in middle-aged to older dogs, with an increased incidence noted in Boxers, Boston terriers, Dachshunds, Poodles, and Scottish terriers.

The hair coat often becomes dry and lusterless, and slowly progressing, bilaterally symmetrical alopecia is common. Alopecia may become generalized, but it usually spares the head and limbs. Remaining hairs are easily epilated, and alopecic skin is often thin, hypotonic, and hyperpigmented. Cutaneous striae and comedones may be seen on the ventral abdomen. The skin may be mildly seborrheic (fine, dry scales), bruise easily, and exhibit poor wound healing. Chronic secondary superficial or deep pyoderma, dermatophytosis, or demodicosis is common and may be the client's primary complaint. Calcinosis cutis (whitish, gritty, firm, bone-like papules and plaques) may develop, especially at the dorsal midline of the neck or ventral abdomen, or in the inguinal area.

Polyuria and polydipsia (water intake >100 mL/kg/day) and polyphagia are common. Muscle wasting or weakness, a pot-bellied appearance (from hepatomegaly, fat redistribution, and weakened abdominal muscles), increased susceptibility to infection (conjunctival, skin, urinary tract, lung), excessive panting, and variable behavioral or neurologic signs (expanding pituitary tumor) are often present.

Top Differentials

Differentials include other causes of endocrine alopecia, follicular dysplasia, alopecia X, superficial pyoderma, demodicosis, and dermatophytosis.

Diagnosis

1. Hemogram: neutrophilia, lymphopenia, and eosinopenia are often seen.
2. Serum biochemistry panel: an elevated alkaline phosphatase enzyme level is typical (90% of cases). Mildly to markedly elevated alanine transaminase activity, as well as elevated cholesterol, triglyceride, or glucose levels, may occur.
3. Urinalysis: the specific gravity is usually low, and bacteriuria, proteinuria, or glucosuria may be present. Subclinical urinary tract infections are common.
4. Urine cortisol/creatinine ratio: usually elevated. A nonspecific screening test that is not diagnostic by itself because false-positive results are common (stress-induced, seen with many other illnesses). To minimize the effects of stress, a home-collected urine sample should be used, instead of one obtained at the veterinary hospital.
5. Dermatohistopathology: often shows nondiagnostic changes consistent with any endocrinopathy. Dystrophic mineralization (calcinosis cutis), thin dermis, and absent erector pili muscles are highly suggestive of hyperadrenocorticism, but these changes are not always present.
6. Abdominal ultrasonography: may demonstrate adrenal hyperplasia or tumor.
7. Computed tomography (CT) or magnetic resonance imaging (MRI): may detect a pituitary mass.
8. Adrenal function tests:
   - ACTH stimulation test (cortisol): an exaggerated poststimulation cortisol level is highly suggestive of endogenous hyperadrenocorticism, but false-negative and false-positive results can occur. In iatrogenic cases, an inadequate response to ACTH stimulation is typical. *Note*: Reconstituted cosyntropin (ACTH solution) can be stored frozen at −20°C in plastic syringes for up to 6 months with no adverse effects on its bioactivity.
   - ACTH stimulation test (17-hydroxyprogesterone): exaggerated basal and poststimulation 17-hydroxyprogesterone levels may be seen in endogenous hyperadrenocorticism, but false-negative and false-positive results can occur. 17-Hydroxyprogesterone, a progestin, is an adrenal gland–produced precursor of cortisol.
   - Low-dose (0.01 mg/kg) dexamethasone suppression test: inadequate cortisol suppression is highly suggestive of endogenous hyperadrenocorticism, but false-negative and false-positive results can occur. Suppression at 4 hours followed by escape from suppression at 8-hour sampling is characteristic of PDH.

- High-dose (0.1 mg/kg) dexamethasone suppression test: used to help differentiate between adrenal neoplasia and pituitary-dependent hyperadrenocorticism. Lack of cortisol suppression is suggestive of adrenal neoplasia, whereas cortisol suppression suggests pituitary disease.
- Endogenous ACTH assay: used to help differentiate between adrenal neoplasia and pituitary-dependent hyperadrenocorticism. An elevated ACTH level is suggestive of pituitary disease, whereas a depressed ACTH level is suggestive of adrenal neoplasia.

Treatment and Prognosis

1. Any concurrent infection (e.g., pyoderma, demodicosis, urinary tract infection) should be treated with appropriate therapy. Any secondary pyoderma, otitis externa, or *Malassezia* dermatitis should be treated with appropriate therapy. Controlling and preventing secondary infection is an essential component of managing atopic dogs. Bathing every 3 to 7 days and treating the ears after every bath helps disinfect the skin and ear canals, preventing the recurrence of secondary infection.

2. The treatment of choice for iatrogenic Cushing's cases is to progressively taper, then discontinue glucocorticoid therapy.

3. Treatment of choice for adrenal neoplasia is adrenalectomy.
   - Dogs with inoperable adrenal tumors or metastases may benefit from mitotane or trilostane therapy.
   - Mitotane for adrenal tumors: one should give 50 mg/kg PO every 24 hours with food for 7 to 14 days. An ACTH stimulation test is performed every 7 days. If inadequate cortisol suppression persists, increase the mitotane dosage to 75–100 mg/kg/day for an additional 7 to 14 days, while monitoring with ACTH stimulation tests weekly. When adequate adrenal suppression is demonstrated, maintenance mitotane therapy is initiated as described below.

4. The traditional (historical) medical treatment of choice for PDH is mitotane 50 mg/kg PO administered every 24 hours with food. The daily dosage is continued until the basal serum or plasma cortisol level normalizes and does not increase after ACTH stimulation. Control is usually achieved within 5 to 10 days of initiation of therapy, so the patient should be closely monitored with ACTH stimulation tests performed every 7 days. Monitoring water and food intake before and during induction may be useful. Water and food intake often markedly decreases when adequate adrenal suppression has been achieved. If signs of adrenal insufficiency (e.g., anorexia, depression, vomiting, diarrhea, ataxia, dis-

orientation) develop, mitotane therapy should be stopped and hydrocortisone 0.5 to 1.0 mg/kg PO every 12 hours administered, until symptoms resolve.
   - To maintain remission after mitotane induction, mitotane PO with food 50 mg/kg administered once weekly, or 25 mg/kg twice weekly. Dogs that relapse during maintenance therapy should be reinduced with daily mitotane for 5 to 14 days or until recontrolled, then maintained with 62 to 75 mg/kg once weekly, or 31 to 37.5 mg/kg twice weekly. A great deal of patient variability occurs, requiring close monitoring.

5. A more recent treatment option and the current recommendation for the medical treatment of PDH is trilostane. At this writing, its optimal dosing regimen has not yet been determined, but many investigators are using the following protocol:
   - Dogs <5 kg: give 30 mg PO with food q 24 hours
   - Dogs between 5 and 20 kg: give 60 mg PO with food q 24 hours
   - Dogs between 20 and 40 kg: give 120 mg PO with food q 24 hours
   - Dogs >40 kg: give 240 mg PO with food q 24 hours

   Assess efficacy by monitoring clinical signs and evaluating results of ACTH stimulation tests 10 days, 4 weeks, and 12 weeks after the start of therapy, then every 3 months thereafter. ACTH stimulation tests should be performed 4 to 6 hours after trilostane dosing. A post-ACTH cortisol level <150 nmol/L (but >20 nmol/L) is usually consistent with good control. However, optimal clinical control has also been reported with post-ACTH cortisol concentrations between 150 and 250 nmol/L, so blood work results should always be interpreted alongside clinical signs. If the dog is not clinically well controlled and post-ACTH cortisol concentrations are >150 nmol/L, the dose of trilostane should be increased. Dose adjustments should be made in increments of 20 to 30 mg/dog. A wide range of trilostane doses to induce and maintain remission have been reported in dogs, with the therapeutic dose for most dogs between 4 and 20 mg/kg/day. Some dogs may require twice-daily dosing if duration of effect is inadequate. Clinical signs such as polydipsia/polyuria/polyphagia often start to improve within the first 10 days of treatment, but alopecia and other skin changes may take 3 or more months to improve. If signs of adrenal insufficiency (depression, inappetence, vomiting, diarrhea) develop at any time during therapy, or if post-ACTH cortisol concentrations (measured 4–6 hours after trilostane dosing) are <20 nmol/L, trilostane should be stopped for 5 to 7 days, then reinstituted at a lower dose. *Note*: Although trilostane appears to be well tolerated

Canine Hyperadrenocorticism—*cont'd*

by most dogs, sudden death has been reported in dogs with concurrent heart problems. Trilostane is also contraindicated in pregnant and lactating dogs, dogs with primary hepatic disease, and dogs with renal insufficiency.

6. Other alternative, but less consistently successful, medical treatments for PDH include the following:
   ■ Ketoconazole 15 mg/kg PO with food q 12 hours
   ■ Selegiline (L-deprenyl) 1–2 mg/kg PO q 24 hours

7. An effective treatment (where available) for PDH is microsurgical transsphenoidal hypophysectomy. This procedure requires a highly skilled neurosurgeon and specialized veterinary facilities that have access to advanced pituitary imaging techniques. Postoperative complications may include hypernatremia, keratoconjunctivitis sicca, diabetes insipidus, and secondary hypothyroidism.

8. For calcinosis cutis, adjunctive topical treatment with dimethyl sulfoxide (DMSO) gel every 24 hours may help resolve the lesions. During DMSO therapy, serum calcium levels should be monitored periodically because hypercalcemia is a potential adverse effect of this treatment.

9. The prognosis ranges from good to poor, depending on the cause and severity of the disease, with the average survival time for dogs with PDH being approximately 2.5 years after diagnosis.

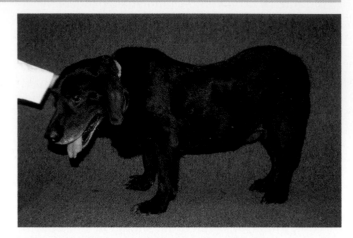

FIGURE 9-29 Canine Hyperadrenocorticism. An adult Labrador with an adrenal tumor, demonstrating severe muscle wasting, which causes the abnormal body confirmation.

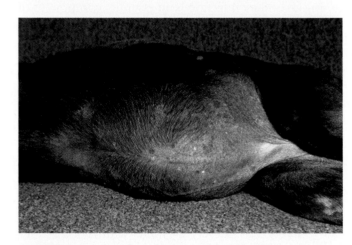

FIGURE 9-30 Canine Hyperadrenocorticism. Same dog as in Figure 9-29. The potbellied appearance and alopecia are apparent.

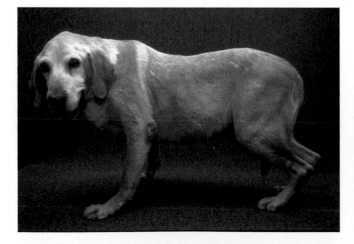

FIGURE 9-28 Canine Hyperadrenocorticism. An adult Labrador demonstrates the typical potbellied appearance. Generalized muscle wasting, which causes the abnormal posture, is also seen. Note that the hair coat is generally in good condition and does not demonstrate bilaterally symmetrical alopecia.

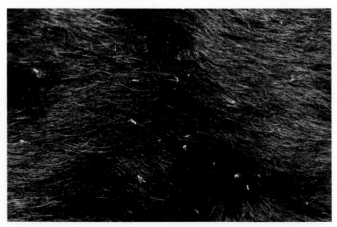

FIGURE 9-31 Canine Hyperadrenocorticism. Same dog as in Figure 9-29. Generalized seborrhea sicca can be secondary to numerous underlying diseases but was caused by hyperadrenocorticism in this dog.

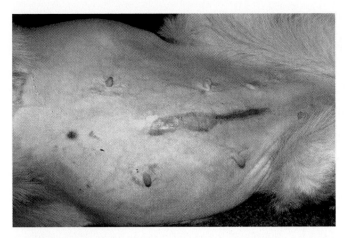

FIGURE 9-32 Canine Hyperadrenocorticism. Severe abdominal distention and alopecia with breakdown of the ovariohysterectomy scar caused by muscle and collagen wasting in this dog with iatrogenic hyperadrenocorticism.

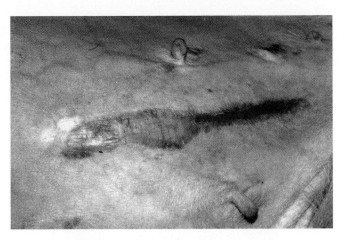

FIGURE 9-33 Canine Hyperadrenocorticism. Close-up of the dog in Figure 9-32. As tissue wasting progressed, the scar became thin and the tissue was pulled apart.

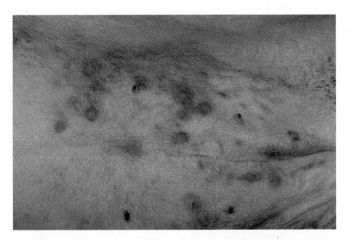

FIGURE 9-34 Canine Hyperadrenocorticism. The papular rash was caused by secondary superficial pyoderma.

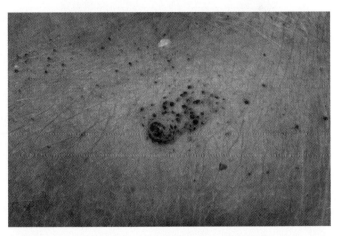

FIGURE 9-35 Canine Hyperadrenocorticism. Numerous comedones on the abdomen of a dog. Comedones are a common feature of Cushing's disease and demodicosis.

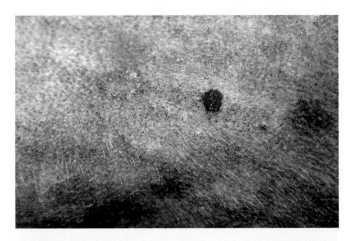

FIGURE 9-36 Canine Hyperadrenocorticism. Phlebectasia (an erythematous papular lesion) is an unusual and unique lesion associated with Cushing's disease.

Canine Hyperadrenocorticism—*cont'd*

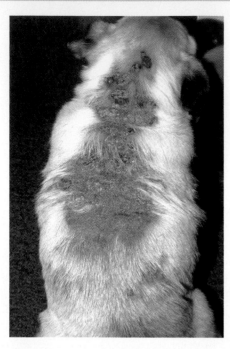

FIGURE 9-37 Canine Hyperadrenocorticism. Extensive calcinosis cutis covering the dorsum of a dog with iatrogenic Cushing's disease.

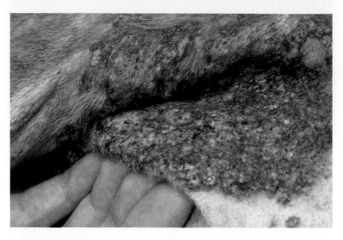

FIGURE 9-38 Canine Hyperadrenocorticism. Calcinosis cutis in the axillary region of a Boxer with iatrogenic hyperadrenocorticism. Note that the entire alopecic, hyperpigmented, papular plaque can be lifted like plate.

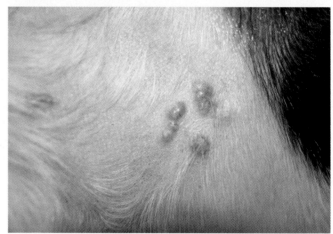

FIGURE 9-40 Canine Hyperadrenocorticism. Mild calcinosis cutis lesions appear as erythematous papules or pustules. At this stage, they can be easily confused with lesions typical of superficial pyoderma.

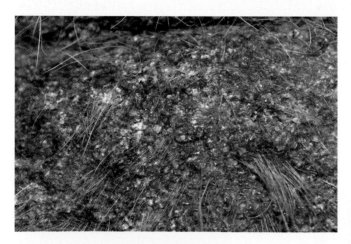

FIGURE 9-39 Canine Hyperadrenocorticism. Calcinosis cutis demonstrating the alopecic, hyperpigmented, papular plaque typical of this syndrome. White papular lesions may appear as pustules, but the calcified material is difficult to express.

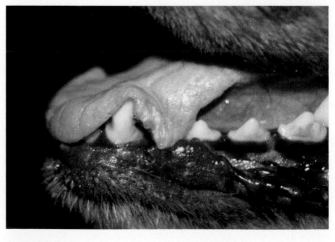

FIGURE 9-41 Canine Hyperadrenocorticism. Calcinosis cutis on the tongue.

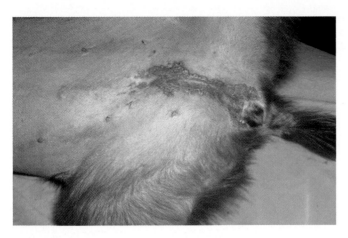

FIGURE 9-42 Canine Hyperadrenocorticism. Calcinosis cutis with a severe inflammatory dermatitis in the inguinal skin fold.

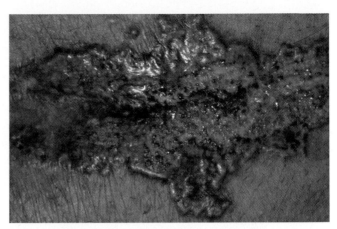

FIGURE 9-43 Canine Hyperadrenocorticism. Close-up of the dog in Figure 9-42. The erythematous, papular plaque was caused by a combination of calcinosis cutis and secondary infection.

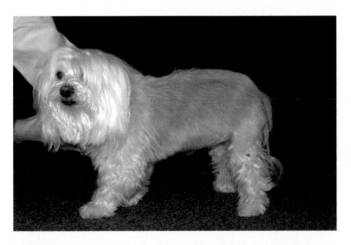

FIGURE 9-44 Canine Hyperadrenocorticism. Symmetrical truncal alopecia in a dog with hyperadrenocorticism.

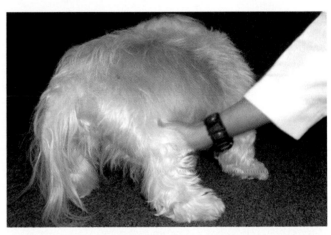

FIGURE 9-45 Canine Hyperadrenocorticism. Same dog as in Figure 9-44. The sparse hair coat was bilaterally symmetrical. This dog was mildly pruritic because of a secondary superficial pyoderma.

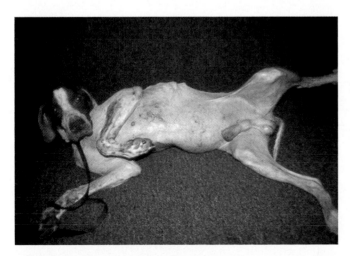

FIGURE 9-46 Canine Hyperadrenocorticism. Ventral alopecia with a distended abdomen in a dog with an adrenal tumor.

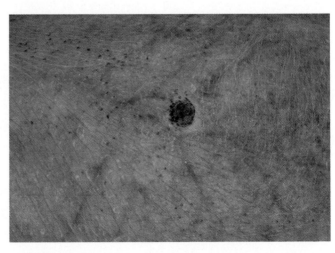

FIGURE 9-47 Canine Hyperadrenocorticism. Phlebectasia (an erythematous papular lesion) on the abdomen of a dog with Cushing's disease.

Canine Hyperadrenocorticism—*cont'd*

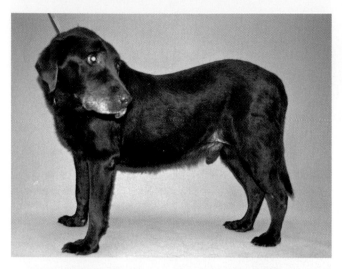

FIGURE 9-48 Canine Hyperadrenocorticism. This Labrador Retriever demonstrates the characteristic body changes typical of premature aging caused by Cushing's disease. This can be caused by long-term steroid administration or endogenous Cushing's disease.

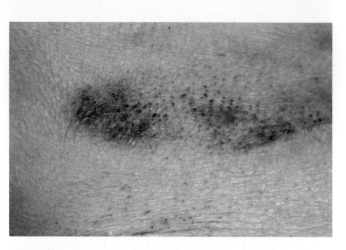

FIGURE 9-49 Canine Hyperadrenocorticism. Comedone formation is a common occurrence with Cushing's disease. Skin scrapes should be performed to rule out demodicosis.

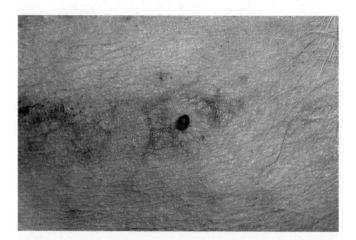

FIGURE 9-50 Canine Hyperadrenocorticism. The vessel showing through extremely thin skin on the abdomen of this dog (around the nipple) is a common feature of Cushing's disease.

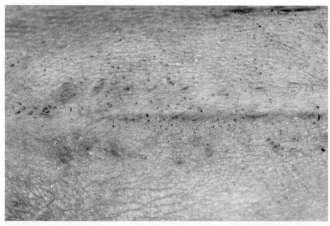

FIGURE 9-51 Canine Hyperadrenocorticism. Cutaneous atrophy and comedone formation are apparent. Note that the spay scar is becoming thinner as the disease progresses.

Postclipping Alopecia

Features

In animals with this condition, hairs fail to regrow in areas that have been clipped (estimated normal regrowth time is 3–4 months). Lack of regrowth may occur after clipping for a surgical procedure or for grooming purposes. It is uncommon in dogs.

Several months post clipping, the affected areas looks as though it has just been clipped. The rest of the hair coat is normal.

Top Differentials

Differentials include other causes of endocrine alopecia, especially hypothyroidism, seasonal timing of normal shed cycles, pyoderma, demodicosis, and dermatophytosis.

Diagnosis

1. Based on history, clinical findings, and rule out other differentials.
2. Dermatohistopathology: may show predominantly catagen hair follicles.

Treatment and Prognosis

1. Spontaneous hair regrowth usually occurs within several months.

2. Short-term treatment with levothyroxine 0.02 mg/kg PO every 12 hours for 4 to 6 weeks may be effective in stimulating hair regrowth within 2 to 3 months.
3. Melatonin (3–12 mg/dog PO q 12–24 hours for 1–2 months) has been used, with variable results.
4. The prognosis is good.

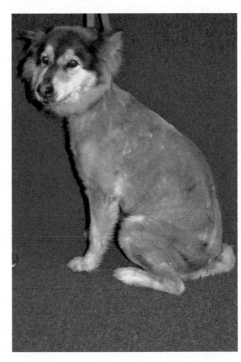

FIGURE 9-53 Postclipping Alopecia. This 6-year-old Alaskan malamute was clipped for summer 5 months earlier. Minimal evidence of hair regrowth can be seen.

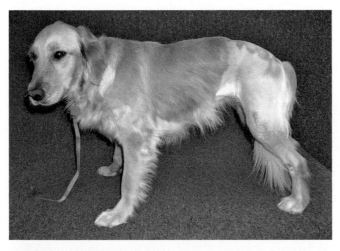

FIGURE 9-52 Postclipping Alopecia. An adult Golden retriever with persistent alopecia several months after orthopedic surgery. No evidence of secondary infection is observed.

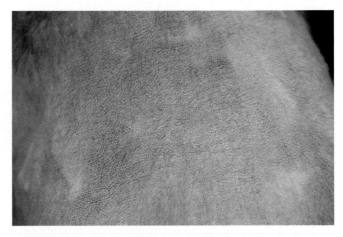

FIGURE 9-54 Postclipping Alopecia. Diffuse alopecia without evidence of secondary infection in an area that was clipped for surgery. Despite the passage of several weeks, no evidence of hair regrowth can be seen.

Alopecia X (adrenal sex hormone imbalance, congenital adrenal hyperplasia, castration-responsive dermatosis, adult-onset hyposomatotropism, growth hormone–responsive dermatosis, pseudo-Cushing's disease, follicular arrest of plush-coated breeds, hair cycle arrest)

Features

The cause of this alopecic condition in dogs is unclear, but several theories have been proposed. One theory is that the disorder is caused by abnormal adrenal steroidogenesis and is a mild variant of pituitary-dependent hyperadrenocorticism. Others have suggested that it may be due to growth hormone deficiency, an adrenal sex hormone imbalance, or excessive production of androgenic steroids by the adrenal glands. Current theories suggest that a local follicular receptor dysregulation may be the underlying disorder. The condition is uncommon in dogs, with the highest incidence in adult dogs 2 to 5 years old, especially Chow Chows, Pomeranians, Keeshonds, Samoyeds, Alaskan malamutes, Siberian huskies, and miniature Poodles.

Gradual loss of primary hairs progresses to complete alopecia of the neck, tail, caudodorsum, perineum, and caudal thighs. Alopecia eventually becomes generalized over the trunk, but the head and front limbs are spared. Hair loss is bilaterally symmetrical, remaining hairs epilate easily, and the alopecic skin may become hyperpigmented, thin, and hypotonic. Mild secondary seborrhea and superficial pyoderma may occur. No systemic signs of illness are noted.

Top Differentials

Differentials include other causes of endocrine alopecia.

Diagnosis

1. Rule out other causes of endocrine alopecia.
2. Dermatohistopathology: nonspecific endocrine changes.
3. ACTH stimulation test (cortisol and sex hormones): basal or poststimulation levels of cortisol, progesterone, 17-hydroxyprogesterone, androstenedione, estradiol, or dehydroepiandrosterone sulfate may be elevated, **but false-positive and false-negative results are common,** and breed-specific normal values have not been established, making the assay's clinical value limited.

Treatment and Prognosis

1. Observation without treatment is reasonable because this disease is purely cosmetic, and affected dogs are otherwise healthy.

2. Neutering of intact dogs may induce permanent or temporary hair regrowth.
3. A variety of medical therapies have been used with inconsistent results to stimulate hair regrowth. These treatments include the following:
   a. Melatonin 3–12 mg/dog PO q 12–24 hours (60% effective) until maximum hair regrowth occurs (approximately 3 months). Then the treatment should be discontinued once the hair regrows so the patient can be retreated if alopecia recurs.
   b. Trilostane may be effective. At this writing, its optimal dosing regimen has not yet been determined:
      ▪ Dogs <2.5 kg were administered 20 mg PO with food q 24 hours.
      ▪ Dogs between 2.5 and 5 kg were administered 30 mg PO with food q 24 hours.
      ▪ Dogs between 5 and 10 kg were administered 60 mg PO with food q 24 hours.
      In most dogs, hair regrowth was evident within 4 to 8 weeks. If no response was seen after 2 months of treatment, the daily dosage of trilostane was doubled. Once full hair regrowth was achieved, the frequency of trilostane administration could be decreased to two to three times per week for maintenance control in some dogs. Therapeutic doses for dogs in this study (all weighing <10 kg) ranged from 5–24 mg/kg/day; at this writing, therapeutic doses for dogs >10 kg have not yet been determined. If signs of adrenal insufficiency (e.g., depression, inappetence, vomiting, diarrhea) develop at any time during therapy, or if post-ACTH cortisol concentrations (measured 4–6 hours after trilostane dosing) are <20 nmol/L, trilostane should be stopped for 5 to 7 days, then reinstituted at a lower dose. *Note:* Although trilostane appears to be well tolerated by most dogs, sudden death has been reported in dogs with concurrent heart problems. Trilostane is also contraindicated in pregnant and lactating dogs, dogs with primary hepatic disease, and dogs with renal insufficiency.
4. Historical medical therapies that may be less effective but have many more adverse effects include the following:
   ▪ Mitotane 15–25 mg/kg PO with food q 24 hours for 5 days. (An ACTH stimulation test on day 7 should show the post-ACTH cortisol level at

between 5 and 7 mg/dL). Then, mitotane 15–25 mg/kg PO should be administered with food q 1–2 weeks for maintenance. Permanent adrenal insufficiency is a potentially serious complication of mitotane therapy.

- Cimetidine 5–10 mg/kg q 8 hours
- Methyltestosterone (neutered dogs) 1 mg/kg (maximum 30 mg) PO q 24 hours until hair regrowth occurs (approximately 1–3 months). Then, 1 mg/kg (maximum 30 mg) should be administered q 48 hours for 2 months, followed by 1 mg/kg (maximum 30 mg) twice per week for 2 months, then once weekly for maintenance. Methyltestosterone is potentially hepatotoxic, and serum liver enzyme levels should be monitored periodically.
- Prednisone 1 mg/kg PO q 24 hours for 1 week, then gradually taper dose to 0.5 mg/kg PO q 48 hours
- Porcine growth hormone 0.15 IU/kg SC twice per week for 6 weeks. Periodic retreatments may be

necessary if relapse occurs. Growth hormone therapy is potentially diabetogenic, and blood glucose levels should be monitored closely during treatment. Porcine growth hormone is difficult to obtain but is preferable to human growth hormone, which may cause death from anaphylaxis.

- Leuprolide acetate (Lupron) 100 mg/kg IM q 4–8 weeks until hair regrowth is seen
- Goserelin (Zoladex) 60 mg/kg SC q 21 days until hair regrowth occurs

5. Regardless of the therapy used, hair regrowth may be incomplete or transient. Initial hair regrowth should be seen within 4 to 8 weeks. If no response is seen after 3 months of treatment, a dosage adjustment or a different therapeutic agent should be considered. The owner should be informed of potential drug risks before any treatment is initiated.

6. The prognosis for hair regrowth is unpredictable. This is a cosmetic disease only that does not affect the dog's quality of life.

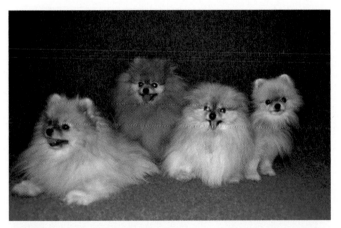

FIGURE 9-55 Alopecia X. A family of Pomeranians demonstrating a range of alopecia and hyperpigmentation typical of this syndrome.

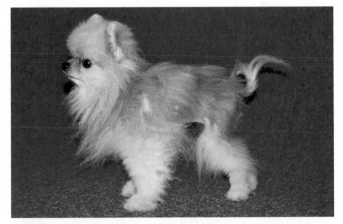

FIGURE 9-57 Alopecia X. Close-up of the dog on the right in Figure 9-56. Alopecia and hyperpigmentation cover the entire trunk, sparing the head and distal extremities. The undercoat is most affected, leaving residual guard hairs.

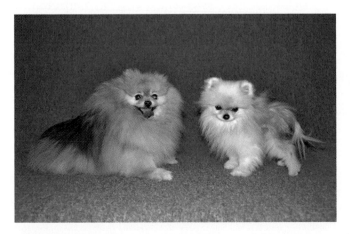

FIGURE 9-56 Alopecia X. Two dogs from Figure 9-55. A normal-coated adult Pomeranian *(left)* and an adult Pomeranian with alopecia X demonstrating characteristic alopecia and hyperpigmentation *(right)*.

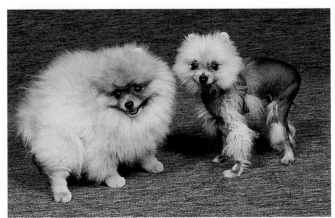

FIGURE 9-58 Alopecia X. These two related male Pomeranians have alopecia X. The dog with a normal fur coat previously had generalized alopecia and hyperpigmentation, similar to the dog on the right.

Alopecia X—*cont'd*

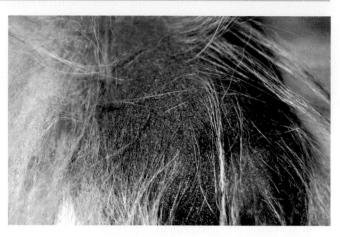

FIGURE 9-59 Alopecia X. Alopecia and hyperpigmentation without a secondary superficial pyoderma are characteristic of this syndrome.

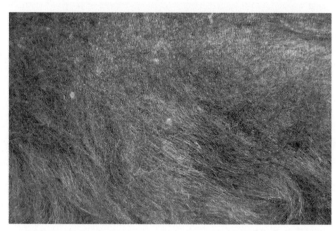

FIGURE 9-60 Alopecia X. Alopecia and hyperpigmentation on the trunk. Note that the undercoat is most affected, leaving a sparse covering of larger guard hairs.

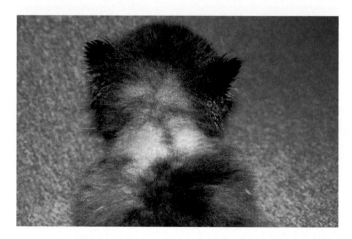

FIGURE 9-61 Alopecia X. Alopecia on the neck and shoulders.

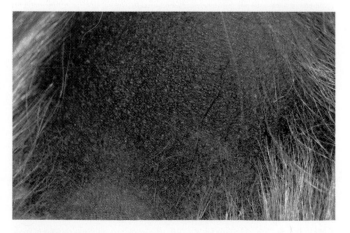

FIGURE 9-62 Alopecia X. Alopecia and hyperpigmentation with abnormal undercoat.

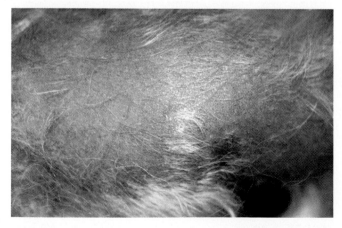

FIGURE 9-63 Alopecia X. Alopecia on the lateral thorax. Note that the typical hyperpigmentation is absent. The red lesion is the site of a skin scrape.

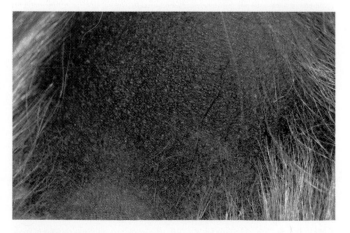

FIGURE 9-64 Alopecia X. The dorsal view demonstrated alopecia and hyperpigmentation without the secondary folliculitis typical of this disease.

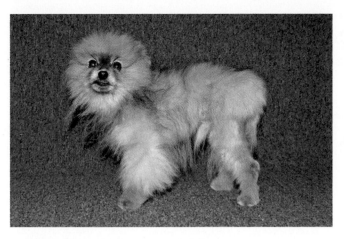

FIGURE 9-65 Alopecia X. This young adult Pomeranian demonstrates the typical pattern with the distal extremities; the head and neck typically are less severely affected.

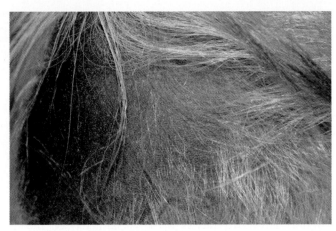

FIGURE 9-66 Alopecia X. Alopecia with hyperpigmentation focusing on the trunk is typical of alopecia X.

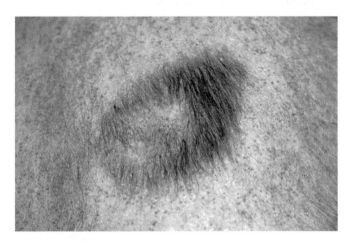

FIGURE 9-67 Alopecia X. Focal regrowth of hair is common with alopecia X. Mechanical stimulation of the hair follicle causes it to become active again, growing new hair.

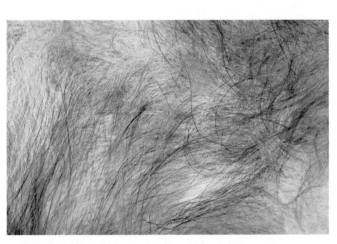

FIGURE 9-68 Alopecia X. Patients with alopecia X usually do not have secondary folliculitis; however, the focal erythematous lesion in this patient is typical of bacterial pyoderma.

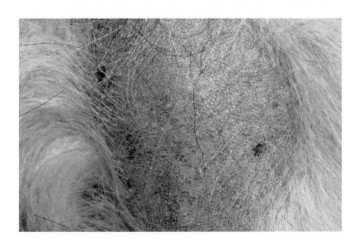

FIGURE 9-69 Alopecia X. Alopecia and hyperpigmentation typical of this disease.

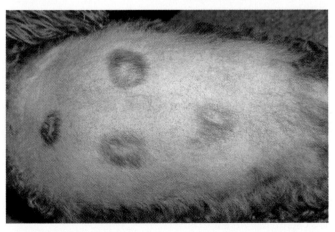

FIGURE 9-70 Alopecia X. Multiple areas of hair regrowth following focal trauma and mechanical stimulation of the follicle, inducing anagen.

Feline Paraneoplastic Alopecia/Dermatitis

Features

Feline paraneoplastic alopecia/dermatitis is a unique dermatosis in aged cats that is a cutaneous marker for an underlying internal malignancy that is due to an adenocarcinoma (often pancreatic or bile duct carcinoma). It is rare, with highest incidence reported in older cats.

Feline paraneoplastic alopecia/dermatitis can mimic allergic dermatitis but is usually characterized by an acute onset of rapidly progressive, bilaterally symmetrical alopecia of the ventrum and limbs. Pruritus is usually a feature and may be related to secondary *Malassezia* dermatitis. The alopecic skin is thin and inelastic, but not fragile, and it has a shiny and glistening appearance. Focal areas of scaling may be present. Hairs in nonalopecic areas epilate easily. In some cats, the footpads are also affected and may be painful, dry, and fissured; soft and translucent; or erythematous and moist. Concurrent systemic signs of illness include anorexia, weight loss, lethargy, vomiting, and diarrhea.

Top Differentials

Differentials include flea allergy dermatitis, dermatophytosis, demodicosis, food allergy, and other causes of self-induced alopecia from ectoparasitism (i.e., cheyletiellosis, flea), cutaneous drug reaction, hyperadrenocorticism, telogen defluxion, or alopecia areata.

Diagnosis

1. Signalment (older patient) with sudden onset of skin disease or with distinctive alopecic, shiny skin and easy epilation of hair; rule out other differentials.
2. Dermatohistopathology: marked follicular miniaturization, atrophy, and telogenation.
3. Radiography, ultrasonography, or exploratory laparotomy: pancreatic or biliary tumor.

Treatment and Prognosis

1. Any secondary pyoderma, otitis externa, and *Malassezia* dermatitis should be treated with appropriate therapies. Controlling and preventing secondary infection is an essential component of managing pruritus.
2. Symptomatic topical therapy for pruritus
3. Supportive care for medical and metabolic problems
4. The treatment of choice is complete surgical excision of the internal malignancy if possible. If surgery is successful, complete hair regrowth should occur within 10 to 12 weeks.
5. The prognosis is poor because widespread tumor metastasis usually has occurred by the time of diagnosis.

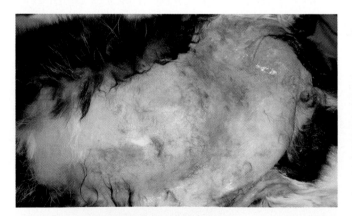

FIGURE 9-71 Feline Paraneoplastic Alopecia/Dermatitis. Almost the entire abdomen of this cat with pancreatic adenocarcinoma became alopecic acutely. Discrete patches of erythematous dermatitis were also observed.

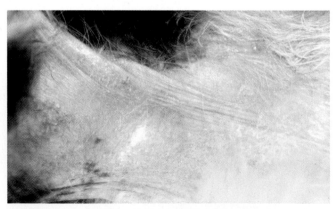

FIGURE 9-72 Feline Paraneoplastic Alopecia/Dermatitis. Same cat as in Figure 9-71. Alopecia in the axillary area reveals smooth, shiny skin, which is typical of this syndrome.

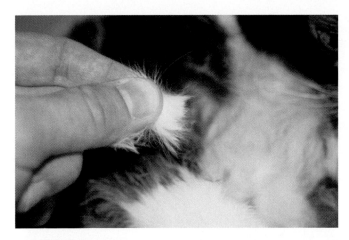

FIGURE 9-73 Same cat as in Figure 9-71. The hair was easily epilated with minimal traction, resulting in large areas of alopecia.

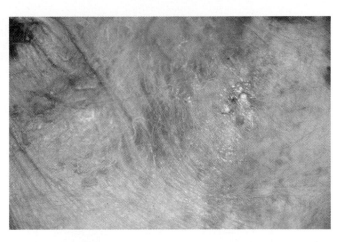

FIGURE 9-74 Feline Paraneoplastic Alopecia/Dermatitis. Same cat as in Figure 9-71. Close-up of multifocal erythematous, macular, papular lesions with areas of crust formation.

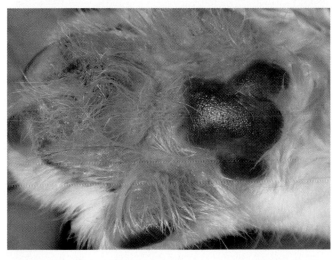

FIGURE 9-75 Feline Paraneoplastic Alopecia/Dermatitis. Severe pododermatitis in a cat with paraneoplastic dermatitis.

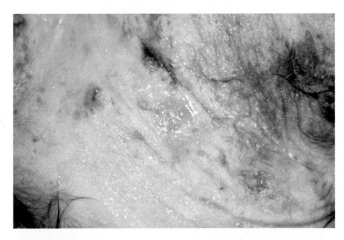

FIGURE 9-76 Feline Paraneoplastic Alopecia/Dermatitis. A large area of alopecia demonstrates the shiny, smooth skin surface typical of this syndrome. The surface was moist because of pruritus and the cat's persistent licking.

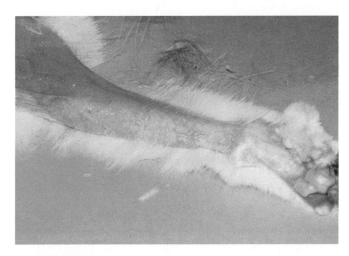

FIGURE 9-77 Feline Paraneoplastic Alopecia/Dermatitis. Generalized alopecia of the distal limb of a cat with pancreatic adenocarcinoma. *(Courtesy K. Campbell.)*

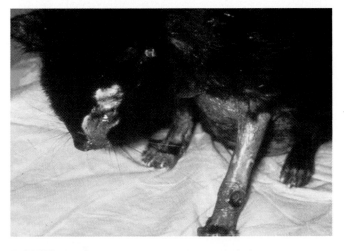

FIGURE 9-78 Feline Paraneoplastic Alopecia/Dermatitis. Diffuse alopecia in a cat with pancreatic adenocarcinoma. Note the smooth, shiny texture of the skin, which is characteristic of this syndrome. *(Courtesy K. Campbell.)*

Feline Paraneoplastic Alopecia/Dermatitis—*cont'd*

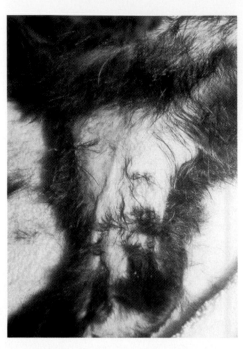

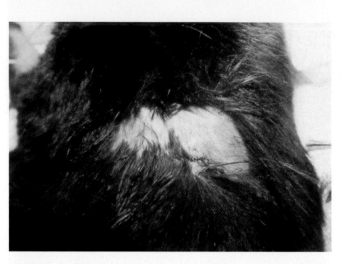

FIGURE 9-80 Feline Paraneoplastic Alopecia/Dermatitis. Same cat as in Figure 9-79. This area of alopecia on the dorsum was caused by normal handling during diagnostic procedures.

FIGURE 9-79 Feline Paraneoplastic Alopecia/Dermatitis. Multifocal alopecia in an adult cat diagnosed with an undifferentiated adenocarcinoma. The hair epilated easily in large sheets.

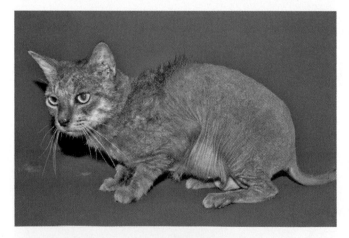

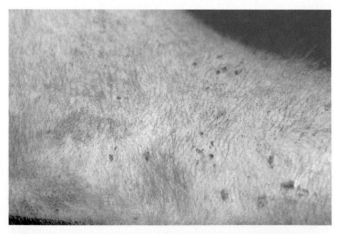

FIGURE 9-81 Feline Paraneoplastic Alopecia/Dermatitis. This elderly cat demonstrates the severe generalized nature of this disease. Often, lesions progress to this severity in only a few weeks.

FIGURE 9-82 Feline Paraneoplastic Alopecia/Dermatitis. Close-up of the alopecic skin demonstrating focal crusting. Inflammatory lesions can be seen, in addition to the more characteristic alopecia associated with this disease.

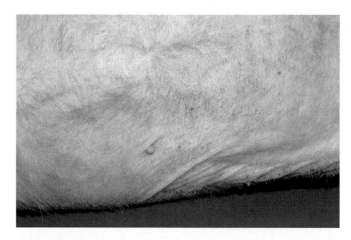

FIGURE 9-83 Feline Paraneoplastic Alopecia/Dermatitis. Generalized alopecia with thin skin and minimal inflammation is characteristic of this disease.

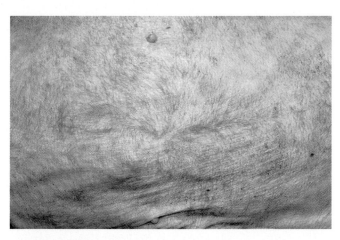

FIGURE 9-84 Feline Paraneoplastic Alopecia/Dermatitis. Close-up of generalized alopecia with mild, focal crusting.

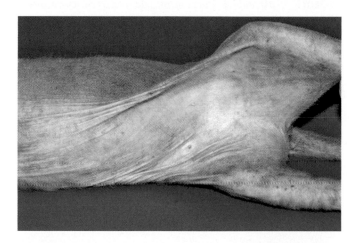

FIGURE 9-85 Feline Paraneoplastic Alopecia/Dermatitis. Generalized alopecia on the abdomen of a geriatric cat.

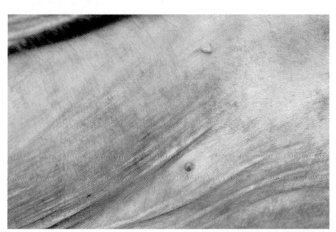

FIGURE 9-86 Feline Paraneoplastic Alopecia/Dermatitis. Close-up of the characteristic alopecia lesion seen with this disease. Note the erythema and mild, focal crusting that can occur. Pruritus may be mild to severe when the inflammatory lesions are present.

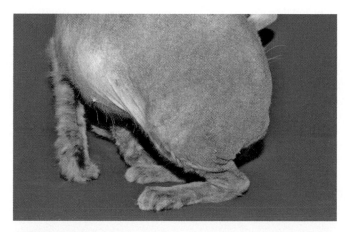

FIGURE 9-87 Feline Paraneoplastic Alopecia/Dermatitis. Close-up of the cat in Figure 9-86. Generalized alopecia that developed rapidly is apparent. This cat was extremely pruritic.

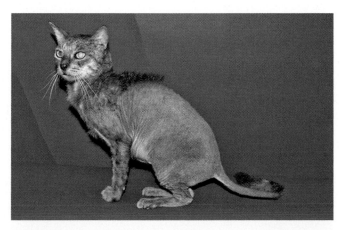

FIGURE 9-88 Feline Paraneoplastic Alopecia/Dermatitis. Generalized alopecia that develops rapidly in an older cat is characteristic of this disease. Inflammation with pruritus may develop as the disease progresses.

Feline Paraneoplastic Alopecia/Dermatitis—*cont'd*

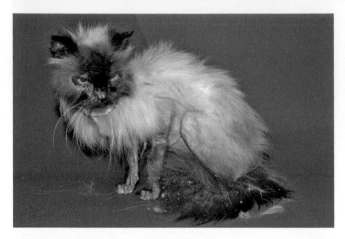

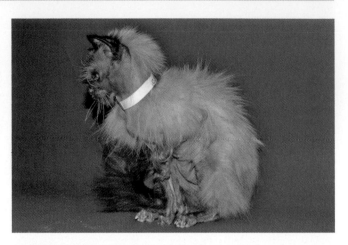

FIGURE 9-89 Feline Paraneoplastic Alopecia/Dermatitis. Generalized alopecia that develops rapidly in an older cat is characteristic of this disease. Inflammation with pruritus may develop as the disease progresses.

FIGURE 9-90 Feline Paraneoplastic Alopecia/Dermatitis. Same cat as in Figure 9-89. The characteristic alopecia is apparent.

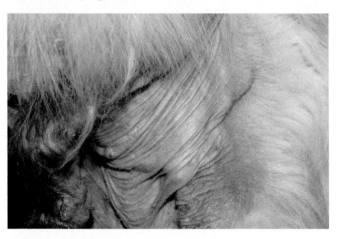

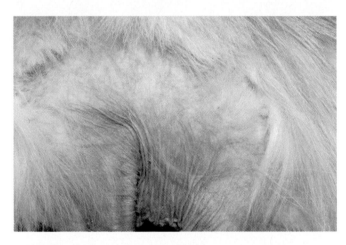

FIGURE 9-91 Feline Paraneoplastic Alopecia/Dermatitis. Same cat as in Figure 9-89. Characteristic alopecia and shiny skin on the cat's abdomen are apparent.

FIGURE 9-92 Feline Paraneoplastic Alopecia/Dermatitis. Generalized alopecia on the abdomen of an elderly cat. Note the mild inflammatory dermatitis that is beginning to form on the ventrum. The cat was becoming progressively more pruritic.

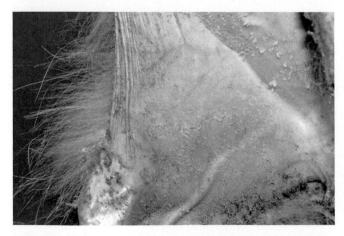

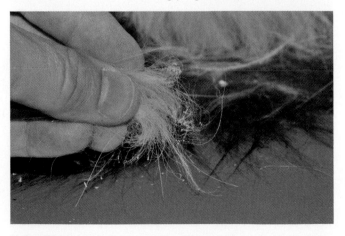

FIGURE 9-93 Feline Paraneoplastic Alopecia/Dermatitis. Severe, generalized alopecia with shiny skin is a unique characteristic of this disease.

FIGURE 9-94 Feline Paraneoplastic Alopecia/Dermatitis. Sudden and profound hair loss is typical of this syndrome. This tuft of hair was easily epilated from the cat.

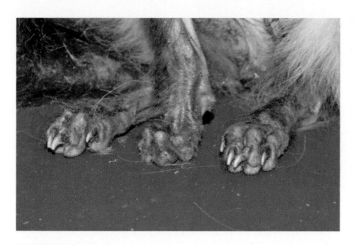

FIGURE 9-95 Feline Paraneoplastic Alopecia/Dermatitis. Generalized alopecia affecting every region is typical.

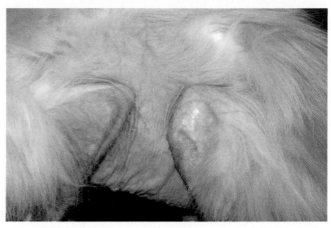

FIGURE 9-96 Feline Paraneoplastic Alopecia/Dermatitis. Generalized alopecia with shiny skin on the flank of an affected cat.

Feline Hyperadrenocorticism

Features

Spontaneously occurring hyperadrenocorticism is associated with excessive production of endogenous steroid hormones by the adrenal cortex. The disease is caused by a hyperfunctioning adrenal tumor that produces excessive quantities of glucocorticoids or sex hormones, or by a pituitary abnormality that results in excessive amounts of ACTH. Iatrogenically induced disease is secondary to excessive administration of exogenous glucocorticoids. Both spontaneously occurring and iatrogenic hyperadrenocorticism are rare in cats, with an increased incidence in middle-aged to older cats.

Polyuria, polydipsia, and polyphagia are common symptoms. These are usually related to concurrent diabetes mellitus, which is common and often insulin-resistant. Depression, lethargy, obesity, anorexia, weight loss, muscle weakness or wasting, hepatomegaly, and a pendulous abdomen also may be present. Skin changes may include a poor, unkempt hair coat; seborrhea sicca; symmetrical alopecia and hyperpigmentation of the trunk, flanks, or ventral abdomen; and thin, fragile skin that tears or bruises easily. Comedones and recurrent abscesses may be seen. Curling of ear tips is often associated with iatrogenic hyperadrenocorticism.

Top Differentials

Differentials include cutaneous asthenia and paraneoplastic alopecia/dermatitis.

Diagnosis

1. Rule out other differentials.
2. Hemogram, serum biochemistry panel, urinalysis: may show changes associated with concurrent diabetes mellitus (hyperglycemia, glucosuria) but otherwise are usually nondiagnostic.
3. Urine cortisol/creatinine ratio: usually elevated, but stress-induced false-positive results are common.
4. Dermatohistopathology: often appears histologically normal, but the amount of dermal collagen may be decreased
5. Abdominal ultrasonography: unilateral or bilateral adrenal enlargement
6. CT or MRI: may detect a pituitary mass
7. Adrenal function tests:
   - ACTH stimulation test (cortisol or sex hormones): an exaggerated poststimulation cortisol response. A poor cortisol response to ACTH stimulation is suggestive of iatrogenic disease. However, false-negative and false-positive results can occur.
   - Low-dose (0.1 mg/kg) dexamethasone suppression test: inadequate cortisol suppression is suggestive of endogenous hyperadrenocorticism, but false-positive and false-negative results can occur.
   - High-dose (1 mg/kg) dexamethasone suppression test: used to help differentiate between adrenal neoplasia and pituitary-dependent hyperadrenocorticism. Lack of cortisol suppression is suggestive of adrenal neoplasia, whereas cortisol suppression suggests pituitary disease.
   - Endogenous ACTH assay: used to help differentiate between adrenal neoplasia and pituitary-dependent hyperadrenocorticism. An elevated ACTH level is suggestive of pituitary disease, whereas a depressed ACTH level is suggestive of adrenal neoplasia.

Treatment and Prognosis

1. Diabetes mellitus and secondary infection, if present, should be treated.
2. The treatment of choice for iatrogenically induced disease is to taper off and stop glucocorticoid therapy.
3. The treatment of choice for adrenal neoplasia is adrenalectomy.
4. An effective treatment (where available) for pituitary-dependent disease is microsurgical transsphenoidal hypophysectomy. This procedure requires a highly skilled neurosurgeon and specialized veterinary facilities that have access to advanced pituitary imaging techniques. Postoperative complications may include soft palate wound dehiscence, transient hypernatremia from decreased water intake, and transient keratoconjunctivitis sicca from impaired tear production.
5. Alternatively, pituitary-dependent disease can be treated with bilateral adrenalectomy followed by lifelong supplementation with replacement doses of glucocorticoids and mineralocorticoids. Because the mortality rate from surgical complications such as sepsis, thromboemboli, and poor wound healing is high, presurgical stabilization with metyrapone (43–65 mg/kg PO q 12 hours) may be helpful, especially in severely affected cats.
6. Medical therapies for pituitary-dependent disease that can be considered but have inconsistent success rates when used alone include the following:
   - Metyrapone 65 mg/kg PO q 12 hours
   - Trilostane 15–30 mg/cat q 12–24 hours

- Ketoconazole 10–15 mg/kg PO with food q 12 hours
7. Mitotane treatment is also inconsistently effective in cats. It does not induce remission when used as directed for canine hyperadrenocorticism, but it may be effective after longer induction periods.

8. The prognosis is fair to poor. Secondary diabetes mellitus in cats often resolves if the underlying hyperadrenocorticism is successfully treated. However, without treatment, concurrent diabetes mellitus may be difficult to control.

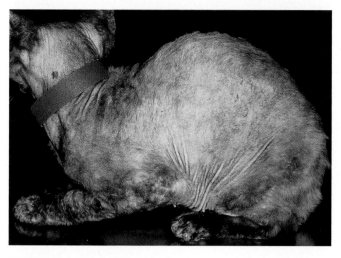

FIGURE 9-97 Feline Hyperadrenocorticism. Generalized alopecia and cutaneous atrophy. *(Courtesy A. Yu.)*

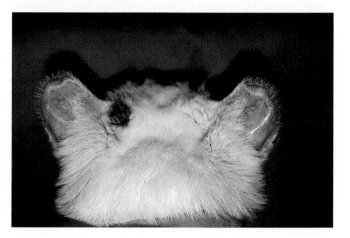

FIGURE 9-99 Feline Hyperadrenocorticism. Alopecia and curling of the ear pinnae are typical of Cushing's syndrome in cats.

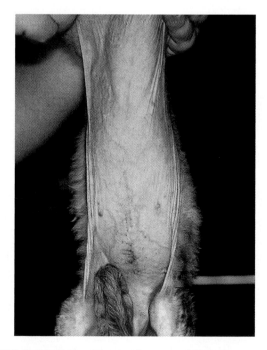

FIGURE 9-98 Feline Hyperadrenocorticism. Same cat as in Figure 9-97. Cutaneous atrophy allows clear visualization of the underlying vessels. The cat's distended abdomen is also apparent. *(Courtesy A. Yu.)*

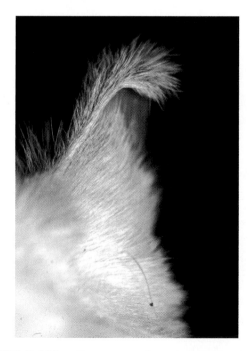

FIGURE 9-100 Feline Hyperadrenocorticism. Close-up of the cat in Figure 9-99. Note curling of the ear pinnae caused by iatrogenic hyperadrenocorticism.

Feline Hyperadrenocorticism—*cont'd*

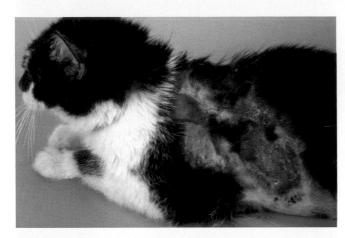

FIGURE 9-101 **Feline Hyperadrenocorticism.** Skin fragility syndrome causing large wounds in a cat. *(Courtesy P. White.)*

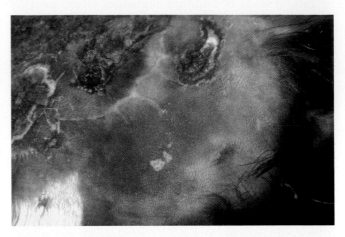

FIGURE 9-102 **Feline Hyperadrenocorticism.** Close-up of the cat in Figure 9-101. Numerous lacerations in the skin with subcutaneous bruising are apparent. *(Courtesy P. White.)*

Sex Hormone Dermatosis—Intact Male Dogs

Features

Sex hormone dermatosis is an endocrinopathy associated with excessive production of sex hormones or precursor sex hormones by the testes (usually caused by testicular tumors). It is common in intact male dogs, with the highest incidence in middle-aged to older dogs.

Sex hormone dermatosis manifests as bilaterally symmetrical alopecia of the neck, rump, perineum, flanks, or trunk that may become generalized but spares the head and limbs. Remaining hairs epilate easily. Alopecic skin may become hyperpigmented. Secondary seborrhea, superficial pyoderma, and yeast dermatitis may be present. Concurrent gynecomastia, pendulous prepuce, galactorrhea, and clinical signs of prostatomegaly or prostatitis may be seen. The testicles may be normal, asymmetrical, or cryptorchid on palpation. The owner may report that the dog is exhibiting abnormal (e.g., attractiveness to other males, standing in a female posture to urinate) or overly aggressive sexual behavior toward other dogs or humans.

Top Differentials

Differentials include other causes of endocrine alopecia.

Diagnosis

1. Rule out other causes of endocrine alopecia.
2. Hemogram: findings are usually unremarkable, but in dogs with concurrent estrogen-induced myelo-toxicosis, nonregenerative anemia, leukopenia, and thrombocytopenia are seen.
3. Dermatohistopathology: nonspecific endocrine changes.
4. Sex hormone assays: serum levels of one or more sex hormones may be elevated, but false-negative and false-positive results are common.
5. Testicular histopathology (castration): may be normal, atrophic, or neoplastic (Sertoli cell tumor, interstitial cell tumor, or seminoma).
6. Response to castration: hair regrowth may occur.

Treatment and Prognosis

1. The treatment of choice is castration (both testicles).
2. Any secondary pyoderma, prostatitis, and yeast dermatitis should be treated with appropriate systemic antibiotics.
3. Fluid therapy, whole blood transfusions, and platelet-rich plasma infusions are also indicated in dogs that have estrogen-induced bone marrow aplasia.
4. The prognosis is excellent for dogs with no tumor metastasis or estrogen-induced myelotoxicity. Hair regrowth should occur within 3 months after castration. Remission followed by relapse may indicate excessive sex hormone production by the adrenal glands (alopecia X) or metastatic testicular neoplasia.

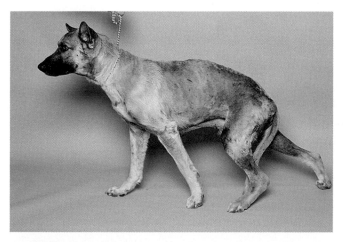

FIGURE 9-103 Sex Hormone Dermatosis—Intact Male Dogs. Generalized alopecia with hyperpigmentation in a male dog with a Sertoli cell tumor.

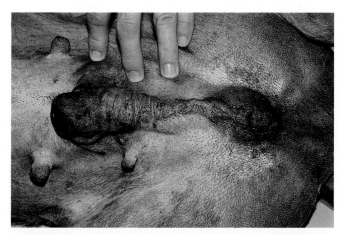

FIGURE 9-104 Sex Hormone Dermatosis—Intact Male Dogs. Close-up of the dog in Figure 9-103. Linear preputial hyperpigmentation in a dog with Sertoli cell tumor. Note the linear preputial macules that are considered unique to and characteristic of Sertoli cell tumors.

Sex Hormone Dermatosis—Intact Male Dogs—*cont'd*

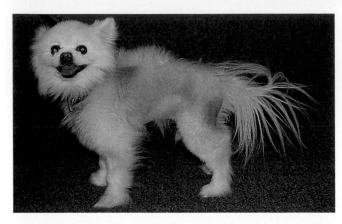

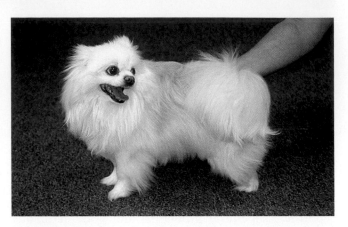

FIGURE 9-105 **Sex Hormone Dermatosis—Intact Male Dogs.** Generalized alopecia in an intact male Pomeranian. The fur coat regrew completely after castration. Note the similarity to alopecia X.

FIGURE 9-106 **Sex Hormone Dermatosis—Intact Male Dogs.** Same dog as in Figure 9-105. After castration, the fur coat regrew completely.

Sex Hormone Dermatosis—Intact Female Dogs

Features

Sex hormone dermatosis is an endocrinopathy that is presumably caused by elevated estrogen or progestin levels. It is rare in intact female dogs, with the highest incidence in middle-aged to older dogs that have cystic ovaries or ovarian neoplasia. It can also occur in neutered female dogs who are receiving exogenous estrogen therapy for urinary incontinence.

Sex hormone dermatosis appears as bilaterally symmetrical, regionalized (flanks, perineum, inguinal) to generalized truncal alopecia that usually spares the head and limbs. Remaining hairs epilate easily. Alopecic skin usually becomes hyperpigmented. Secondary lichenification, seborrhea, and superficial pyoderma may occur. Concurrent gynecomastia and vulvar enlargement are usually present. Some dogs have a history of estrus cycle abnormalities, prolonged pseudopregnancies, or nymphomania.

Top Differentials

Differentials include other causes of endocrine alopecia.

Diagnosis

1. Rule out other causes of endocrine alopecia.
2. Hemogram: findings are usually unremarkable, but in dogs with concurrent estrogen-induced myelotoxicosis, nonregenerative anemia, leukopenia, and thrombocytopenia are seen.
3. Dermatohistopathology: nonspecific endocrine changes.
4. Sex hormone assays: estrogen/progestin levels may be elevated, but false-negative and false-positive results are common.
5. Response to ovariohysterectomy/cessation of estrogen therapy: hair regrowth occurs.

Treatment and Prognosis

1. Any secondary seborrhea, pyoderma, and yeast dermatitis should be treated with appropriate therapies. Fluid therapy, whole blood transfusion, and platelet-rich plasma infusion are also indicated in dogs that have estrogen-induced bone marrow aplasia.
2. If the condition is iatrogenically induced, estrogen therapy should be stopped.
3. Ovariohysterectomy is the treatment of choice for intact females.
4. The prognosis is good. Resolution of clinical signs and hair regrowth usually occur in 3 to 4 months, but in some dogs, this may take as long as 6 months.

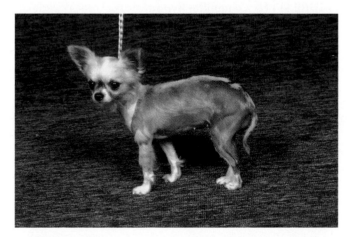

FIGURE 9-107 Sex Hormone Dermatosis—Intact Female Dogs. Generalized alopecia in an adult intact female Chihuahua with an ovarian cyst. The hair regrew after an ovariohysterectomy.

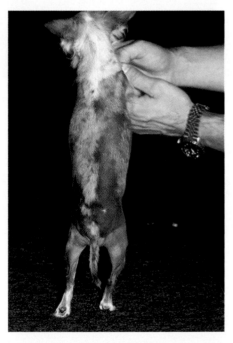

FIGURE 9-108 Sex Hormone Dermatosis—Intact Female Dogs. Same dog as in Figure 9-107. Alopecia and hyperpigmentation extend from the neck to the distal rear limbs.

Congenital Hypotrichosis

Features

Congenital hypotrichosis is a developmental non–color-linked alopecic disorder. It is rare in dogs and cats. One or more animals in the litter may be affected.

Affected animals may be born with alopecia or may appear normal at birth, but they begin to lose hair at around 1 month of age. Hair loss is symmetrical and usually involves the head, trunk, or ventrum. Regionalized or generalized alopecia may be seen. Alopecic skin often becomes secondarily hyperpigmented and seborrheic. Abnormal dentition may be present.

Top Differentials

Differentials include demodicosis, dermatophytosis, and superficial pyoderma.

Diagnosis

1. Based on history, clinical findings, and rule out other differentials.
2. Dermatohistopathology: hair follicles are completely absent or atrophic and decreased in number in affected skin.

Treatment and Prognosis

1. No treatment is known.
2. The prognosis is good; this is a cosmetic problem only that does not affect the animal's quality of life. Affected animals should not be bred.

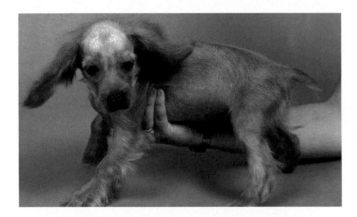

FIGURE 9-109 Congenital Hypotrichosis. This young puppy was born with alopecia on the head and trunk. *(Courtesy D. Angarano.)*

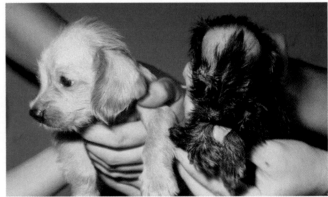

FIGURE 9-110 Congenital Hypotrichosis. Focal alopecia on the face and ears of two puppies from the same litter as the dog in Figure 9-109. *(Courtesy D. Angarano.)*

Color Dilution Alopecia (color mutant alopecia)

Features

Color dilution alopecia is a follicular dysplasia of color-dilute hairs that is associated with defective hair pigmentation and formation. An autosomal recessive mode of inheritance is suspected. It is common in color-dilute dogs such as those bred to be blue (dilution of black) or fawn (dilution of brown). The disorder is especially common in Dobermann pinschers but also occurs in other breeds, including Yorkshire terriers, miniature pinschers, Great Danes, Whippets, Italian greyhounds, Salukis, Chow Chows, Dachshunds, Silky terriers, Boston terriers, Newfoundlands, Bernese mountain dogs, Shetland Sheep dogs, Schipperkes, Chihuahuas, Poodles, and Irish setters.

Affected dogs appear normal at birth but usually begin to lose hair over the dorsum of the trunk at between 6 months and 2 years of age. Although hair coat thinning often progresses to partial or complete alopecia, only the color-diluted hairs are lost. The dog's normal-colored markings are not affected. Secondary superficial pyoderma is common.

Top Differentials

Differentials include dermatophytosis, demodicosis, superficial pyoderma, and causes of endocrine alopecia (e.g., hypothyroidism, hyperadrenocorticism, sex hormone dermatosis).

Diagnosis

1. Signalment, history, clinical findings, and rule out other differentials.
2. Trichogram of affected hairs (microscopic examination of plucked hairs): hair cortices and medullas contain numerous large melanin clumps, and hair cuticles have defects and fractures.
3. Dermatohistopathology: dilated, cystic, keratin-filled hair follicles. Abnormal clumps of melanin are present in epidermal and follicular basal cells, hair, and peribulbar melanophages with pigmentary incontinence.

Treatment and Prognosis

1. No specific treatment is known that reverses or prevents further hair loss.
2. Treat symptomatically with comedolytic or antibacterial shampoos (benzoyl peroxide) and conditioners as needed.
3. Give appropriate systemic antibiotics for 3 to 4 weeks if secondary pyoderma is present.
4. Prognosis is good. Although hair loss is irreversible, and routine symptomatic skin care may be needed, this is a cosmetic problem only that does not affect the dog's quality of life.

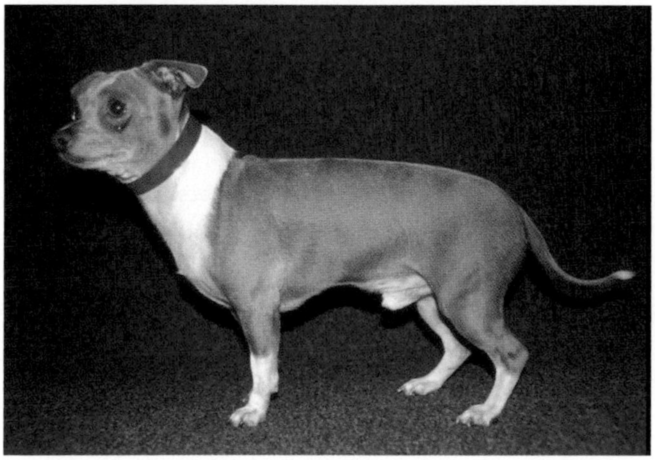

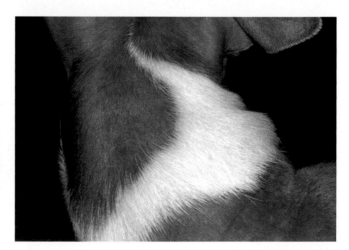

FIGURE 9-111 **Color Dilution Alopecia.** Generalized alopecia affecting only the pigmented patches of hair.

FIGURE 9-112 **Color Dilution Alopecia.** Close-up of the dog in Figure 9-111. Generalized alopecia affecting the pigmented patches of hair. The patches of white hair are completely normal, which is characteristic of this syndrome.

Color Dilution Alopecia—*cont'd*

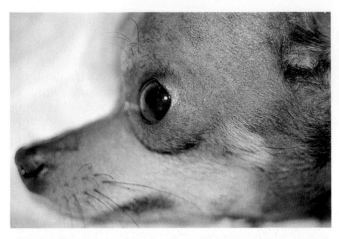

FIGURE 9-113 Color Dilution Alopecia. Areas of color-diluted hair were partially alopecic in this Chihuahua. The adjacent area of normal-colored brown hair was unaffected.

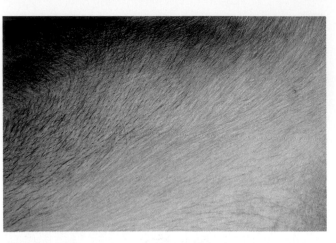

FIGURE 9-114 Color Dilution Alopecia. Areas of color-diluted hair were alopecic. The adjacent area of normal-colored brown hair was unaffected.

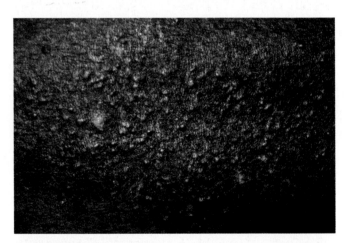

FIGURE 9-115 Color Dilution Alopecia. Numerous comedones and milia are common on the areas of affected skin. As the dog ages, the hair follicles become obstructed, forming comedones and eventually milia. Note the similarity with alopecic breeds.

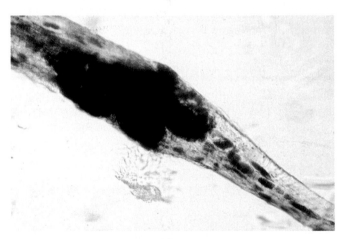

FIGURE 9-116 Color Dilution Alopecia. Microscopic image of a hair, demonstrating clumped pigment as seen with a 10× objective. Clumping of pigment causes a defect in the hair, which eventually breaks, resulting in alopecia.

Black Hair Follicular Dysplasia

Features

Black hair follicular dysplasia is a color-linked follicular dysplasia of black hairs that is associated with defective hair pigmentation and formation. An autosomal recessive mode of inheritance is suspected. It is rare in young bicolored and tricolored dogs.

Affected puppies appear normal at birth but begin to lose hair at around 1 month of age. Only black hairs are affected, with alopecia progressing until all black hairs have been lost.

Top Differentials

Differentials include dermatophytosis, demodicosis, superficial pyoderma, and causes of endocrine alopecia.

Diagnosis

1. Based on history, clinical findings, and rule out other differentials.

2. Trichogram of affected hairs (microscopic examination of plucked hairs): hair cortices and medullas contain numerous large melanin clumps, and hair cuticles have defects and fractures.
3. Dermatohistopathology: non–black-haired skin is normal. Black-haired skin has dilated hair follicles filled with keratin, hair shaft fragments, and free melanin. Abnormal clumps of melanin are present in follicular and epidermal basal cells and in hair matrix cells.

Treatment and Prognosis

1. No treatment is known.
2. Treat symptomatically with comedolytic or antibacterial shampoos (benzoyl peroxide) and conditioners as needed.
3. Give appropriate systemic antibiotics for 3 to 4 weeks if secondary pyoderma is present.
4. The prognosis is good. Although the alopecia is irreversible, this is a cosmetic problem only that does not affect the dog's quality of life.

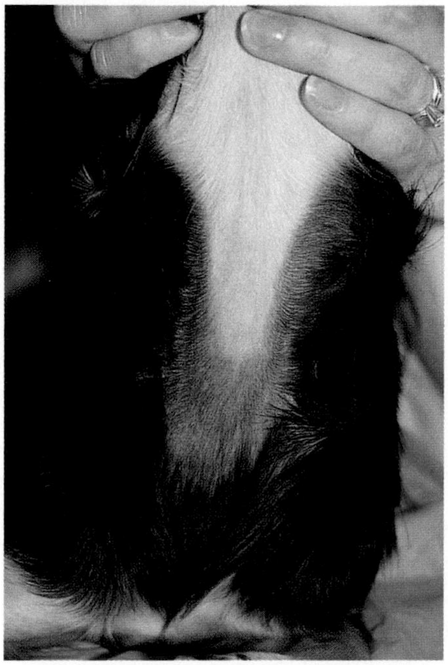

FIGURE 9-117 **Black Hair Follicle Dysplasia.** Partial alopecia affecting only the areas of black hair.

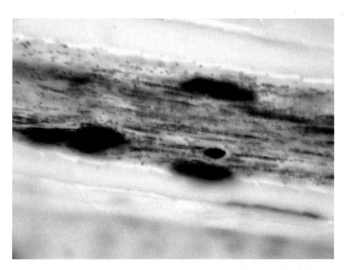

FIGURE 9-118 **Black Hair Follicle Dysplasia.** Microscopic image of clumping pigment within the hair shaft as seen with a 40× objective. Clumping of pigment causes a defect in the hair, which eventually breaks, resulting in alopecia.

Canine Pattern Baldness

Features

Canine pattern baldness is an idiopathic alopecic disorder that is most common in Dachshunds, but it can occur in other short-coated breeds such as Chihuahuas, Whippets, Manchester terriers, Boston terriers, Boxers, and Greyhounds (see also "Idiopathic Bald Thigh Syndrome of Greyhounds"). Pattern baldness often begins during late puberty or early adulthood.

Gradual thinning of hairs usually progresses to complete alopecia as the dog gets older. Hair loss is symmetrical, but remaining hairs do not easily epilate. Alopecia may involve the lateral aspects of the ear pinnae, postauricular regions, and caudomedial thighs, and the ventral aspect of the neck, chest, and abdomen. Alopecic skin becomes secondarily hyperpigmented over time.

Top Differentials

Differentials include dermatophytosis, demodicosis, superficial pyoderma, and causes of endocrine alopecia (hyperadrenocorticism, hypothyroidism, sex hormone dermatosis).

Diagnosis

1. Rule out other differentials.
2. Dermatohistopathology: hair follicles are smaller than normal.

Treatment and Prognosis

1. No specific treatment is known.
2. In some dogs, hair regrowth may occur with melatonin. Both sustained-release melatonin (1–3) (12-mg implants/dog SC once) and melatonin (3–12 mg/dog PO q 12–24 hours for 3 months) have been used, with variable results. Improvement, if any, should occur within 3 months after treatment.
3. The prognosis is good. Although hair loss is usually irreversible, this is a cosmetic problem only that does not affect the dog's quality of life.

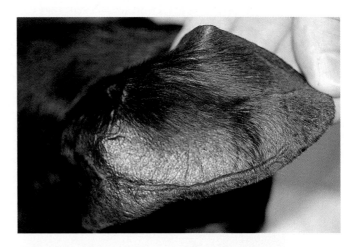

FIGURE 9-120 Canine Pattern Baldness. Diffuse alopecia on the ear pinna of an adult Dachshund.

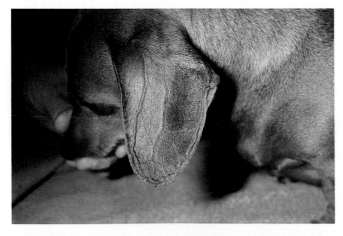

FIGURE 9-119 Canine Pattern Baldness. Complete alopecia on this Dachshund's ear pinna is typical of this syndrome. *(Courtesy J. MacDonald.)*

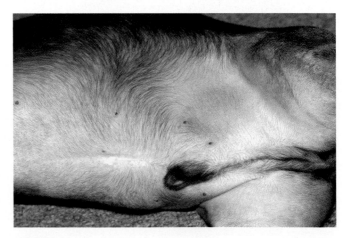

FIGURE 9-121 Canine Pattern Baldness. Diffuse alopecia on the chest and abdomen. Note the lack of evidence of a papular rash, which would suggest a superficial pyoderma.

Idiopathic Bald Thigh Syndrome of Greyhounds

Features

Idiopathic bald thigh syndrome of Greyhounds is an alopecic disorder of unknown cause that is common in Greyhound dogs. Alopecia may begin during late puberty or early adulthood, and it often slowly progresses as the dog ages.

Gradual, bilaterally symmetrical thinning of hairs on the lateral and caudal aspects of the thighs often extends to the ventral abdomen. Remaining hairs do not epilate easily. Except for the alopecia, affected skin appears normal. No systemic signs of illness are noted.

Top Differentials

Differentials include demodicosis, dermatophytosis, superficial pyoderma, and causes of endocrine alopecia (hypothyroidism, hyperadrenocorticism, sex hormone dermatosis).

Diagnosis

1. Based on signalment, history, clinical findings, and rule out other differentials.
2. Dermatohistopathology (nondiagnostic): findings are nonspecific and similar to those seen with endocrinopathies.

Treatment and Prognosis

1. No specific treatment reverses or prevents further hair loss.
2. The prognosis is good. Although hair loss is usually permanent, this is a cosmetic disease only that does not affect the dog's quality of life.

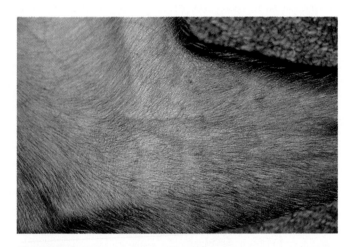

FIGURE 9-123 Idiopathic Bald Thigh Syndrome of Greyhounds. Diffuse alopecia on the rear legs of an adult Greyhound. No evidence of secondary infection is seen.

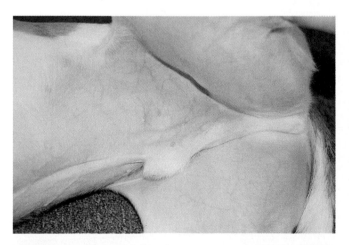

FIGURE 9-122 Idiopathic Bald Thigh Syndrome of Greyhounds. Complete alopecia on the abdominal and inguinal regions of an adult Greyhound. No evidence of secondary infection is seen.

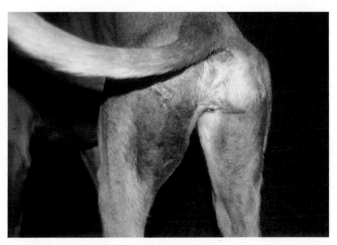

FIGURE 9-124 Idiopathic Bald Thigh Syndrome of Greyhounds. Diffuse alopecia and hyperpigmentation on the caudal thighs of an adult Greyhound.

Canine Recurrent Flank Alopecia (seasonal flank alopecia, cyclic flank alopecia, cyclic follicular dysplasia)

Features

Canine recurrent flank alopecia is a seasonally recurring follicular dysplasia. The exact cause is unknown, but photoperiod control of melatonin and prolactin secretion may be involved. Onset of alopecia in the Northern hemisphere usually occurs between November and March. Most dogs regrow their hair spontaneously 3 to 8 months later. Episodes of hair loss may occur sporadically only once or twice, or regularly each year. With repeated episodes, a progressive increase in the amount and duration of hair loss may be seen. It is uncommon in dogs, with highest incidence in young adult Boxers, bulldogs, Airedales, and Schnauzers.

Canine recurrent flank alopecia manifests as nonpruritic, noninflamed, well-demarcated alopecia limited to the thoracolumbar region that is usually bilaterally symmetrical but may be asymmetrical or may involve only one side. Affected skin may become secondarily hyperpigmented. No systemic signs of illness are noted.

Top Differentials

Differentials include superficial pyoderma, demodicosis, dermatophytosis, other endocrinopathies especially hypothyroidism, alopecia areata, and topical steroid reaction.

Diagnosis

1. History and clinical findings: rule out other differentials.

2. Dermatohistopathology: dysplastic, atrophic, and keratin-filled hair follicles with finger-like projections into the underlying dermis. Increased melanin may be seen in sebaceous ducts and in hair follicles.

Treatment and Prognosis

1. Observation without treatment is reasonable because this disease is purely cosmetic and affected dogs are otherwise healthy.
2. Treatment with melatonin may be effective. Protocols include the following:
   ■ Melatonin 3–12 mg/dog PO q 12–24 hours for 3 months and several weeks before the onset of the next occurrence because this disorder is recurrent.
3. The prognosis for hair regrowth is variable. Spontaneous hair regrowth often occurs within 3 to 8 months, even without treatment. However, regrowth may be incomplete, and new hairs may be duller in color and drier in texture. Reinitiating melatonin therapy each year 4 to 6 weeks before anticipated recurrences may prevent future episodes. This is a cosmetic disease that does not affect the dog's quality of life.

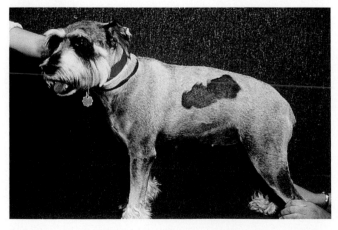

FIGURE 9-125 Canine Recurrent Flank Alopecia. Well-demarcated alopecia and hyperpigmentation on the lateral flank of a 2-year-old Schnauzer. The lesion recurred every spring and resolved in the winter.

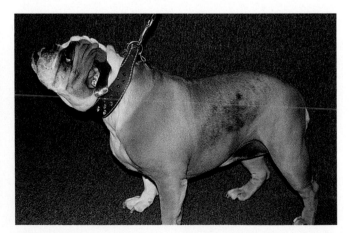

FIGURE 9-126 Canine Recurrent Flank Alopecia. Alopecia on the flank of an adult bulldog.

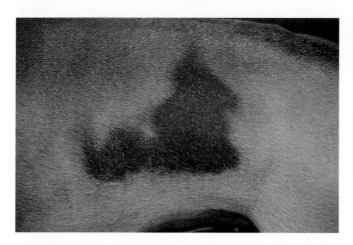

FIGURE 9-127 Canine Recurrent Flank Alopecia. Alopecia and hyperpigmentation on the lateral flank of an adult Boxer. Lesions waxed and waned with the seasons but never completely resolved. Note the well-demarcated margin and lack of secondary infection.

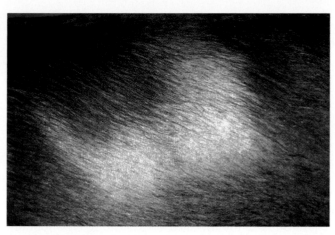

FIGURE 9-128 Canine Recurrent Flank Alopecia. Alopecia on the flank. Note no evidence of secondary infection can be seen.

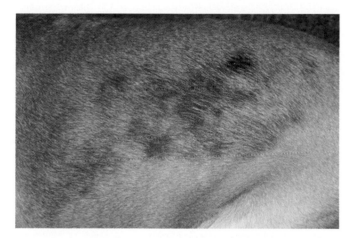

FIGURE 9-129 Canine Recurrent Flank Alopecia. Alopecia and hyperpigmentation with no evidence of secondary superficial pyoderma.

Miscellaneous Canine Follicular Dysplasias

Features

This section discusses a group of poorly understood follicular dysplasias that are not endocrine-related. Alopecia, which results from abnormal hair follicle development or structural abnormalities, is neither color-linked nor seasonal. In most cases, an autosomal recessive mode of inheritance is suspected. It is rare in young adult to middle-aged dogs, although it is sporadically reported in many breeds; its highest incidence is documented in Irish water spaniels, Portuguese water dogs, Pont-Audemer spaniels, black or red Dobermann pinschers, and Weimaraners.

Irish Water Spaniels

Although alopecia of the ventral neck and distal tail is normal and is considered a special characteristic of this breed, affected dogs also develop focal to diffuse areas of alopecia involving the lateral neck, flanks, trunk, rump, and thighs. In males, hair loss usually begins during middle age, is nonseasonal, and progressively worsens with age. In females, hair loss tends to begin after the first or second estrus cycle. Typically, hair loss develops 6 to 8 weeks after estrus; hair initially regrows 3 to 4 weeks later, but loss becomes more progressive, often bilaterally symmetrical, and permanent with each subsequent estrus cycle. Secondary superficial pyoderma (i.e., papules, pustules, and epidermal collarettes) is common.

Portuguese Water Dogs

Alopecia is symmetrical and affects the flanks, caudodorsum of the trunk, and periocular region. A waxing and waning course is characteristic, and spontaneous hair regrowth occurs in most dogs , but regrown hairs are abnormally dull, dry, and fragile. With each subsequent episode of hair loss, less hair regrows until eventually, the hair loss becomes permanent.

Pont-Audemer Spaniels

Alopecia is restricted to brown-haired areas of the trunk and ears.

Black or Red Dobermann Pinschers

Affected dogs develop a slowly progressive alopecia over the dorsolumbar region and flanks. Remaining hairs do not epilate easily. Recurring superficial bacterial folliculitis is common.

Weimaraners

Progressive, bilaterally symmetrical alopecia of the trunk occurs. Remaining hairs are dry and brittle but do not epilate easily. The trunk eventually may become almost completely hairless, but the head and limbs are spared. Recurrent bouts of bacterial folliculitis and furunculosis are common.

Top Differentials

Differentials include dermatophytosis, demodicosis, superficial pyoderma, causes of endocrine alopecia, and topical steroid reaction.

Diagnosis

1. Based on history, clinical findings, and rule out other differentials.
2. Trichogram of affected hairs (microscopic examination of plucked hairs): hair cortices and medullas contain numerous large melanin clumps, and hair cuticles have defects and fractures.
3. Dermatohistopathology: dilated hair follicles are filled with keratin, hair shaft fragments, and free melanin. Abnormal clumps of melanin are present in follicular and epidermal basal cells and in hair matrix cells. Apoptosis of keratinocytes in the external and internal root sheaths and vacuolation of hair matrix cells may also be seen.

Treatment and Prognosis

1. The animal should be treated symptomatically with mild antiseborrheic or antibacterial shampoos and conditioners as needed.
2. Appropriate systemic antibiotics should be administered for 3 to 4 weeks if secondary pyoderma is present.
3. No specific treatment is known, but fatty acid supplementation has been reported to improve coat condition or result in hair regrowth in some Irish water spaniels.
4. The prognosis is good. Although hair loss is usually irreversible, and routine symptomatic skin care may be needed, this is a cosmetic problem only that does not affect the dog's quality of life. Affected dogs should not be bred.

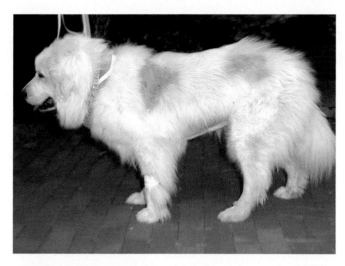

FIGURE 9-130 **Miscellaneous Canine Follicular Dysplasias.** Multifocal alopecia on the shoulder and flank.

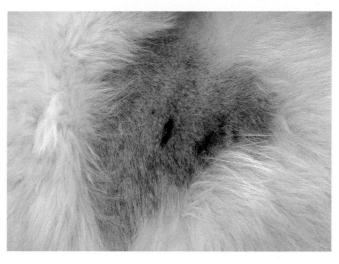

FIGURE 9-131 **Miscellaneous Canine Follicular Dysplasias.** Close-up of the dog in Figure 9-130. The well-demarcated area of alopecia lacked evidence of secondary infection.

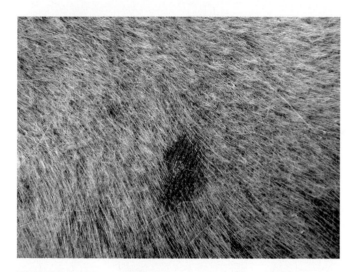

FIGURE 9-132 **Miscellaneous Canine Follicular Dysplasias.** Close-up of the dog in Figure 9-130. Diffuse alopecia with no evidence of secondary infection.

Feline Preauricular and Pinnal Alopecias

Features

Preauricular alopecia is a common and normal finding in cats. It is characterized by sparsely haired skin on the head between the ears and eyes that is not usually noticeable in long-haired cats but is more readily apparent in short-haired cats. No skin lesions are present.

Pinnal alopecia is uncommon in cats and is characterized by periodic episodes of nonpruritic pinnal alopecia. Siamese cats are predisposed. The alopecia may be patchy or may involve most of the pinna, and both ears are usually involved. Except for alopecia, the skin is otherwise normal.

Top Differentials

Differentials include dermatophytosis, flea allergy dermatitis, food allergy, atopy, demodicosis, and pyoderma.

Diagnosis

1. Based on history, clinical findings, and rule out other differentials.

Treatment and Prognosis

1. No treatment is known.
2. The prognosis is good. Preauricular alopecia is a normal finding in cats. Cats with pinnal alopecia usually regrow hair within several months.

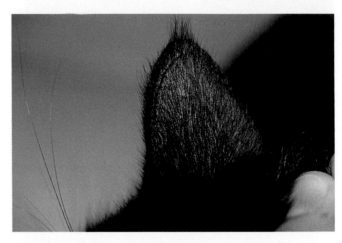

FIGURE 9-134 Feline Preauricular and Pinnal Alopecia. Close-up of the cat in Figure 9-133. Partial alopecia on the ear pinna with no evidence of secondary infection.

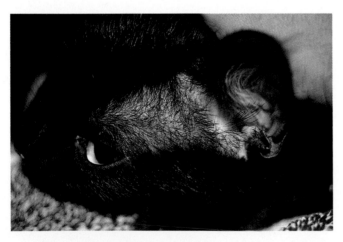

FIGURE 9-133 Feline Preauricular and Pinnal Alopecia. Diffuse alopecia on the preauricular skin of a cat.

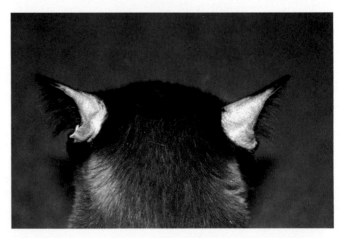

FIGURE 9-135 Feline Preauricular and Pinnal Alopecia. Total bilaterally symmetrical alopecia of the ear pinnae.

Anagen and Telogen Defluxion

Features

Alopecia develops when normal hair growth and cycle are adversely affected by underlying disease or stress such as chemotherapy drug administration, infection, metabolic disease, fever, pregnancy, shock, surgery, and anesthesia. It occurs rarely in dogs and cats.

This condition begins as an acute onset of hair loss within days of the insult (anagen defluxion) or 1 to 3 months after the insult (telogen defluxion). Except for alopecia, affected skin appears otherwise normal. In telogen defluxion, hair loss usually is widespread, progresses rapidly over a few to several days, and tends to spare the head. In anagen defluxion, hair loss is less dramatic and is characterized by excessive shedding.

Top Differentials

Differentials include other causes of endocrine alopecia, pyoderma, demodicosis, dermatophytosis, and excessive shedding.

Diagnosis

1. Based on history, clinical findings, and rule out other differentials.
2. Dermatohistopathology (rarely diagnostic): usually reveals normal skin, but hairs diffusely in telogen may be seen in telogen defluxion, and abnormal hair matrix cells with dysplastic hair shafts may be seen in anagen defluxion.

Treatment and Prognosis

1. The underlying cause should be corrected.
2. The prognosis is good. Spontaneous hair regrowth occurs after resolution or cessation of the cause.

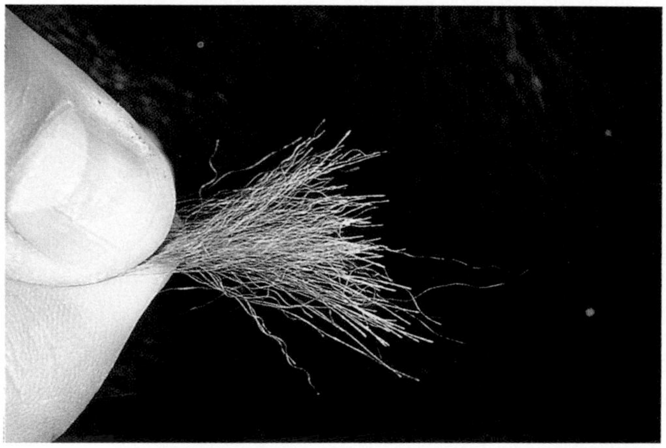

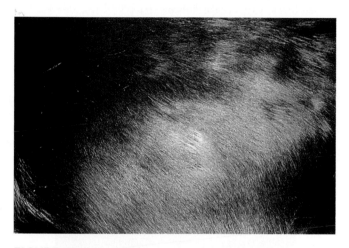

FIGURE 9-137 Anagen and Telogen Defluxion. The moth-eaten alopecia on this dog's body was caused by telogen defluxion. *(Courtesy A. Yu.)*

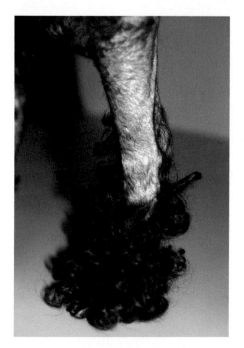

FIGURE 9-138 Anagen and Telogen Defluxion. Diffuse alopecia affecting the distal extremities of a Poodle.

FIGURE 9-136 Anagen and Telogen Defluxion. Large clumps of hair can be easily epilated in dogs with this syndrome. *(Courtesy A. Yu.)*

Traction Alopecia

Features

Traction alopecia is an alopecia that occurs when hair clips or rubber bands used to hold hair in place are fastened too tightly or for too long. It is uncommon in dogs.

Initially, an erythematous plaque appears at the site of the hair device. It may progress into a localized patch of scarred alopecia. The lesion most commonly occurs on the top of or on the lateral aspect of the head.

Top Differentials

Differentials include demodicosis, dermatophytosis, superficial pyoderma, alopecia areata, and topical steroid reaction.

Diagnosis

1. Usually based on history and clinical findings.
2. Dermatohistopathology: variable mononuclear cell infiltrates, edema, vasodilatation, pilosebaceous atrophy, fibrosing dermatitis, or scarring alopecia.

Treatment and Prognosis

1. The hair device should be removed.
2. As a preventive, hair devices should be applied properly so that excessive traction on hairs is not produced.
3. The prognosis depends on the duration of the lesion. Early lesions should resolve spontaneously after the hair device has been removed. Chronic, scarred lesions may be permanent.

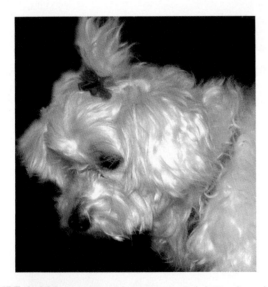

FIGURE 9-139 Traction Alopecia. An adult Toy breed demonstrating the typical bow-bound hairstyle.

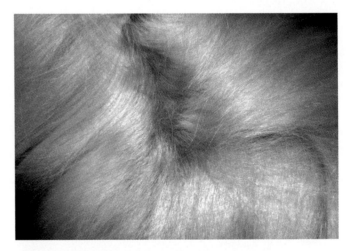

FIGURE 9-140 Traction Alopecia. Same dog as in Figure 9-139. Focal alopecia and erythema caused by persistent traction.

Alopecia Areata

Features

Alopecia areata is an immune-mediated reaction to follicular wall antigens. Hair loss appears to result from cellular and humoral immune responses against hair follicle antigens. It is rare in dogs and cats, with highest incidence in adult animals.

Alopecia areata is a spontaneously occurring, nonpruritic, focal to multifocal, usually well-demarcated patchy area of alopecia that may gradually enlarge. Lesions may appear anywhere on the body but are most common on the head (muzzle, periocular area, ears, chin, forehead) neck, and legs. Facial lesions are often bilaterally symmetrical. In some dogs with multicolored hair coats, the alopecic lesions appear first in pigmented areas. The alopecic skin may gradually develop melanoderma (hyperpigmentation) but otherwise appears normal. Leukotrichia may also be seen.

Top Differentials

Differentials include dermatophytosis, demodicosis, superficial pyoderma, injection reaction, topical steroid reaction, and traction alopecia.

Diagnosis

1. Rule out other differentials.
2. Dermatohistopathology: findings vary according to the stage of the lesion. Early lesions have peribulbar and intrabulbar accumulations of lymphocytes, histiocytes, and plasma cells that affect almost exclusively anagen hair follicles. Older lesions show a predominance of catagen, telogen, and atrophic hair follicles. In chronic lesions, absence of hair follicles is noted, along with residual fibrous tracts.

Treatment and Prognosis

1. No specific treatment is known.
2. Spontaneous and complete hair regrowth may be seen in some cases, but this can take months to years to occur.
3. Topical treatment with steroids or tacrolimus may be effective (apply every 12–24 hours until hair regrows).
4. Systemic therapy with systemic cyclosporine or immunosuppressive doses of glucocorticoids can be attempted, but hair regrowth does not always occur. The adverse effects of high-dose steroid therapy may be worse than the disease itself.
5. The prognosis for hair regrowth is fair to guarded; hairs that regrow may be nonpigmented and may permanently remain white thereafter. This is a cosmetic disease only that does not affect the animal's quality of life.

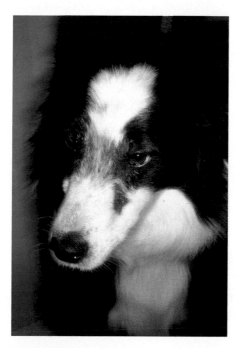

FIGURE 9-141 Alopecia Areata. Focal alopecia on the face of an adult dog. *(Courtesy A. Yu.)*

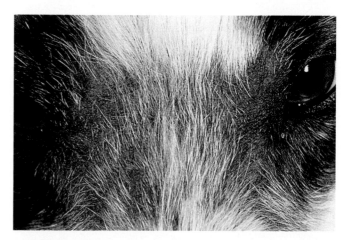

FIGURE 9-142 Alopecia Areata. Close-up of the dog in Figure 9-141. Alopecia with no evidence of secondary infection. *(Courtesy A. Yu.)*

Alopecia Areata—*cont'd*

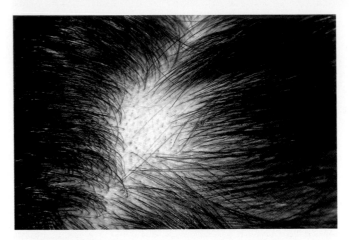

FIGURE 9-143 Alopecia Areata. Focal area of alopecia with well-demarcated margins typical of this syndrome. Note that no evidence of inflammation or secondary infection can be seen.

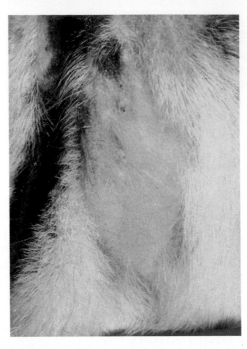

FIGURE 9-144 Alopecia Areata. Alopecia and erythema on the chin and ventral neck. Note the erythema may indicate an active inflammatory phase of this syndrome. *(Courtesy A. Yu.)*

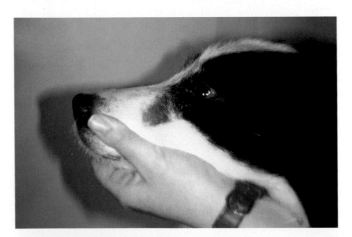

FIGURE 9-145 Alopecia Areata. Well-demarcated areas of alopecia on the face are typical of this syndrome. *(Courtesy A. Yu.)*

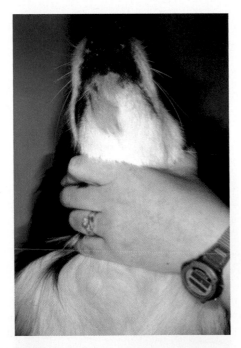

FIGURE 9-146 Alopecia Areata. Alopecic lesions on the chin and ventral neck are apparent. *(Courtesy A.Yu.)*

Feline Psychogenic Alopecia (neurodermatitis)

Features

Feline psychogenic alopecia is extremely overdiagnosed. Behavioral causes of alopecia and dermatitis in cats are very rare but usually manifest as self-induced depilation and alopecia resulting from excessive or inappropriate grooming, licking, chewing, or hair pulling. Excessive and out-of-context grooming is thought to be an obsessive-compulsive behavior that is triggered by environmental stresses and anxiety. Because most cats spend a great part of each day grooming themselves, the owner of a cat with psychogenic alopecia may not realize that the cat's alopecia is self-created. The condition is uncommon in cats, with purebred cats that have high-strung, nervous temperaments (e.g., Siamese, Burmese, Himalayans, Abyssinians) being possibly predisposed. Psychogenic alopecia is overdiagnosed; flea hypersensitivity, food allergy, atopy, and other ectoparasites are more common causes of feline alopecia.

Alopecia is produced when the cat grooms hard enough to remove hairs but not vigorously enough to damage the skin. Regional, multifocal, or generalized hair loss occurs. Alopecia may occur anywhere on the body where the cat can lick, but it most commonly involves the medial forelegs, inner thighs, perineum, and ventral abdomen. Hair loss is often bilaterally symmetrical, but remaining hairs do not epilate easily. Careful inspection of the alopecic skin reveals that the hairs have not actually fallen out; they are still present but are broken off near the surface of the skin. Rarely, overly aggressive grooming may result in an area of abraded, excoriated skin. Hair in the feces and vomited hairballs may be seen.

Top Differentials

Differentials include flea allergy dermatitis, food allergy, dermatophytosis, ectoparasites (fleas, demodicosis, cheyletiellosis), and hypersensitivity (atopy).

Diagnosis

1. Rule out ectoparasitism and other hypersensitivities.
2. Failure to respond to aggressive flea control (nitenpyram administered every other day for 1 month).
3. Usually based on history that the onset of overgrooming behavior followed a stressful event or a change in environment, the clinical findings, and rule out all other differentials (failure to respond to aggressive flea control, lime sulfur dips, and steroid therapy).
4. Trichogram (microscopic examination of plucked hairs): hairs are broken off.
5. Dermatohistopathology: normal, noninflamed skin.

Treatment and Prognosis

1. The underlying cause of the psychological stress (e.g., separation from owner, moved to a new house, animal companion died, new pet in household, formerly outdoor cat denied access to outdoors) must be identified and appropriate environmental modifications made, if possible.
2. A good flea control program should be instituted to prevent fleas from aggravating the symptoms.
3. Use of a mechanical barrier (e.g., Elizabethan collar, T-shirt) for 1 to 2 months to prevent grooming may help break the habit.
4. Behavior-modifying drugs may help stop the abnormal grooming behavior. In some cases, treatment may be discontinued after 30 to 60 days of therapy; in others, lifelong therapy is required for control. Drugs that may be effective include the following:
   - Amitriptyline 5–10 mg/cat PO q 12–24 hours
   - Clomipramine 1.25–2.5 mg/cat PO q 24 hours
   - Buspirone 1.25–5 mg/cat q 12 hours
   - Phenobarbital 4–8 mg/cat PO q 12 hours
   - Diazepam 1–2 mg/cat PO q 12–24 hours
   - Naloxone 1 mg/kg SC q several weeks as needed
5. The prognosis for hair regrowth is variable, depending on whether the underlying cause can be identified and corrected. Some cats respond completely to behavior-modifying drugs. Psychogenic alopecia is essentially a cosmetic disease; observation without treatment may be reasonable because long-term use of behavioral-modifying drugs may result in serious adverse effects.

Feline Psychogenic Alopecia—*cont'd*

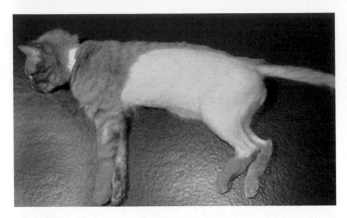

FIGURE 9-147 **Psychogenic Alopecia.** Alopecia on the lateral flank caused by excessive grooming. The hair at the dorsal midline was difficult for the cat to reach; therefore, it remained normal. *(Courtesy T. Manning.)*

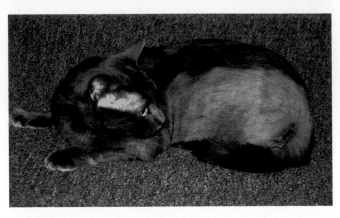

FIGURE 9-148 **Psychogenic Alopecia.** Alopecia on the lateral trunk caused by excessive grooming *in a food-allergic cat*. Note the similarity to Figure 9-147.

CHAPTER 10

Congenital Diseases

- Epidermolysis Bullosa
- Familial Canine Dermatomyositis
- Ichthyosis
- Ehlers-Danlos Syndrome (cutaneous asthenia, dermatosparaxis)

- Cutaneous Mucinosis
- Dermoid Sinus
- Canine Juvenile Cellulitis (juvenile pyoderma, puppy strangles)

Epidermolysis Bullosa

Features

Epidermolysis bullosa refers to a group of hereditary mechanobullous diseases in which minor trauma results in blister formation. Structural defects in the basement membrane zone are responsible for incomplete cohesion between the epidermis and the dermis. The condition is rare in dogs and cats, with affected animals usually developing lesions shortly after birth.

Vesicles, bullae, erosions, crusts, and ulcers appear at sites of frictional trauma such as on the footpads, lips, gingiva, tongue, and palate, and over bony prominences of the limbs. Lesions may also involve the face, trunk, tail, or ventral abdomen. Claw sloughing and secondary bacterial paronychia may be seen. In some forms of the disease, in addition to oral vesicles and ulcers, other parts of the upper digestive tract (e.g., esophagus) are similarly affected.

Top Differentials

Differentials include dermatomyositis, pemphigus vulgaris, bullous pemphigoid, systemic lupus erythematosus, cutaneous vesicular lupus erythematosus, erythema multiforme/toxic epidermal necrolysis, drug eruption, and vasculitis.

Diagnosis

1. Rule out other differentials.
2. Dermatohistopathology: subepidermal clefting and vesicle formation with minimal inflammation.
3. Electron microscopy (skin biopsy specimens): depending on the subtype of epidermolysis bullosa, clefting may be intraepidermal from cytolysis of basal cells, below the lamina densa, or within the lamina lucida of the basement membrane zone.

Treatment and Prognosis

1. No specific treatment is known.
2. Trauma should be avoided by keeping the affected animal indoors, away from other animals, and handling it carefully.
3. Appropriate systemic antibiotics should be administered as needed for secondary bacterial infection.
4. The prognosis for severely affected animals is poor. With proper environmental management, mildly affected animals may enjoy a reasonable quality of life. Affected animals should not be bred.

Epidermolysis Bullosa—*cont'd*

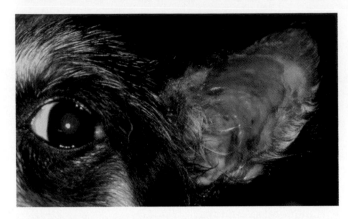

FIGURE 10-1 Epidermolysis Bullosa. Ulceration of the ear pinna. *(Courtesy P. Rakich.)*

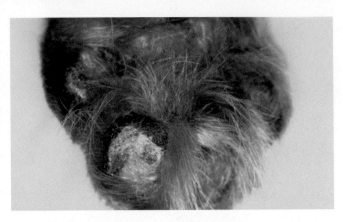

FIGURE 10-2 Epidermolysis Bullosa. Sloughing of the foot-pads. The superficial epidermis is peeling off. *(Courtesy P. Rakich.)*

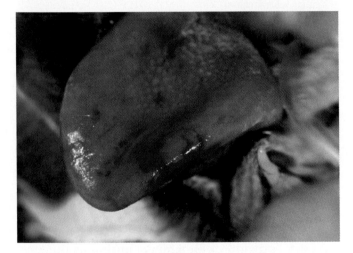

FIGURE 10-3 Epidermolysis Bullosa. Ulcerations on the tongue of the young kitten. The primary lesions are vesicles, which easily rupture, leaving ulcers. *(Courtesy A. Wolf.)*

Familial Canine Dermatomyositis

Features

Familial canine dermatomyositis is an inherited inflammatory disorder of the skin and muscles in which a microvascular vasculopathy is thought to play a role. The cause is unclear, but a genetic predisposition followed by a trigger (e.g., infection, other environmental factor) that initiates an immune-mediated process and the clinical signs has been proposed. It is uncommon in dogs, with the highest incidence in collies, Shetland Sheep dogs, and their cross-breeds. Lesions usually first appear in puppies at between 2 and 6 months of age. Several littermates may be affected, but the severity of the disease often varies significantly among puppies.

Skin lesions are nonpruritic, vary in severity, and may wax and wane. They are characterized by variable degrees of erythema, alopecia, scaling, crusting, erosion, ulceration, and scarring and, rarely, by papules and vesicles. Skin lesions occur on the bridge of the nose, around the eyes and lips, in the inner ear pinnae, on the tail tip, and over bony prominences of the distal extremities. Rarely, footpad ulcers are seen. Signs of muscle involvement are variable. Dogs may appear to be unaffected, to have bilaterally symmetrical atrophy of the masseter or temporalis muscle, or to have generalized symmetrical muscle atrophy. Dogs with masseter muscle involvement may have difficulty eating, drinking, and swallowing. Severely affected dogs may be weak, lethargic, stunted, lame, and infertile. If the leg muscles atrophy, affected dogs may exhibit an abnormal "high-stepping" gait. When the esophageal muscles are affected, megaesophagus may develop.

Top Differentials

Differentials include demodicosis, dermatophytosis, superficial pyoderma, autoimmune skin disease, vasculitis, and polymyositis.

Diagnosis

1. Rule out other differentials.
2. Dermatohistopathology (may be nondiagnostic): scattered epidermal basal cell degeneration; perifollicular inflammatory infiltrates of lymphocytes, histiocytes, and variable numbers of mast cells and neutrophils; follicular basal cell degeneration; and follicular atrophy are highly suggestive findings but may not be present, especially in chronic or scarred lesions.
3. Electromyography: fibrillation potentials, bizarre high-frequency discharges, and sharp waves are seen in affected muscles.
4. Histopathology (muscle biopsies): variable multifocal accumulations of inflammatory cells, including lymphocytes, macrophages, plasma cells, neutrophils, and eosinophils; myofibril degeneration; and myofiber atrophy and regeneration.

Treatment and Prognosis

1. Symptomatic shampoo therapy may be helpful for removing crusts.
2. Any secondary superficial pyoderma should be treated with appropriate systemic antibiotics.
3. Activities that may traumatize the skin should be avoided.
4. Intact females should be spayed because estrus, pregnancy, and lactation exacerbate the disease. Affected males should be neutered so they cannot reproduce.
5. Daily supplementation with oral essential fatty acids and treatment with vitamin E 400 to 800 IU PO every 24 hours may be beneficial for the skin lesions. Improvement should be seen after 2 to 3 months of therapy (see Table 8-2).
6. Treatment with pentoxifylline (Trental) 25 mg/kg PO every 12 hours with food may be beneficial in some dogs. Improvement should be seen within 1 to 3 months of therapy.
7. Cyclosporine (Atopica) 5–10 mg/kg PO administered every 24 hours may be beneficial (effects are seen in approximately 4–6 weeks). Then, dosage frequency should be tapered down to every 48 to 72 hours. Glucocorticoids can be used initially to speed response. As of this writing, no statistically significant increase in tumor risk or severe infection is known to result from the immune effects of cyclosporine.
8. Prednisone 1 mg/kg PO every 24 hours until lesions improve (approximately 7–10 days), then tapered off, may be used for acute flare-ups; however, prolonged steroid usage may exacerbate muscle atrophy.
9. The prognosis is variable, depending on the severity of the disease. Skin lesions in minimally affected dogs tend to resolve spontaneously, with no scarring. Skin lesions in mildly to moderately affected dogs usually resolve eventually, but residual scarring is common. Even when lesions resolve, however, relapses may occur later on, when the dog is an adult. In severely affected dogs, dermatitis and myositis do not resolve, and the prognosis for long-term survival is poor. Regardless of disease severity, affected dogs should not be bred.

Familial Canine Dermatomyositis—cont'd

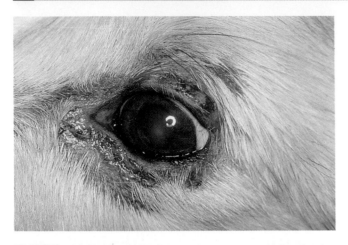

FIGURE 10-4 Familial Canine Dermatomyositis. Erosive lesions on the periocular skin are characteristic of active lesions. As the dog ages and active lesions resolve, the skin may become scarred and remain alopecic. *(Courtesy M. Mahaffey.)*

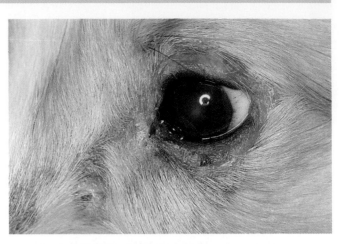

FIGURE 10-5 Familial Canine Dermatomyositis. The same dog as in Figure 10-4. Active lesions have resolved, leaving alopecic, scarred skin. *(Courtesy M. Mahaffey.)*

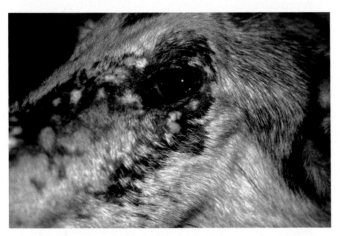

FIGURE 10-6 Familial Canine Dermatomyositis. Alopecia and scarring on the face of an adult collie. The erythematous macules were active lesions.

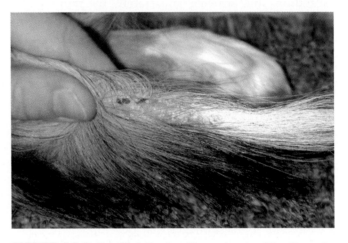

FIGURE 10-7 Familial Canine Dermatomyositis. Alopecic, erythematous, crusting dermatitis on the tail of a collie with dermatomyositis.

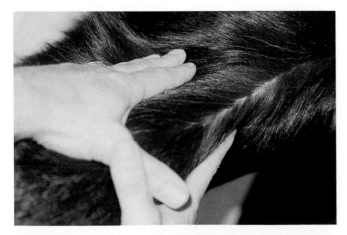

FIGURE 10-8 Familial Canine Dermatomyositis. Severe muscle atrophy on the lumbar musculature in an infected dog. The lateral processes of the vertebrae can be easily palpated. *(Courtesy D. Angarano.)*

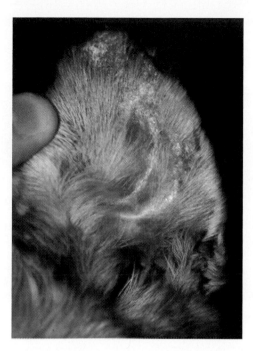

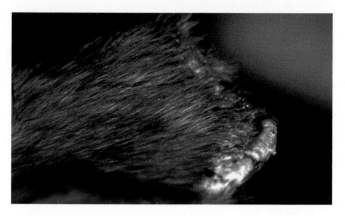

FIGURE 10-10 Familial Canine Dermatomyositis. Crusting lesions on the ear margin waxed and waned for several years. Note the similarity to vasculitis and other autoimmune skin diseases.

FIGURE 10-9 Familial Canine Dermatomyositis. Crusting, erosive lesions on the ear pinna of an adult collie with chronic lesions.

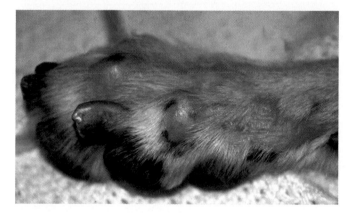

FIGURE 10-11 Familial Canine Dermatomyositis. Alopecia and scarring typical of chronic lesions.

Ichthyosis

Features

Ichthyosis is a congenital keratinization disorder. It is rare in dogs, with West Highland White terriers, Golden retrievers, Cavalier King Charles spaniels, Doberman pinschers, Jack Russell terriers, Norfolk terriers, and Yorkshire terriers possibly predisposed. Dogs are abnormal at birth, and one or more puppies in the litter may be affected.

Most of the body is covered with tightly adhering scales, which may flake off in large sheets or accumulate as seborrheic debris on the surface of the skin. The skin may be erythematous and alopecic. Marked hyperkeratosis of the nasal planum and footpads, especially at the margins of the pads, is typical. The feet may be swollen and painful.

Top Differentials

Differentials include primary seborrhea and epidermal dysplasia.

Diagnosis

1. Dermatohistopathology: marked orthokeratotic hyperkeratosis, hypergranulosis, and numerous mitotic figures in keratinocytes are usually seen. Follicular keratosis and plugging are common. Reticular degeneration may be seen.

Treatment and Prognosis

1. No specific treatment is known.
2. Therapeutic trials with isotretinoin have not been effective.
3. Any secondary bacterial or *Malassezia* skin infections should be treated with appropriate systemic medications.
4. For mild cases, daily oral essential fatty acid supplementation (180 mg EPA/10 lb) and topical therapy with antiseborrheic shampoos, emollient rinses, and humectants applied every 2 to 4 days or as needed may effectively control symptoms. Essential fatty acid supplementation may be effective.
5. The prognosis is poor. This is a chronic and incurable disease that is difficult to manage symptomatically. Affected dogs should not be bred.

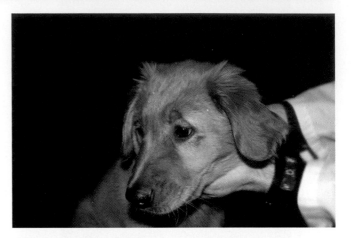

FIGURE 10-12 Ichthyosis. Large cornflake-like flakes on the head of a young Golden retriever.

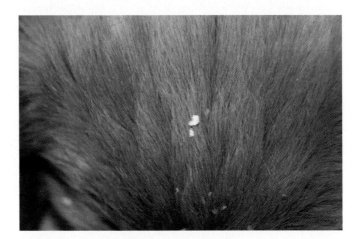

FIGURE 10-13 Ichthyosis. Close-up of the dog in Figure 10-12. Large flakes are apparent.

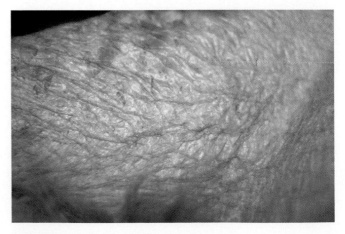

FIGURE 10-14 Ichthyosis. Rice paper–like skin on the ventral abdomen of a puppy with ichthyosis.

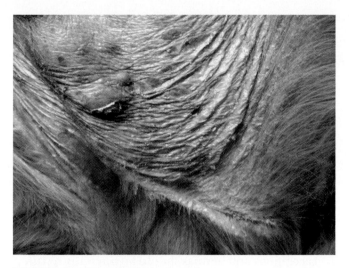

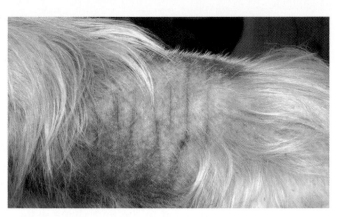

FIGURE 10-16 **Ichthyosis.** Alopecia, erythema, and scaling in a female spayed West Highland White terrier.

FIGURE 10-15 **Ichthyosis.** Rice paper–like skin on the ventral abdomen. The crinkled effect is unique.

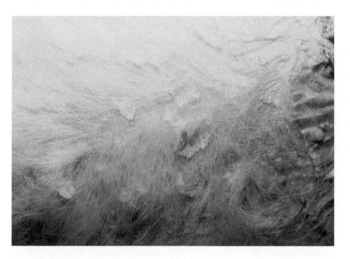

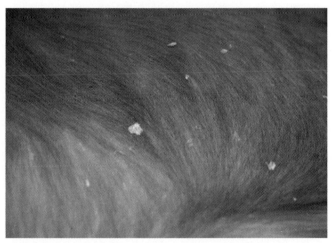

FIGURE 10-17 **Ichthyosis.** Alopecia and large, tightly adherent scales are typical. *(Courtesy K. Credille and R. Dunstan.)*

FIGURE 10-18 **Ichthyosis.** Large cornflake-like flakes on the lateral thorax in a Golden retriever puppy.

Ehlers-Danlos Syndrome (cutaneous asthenia, dermatosparaxis)

Features

Ehlers-Danlos syndrome is a group of inherited collagenopathies that are characterized by defective collagen synthesis or fiber formation that results in abnormal skin extensibility and fragility. It is rare in dogs and cats.

Cutaneous signs are characterized by skin hyperextensibility or skin that is thin and fragile. Hyperextensible skin is loosely attached to the underlying tissues, can be stretched to extreme lengths, and may hang in folds, especially on the limbs and the ventral aspect of the neck. Fragile skin easily or spontaneously tears with little to no bleeding; wound healing results in highly visible "cigarette paper" scars. Concurrent widening of the bridge of the nose, hygromas, joint laxity and dislocation, corneal changes, lens luxation, and cataracts may be present. Nontraumatic hernias (inguinal, perineal, and diaphragmatic) may rarely occur.

Top Differentials

Dogs

No differentials in dogs are known. This is a clinically distinct syndrome.

Cats

In cats, the differential is acquired skin fragility (from spontaneous hyperadrenocorticism, diabetes mellitus, hepatic lipidosis, or administration of corticosteroids or progestins).

Diagnosis

1. History and clinical findings.
2. Skin extensibility index ([vertical height of dorsal lumbar skin fold when extended divided by body length from occipital crest to tail base] × 100): affected dogs and cats have values above 14.5% and 19%, respectively.
3. Dermatohistopathology (often nondiagnostic): dermal collagen may appear to be architecturally normal or may be fragmented, disoriented, and abnormally organized.
4. Electron microscopy (skin biopsy): abnormal structure or amount of collagen.

Treatment and Prognosis

1. No specific treatment is known.
2. Trauma should be avoided by keeping the affected animal indoors and away from other animals. Objects with sharp or rough edges and surfaces should be padded or removed. Dogs should be leash-walked in well-groomed areas.
3. The animal should be handled and restrained carefully to avoid tearing the skin.
4. Cats should be declawed to prevent self-trauma from scratching.
5. Bedding and resting areas should be well padded to prevent hygromas.
6. Routine flea control should be practiced, and other skin conditions should be promptly addressed and treated to prevent self-trauma from pruritus.
7. Lacerations and hernias should be surgically repaired as they occur.
8. The prognosis is poor, especially for animals with joint laxity. Affected animals should not be bred.

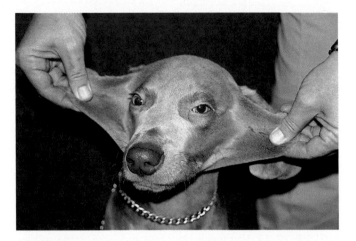

FIGURE 10-19 Ehlers-Danlos Syndrome. This 5-month-old weimaraner has the characteristic skin elasticity associated with the syndrome.

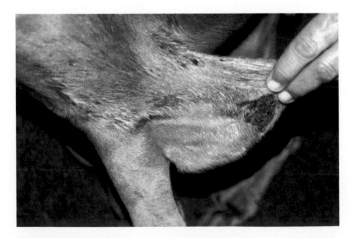

FIGURE 10-20 Ehlers-Danlos Syndrome. Close-up of the dog in Figure 10-19. The remarkable elasticity of the skin is demonstrated on the elbow.

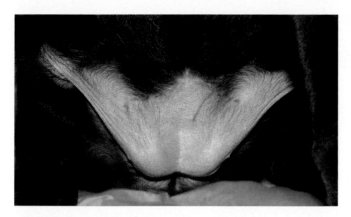

FIGURE 10-21 Ehlers-Danlos Syndrome. The sagging abdominal skin just cranial to the vulva in this young female Labrador is typical of Ehlers-Danlos syndrome.

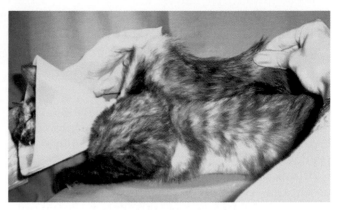

FIGURE 10-22 A young cat with extremely distensible dorsal skin. The skin can be tented well beyond normal limits because of the collagen defect. *(Courtesy E. Kish.)*

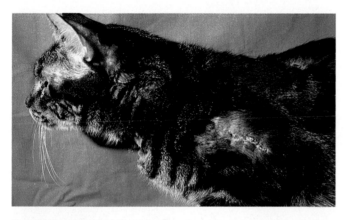

FIGURE 10-23 Ehlers-Danlos Syndrome. A healing laceration on the lateral shoulder of a cat. Wound prevention and management are the most significant clinical concerns for these patients. *(Courtesy J. MacDonald.)*

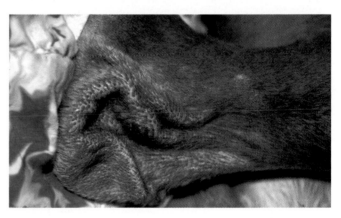

FIGURE 10-24 Ehlers-Danlos Syndrome. The collagen defect caused the skin to loosen, producing these wrinkles.

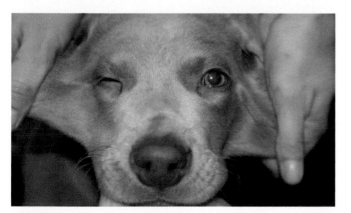

FIGURE 10-25 Ehlers-Danlos Syndrome. The skin on the face is easily stretched beyond normal limits.

Cutaneous Mucinosis

Features

Cutaneous mucinosis is an idiopathic condition characterized by an excessive accumulation or deposition of dermal mucin. It is rare in dogs, except for Chinese Shar pei dogs.

It appears as mild, moderate, or severe exaggeration of skin folds, especially on the head, ventrum, and distal extremities. Affected skin is puffy, thickened, and non-pitting. Clear vesicles and bullae that contain a viscous, sticky fluid (mucin) may be present. If the oropharynx is involved, upper respiratory stridor may be present.

Top Differentials

Differentials include myxedema with hypothyroidism, and autoimmune and immune-mediated skin disorders for vesicular lesions.

Diagnosis

1. Signalment, history, clinical findings, and rule out other differentials.
2. Cytology (vesicle, bulla): amorphous, acellular, basophilic substance (mucin).
3. Dermatohistopathology: excessive dermal mucin, with no other histologic abnormalities.

Treatment and Prognosis

1. Any concurrent skin disease, such as atopy, food hypersensitivity, pyoderma, or yeast dermatitis, should be identified and treated because it may contribute to the development of vesicles.
2. For dermal mucinosis, observation with no treatment is reasonable because skin changes resolve spontaneously by 2 to 5 years of age in most Chinese Shar pei dogs.
3. For severely affected dogs, treatment with prednisolone 1–2 mg/kg PO every 24 hours for 7 days, followed by a gradual reduction in dosage over 30 days, may reduce mucin accumulation. Most dogs need only one course of treatment, but some may require repeated treatments or continuous low-dose maintenance therapy.
4. The prognosis is good. This is primarily a cosmetic problem, which most dogs eventually outgrow. Dogs with oropharyngeal mucinosis are anesthetic risks and should be monitored carefully during administration of anesthesia to prevent respiratory arrest.

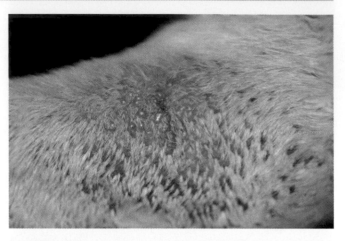

FIGURE 10-26 Cutaneous Mucinosis. Close-up of the skin showing clear vesicles filled with mucin.

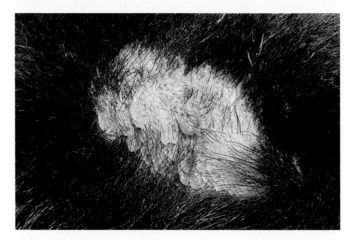

FIGURE 10-27 Cutaneous Mucinosis. Multiple mucin-filled vesicles on the back of an adult Shar pei.

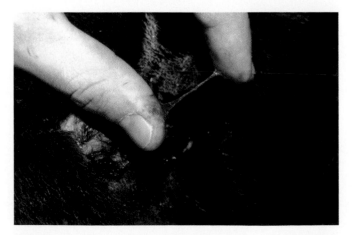

FIGURE 10-28 Cutaneous Mucinosis. Same dog as in Figure 10-27. The vesicle has ruptured. Note the viscosity of the mucin.

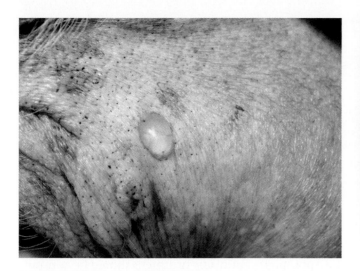

FIGURE 10-29 Cutaneous Mucinosis. A focal vesicle filled with mucin on the skin of a Shar Pei.

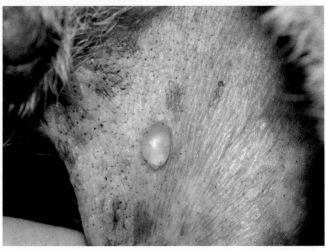

FIGURE 10-30 Cutaneous Mucinosis. A focal vesicle filled with mucin on the skin of a Shar Pei. The surrounding skin is very swollen with mucin without forming vesicles.

Dermoid Sinus

Features

Dermoid sinus is a defect in embryonic development that results in an incomplete separation between the skin and the neural tube. A sinus forms that either extends from the skin to the dura mater, or ends as a blind sac in the subcutaneous tissue. A dorsal dermoid sinus is an incomplete separation between the skin and the spinal cord. It can occur anywhere along the dorsal midline between the cervical and sacrococcygeal regions. A nasal dermal sinus cyst is an incomplete obliteration of neuroectodermal tissue in the prenasal space, which may extend intracranially. Dorsal dermoid sinuses are rare in dogs, with highest incidence in Rhodesian Ridgebacks. Nasal dermoid sinus cysts are also rare in dogs; however, Golden retrievers and spaniel breeds are possibly predisposed.

Dorsal Dermoid Sinus

The sinus has single or multiple small openings that may have tufts of hair protruding from them. This opening may be found anywhere along the dorsal midline but is most common over the cervical spine. A cord of tissue that extends from the cutaneous opening toward the spinal cord may be palpable. The sinus may contain sebum, keratin, debris, and hair. Sinuses may become inflamed, secondarily infected, or cystic, and may drain; if they extend to the spinal cord, this may lead to bacterial meningoencephalitis.

Nasal Dermoid Sinus Cyst

A nasal dermoid sinus cyst is a fluctuant, usually non-painful swelling that occurs on the dorsal aspect of the nose. It is characterized by a small opening ("nasal pit") on the dorsal midline at or just caudal to the junction between the haired skin of the bridge of the nose and the nasal planum. This opening intermittently discharges sebaceous or purulent material, and the swelling may become painful if secondary infection develops.

Top Differentials

Differentials include foreign body, deep infection (bacterial, fungal), and epidermal inclusion cyst.

Diagnosis

1. Signalment, history, and clinical findings.
2. Radiography, computed tomography (CT), or magnetic resonance imaging (MRI): detection of a tract that extends from the skin toward the spine, or a nasal sinus tract with an intracranial extension.

Treatment and Prognosis

1. For quiescent sinuses, observation without treatment is acceptable.
2. For draining or cystic tracts, complete surgical removal of the sinus is the treatment of choice. Incomplete surgical excision results in recurrence, usually within 1 month of surgery.
3. Appropriate antibiotic treatment should be administered to treat secondary bacterial infection, if present.
4. The prognosis is good because complete surgical excision is curative. Affected dogs should not be bred.

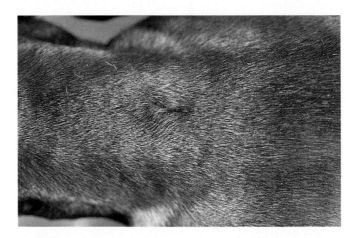

FIGURE 10-31 Dermoid Sinus. A sinus on the back of a Rhodesian Ridgeback appears as a small cutaneous defect.

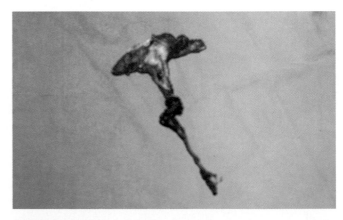

FIGURE 10-32 Dermoid Sinus. The sinus has been surgically removed from the dog in Figure 10-31. The deep extension of the lesion is apparent.

Canine Juvenile Cellulitis (juvenile pyoderma, puppy strangles)

Features

The cause and pathogenesis of this disease are unknown. It is uncommon in dogs, with highest incidence in puppies between 3 weeks and 6 months of age. Dachshund, Golden retriever, Labrador retriever, Gordon setter, Beagle, and Pointer puppies may be predisposed. More than one puppy in a litter may be affected.

Vesicles, pustules, serous to purulent exudate, crusts, cellulitis, and alopecia develop on the lips, muzzle, and eyelid margins. The ear pinnae may be swollen and exudative. In some dogs, lesions may also involve the anus and prepuce. Lesions may be mild to severe and are often painful but are not pruritic. Marked regional to diffuse lymphadenomegaly is common, and lymph node abscessation can occur. Severely affected puppies are usually depressed and often anorectic and febrile.

Top Differentials

Differentials include chin pyoderma, demodicosis, deep pyoderma, dermatophytosis, angioedema, and distemper.

Diagnosis

1. Signalment, history, clinical findings, and rule out other differentials.
2. Cytology (skin or ear exudate): purulent to pyogranulomatous inflammation. Secondary infections, bacteria, or yeasts may be seen.
3. Cytology (lymph node aspirate): suppurative, pyogranulomatous, or granulomatous inflammation. No infectious agents are seen.
4. Dermatohistopathology: diffuse (pyo)granulomatous dermatitis and panniculitis. Infectious agents are not seen.
5. Bacterial culture (exudate): usually sterile, but bacteria may be isolated if secondary infections are present. However, little to no improvement is seen with systemic antibiotic therapy alone.

Treatment and Prognosis

1. Treat any secondary bacterial infection; systemic antibiotics (minimum 3–4 weeks) should be administered and continued 1 week beyond complete clinical and cytologic resolution (see Box 3-2).
2. Daily, gentle, topical warm water soaks should be used to remove crusts and exudate.
3. Prednisone 2 mg/kg PO administered every 24 hours until lesions resolve (approximately 1–4 weeks); then, 2 mg/kg PO administered every 48 hours for 2–3 weeks, tapering completely over the next few weeks. If prednisone therapy is tapered or discontinued too soon, a relapse may occur.
4. Cyclosporine (Atopica) 5–10 mg/kg PO administered every 24 hours may be beneficial (effects are seen in approximately 4–6 weeks). Then, dosage frequency should be tapered down to every 48 to 72 hours. Glucocorticoids can be used initially to speed response. As of this writing, no statistically significant increase in tumor risk or severe infection is known to result from the immune effects of cyclosporine.
5. The prognosis is good if response to therapy is seen within 4 to 5 days. In severe cases, even with treatment, permanent scarring may be a sequela. Death may occur in puppies if the disease is not treated.

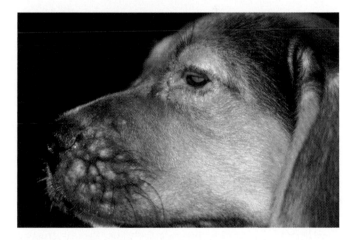

FIGURE 10-33 Canine Juvenile Cellulitis. Papular rash with pustules and moist exudates on the muzzle and periocular region of a puppy.

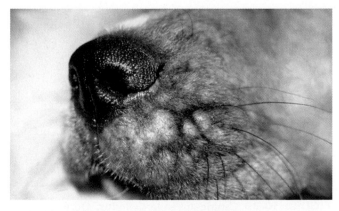

FIGURE 10-34 Canine Juvenile Cellulitis. Close-up of the dog in Figure 10-33. Alopecic, erythematous, papular dermatitis and tissue swelling are typical of juvenile cellulitis.

Canine Juvenile Cellulitis—*cont'd*

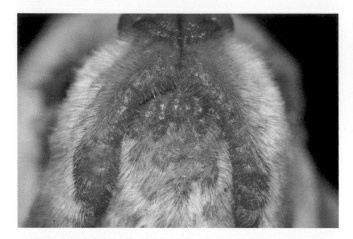

FIGURE 10-35 Canine Juvenile Cellulitis. Moist, erythematous papular lesions with alopecia on the muzzle and chin.

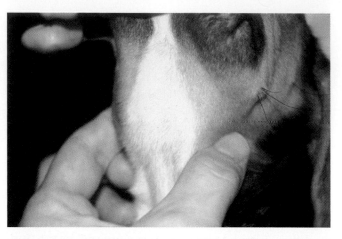

FIGURE 10-36 Canine Juvenile Cellulitis. Profound lymphadenopathy is a classic feature of juvenile cellulitis. The lymph nodes are readily apparent and are easily palpated in this puppy.

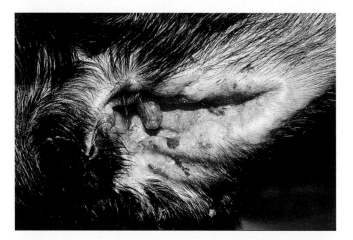

FIGURE 10-37 Canine Juvenile Cellulitis. Papular crusting lesions on the ear pinnae.

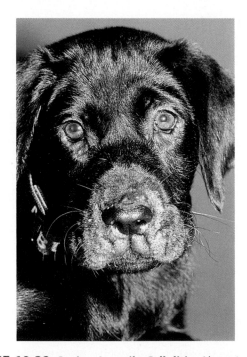

FIGURE 10-38 Canine Juvenile Cellulitis. Alopecic papular lesions on the nose and face. Note that this dog is somewhat older than the typical puppy in which onset occurs.

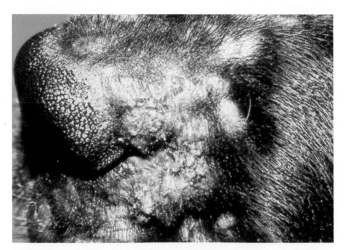

FIGURE 10-39 Canine Juvenile Cellulitis. Close-up of the dog in Figure 10-38. Papular crusting lesions on the nose indicate partial resolution of the typical moist dermatitis associated with juvenile cellulitis.

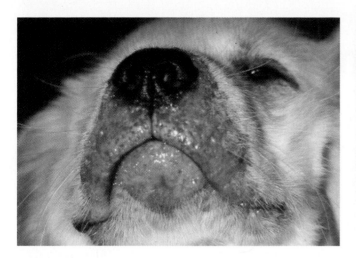

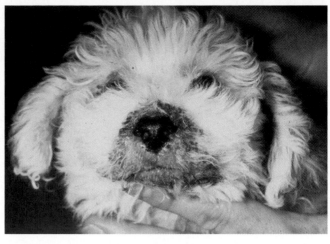

FIGURE 10-40 Canine Juvenile Cellulitis. Moist, erythematous papular lesions on the chin and muzzle. *(Courtesy D. Angarano.)*

FIGURE 10-41 Canine Juvenile Cellulitis. Moist, alopecic papular dermatitis on the muzzle typical of the syndrome.

CHAPTER | 11
Pigmentary Abnormalities

- Lentigo
- Postinflammatory Hyperpigmentation
- Nasal Depigmentation (Dudley nose, snow nose)

- Vitiligo
- Canine Uveodermatologic Syndrome (Vogt-Koyanagi-Harada–like syndrome, VKH)

Lentigo

Features

Lentigo is an asymptomatic condition characterized by one (lentigo) or more (lentigines) flat macule(s) or patch(es) of black skin. It is common in dogs, with highest incidences reported in middle-aged to older dogs. It is uncommon in cats, with the highest incidence in young orange cats.

Dogs

In dogs, lentigo appears as one or more macular to patchy areas of hyperpigmented skin. Lesions are most commonly found on the ventral abdomen and chest.

Cats

In cats, multiple 1- to 10-mm-diameter black macules may coalesce on the lips, gingiva, pinnae, or eyelids.

Top Differential

Melanoma is the differential.

Diagnosis

1. History and clinical findings.
2. Dermatohistopathology: epidermal hyperplasia, hyperpigmentation, and increased numbers of melanocytes.

Treatment and Prognosis

1. No medical treatment is known.
2. The prognosis is good as lentigines are benign skin changes and a cosmetic problem only.

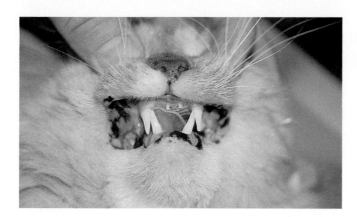

FIGURE 11-1 Lentigo. Multiple pigmented macules on the lips of a young adult cat.

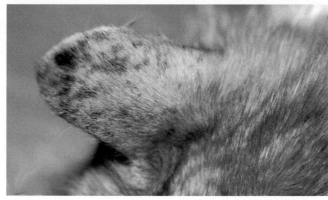

FIGURE 11-2 Lentigo. Multiple pigmented macules on the ear pinna of a young adult cat.

Postinflammatory Hyperpigmentation

Features

In postinflammatory hyperpigmentation, skin (melanoderma) or hairs (melanotrichia) become hyperpigmented as a sequela to an underlying skin disease such as pyoderma, demodicosis, dermatophytosis, or hypersensitivity. This hyperpigmentation may be focal and circumscribed, patchy, or diffuse. It is common in dogs and uncommon in cats.

Top Differentials

Differentials include lentigo and melanoma.

Diagnosis

1. History, clinical findings, and identification of underlying diseases.

Treatment and Prognosis

1. The underlying cause should be identified and treated.
2. The prognosis is good. Melanoderma usually resolves slowly after the underlying cause has been treated. Melanotrichia usually resolves at the next shedding cycle.

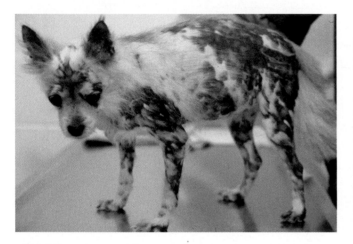

FIGURE 11-3 Postinflammatory Hyperpigmentation. Generalized hyperpigmentation associated with resolving erythema multiforme.

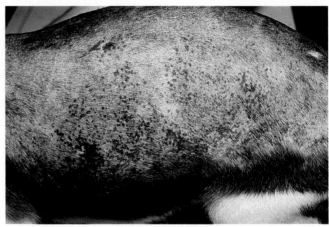

FIGURE 11-4 Postinflammatory Hyperpigmentation. Multiple pigmented macules on the lateral flank of a dog. The initial papular dermatitis was caused by contact dermatitis associated with a medicated shampoo.

Nasal Depigmentation (Dudley nose, snow nose)

Features

Nasal depigmentation is an idiopathic disorder in which affected dogs are born with a pigmented nose, which later in life lightens to a light brown or whitish color. Nasal depigmentation may wax and wane, may be seasonal, may resolve spontaneously, or may be a permanent change. Only the nose is affected, and the normal cobble texture of the nose is preserved (autoimmune skin diseases destroy the normal architecture). It is common in dogs, with the highest incidence in Golden retrievers, yellow Labrador retrievers, Siberian huskies, and Alaskan malamutes.

Dudley nose usually describes a permanent pigmentary defect (undesirable show fault), whereas snow nose describes transient, seasonal depigmentation changes.

Top Differentials

Differentials include uveodermatologic syndrome, vitiligo, nasal solar dermatitis, autoimmune skin diseases, and cutaneous lymphoma.

Diagnosis

1. History and clinical findings.
2. Dermatohistopathology: marked reduction of epidermal melanocytes and melanin.

Treatment and Prognosis

1. No treatment is known.
2. The prognosis is good, as this is a cosmetic problem only. However, it is considered a defect in show dogs.

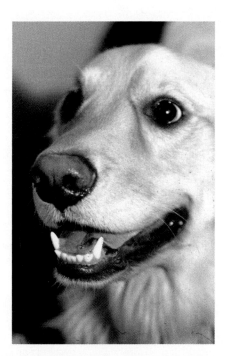

FIGURE 11-5 Nasal Depigmentation. Nasal depigmentation in a Golden retriever that occurred during the winter.

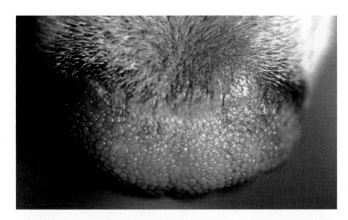

FIGURE 11-6 Nasal Depigmentation. Close-up of the dog in Figure 11-5. Seasonal depigmentation on the nose of a Golden retriever. The nose repigmented completely during the spring and summer.

Vitiligo

Features

Vitiligo is an asymptomatic condition that is characterized by one or more macular areas of depigmented skin (leukoderma) or depigmented hair (leukotrichia). Lesions are usually first noted in young adulthood and often affect the nose, lips, face, buccal mucosa, and footpads. It is uncommon in dogs, with the highest incidence in Belgian Tervurens, German shepherds, Rottweilers, and Dobermann pinschers. It is rare in cats, with the highest incidence in Siamese cats.

Top Differentials

Differentials include uveodermatologic syndrome, nasal depigmentation, autoimmune skin diseases, and cutaneous lymphoma.

Diagnosis

1. Dermatohistopathology: essentially normal skin, except no melanocytes are seen. A transient inflammatory phase may be observed.

Treatment and Prognosis

1. No treatment has been consistently documented in veterinary species; however, treatments used for autoimmune skin diseases (pemphigus and lupus) may be beneficial.
2. The prognosis is good. This is a cosmetic disease that does not affect the animal's quality of life. The depigmentation is usually permanent, but in some animals, spontaneous repigmentation eventually may occur.

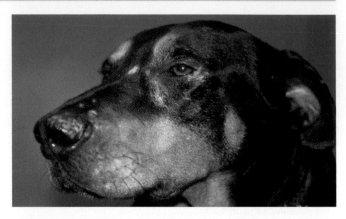

FIGURE 11-8 Vitiligo. Multifocal areas of depigmentation on the nasal planum and face of an adult Dobermann pinscher.

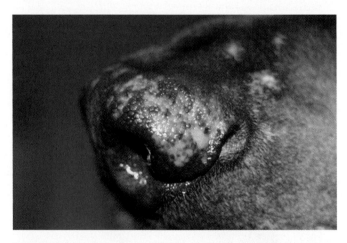

FIGURE 11-9 Vitiligo. Close-up of the dog in Figure 11-8. The spotty depigmentation of the nasal planum and hair is apparent.

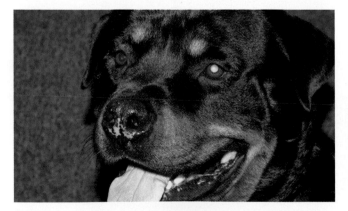

FIGURE 11-7 Vitiligo. Depigmentation on the nose of an adult Rottweiler typical of this syndrome. Note the spotty pattern, which differentiates this disease from seasonal nasal depigmentation and most autoimmune skin disorders.

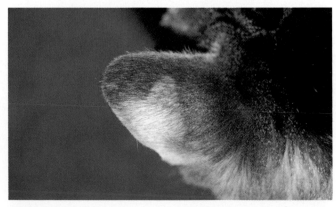

FIGURE 11-10 Vitiligo. Well-demarcated depigmentation on the ear pinna of a cat. Note the unusual asymmetrical pattern.

Canine Uveodermatologic Syndrome (Vogt-Koyanagi-Harada–like syndrome, VKH)

Features

The cause of this disorder is not completely understood, but immune-mediated and hereditary factors appear to be involved. The production of autoantibodies against melanocytes results in granulomatous panuveitis, leukoderma (skin depigmentation), and leukotrichia (hair depigmentation). It is rare in dogs, with the highest incidence in young adult and middle-aged dogs, especially Akitas. Other affected breeds include Siberian husky, Samoyed, Chow Chow, Irish setter, Dachshund, Fox terrier, Shetland Sheep dog, St. Bernard, Old English sheepdog, and Brazilian Fila dog.

An acute onset of ophthalmic signs may include diminished or absent pupillary light reflexes, blepharospasm, photophobia, anterior uveitis, keratic precipitates, hyphema, chorioretinitis, conjunctivitis, serous ocular discharge, and sometimes retinal detachment; cataracts, iris bombe, secondary glaucoma, and blindness may ensue. Ocular signs develop shortly before, concurrently with, or subsequent to well-demarcated symmetrical depigmentation of the nose, lips, and eyelids. Occasionally, the scrotum or vulva, anus, footpads, and hard palate also are depigmented. Rarely, skin lesions become eroded, ulcerated, and crusted. In some dogs, generalized skin and hair coat depigmentation may develop.

Top Differential

Bilateral Uveitis

For bilateral uveitis, differentials include toxins, infection, trauma, neoplasia, and immune-mediated disease.

Skin Depigmentation

For skin depigmentation, differentials include vitiligo, other autoimmune skin diseases, and cutaneous lymphoma.

Diagnosis

1. History, clinical findings, and ruling out of other differentials.
2. Ophthalmic findings: sterile uveitis and chorioretinitis.
3. Dermatohistopathology: pigmentary incontinence and lichenoid interface dermatitis composed of large histiocytes, small mononuclear cells, and multinucleated giant cells. Occasionally, plasma cells and lymphocytes may predominate.

Treatment and Prognosis

1. To prevent blindness, early and aggressive treatment is essential.
2. The eyes should be treated with topical or subconjunctival glucocorticoids until uveitis has resolved. Effective therapies include the following:
   - 0.1% dexamethasone ophthalmic solution OU q 4 hours
   - 1% prednisone ophthalmic solution OU q 4 hours
   - Dexamethasone 1 to 2 mg subconjunctivally OU
   - Triamcinolone 10 to 20 mg subconjunctivally OU once
   - Depot betamethasone 6 mg subconjunctivally OU once
3. Also, a topical cycloplegic (1% atropine ophthalmic solution) should be instilled OU every 6 to 24 hours or to effect.
4. Immunosuppressive doses of oral prednisone or methylprednisolone should be given (see Table 8-1). After ocular lesions have resolved (approximately 4–8 weeks), dosage should be gradually tapered over a period of several (8–10) weeks until the lowest possible alternate-day dose that maintains remission is being given. If no significant improvement is seen within 2 weeks of initiation of therapy, one should consider alternate or additional immunosuppressive medications.
5. Alternative glucocorticoids for refractory cases include triamcinolone and dexamethasone (see Table 8-1).
6. If systemic glucocorticoid therapy alone is ineffective, or if undesirable adverse effects develop, treatment with cyclosporine, oral azathioprine, combination tetracycline and niacinamide, or cyclophosphamide may have a steroid-sparing effect (see Table 8-2). A beneficial response should be noted within 8 to 12 weeks of initiation of treatment. Once remission has been achieved, attempt to taper or discontinue steroid administration, then taper azathioprine, tetracycline/niacinamide, or cyclophosphamide dose and frequency of administration for long-term maintenance therapy (see Table 8-2).
7. The prognosis is guarded to fair. Lifelong therapy is usually needed, and control may be difficult to maintain. If uveitis is not treated early and aggressively, or if it is poorly controlled, glaucoma, cataracts, and blindness are likely sequelae. Cutaneous depigmentation is usually a cosmetic problem only, and it may become permanent or may be incompletely improved in some cases.

Canine Uveodermatologic Syndrome—*cont'd*

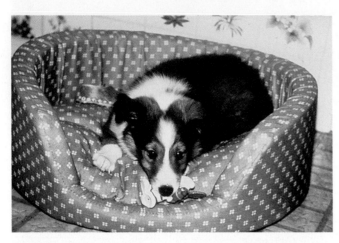

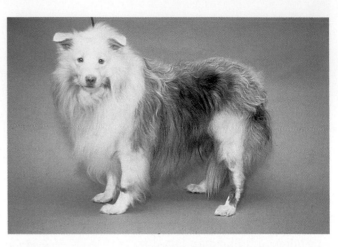

FIGURE 11-11 **Canine Uveodermatologic Syndrome.** This young sheltie was diagnosed early. As the disease progresses, the cutaneous pigmentation is lost. *(Courtesy Campbell K, McLaughlin S: Generalized leukoderma and poliosis following uveitis in a dog,* J Am Anim Hosp Assoc *22:121, 1986.)*

FIGURE 11-12 **Canine Uveodermatologic Syndrome.** The same dog as in Figure 11-11. The depigmentation has progressed over several years. *(Courtesy Campbell K, McLaughlin S: Generalized leukoderma and poliosis following uveitis in a dog,* J Am Anim Hosp Assoc *22:121, 1986.)*

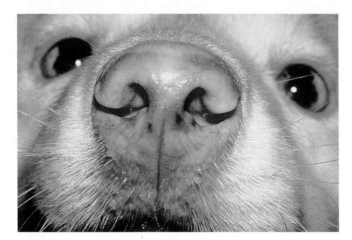

FIGURE 11-13 **Canine Uveodermatologic Syndrome.** Close-up of the dog in Figure 11-12. The nasal depigmentation has progressed and is almost complete. *(Courtesy Campbell K, McLaughlin S: Generalized leukoderma and poliosis following uveitis in a dog,* J Am Anim Hosp Assoc *22:121, 1986.)*

CHAPTER 12

Keratinization and Seborrheic Disorders

- Callus
- Feline Acne
- Idiopathic Nasodigital Hyperkeratosis
- Hereditary Nasal Parakeratosis of Labrador Retrievers
- Parasympathetic Nasal Hyperkeratosis (xeromycteria: dry nose)
- Canine Primary Seborrhea
- Vitamin A–Responsive Dermatosis
- Schnauzer Comedo Syndrome (Schnauzer bumps)
- Canine Ear Margin Dermatosis

- Zinc-Responsive Dermatosis
- Tail Gland Hyperplasia (stud tail)
- Epidermal Dysplasia of West Highland White Terriers
- Sebaceous Adenitis
- Hepatocutaneous Syndrome (superficial necrolytic dermatitis, superficial necrolytic migratory erythema [SNME], metabolic epidermal necrosis, diabetic dermatopathy)
- Familial Footpad Hyperkeratosis
- Facial Dermatitis of Persian Cats

Callus

Features

Callus occurs as a localized, hyperplastic skin reaction to trauma caused by pressure or friction. It is common in dogs, with highest incidences noted in large and giant-breed dogs.

A round to oval, alopecic, hyperpigmented, hyperkeratotic, hyperplastic plaque forms over a bony pressure point. The elbow, hock, or sternum (deep-chested dogs) is most commonly affected. Lesions may become ulcerated, fistulated, and exudative from secondary bacterial infection. Impacted follicles ("ingrown hairs") can become dilated and cystic over time.

Top Differentials

Differentials include dermatophytosis, demodicosis, pyoderma, and neoplasia.

Diagnosis

1. Usually based on history and clinical findings.
2. Cytology (exudate): keratin debris; purulent or pyogranulomatous inflammation, free hair shafts, and bacteria may be seen.
3. Dermatohistopathology: marked epidermal hyperplasia, orthokeratotic to parakeratotic hyperkeratosis, follicular keratosis, and dilated follicular cysts.

Treatment and Prognosis

1. Observation without treatment is appropriate for noninfected lesions.
2. If lesion is secondarily infected, long-term systemic antibiotics (minimum, 4–6 weeks) should be administered. Alternatively, topical dimethyl sulfoxide (DMSO) combined with enrofloxacin (to make a

355

Callus—*cont'd*

10-mg/mL solution) could be applied every 12 to 72 hours until lesions resolve.

3. Special efforts should be taken to remove the "ingrown hairs" from the callus as these will eventually lead to furunculosis and infection. Scrub the hairs out frequently (every 2–7 days) using a cloth, brush, or sponge in the direction of hair growth. Tape-strip the hairs using a very sticky tape product; typically, only the ingrown hairs are removable, leaving the healthy and active hairs intact.

4. Bedding and other sleeping/resting areas should be padded, and padded bandages should be used to prevent trauma to the affected area.

5. Moisturizers, antibiotic ointments (mupirocin), 2.5% benzoyl peroxide gel, or salicylic acid/sodium lactate/urea gel should be applied to the affected area every 12 to 24 hours to soften the skin. However, secondary infections are likely to occur if moisturizers are used without the implementation of protective padding measures.

6. Surgical excision usually is not recommended because wound dehiscence is a possible postoperative complication.

7. The prognosis is good for noninfected lesions. This is a cosmetic disease that does not affect the dog's quality of life.

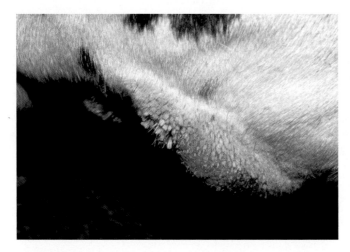

FIGURE 12-1 Callus. Thickening of the skin over the elbow of a dog. The hair is clumped, and skin appears partially alopecic, which is typical of a callus.

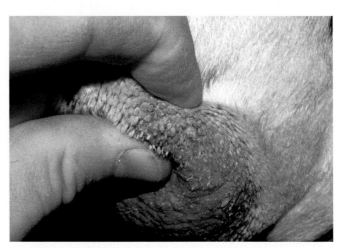

FIGURE 12-3 Callus. Close-up of the lesion in Figure 12-1. The clinician is gently squeezing the callus to express the impacted hairs, which are now exuding from the surface of the skin. These hairs serve as a nidus for recurrent infection.

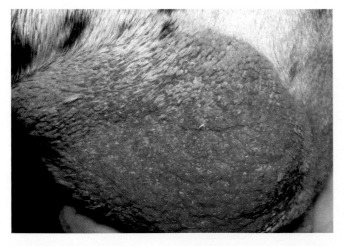

FIGURE 12-2 Callus. Close-up of the lesion in Figure 12-1. The large alopecic area of thickened skin over the elbow is typical of this syndrome. Often in short-coated dogs, the hairs become impacted within the follicles and callus.

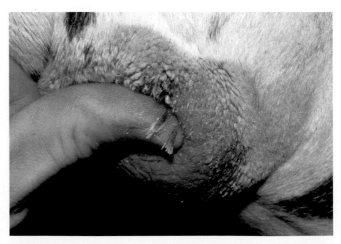

FIGURE 12-4 Callus. Close-up of the lesion in Figure 12-1. The exuded hairs are apparent. This technique is not recommended because forcing the hairs to rupture internally could result in cellulitis and scarring.

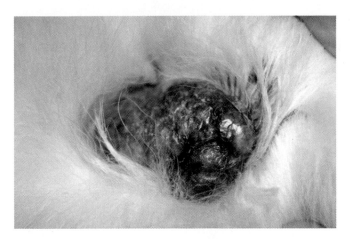

FIGURE 12-5 Callus. A focal area of alopecia and thickened skin over the elbow. The large cystic structures are hair follicles that became obstructed and filled with keratin debris.

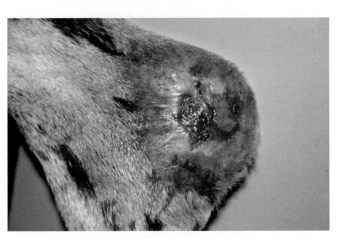

FIGURE 12-6 Callus. Severe alopecia and thickening of the skin with ulceration over the hock of a dog. The chronic pressure that causes callus formation can also lead to decubital ulcers.

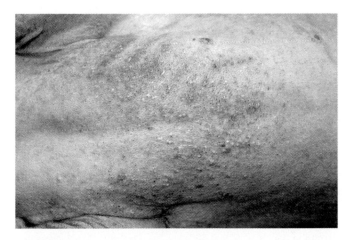

FIGURE 12-7 Callus. A sternal plaque demonstrating the focal area of alopecia and comedo formation caused by chronic pressure and friction in deep-chested dogs. This is most often seen in Dachshunds.

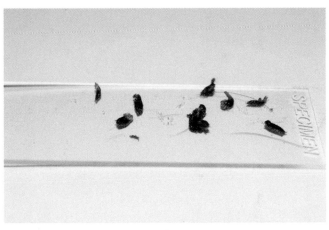

FIGURE 12-8 Callus. Keratin material has been expressed from the comedones of the sternal plaque of a Dachshund. Note the large keratin plugs that were formed by persistent pressure produced when the dog rests in a sternal position.

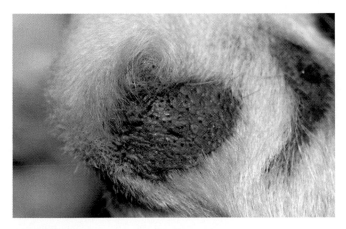

FIGURE 12-9 Callus. The ingrown, dead hairs have been removed. Note the unexpected length of the hair shaft, which was embedded in the callus.

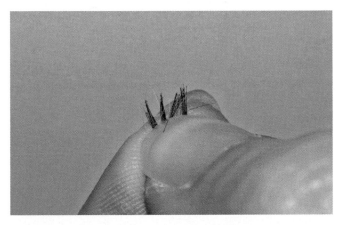

FIGURE 12-10 Callus. Ingrown hairs that have been removed from a callus.

Callus—*cont'd*

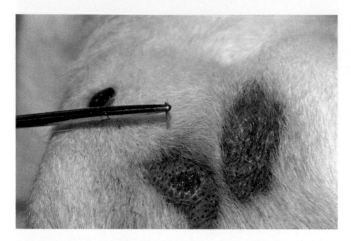

FIGURE 12-11 Callus. A focal callus with ulceration resulting from extreme focal pressure and secondary infection. Embedded hairs have been removed.

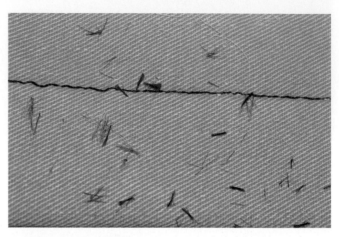

FIGURE 12-12 Callus. Numerous embedded hairs that were removed from a chronic callus.

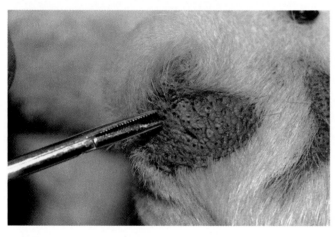

FIGURE 12-13 Callus. Embedded hairs are being removed from a chronic callus. Note how little of the hair shaft is exposed above the surface of the callus.

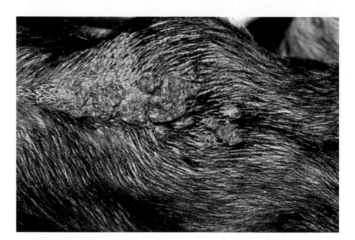

FIGURE 12-14 Callus. A chronic callus demonstrating the dilated cystic follicles that develop from chronic pressure and subsequent obstruction of the follicular opening. Note the lack of active infection despite the large cystic follicles.

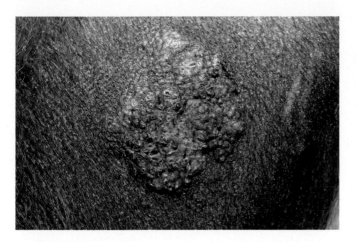

FIGURE 12-15 Callus. A chronic callus demonstrating the dilated cystic follicles that develop from chronic pressure and subsequent obstruction of the follicular opening. Note the lack of active infection despite the large cystic follicles.

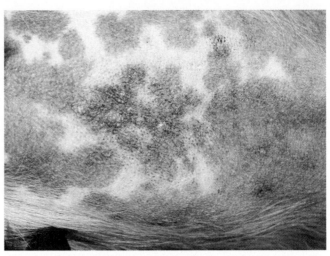

FIGURE 12-16 Callus. The comedones create dilated follicles that often become secondarily infected and may rupture, resulting in furunculosis. The follicles are plugged (comedones) as a result of the constant pressure applied when the deep-chested dog rests in a sternal position.

Feline Acne

Features

Feline acne is a disorder of follicular keratinization and glandular hyperplasia. It is common in cats.

Asymptomatic comedones (blackheads) form on the chin, the lower lip, and occasionally, the upper lip. Papules and pustules and, rarely, furunculosis and cellulitis may develop if lesions become secondarily infected. In severe cases, affected skin may become edematous, thickened, cystic, or scarred.

Top Differentials

Differentials include demodicosis, dermatophytosis, *Malassezia* dermatitis, and eosinophilic granuloma (if edematous).

Diagnosis

1. History, clinical findings, and rule out other differentials.
2. Dermatohistopathology: follicular keratosis, plugging, and dilation. Glandular hyperplasia, perifolliculitis, folliculitis, furunculosis, or cellulitis may be seen if secondary bacterial infection is present.

Treatment and Prognosis

1. Any secondary bacterial infection should be treated with appropriate systemic antibiotics for at least 2 to 3 weeks. *Malassezia* infections should be treated with fluconazole 10 mg/kg daily for 30 days.
2. Hairs around lesions should be clipped, warm water compresses applied, and affected areas cleansed with human alcohol free acne pads, or with benzoyl peroxide–, sulfur-salicylic acid–, or ethyl lactate–containing shampoo every 1 to 2 days until lesions resolve, then as needed for maintenance control. Often frequent chin cleaning (every 2–3 days) is needed to prevent relapses.
3. Alternative topical products that may be effective when used every 1 to 3 days, or on an as-needed basis, include the following:
   - Mupirocin ointment or cream
   - 2.5% benzoyl peroxide gel (*Note*: may be irritating in some cats)
   - 0.01% to 0.025% tretinoin cream or lotion
   - 0.75% metronidazole gel
   - Clindamycin-, erythromycin-, or tetracycline-containing topicals
4. For severe refractory cases, systemic vitamin A therapy may be effective.
5. The prognosis is good, but lifelong symptomatic treatment is often necessary for control. Unless secondary infection occurs, this is a cosmetic disease that does not affect the animal's quality of life.

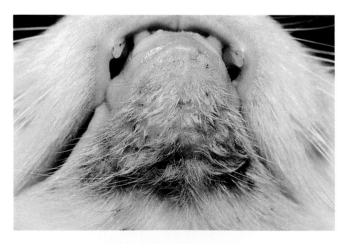

FIGURE 12-17 Feline Acne. Moist, draining papular lesions on the chin of an adult cat. Furunculosis and cellulitis caused the tissue swelling and exudate.

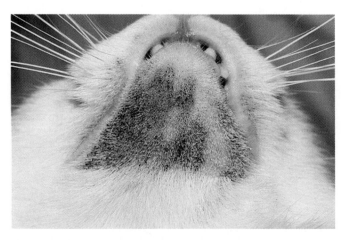

FIGURE 12-18 Feline Acne. The hair has been clipped to provide better visualization of the erythema, hyperpigmentation, and comedones.

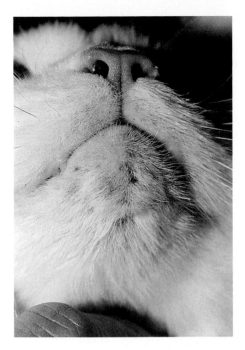

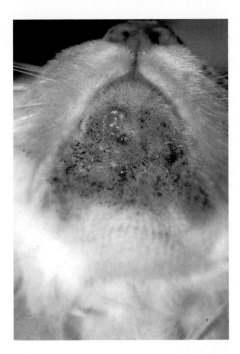

FIGURE 12-19 Feline Acne. Alopecia and scarring remained as sequelae after treatment with topical mupirocin ointment.

FIGURE 12-20 Feline Acne. The hair has been clipped, allowing better visualization of the comedones, papules, and draining lesions in this severe case of feline acne, which usually is limited to the chin.

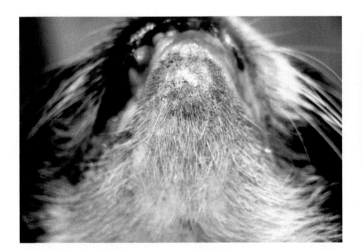

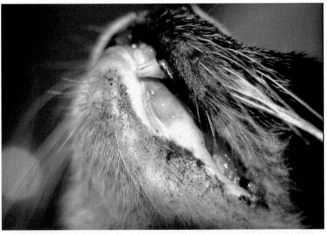

FIGURE 12-21 Feline Acne. The brown discoloration is typical of comedo formation associated with feline acne.

FIGURE 12-22 Feline Acne. Close-up of the cat in Figure 12-21. The lesions extended along the lateral lip surface. This is unusual for feline acne.

Idiopathic Nasodigital Hyperkeratosis

Features

Idiopathic nasodigital hyperkeratosis is an idiopathic condition that is characterized by the excessive formation of nasal or footpad keratin. It is common in older dogs, especially Cocker spaniels.

Thickened, hard, dry keratin accumulates on the nasal planum, footpads, or both. Accumulated keratin usually is most prominent on the dorsum of the nose and at the edges of the footpads. Secondary erosions, ulcers, and fissures may suggest an autoimmune skin disease. Excessive digital hyperkeratosis may result in horny growths, which can cause pain from pressure against adjacent footpads. Nasolacrimal duct blockage may present a contributing factor.

Top Differentials

Differentials include distemper, zinc-responsive dermatosis, superficial necrolytic dermatitis, hereditary nasal parakeratosis, familial footpad hyperkeratosis, pemphigus foliaceus, systemic or discoid lupus erythematosus, and leishmaniasis.

Diagnosis

1. History, clinical findings, and rule out other differentials.
2. Dermatohistopathology: epidermal hyperplasia with marked orthokeratotic or parakeratotic hyperkeratosis.

Treatment and Prognosis

1. The intensity of therapy depends on the severity of the lesions.
2. The nasolacrimal ducts should be flushed.
3. For mild, asymptomatic cases, benign neglect and observation without treatment may be appropriate.
4. For moderate to severe cases, affected areas should be hydrated with a warm water soak or compressed for 5 to 10 minutes. Then, a softening agent should be applied every 24 hours until excessive keratin has been removed (approximately 7–10 days). Treatment should be continued on an as-needed basis for control. Effective softening agents include the following:
   - Petroleum jelly
   - A&D ointment
   - Ichthammol ointment
   - Salicylic acid/sodium lactate/urea gel
   - Tretinoin gel
5. For horny growths, excessive keratin should be trimmed away before hydration and softening therapy are begun.
6. For fissured lesions, combination antibiotic/glucocorticoid ointment may be applied to lesions every 8 to 12 hours until healed.
7. The prognosis is good. Although it is incurable, this is a cosmetic disease that usually can be managed symptomatically.

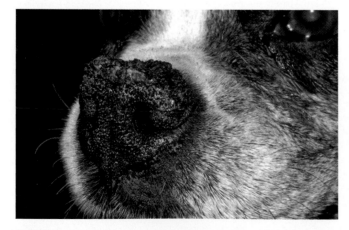

FIGURE 12-23 Idiopathic Nasodigital Hyperkeratosis. Severe frondlike hyperkeratotic projections with crust formation on the nose of an old Boxer.

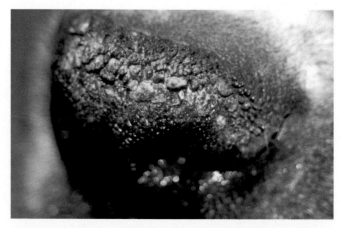

FIGURE 12-24 Idiopathic Nasodigital Hyperkeratosis. Severe crusting and frondlike projections on the nose.

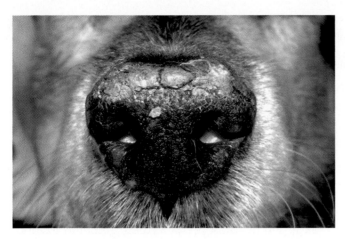

FIGURE 12-25 Idiopathic Nasodigital Hyperkeratosis. Thick, adherent crusts cover most of the nasal planum in this dog.

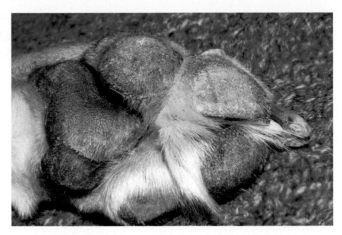

FIGURE 12-26 Idiopathic Nasodigital Hyperkeratosis. Mild hyperkeratosis of the footpads without other lesions (which would be more typical of autoimmune skin disease or hepatocutaneous syndrome).

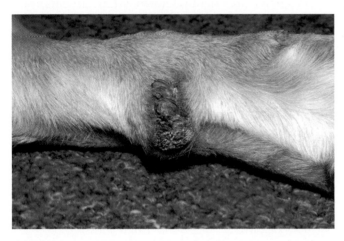

FIGURE 12-27 Idiopathic Nasodigital Hyperkeratosis. Hyperkeratosis and crusting of the metacarpal pad.

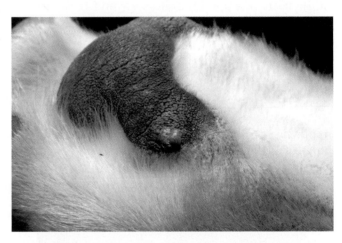

FIGURE 12-28 Idiopathic Nasodigital Hyperkeratosis. A focal area of hyperkeratosis on the central pad of a Greyhound (Greyhound corns).

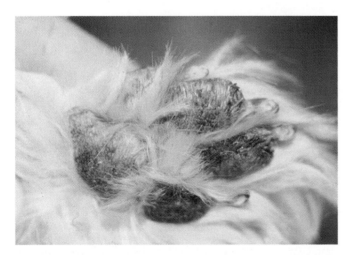

FIGURE 12-29 Idiopathic Nasodigital Hyperkeratosis. Hyperkeratosis and crusting on the footpads.

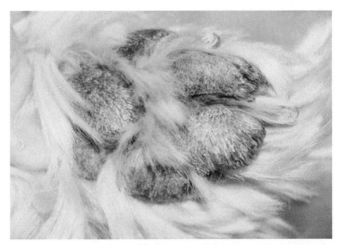

FIGURE 12-30 Idiopathic Nasodigital Hyperkeratosis. Hyperkeratosis and crusting with frondlike projections on the footpads.

Hereditary Nasal Parakeratosis of Labrador Retrievers

Features

Hereditary nasal parakeratosis of Labrador retrievers is a clinically manageable but incurable familial dermatosis that becomes apparent between 6 and 12 months of age. An autosomal recessive mode of inheritance is suspected. It is uncommon in Labrador retrievers and their crosses.

Grayish or brownish adherent keratinaceous debris accumulates on the dorsal aspect of the nasal planum. Crusting, erosions, ulcerations, fissures, or depigmentation may develop, but the nose is not pruritic or painful. The dermatosis may remain stable, may wax and wane, or may progressively worsen. Lesions are usually limited to the nasal planum, but mild scaly and crusty lesions on the hairy part of the bridge of the nose and hyperkeratotic footpads may also be seen. Affected dogs are otherwise healthy.

Top Differentials

Differentials include distemper, ichthyosis, zinc-responsive dermatosis, pemphigus erythematosus, pemphigus foliaceus, systemic or discoid lupus erythematosus, leishmaniasis, idiopathic nasal hyperkeratosis, and primary seborrheic dermatitis.

Diagnosis

1. Rule out other differentials.
2. Dermatohistopathology (nasal planum): moderate to marked parakeratosis, multifocal accumulations of proteinaceous fluid between keratinocytes within the stratum corneum and superficial stratum spinosum, mild to moderate superficial interstitial to interfacial lymphoplasmacytic dermatitis, lymphocytic and neutrophilic exocytosis, and mild to moderate pigmentary incontinence.

Treatment and Prognosis

1. No specific treatment is known, but treatments as for idiopathic nasodigital hyperkeratosis may be effective. (See previous section.)
2. Alternatively, improvement is usually obtained with topical propylene glycol (diluted 50:50 in water), topical petroleum jelly, or topical vitamin E. Initially, treatment should be applied to lesions every 12 hours until a satisfactory response is seen, then used as needed for lifelong control.
3. Immunosuppressive doses of oral prednisone (2 mg/kg q 24 hours) may be effective, but long-term daily dosing is required to maintain control. Therefore, the likelihood of unacceptable steroid adverse effects makes this an inappropriate treatment option in most cases.
4. The prognosis for cure is poor, but dogs enjoy a good quality of life with routine symptomatic therapy. Affected dogs should not be bred.

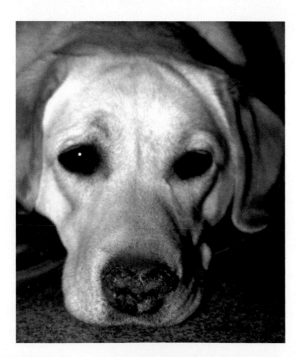

FIGURE 12-31 Hereditary Nasal Parakeratosis of Labrador Retrievers. Hyperkeratosis and crusting on the nose of a young adult Labrador. *(Courtesy M. Paradis.)*

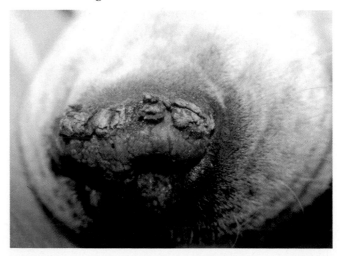

FIGURE 12-32 Hereditary Nasal Parakeratosis of Labrador Retrievers. Severe crusting and hyperkeratosis covering almost the entire nasal planum. *(Courtesy M. Paradis.)*

Parasympathetic Nasal Hyperkeratosis (xeromycteria: dry nose)

Features

Parasympathetic dysfunction may result in loss of function of the normal nasal gland, which is located in the lateral mucosa of the nose. The gland has parasympathetic innervation via the facial nerve. If concurrent keratoconjunctivitis sicca (KCS) is present, damage to the preganglionic parasympathetic fibers proximal to the pterygopalatine ganglion may have occurred in association with possible concurrent otitis, damaging the nerve fibers as they course through the temporal bone.

Lesion may be unilateral or bilateral. Grayish or brownish adherent keratinaceous debris accumulates on the dorsal aspect of the nasal planum. The dermatosis may remain stable, may wax and wane, or may progressively worsen. Lesions are usually limited to the nasal planum, but mild scaly and crusty lesions may appear on the hairy part of the bridge of the nose. Affected dogs should be evaluated for KCS and otitis.

Top Differentials

Differentials include idiopathic nasal parakeratosis, autoimmune skin disease (pemphigus foliaceus, systemic or discoid lupus erythematosus), distemper, zinc-responsive dermatosis, superficial necrolytic dermatitis, and leishmaniasis.

Diagnosis

1. History, clinical findings, and rule out other differentials; concurrent KCS and otitis may provide supporting evidence.

2. Dermatohistopathology: epidermal hyperplasia with marked orthokeratotic or parakeratotic hyperkeratosis.

Treatment and Prognosis

1. The intensity of therapy depends on the severity of the lesions.
2. Pilocarpine may be helpful.
3. Treatment as for idiopathic nasal hyperkeratosis should be used:
   a. The nasolacrimal ducts should be flushed.
   b. For mild, asymptomatic cases, benign neglect and observation without treatment may be appropriate.
   c. For moderate to severe cases, affected areas should be hydrated with a warm water soak or compressed for 5 to 10 minutes. Then, a softening agent should be applied every 24 hours until excessive keratin has been removed (approximately 7–10 days). Treatment should be continued on an as-needed basis for control. Effective softening agents include the following:
      - Petroleum jelly
      - A&D ointment
      - Salicylic acid/sodium lactate/urea gel
4. The prognosis is good.

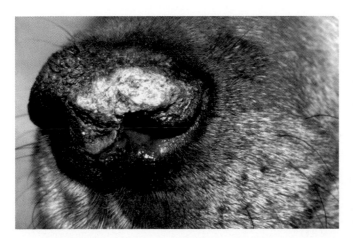

FIGURE 12-33 Parasympathetic Nasal Hyperkeratosis. Hyperkeratosis and crusting asymmetrically affecting the nasal planum.

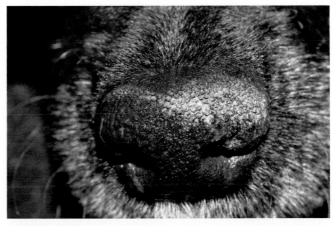

FIGURE 12-34 Parasympathetic Nasal Hyperkeratosis. Close-up of the dog in Figure 12-33. The asymmetrical (only half) pattern of crusting is apparent.

Parasympathetic Nasal Hyperkeratosis—*cont'd*

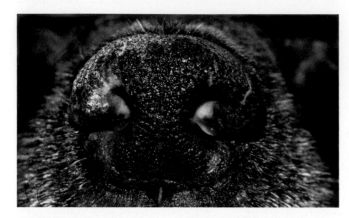

FIGURE 12-35 **Parasympathetic Nasal Hyperkeratosis.** A symmetrical hyperkeratosis of the nasal planum.

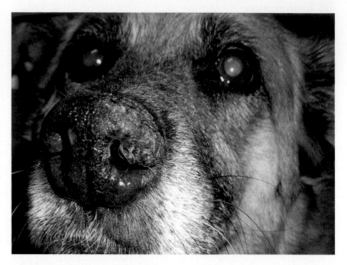

FIGURE 12-36 **Parasympathetic Nasal Hyperkeratosis.** The nasal planum is dry and crusted from the lack of normal nasal gland secretions. The normal cobblestone surface remains intact, making a diagnosis of autoimmune skin disease less likely.

Canine Primary Seborrhea

Features

Canine primary seborrhea is a hereditary disorder of keratinization. It is common in dogs, with the highest incidence in American Cocker spaniels, English Springer spaniels, West Highland White terriers, and Basset hounds. Clinical symptoms initially appear during puppyhood and may be mild at first but worsen with age. Symptoms may become apparent or worsen as an adult if underlying concurrent diseases develop.

Clinical signs may include a dull, dry, lusterless hair coat, excessive scaling (dandruff), follicular casts, scaly and crusty seborrheic patches and plaques, and greasy, malodorous skin. Most of the body is involved to some degree, with interdigital areas, perineum, face, axillae, ventral neck, abdomen, and skin folds usually most severely affected. Pruritus is mild to intense, and ceruminous otitis externa is common. Secondary skin and ear infections with bacteria and *Malassezia* are often present.

Top Differentials

Differentials include vitamin A–responsive dermatosis and other causes of secondary seborrhea (Box 12-1).

Diagnosis

1. Based on early age of onset and rule out other causes of seborrhea.
2. Dermatohistopathology (nonspecific): hyperplastic, superficial, perivascular dermatitis with orthokeratotic or parakeratotic hyperkeratosis, follicular keratosis, and variable dyskeratosis. Bacteria and yeast may be seen within surface and follicular keratin. Secondary bacterial folliculitis and yeast dermatitis are common.

Treatment and Prognosis

1. Ensure good nutrition. A commercially balanced dog food that meets Association of American Feed Control Officials (AAFCO) requirements should be fed.
2. Any secondary bacterial and *Malassezia* skin and ear infection should be treated with appropriate topical and systemic therapies. Periodic retreatments or long-term, low-dose maintenance therapy may be needed because these dogs are susceptible to recurring infection.
3. For symptomatic control of ceruminous otitis, long-term maintenance ear care is necessary. Ear treatments with a multimodal therapy or ear cleaner

should be administered AU every 1 to 7 days to control cerumen accumulation.

4. For symptomatic control of seborrhea, antiseborrheic shampoos and emollients may be used every 2 to 7 days until the skin condition is improved (approximately 2–3 weeks); then, bathing frequency

BOX 12-1 Causes of Secondary Seborrhea in Dogs

Infectious
- Pyoderma
- Dermatophytosis
- *Malassezia* dermatitis
- Leishmaniasis

Allergic
- Flea allergy dermatitis
- Atopy
- Food hypersensitivity
- Contact dermatitis

Endocrine
- Hypothyroidism
- Hyperadrenocorticism
- Sex hormone imbalance
- Diabetes mellitus

Parasitic
- Demodicosis
- Scabies
- Cheyletiellosis
- Pediculosis
- *Otodectes* spp.

Nutritional
- Vitamin A–responsive dermatosis
- Zinc-responsive dermatosis
- Dietary imbalance

Immune-mediated
- Pemphigus foliaceus
- Pemphigus erythematosus
- Discoid lupus erythematosus
- Systemic lupus erythematosus
- Cutaneous drug reaction
- Sebaceous adenitis

Metabolic
- Malabsorption/maldigestion
- Superficial necrolytic dermatitis

Neoplastic
- Cutaneous epitheliotropic lymphoma

Canine Primary Seborrhea—cont'd

should be decreased to every 1 to 2 weeks or as needed for maintenance.

5. Daily oral fatty acid supplementation may be helpful as an adjunct therapy (180 mg EPA/10 lb).

6. Vitamin A 8000 to 10,000 IU per 20 lb PO administered with a fatty meal every 24 hours. Improvement should be seen within 4 to 6 weeks.

7. Historical therapies varied; they were often ineffective and caused numerous adverse effects but included the following:
   a. For dogs with severe, greasy, malodorous, pruritic seborrhea, treatment with systemic corticosteroids may be helpful. Prednisone 1–2 mg/kg PO administered every 24 hours until symptoms are controlled (approximately 2 weeks), then tapered to the lowest possible alternate-day dosage if maintenance therapy is needed. However, unacceptable steroid adverse effects and recurrent skin and ear infections are potential sequelae if long-term steroid therapy is used.
   b. Acitretin (a retinoid) 0.5–1 mg/kg PO administered every 24 hours may be helpful in some dogs.
   c. Calcitriol (vitamin D) 10 mg/kg/day PO may be helpful in some cases. Serum calcium levels should be closely monitored.

8. The prognosis is variable, depending on the severity of the seborrhea. This is an incurable condition that requires lifelong therapy for control. Affected dogs should not be bred.

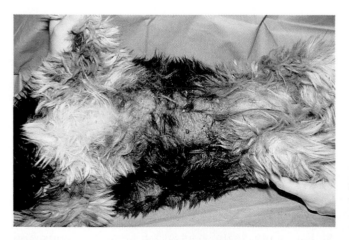

FIGURE 12-37 Canine Primary Seborrhea. Greasy, poor-quality fur coat in a 4-year-old female spayed Cocker spaniel. *(Courtesy A. Yu.)*

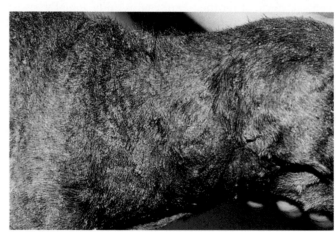

FIGURE 12-39 Canine Primary Seborrhea. Close-up of the dog in Figure 12-37. The fur coat has been clipped, revealing generalized seborrhea, scales, crusts, and erythema. *(Courtesy A. Yu.)*

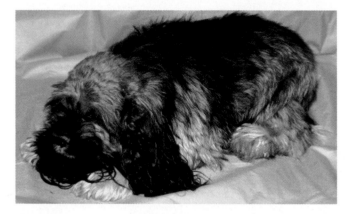

FIGURE 12-38 Canine Primary Seborrhea. Close-up of the dog in Figure 12-37. Partial alopecia and seborrheic dermatitis on the ventral abdomen. *(Courtesy A. Yu.)*

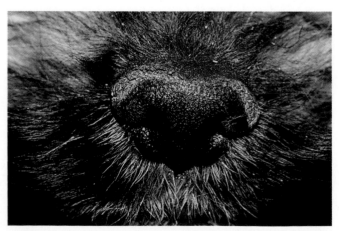

FIGURE 12-40 Canine Primary Seborrhea. Crusting around the nose is characteristic of this disease. *(Courtesy A. Yu.)*

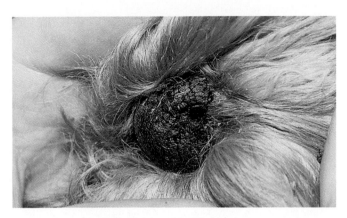

FIGURE 12-41 Canine Primary Seborrhea. Hyperkeratosis of the footpads. *(Courtesy A. Yu.)*

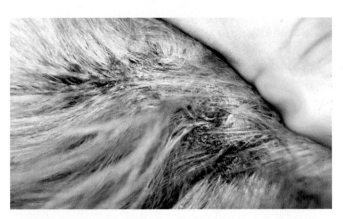

FIGURE 12-42 Canine Primary Seborrhea. Waxy seborrheic dermatitis causing discoloration and clumping of the hairs.

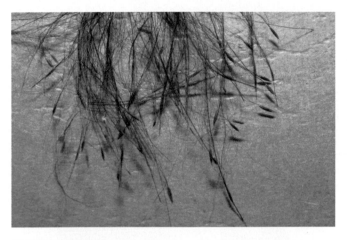

FIGURE 12-43 Canine Primary Seborrhea. Follicular casts are apparent after the hair was epilated. Follicular casts are a characteristic finding in several primary keratinization disorders (primary seborrhea, vitamin A–responsive dermatosis, sebaceous adenitis).

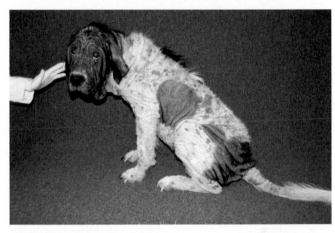

FIGURE 12-44 Canine Primary Seborrhea. Generalized alopecia and lichenification affecting the entire cutaneous surface area.

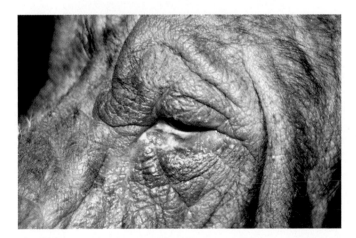

FIGURE 12-45 Canine Primary Seborrhea. Same dog as in Figure 12-44. Alopecia and lichenification affect the entire cutaneous surface, including the eyelid margins.

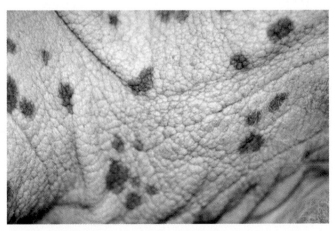

FIGURE 12-46 Canine Primary Seborrhea. Close-up of the dog in Figure 12-44. Alopecic, lichenified skin is typical of a secondary *Malassezia* dermatitis associated with primary seborrhea.

Canine Primary Seborrhea—cont'd

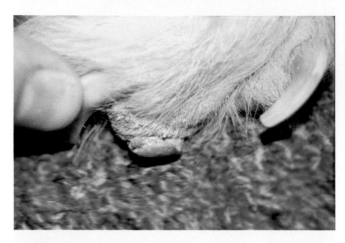

FIGURE 12-47 **Canine Primary Seborrhea.** Cutaneous horn forming on the margin of a footpad associated with primary seborrhea.

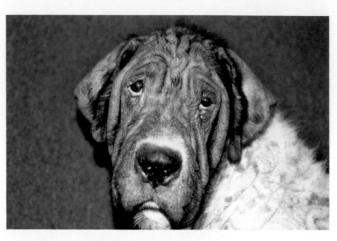

FIGURE 12-48 **Canine Primary Seborrhea.** Alopecia and lichenification caused by secondary *Malassezia* dermatitis associated with primary seborrhea.

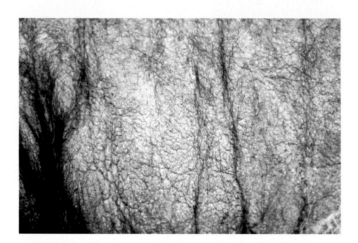

FIGURE 12-49 **Canine Primary Seborrhea.** Alopecia and lichenification affecting the entire cutaneous surface are apparent.

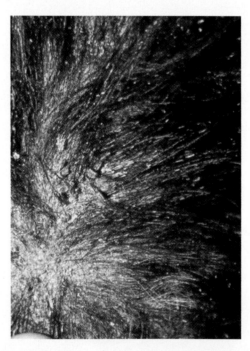

FIGURE 12-50 **Canine Primary Seborrhea.** Alopecia, erythema, scale, and crusts are typical of this disease. Lesions may be focal or generalized. *(Courtesy A. Yu.)*

Vitamin A–Responsive Dermatosis

Features

Vitamin A–responsive dermatosis is an incompletely understood disorder of keratinization that that is most likely a mild variant of canine primary seborrhea. This disorder responds completely to treatment with high doses of vitamin A. It is rare in dogs, with highest incidences reported in young (2- to 3-year-old) American Cocker spaniels.

Marked follicular plugging, focal areas of crusting, and hyperkeratotic plaques have keratinaceous frond-like plugs. Lesions are most commonly found on the ventral and lateral aspects of the chest and abdomen. Mild to moderate pruritus, a dull dry hair coat that epilates easily, a rancid body odor, and generalized scaling may be present. Concurrent ceruminous otitis externa is common.

Top Differentials

Differentials include primary seborrhea, sebaceous adenitis, zinc-responsive dermatosis, and other causes of secondary seborrhea (see Box 12-1).

Diagnosis

1. Rule out other differentials.
2. Dermatohistopathology: marked, disproportionate follicular orthokeratotic hyperkeratosis with minimal epidermal hyperkeratosis.
3. Response to vitamin A.

Treatment and Prognosis

1. Ensure good nutrition. A commercially balanced dog food that meets Association of American Feed Control Officials (AAFCO) requirements should be fed.
2. Any secondary bacterial and *Malassezia* skin and ear infection should be treated with appropriate topical and systemic therapies. Periodic retreatments or long-term, low-dose maintenance therapy may be needed because these dogs are susceptible to recurring infection.
3. For symptomatic control of ceruminous otitis, long-term maintenance ear care is necessary. Ear treatments with a multimodal therapy or ear cleaner should be administered AU every 1 to 7 days to control cerumen accumulation.
4. For symptomatic control of seborrhea, antiseborrheic shampoos and emollients may be used every 2 to 7 days until the skin condition is improved (approximately 2–3 weeks); then, bathing frequency should be decreased to every 1 to 2 weeks or as needed for maintenance.
5. Daily oral fatty acid supplementation may be helpful as an adjunct therapy (180 mg EPA/10 lb).
6. Vitamin A 8000 to 10,000 IU per 20 lb PO administered with a fatty meal every 24 hours. Improvement should be seen within 4 to 6 weeks and complete clinical remission within 8 to 10 weeks.
7. The prognosis is good, but lifelong vitamin A therapy is usually necessary to maintain remission.

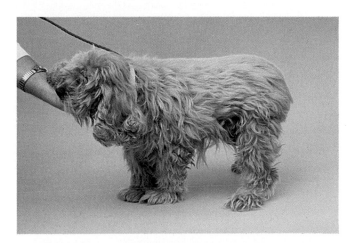

FIGURE 12-51 Vitamin A–Responsive Dermatosis. Greasy, poor-quality fur coat in an adult Cocker spaniel. Note the similarity to canine primary seborrhea. *(Courtesy A. Yu.)*

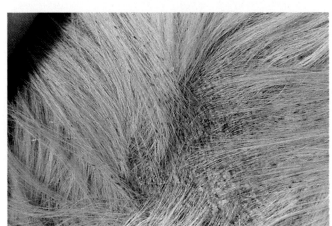

FIGURE 12-52 Vitamin A–Responsive Dermatosis. Close-up of the dog in Figure 12-51. Scale and follicular casts can be seen. The skin lesions are generalized. *(Courtesy A. Yu.)*

Schnauzer Comedo Syndrome (Schnauzer bumps)

Features

Schnauzer comedo syndrome is a common acne-like disorder of follicular keratinization that occurs in miniature Schnauzers.

Few to many nonpainful, nonpruritic comedones (blackheads) and crusted papules are found on the dorsal midline of the back between the shoulders and the sacrum. If lesions become secondarily infected, a widespread papular eruption and pruritus may develop.

Top Differentials

Differentials include demodicosis, superficial pyoderma, and dermatophytosis.

Diagnosis

1. Signalment, history, clinical findings, and rule out other differentials.
2. Dermatohistopathology: superficial portion of the hair follicle is distended with keratin. The keratin-dilated infundibulum may have a cystic appearance. Secondary bacterial folliculitis and furunculosis with comedone rupture may be present.

Treatment and Prognosis

1. For any secondary pyoderma, appropriate systemic antibiotics should be administered for 3 to 4 weeks.
2. For mild to moderate lesions, affected areas should be cleansed with human acne pads, chlorhexidine/miconazole pledgets, or 2½% benzoyl peroxide gel every 1 to 2 days until comedones have resolved (approximately 1–3 weeks). Then, these areas should be cleansed every 2 to 7 days or as needed for maintenance control.
3. For moderate to severe lesions, affected areas should be cleansed with a sulfur and salicylic acid, ethyl lactate, tar and sulfur, or benzoyl peroxide– and sulfur-containing shampoo every 2 to 3 days until comedones have resolved (approximately 1–3 weeks). Then, these areas should be cleansed as needed for long-term control.
4. Vitamin A 8000–10,000 IU/20 lb PO q 24 hours may be beneficial.
5. The prognosis is good. Unless lesions are secondarily infected, this is a cosmetic disease that does not affect the dog's quality of life and is usually readily controlled with routine symptomatic therapy.

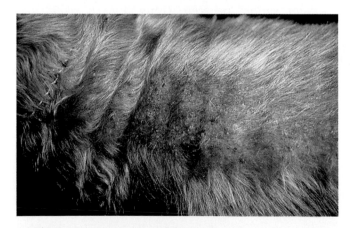

FIGURE 12-53 Schnauzer Comedo Syndrome. Comedones are visible through the partial alopecia. *(Courtesy W. Miller.)*

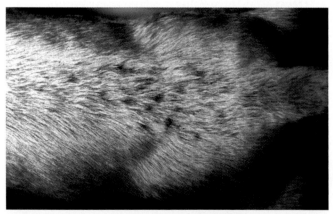

FIGURE 12-54 Schnauzer Comedo Syndrome. This moth-eaten alopecia was caused by numerous comedones on the lumbar area of this Schnauzer. *(Courtesy L. Frank.)*

Canine Ear Margin Dermatosis

Features

Canine ear margin dermatosis is a common idiopathic seborrheic condition of ear margins in dogs with pendulous ears, especially Dachshunds. Many dogs progress over time to demonstrate symptoms typical of vascular disease (vasculitis).

Initially, an asymptomatic accumulation of soft, greasy, keratinaceous debris occurs along the edges of the ears. With chronicity, the ear margins may become alopecic, crusted, cracked, ulcerated, and fissured. Fissured lesions may be painful and may induce head shaking, which further exacerbates the fissuring and pain. Except for the ear margins, the skin is otherwise normal. If the lesions progress and notch defects develop, or if other body regions are affected (e.g., nose, nails, oral cavity), autoimmune skin disease or vasculitis should be considered.

Top Differentials

Differentials include scabies, vasculitis, neoplasia, autoimmune skin disease, and causes of secondary seborrhea (see Box 12-1).

Diagnosis

1. Signalment, history, clinical findings, and rule out other differentials.
2. Dermatohistopathology: marked orthokeratotic or parakeratotic hyperkeratosis and follicular keratosis.

Treatment and Prognosis

1. No specific treatment is known.
2. The dog should be kept away from dry heat sources (e.g., wood stoves, fireplaces, forced air ducts) because dry heat aggravates the dermatosis.
3. To remove accumulated debris, gently cleanse ear margins with a sulfur and salicylic acid– or benzoyl peroxide–containing shampoo every 1 to 2 days until all debris is eliminated (approximately 5–14 days, depending on severity). Continue cleansing ear margins on an as-needed basis for maintenance control.
4. If accumulated crusts are tightly adherent and hardened, the first few shampoo applications should be preceded by a 5- to 10-minute warm water soak.
5. A moisturizer may be applied to ear margins after each shampoo therapy.
6. If ear margins are mildly to moderately inflamed, topical therapy with a steroid-containing ointment should be provided every 24 hours for the first 5 to 10 days.
7. Daily supplementation with oral essential fatty acids (180 mg EPA/10 lb), vitamin A (8000–10,000 IU), or zinc (zinc methionine or zinc sulfate 2–3 mg/kg/day of elemental zinc) may be beneficial for the skin lesions. Improvement should be seen after 1 to 2 months of therapy.
8. Treatment with vitamin E, tetracycline, doxycycline, or niacinamide may be beneficial (see Table 8-2).
9. Treatment with pentoxifylline 25 mg/kg PO every 12 hours with food may be beneficial in some dogs. Improvement should be seen within 1 to 3 months of therapy.
10. If ear margins are severely inflamed and if evidence of vasculitis is present, the patient should be evaluated and treated for vasculitis and autoimmune skin disease.
11. If ear margins are extensively fissured and respond poorly to topical therapy, a cosmetic ear crop to remove the fissured tissue may be considered. Lesions may recur at the surgical site.
12. The prognosis is variable, depending on severity. This condition is incurable, but most cases can be controlled symptomatically.

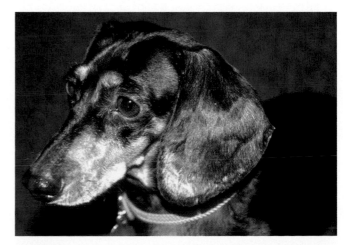

FIGURE 12-55 Canine Ear Margin Dermatosis. Alopecia with a crusting dermatitis on the ear margin of an adult Dachshund.

Canine Ear Margin Dermatosis—*cont'd*

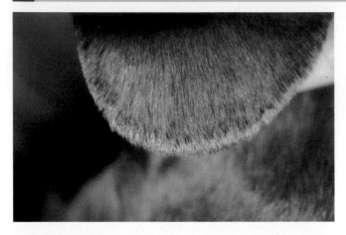

FIGURE 12-56 **Canine Ear Margin Dermatosis.** Alopecia and crusting on the distal ear margin of a young adult Dachshund.

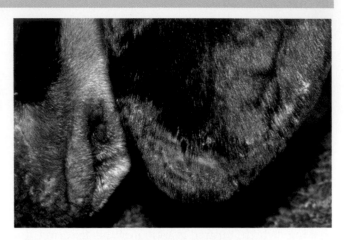

FIGURE 12-57 **Canine Ear Margin Dermatosis.** More severe alopecia extending onto the lateral ear pinna.

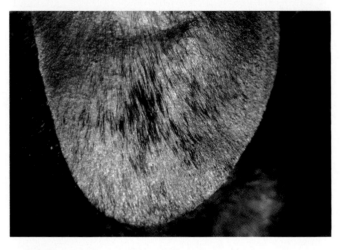

FIGURE 12-58 **Canine Ear Margin Dermatosis.** Diffuse alopecia covering almost the entire ear pinna.

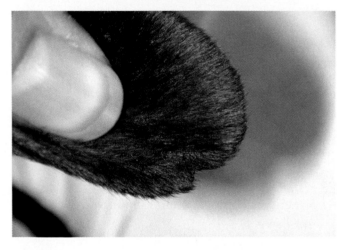

FIGURE 12-59 **Canine Ear Margin Dermatosis.** Alopecia and crusting on the ear margin with a notch defect. The notch is typical of a vasculitis lesion.

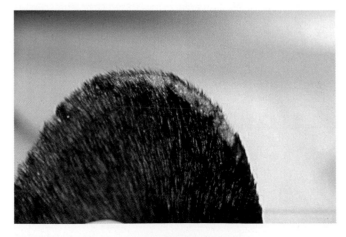

FIGURE 12-60 **Canine Ear Margin Dermatosis.** Alopecia and scaling affected only the distal margin of this adult Dachshund's ear pinna. The lesions are not pruritic.

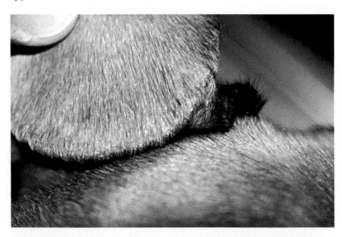

FIGURE 12-61 **Canine Ear Margin Dermatosis.** Alopecic crusting dermatitis on the ear margin.

Zinc-Responsive Dermatosis

Features

Zinc-responsive dermatosis is a zinc deficiency–induced disorder of keratinization. An inherent diminished ability to absorb zinc from the intestinal tract, a diet low in absolute zinc concentration, or mineral antagonisms that prevent zinc absorption from the food (e.g., diets high in phytate [plant protein], a cereal- or soy-based diet, excessive calcium supplementation) can cause zinc deficiency. It is rare in dogs, with the highest incidence in young adult Northern breed dogs (Siberian huskies, Samoyeds, and Alaskan malamutes) and in young, rapidly growing puppies of any breed.

Crusting, scaling, erythema, and alopecia typically develop around the eyes and mouth; the muzzle, nasal planum, ear pinnae, and genitalia may also be involved. Hyperkeratotic or thick, crusty plaques may be present on the elbows, stifles, and other pressure points, and at sites of trauma. The footpads may be hyperkeratotic and fissured. Lesions may be asymmetrical and mildly to moderately pruritic in some dogs. Secondary bacterial and *Malassezia* skin infections are common. Concurrent depression, anorexia, lymphadenomegaly, and pitting edema of the distal extremities may be seen. Severely affected puppies may have stunted growth.

Top Differentials

Differentials include primary seborrhea, autoimmune skin disease, and other causes of secondary seborrhea (see Box 12-1).

Diagnosis

1. Rule out other differentials.
2. Dermatohistopathology: marked, diffuse epidermal and follicular parakeratosis and superficial perivascular dermatitis. Papillomatosis, spongiosis, and evidence of secondary infection (intraepidermal pustules, folliculitis) are common.
3. Response to zinc therapy.

Treatment and Prognosis

1. Any secondary bacterial or *Malassezia* skin infection should be treated with appropriate medical therapy for at least 3 to 4 weeks.
2. For dogs with diet-induced zinc deficiency, the dietary imbalance should be identified and corrected. Only Association of American Feed Control Officials (AAFCO)-approved dog foods should be fed. Skin lesions should resolve within 2 to 6 weeks of the dietary change.
3. Zinc supplementation may be needed in some dogs, either initially for the first few weeks of the dietary change or lifelong if there is a diminished ability to absorb zinc. Zinc methionine or zinc sulfate (2–3 mg/kg/day of elemental zinc) PO should be administered with food. Improvement should occur within 6 weeks. If no response is seen, the zinc dosage can be doubled or a different zinc product tried. Signs of zinc toxicosis include depression, anorexia, vomiting, and diarrhea. Cutaneous lesions of zinc toxicosis can mimic zinc deficiency; therefore blood levels should be monitored.
4. Initiating oral essential fatty acid therapy may allow for a reduction in zinc dosage or may eliminate the need for zinc supplementation altogether in some dogs.
5. Concurrent symptomatic therapy with warm water soaks, antiseborrheic shampoos, and topical applications of ointments on the lesions may be helpful.
6. Intact females who are not well controlled with zinc supplementation should be neutered because estrus may exacerbate the disease.
7. The prognosis is good for most dogs, although lifelong zinc supplementation sometimes is needed.

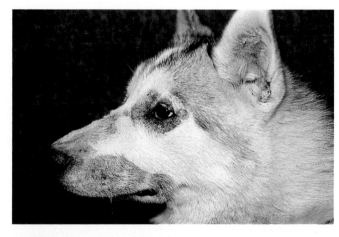

FIGURE 12-62 Zinc-Responsive Dermatosis. Alopecia and hyperkeratotic plaques on the face of a young adult Siberian husky.

Zinc-Responsive Dermatosis—*cont'd*

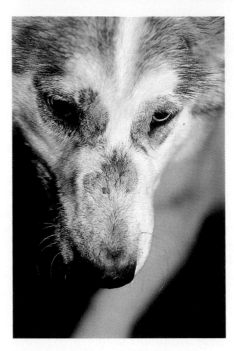

FIGURE 12-63 **Zinc-Responsive Dermatosis.** Same dog as in Figure 12-62. Alopecia and crusting around the nose and eyes resolved with zinc supplementation.

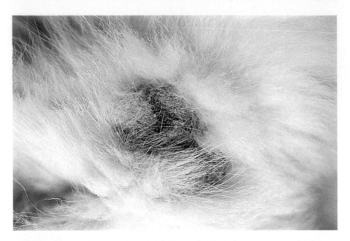

FIGURE 12-64 **Zinc-Responsive Dermatosis.** An alopecic, seborrheic plaque on the abdomen.

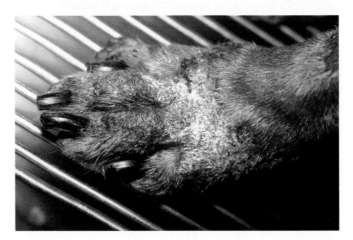

FIGURE 12-65 **Zinc-Responsive Dermatosis.** Alopecia with scale and crust formation on the foot of a dog with dietary zinc deficiency.

Tail Gland Hyperplasia (stud tail)

Features

Tail gland hyperplasia is a seborrheic condition that is associated with hyperplastic sebaceous glands in the tail gland area (dogs, cats) or the perianal region (dogs). In cats, it occurs as a localized idiopathic condition. In dogs, it may be localized or may be associated with a generalized primary or secondary seborrheic disorder. It is common in dogs, with intact males possibly predisposed. The condition is uncommon in cats, with the highest incidence in cage-confined cattery cats or in cats with poor grooming habits. Intact male cats may be predisposed.

Dogs

In dogs, the lesion is a slowly enlarging, asymptomatic, oval, raised area of hair loss on the dorsum of the tail approximately 2.5 to 5.0 cm distal to the tail head. Affected skin may be scaly, greasy, and hyperpigmented. Pustules from secondary bacterial infection may be seen. In dogs with primary or secondary seborrhea, other skin lesions are present.

Cats

A bandlike strip of matted hair or an accumulation of waxy, seborrheic debris occurs along the dorsum of the tail. Affected skin may become hyperpigmented or partially alopecic. Lesions are asymptomatic, and no other skin involvement is noted.

Top Differentials

Differentials include demodicosis, dermatophytosis, superficial pyoderma, and neoplasia.

Diagnosis

1. History, clinical findings, and rule out other differentials.
2. Dermatohistopathology: sebaceous gland hyperplasia.

Treatment and Prognosis

1. In dogs, if generalized skin disease is present, the underlying cause of the seborrhea should be identified and controlled.
2. Appropriate systemic antibiotics should be administered for 3 to 4 weeks if lesions in dogs are secondarily infected.
3. Clinical improvement in dogs and cats may be seen with localized topical antiseborrheic therapy applied on an as-needed basis.
4. In cats, self-grooming should be encouraged by minimizing cage confinement. Regular grooming and combing by the owner may be necessary in cats that are poor groomers.
5. In intact male dogs, castration may induce partial to complete lesion regression or may prevent further lesion enlargement. Improvement should be seen within 2 months of castration. In intact male cats, castration may not induce lesion resolution but may help prevent further progression.
6. For cosmetically unacceptable lesions in dogs, excess glandular tissue can be surgically resected. Without concurrent castration, however, lesion recurrence within 1 to 3 years is likely. Wound closure may be extremely difficult.
7. The prognosis is good. This is a cosmetic disease that does not affect the animal's quality of life.

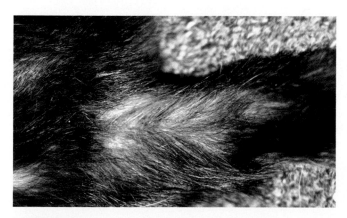

FIGURE 12-66 Tail Gland Hyperplasia. Focal alopecia and seborrhea oleosa over the dorsal tail head are typical of this disease.

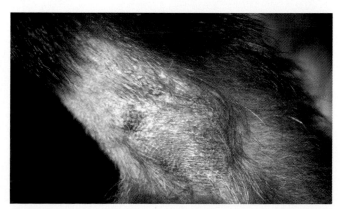

FIGURE 12-67 A focal area of alopecia with a crusting dermatitis developed over the area of the tail gland.

Tail Gland Hyperplasia—*cont'd*

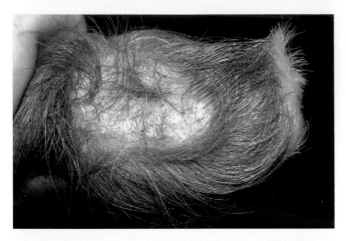

FIGURE 12-68 **Tail Gland Hyperplasia.** Alopecic dermatitis with cystlike structures over the tail gland in an adult Brittany spaniel.

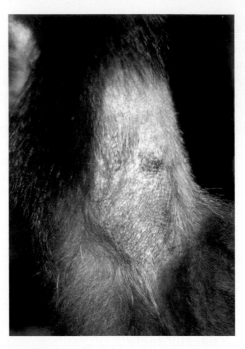

FIGURE 12-69 **Tail Gland Hyperplasia.** Alopecic dermatitis over the tail gland.

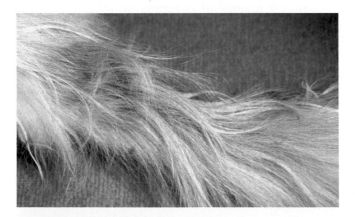

FIGURE 12-70 **Tail Gland Hyperplasia.** Partial alopecia with a focal, greasy, poor-quality fur coat on the dorsal tail region is characteristic of this disorder. *(Courtesy D. Angarano.)*

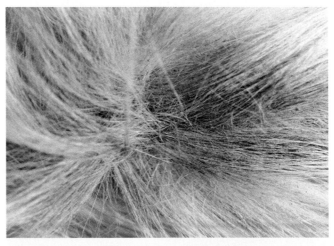

FIGURE 12-71 **Tail Gland Hyperplasia.** Close-up of the cat in Figure 21-68. Discoloration of the skin and hair is due to abnormal glandular secretion. *(Courtesy D. Angarano.)*

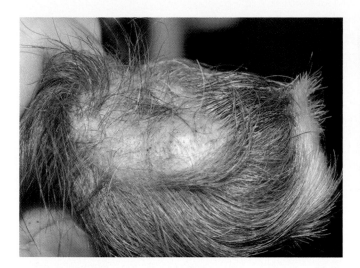

FIGURE 12-72 **Tail Gland Hyperplasia.** Alopecia and comedone formation caused by hypertrophy of the tail gland.

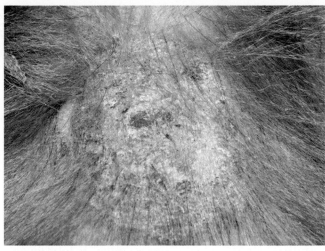

FIGURE 12-73 **Tail Gland Hyperplasia.** Alopecia and crusting of the skin over the tail gland caused by hypertrophy of the gland and resulting dermatitis.

Epidermal Dysplasia of West Highland White Terriers

Features

This severe chronic dermatosis is characterized by pruritus, seborrhea, and lichenification; it occurs in West Highland White terriers. This disorder is presumed by many dermatologists to be an inherited disorder of keratinization in which a dysplastic epidermis is predisposed to secondary *Malassezia* infection. However, recent investigators have suggested that the epidermal dysplasia may actually be an inflammatory or hypersensitivity reaction to the *Malassezia* infection, which, in turn, is secondary to underlying atopy or food hypersensitivity. It is uncommon in West Highland White terriers, with clinical signs usually appearing at between 6 and 12 months of age.

The development of a greasy hair coat is followed by mild to moderate pruritus of the face, ears, limbs, feet, and ventrum. With chronicity, the pruritus becomes intense, and widespread areas of erythema, alopecia, scaling, crusting, lichenification, hyperpigmentation, and greasy, malodorous skin exudate develop. Concurrent otitis externa with greasy ceruminous exudate and scaling is common.

Top Differentials

Differentials include primary seborrhea, ichthyosis, and causes of secondary seborrhea (see Box 12-1).

Diagnosis

1. Rule out other differentials.
2. Cytology (skin imprints, ear swabs): yeast organisms are seen. Bacterial cocci may also be present.
3. Dermatohistopathology: epidermal hyperplasia and dysplasia (frequent keratinocyte mitotic figures, crowding of epidermal basal cells, and loss of polarity). Parakeratotic hyperkeratosis, follicular hyperkeratosis, and surface yeasts are usually seen.

Treatment and Prognosis

1. Any underlying allergies (atopy, food, flea allergy) should be identified and treated.
2. Any endocrinopathy should be identified and treated (hypothyroidism, Cushing's disease).
3. Any secondary pyoderma should be treated with appropriate systemic antibiotics for at least 3 to 4 weeks.
4. Secondary *Malassezia* infection should be treated for at least 30 to 60 days to determine the response to eliminating the yeast infection. Treatment with other topical antifungal therapies (e.g., miconazole/chlorhexidine, ketoconazole/chlorhexidine shampoo) is beneficial, speeds resolution, and helps to prevent recurrence.
5. The prognosis for control is poor if no underlying allergies are found. Affected dogs should not be bred.

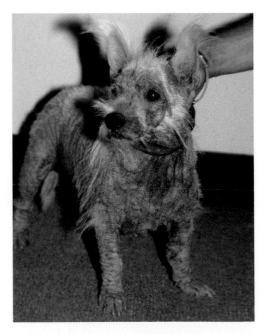

FIGURE 12-74 Epidermal Dysplasia of West Highland White Terriers. Generalized alopecia, lichenification, and hyperpigmentation are characteristic of this disorder. Secondary *Malassezia* dermatitis worsens the lichenification.

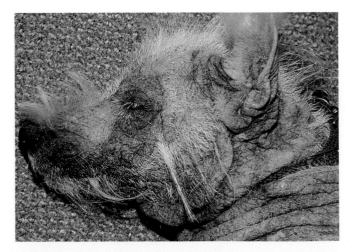

FIGURE 12-75 Epidermal Dysplasia of West Highland White Terriers. Close-up of the dog in Figure 12-74. Generalized alopecia, lichenification, and hyperpigmentation affect the face. Secondary *Malassezia* and bacterial infections worsen the pruritus, alopecia, and lichenification.

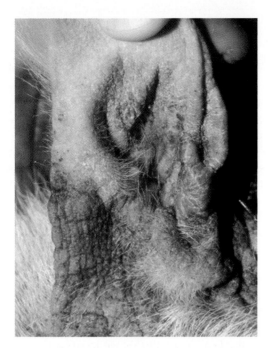

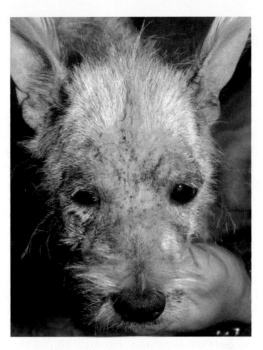

FIGURE 12-76 Epidermal Dysplasia of West Highland White Terriers. Alopecia, lichenification, and hyperpigmentation on the ear. Note that the entire cutaneous surface is affected, similar to primary seborrhea.

FIGURE 12-77 Epidermal Dysplasia of West Highland White Terriers. Alopecia, lichenification, and hyperpigmentation affecting the face. Crusting papular dermatitis was caused by a secondary superficial pyoderma.

Sebaceous Adenitis

Features

Sebaceous adenitis is a destructive inflammatory disease of sebaceous glands. It is uncommon in dogs, with the highest incidence reported in young adult to middle-aged Standard Poodles, Hungarian vizslas, Akitas, and Samoyeds. An autosomal recessive mode of inheritance is suspected in Standard Poodles and Akitas.

Mild to severe scaling most often involves the dorsum of the back and neck, top of the head, face (dorsal planum of nose), ears (pinnae or external canals), and tail. The skin disease may remain localized, become multifocal, or be generalized over the trunk. In short-coated dogs, the scales are usually fine and nonadherent. In longer-coated dogs, the scales tightly adhere to the hairs, and the hair coat may be dull, dry, or matted; follicular casts are common. Annular to patchy (short-haired dogs) or diffuse (long-haired dogs) alopecia occurs frequently. In long-haired dogs, the undercoat tends to be lost while the primary hairs are usually spared. Akitas may also have a greasy skin and hair coat, with papules and pustules; they may be concurrently febrile and depressed, and may lose weight. Pruritus is not usually seen unless there is a secondary bacterial or *Malassezia* infection, which is common. Subclinical disease (histologic lesions without clinical symptoms) has also been documented in Standard Poodles.

Top Differentials

Differentials include primary seborrhea and causes of secondary seborrhea (see Box 12-1).

Diagnosis

1. Rule out other differentials.
2. Dermatohistopathology (from dorsum of neck in suspected subclinical cases): in early lesions, there are discrete granulomas in areas of the sebaceous glands, with no involvement of other adnexa. In chronic lesions, the sebaceous glands are absent and are replaced by fibrosis. Follicular plugging and hyperkeratosis may be seen.

Treatment and Prognosis

1. Any secondary bacterial or *Malassezia* skin infections should be treated with appropriate systemic medications.
2. For mild cases, daily oral essential fatty acid supplementation and topical therapy with antiseborrheic shampoos, emollient rinses, and humectants applied every 2 to 4 days or as needed may effectively control symptoms. Essential fatty acid supplementation may be effective.
3. For more severe cases, daily treatments with high doses of oral fatty acids and topical spray applications of 50% to 75% propylene glycol in water or water-based moisturizing spray may be helpful.
4. Systemic therapy may be effective in preventing further sebaceous gland destruction and even in restoring more normal glandular function in some dogs. Dogs should be treated using the following:
   - Vitamin A 8000–10,000 IU/20 lb PO q 24 hours
   - Cyclosporine (Atopica) 5–10 mg/kg PO q 24 hours for 6 to 8 weeks or until improvement occurs; then the cyclosporine should be tapered to the lowest possible dose to prevent recurrence of the disease (usually every other day).
5. Historically, many drugs have been used with variable results; these include the following, as well as drugs typically used for autoimmune skin disorders:
   - Tetracycline and niacinamide (as described in Table 8-2)
   - Prednisone 2 mg/kg PO q 24 hours until lesions are controlled, then tapered to the lowest possible alternate-day dosage that controls signs
   - Isotretinoin 1 mg/kg PO q 12–24 hours until lesions improved (approximately 6 weeks), then 1 mg/kg PO q 24–48 hours for 6 weeks, then 1 mg/kg PO q 48 hours or 0.5 mg/kg PO q 24 hours for maintenance; liver adverse effects are common
   - Acitretin 1 mg/kg PO q 12–24 hours until lesions improve (approximately 6 weeks), then 1 mg/kg PO q 24–48 hours for 6 weeks, then 1 mg/kg PO q 48 hours or 0.5 mg/kg PO q 24 hours for maintenance
   - Asparaginase 10,000 IU IM q 7 days for two or three treatments, then as needed
6. The prognosis is variable, depending on disease severity. This is an incurable disease, but early diagnosis and treatment improve the prognosis for long-term control. Short-coated dogs, which tend to have milder symptoms, may have a more favorable prognosis than longer-coated dogs. Standard Poodles and Akitas have the greatest tendency to develop progressive, refractory disease, and if hair regrowth does occur in Standard Poodles, the hair may be straight rather than curled. Affected dogs should not be bred.

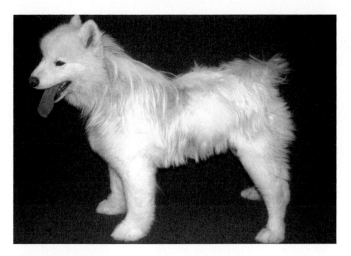

FIGURE 12-78 Sebaceous Adenitis. Generalized alopecia and erythema caused by sebaceous adenitis.

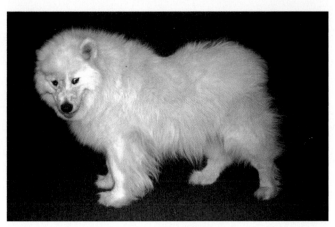

FIGURE 12-79 Sebaceous Adenitis. Same dog as in Figure 12-78. After therapy with vitamin A and topical therapies, the alopecia and dermatitis are much improved.

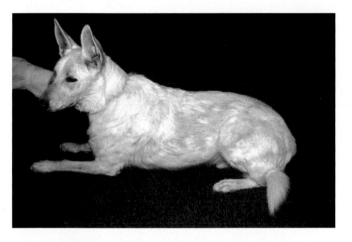

FIGURE 12-80 Sebaceous Adenitis. Generalized alopecia, erythema, and scaling typical of sebaceous adenitis.

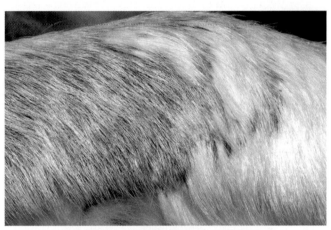

FIGURE 12-81 Sebaceous Adenitis. Alopecia and crusting dermatitis are caused by the lack of sebum production, which results in abnormal moisture and barrier function. This often leads to secondary infection.

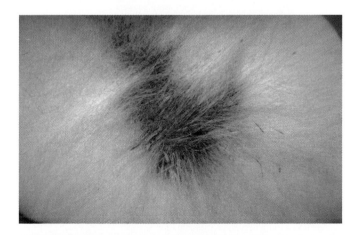

FIGURE 12-82 Sebaceous Adenitis. Clumping of hairs at the face, typical of primary keratinization defects.

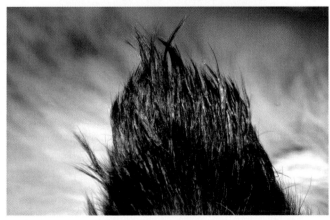

FIGURE 12-83 Sebaceous Adenitis. The poor-quality hair coat with adherent scales and crusts on the ear pinna is typical of this disease.

Sebaceous Adenitis—*cont'd*

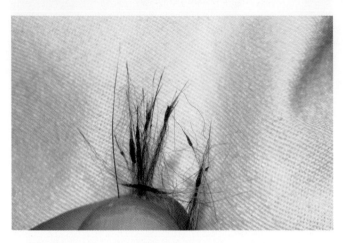

FIGURE 12-84 Sebaceous Adenitis. When the hairs are epilated, follicular casts adhere to the hair shaft, which is classic for primary keratinization defects such as sebaceous adenitis, primary seborrhea, and vitamin A–responsive dermatosis.

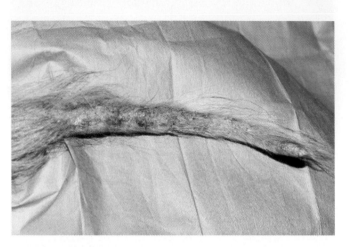

FIGURE 12-85 Sebaceous Adenitis. Alopecia and crusting on the distal tail of a dog with generalized lesions.

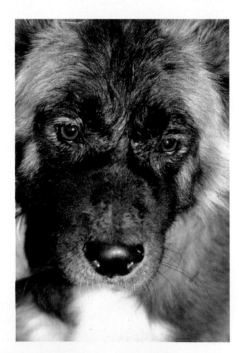

FIGURE 12-86 Sebaceous Adenitis. Crusts on the bridge of the nose and clumping of the fur on the face are apparent.

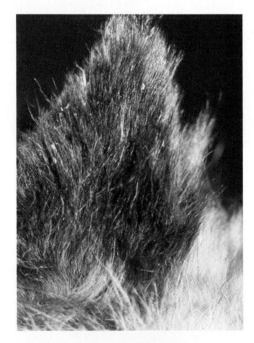

FIGURE 12-87 Sebaceous Adenitis. The poor-quality hair coat and clumping of hairs are apparent on the ear pinna of this dog. These lesions are most often found in a generalized pattern.

Hepatocutaneous Syndrome (superficial necrolytic dermatitis, superficial necrolytic migratory erythema [SNME], metabolic epidermal necrosis, diabetic dermatopathy)

Features

Hepatocutaneous syndrome/superficial necrolytic dermatitis is a unique skin disease in animals that have chronic liver disease or glucagon-secreting pancreatic tumors. The exact pathogenesis is unknown, but increased gluconeogenesis triggered by hyperglucagonemia (pancreatic tumor) or increased hepatic catabolism of amino acids (chronic liver disease) is thought to result in low plasma amino acid concentrations and epidermal protein depletion, which causes the skin lesions of superficial necrolytic dermatitis. It is uncommon in dogs and rare in cats, with the highest incidence in older animals. Among dogs, Shetland Sheep dogs, West Highland White terriers, Cocker spaniels, and Scottish terriers may be predisposed.

Skin lesions are characterized by minimally to intensely pruritic, bilaterally symmetrical erythema; scaling; crusting; erosions; and ulcers on the distal limbs and around the mouth and eyes. Lesions also may involve the ear pinnae, elbows, hocks, external genitalia, ventrum, and oral cavity. The footpads are usually mildly to markedly hyperkeratotic, fissured, and ulcerated. Lameness secondary to footpad lesions may be evident. Polydipsia and polyuria may be present if there is concurrent diabetes mellitus. Otherwise, systemic signs of underlying metabolic disease are rarely evident at initial presentation but usually become apparent a few to several months later.

Top Differentials

Differentials include cutaneous epitheliotropic lymphoma, pemphigus foliaceus or vulgaris, systemic lupus erythematosus, drug eruption, severe furunculosis (demodicosis, dermatophytosis, pyoderma), and zinc-responsive dermatosis.

Diagnosis

1. Hemogram: neutrophilia or normocytic, normochromic, nonregenerative anemia may be present.
2. Serum biochemistry panel (liver failure): findings usually include mild to moderate increases in serum alkaline phosphatase (ALP) and alanine aminotransferase (ALT) activities, total bilirubin, and bile acids. Hypoalbuminemia and decreased blood urea nitrogen (BUN) are also common. Hyperglycemia may be present.
3. Plasma amino acid concentrations: markedly decreased (hypoaminoacidemia).
4. Serum glucagon concentrations: elevated with glucagonoma, may or may not be elevated with hepatopathy.
5. Abdominal ultrasonography: evidence of chronic liver disease (small liver with hyperechoic, reticular pattern surrounding hypoechoic areas in a "honeycombed" pattern), pancreatic tumor, or metastasis to liver (hyperechoic or hypoechoic foci in liver parenchyma).
6. Histopathology (liver biopsy): chronic liver disease is usually characterized by a distinctive vacuolar hepatopathy with parenchymal collapse, or by extensive liver fibrosis (cirrhosis).
7. Dermatohistopathology: early lesions show the diagnostic findings of marked, diffuse parakeratotic hyperkeratosis with striking intercellular and intracellular edema, keratinocyte degeneration in the upper epidermis, and hyperplastic basal cells, which give the characteristic "red, white, and blue" histologic appearance of a striatonigral degeneration (SND) lesion. Mild, superficial, perivascular dermatitis with evidence of secondary bacterial, dermatophyte, or yeast infection may be present. Chronic lesions usually reveal nonspecific changes that are rarely diagnostic.

Treatment and Prognosis

1. Any secondary bacterial or yeast skin infection should be treated with appropriate antimicrobial therapies.
2. If the underlying cause is a resectable glucagonoma, surgical excision of the tumor is curative.
3. If the underlying problem is liver disease, its cause should be identified and corrected (e.g., anticonvulsant drug hepatotoxicity). To symptomatically improve liver function, therapy with one of the following antioxidants may be helpful:
   - S-adenosylmethionine (sAME) denosyl 18–22 mg/kg PO daily (90 mg small animals, 225 mg larger animals)
   - Ursodiol (Actigall) 10 mg/kg PO daily
   - Vitamin E 400 IU PO q 12 hours
4. In dogs with liver fibrosis, colchicine 0.03 mg/kg PO administered every 24 hours may help slow the progression of fibrosis. Potential adverse effects of long-term colchicine use include vomiting, hyperperistalsis, and diarrhea.
5. Parenteral amino acid supplementation is the symptomatic treatment of choice for improving skin lesions in animals with chronic liver disease and

Hepatocutaneous Syndrome—*cont'd*

may prolong survival time by several months. A 10% crystalline amino acid solution (Aminosyn, Abbott Laboratories, Abbott Park, IL) 25 mL/kg IV can be administered via jugular catheterization over 6 to 8 hours, or a 3% amino acid and electrolyte solution (Procalamine, Braun Medical Inc., Bethlehem, PA) 25 mL/kg IV can be administered via peripheral catheterization over 8 hours. Treatments may be repeated every 7 to 10 days or as needed. Marked improvement in skin lesions should be seen within 1 to 3 weeks.

6. Oral administration of amino acid solutions works well. Alternatively, oral supplementation with three to six raw egg yolks per day, zinc, and essential fatty acids may help improve skin lesions in some animals, but these treatments are usually not as effective as intravenous amino acid therapy.

7. Treatment with anti-inflammatory doses of prednisone may temporarily improve skin lesions, but some dogs are susceptible to diabetes or additional liver disease after glucocorticoid use.

8. Symptomatic topical therapies (keratolytic or moisturizing shampoos) may help improve skin lesions.

9. The prognosis for animals with chronic hepatic disease or metastatic pancreatic neoplasia is poor, and survival time after the onset of skin lesions may be only a few months.

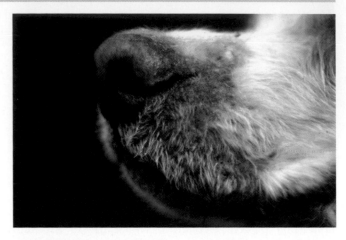

FIGURE 12-89 Hepatocutaneous Syndrome. Same dog as in Figure 12-88. Alopecic, crusting dermatitis on the nasal planum and muzzle.

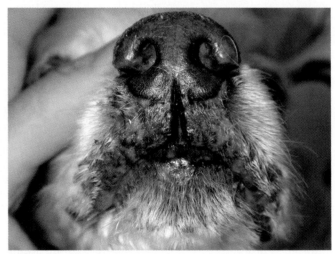

FIGURE 12-90 Hepatocutaneous Syndrome. Close-up of the dog in Figure 12-88. Alopecic crusting dermatitis on the lips and nasal planum is similar to lesions found in autoimmune skin disease.

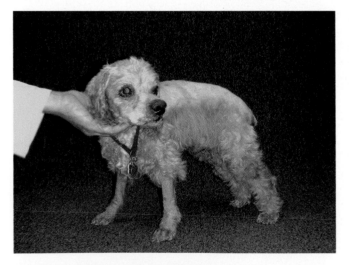

FIGURE 12-88 Hepatocutaneous Syndrome. A debilitated old dog with gross evidence of systemic disease. Crusting lesions on the nasal planum and periocular areas are typical of this syndrome. Note the similarity to autoimmune skin disease, which usually occurs in younger dogs.

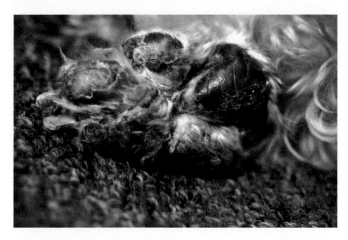

FIGURE 12-91 **Hepatocutaneous Syndrome.** Severe hyperkeratosis and crusting of the footpads are common findings in hepatocutaneous syndrome. Note the similarity to autoimmune skin disease.

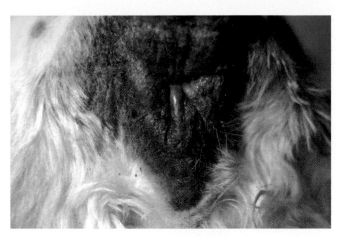

FIGURE 12-92 **Hepatocutaneous Syndrome.** Lesions around the mucous membrane are common in hepatocutaneous syndrome. Perianal dermatitis is apparent.

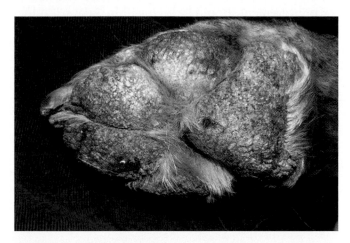

FIGURE 12-93 **Hepatocutaneous Syndrome.** Severe crusting of the footpads of a dog with hepatocutaneous syndrome.

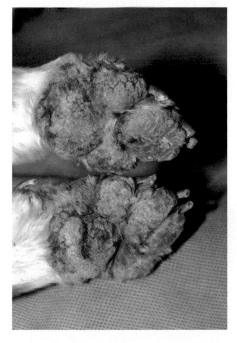

FIGURE 12-95 **Hepatocutaneous Syndrome.** Severe crusting and hyperkeratosis of the footpads developed over several months in this older mixed-breed dog. *(Courtesy A. Yu.)*

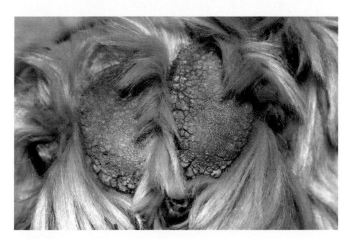

FIGURE 12-94 **Hepatocutaneous Syndrome.** Footpad hyperkeratosis and crusting. Note the similarities to autoimmune skin disease.

Familial Footpad Hyperkeratosis

Features

Familial footpad hyperkeratosis is a familial disorder that results in severe digital hyperkeratosis by 5 to 6 months of age. It is rare in dogs, with the highest incidence in Irish terriers, Dogues de Bordeaux, and Kerry blue terriers. An autosomal recessive mode of inheritance is suspected in Irish terriers.

At birth, the footpads appear to be normal, but by 4 to 6 months of age, affected dogs begin to develop marked hyperkeratotic, thickened, hard, and cracked footpads. The entire surfaces of all footpads are involved, and subsequent formation of horny growths, expanding fissures, and secondary bacterial infection usually result in severe, intermittent lameness. No other skin involvement occurs, but concurrent abnormal nail development, characterized by slightly faster growth and round profiles instead of the normal U-shaped ones, may be seen in Irish terriers.

Top Differentials

Differentials include distemper, zinc-responsive dermatosis, autoimmune skin disease, and superficial necrolytic dermatitis.

Diagnosis

1. Rule out other differentials.
2. Dermatohistopathology: marked orthokeratotic hyperkeratosis with mild to severe epidermal hyperplasia.

Treatment and Prognosis

1. No specific treatment is known, but treatments as for idiopathic nasodigital hyperkeratosis may be effective.
2. Symptomatically treat with daily foot soaks in 50% propylene glycol combined with frequent filing of the footpads to remove surplus keratin. Significant improvement should be seen within 5 days, but life-long maintenance therapy is required for control.
3. For fissured lesions, a combination antibiotic/glucocorticoid ointment may be applied every 8 to 12 hours until lesions are healed; appropriate systemic antibiotics should be administered for 3 to 4 weeks if footpads are secondarily infected.
4. Fast-growing nails should be trimmed frequently.
5. The prognosis for cure is poor, but most dogs enjoy a good quality of life with routine symptomatic therapy. Affected dogs should not be bred.

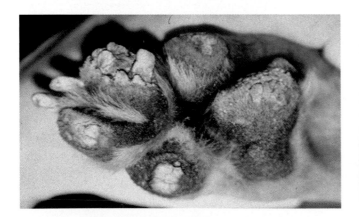

FIGURE 12-96 Familial Footpad Hyperkeratosis. Severe hyperkeratosis and crusting of the pads are characteristic of this disorder. *(Courtesy Paradis M: Footpad hyperkeratosis in a family of Dogues de Bordeaux, Vet Dermatol 3:75, 1992, Blackwell Science Ltd.)*

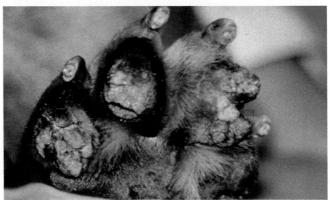

FIGURE 12-97 Familial Footpad Hyperkeratosis. Severe hyperkeratosis resulted in footpad disfigurement. *(Courtesy Paradis M: Footpad hyperkeratosis in a family of Dogues de Bordeaux, Vet Dermatol 3:75, 1992, Blackwell Science Ltd.)*

Facial Dermatitis of Persian Cats

Features

Facial dermatitis of Persian cats is a facial skin disease of unclear cause. It is uncommon to rare in Persian and Himalayan cats, with highest incidence in older kittens and young adult cats.

Black, waxy debris that mats the hair accumulates symmetrically around the eyes or mouth, or on the chin. Initially, lesions are not pruritic, but as they progress and become inflamed, moderate to severe pruritus develops. Exudative and erythematous facial folds, a mucoid ocular discharge, erythema of the preauricular skin, and otitis externa with black, waxy debris in the ear canals may also be present. Secondary bacterial and *Malassezia* skin infections are common. Submandibular lymphadenomegaly may be seen.

Top Differentials

Differentials include demodicosis, dermatophytosis, *Malassezia* dermatitis, bacterial folliculitis, and other causes of secondary seborrhea (see Box 12-1).

Diagnosis

1. Signalment, history, clinical findings, and rule out other differentials.
2. Cytology (skin imprints, ear swab): waxy debris. Bacteria or yeast may be seen.
3. Dermatohistopathology: findings include marked acanthosis, superficial crusts that often contain sebum, hydropic degeneration of basal cells, and occasional dyskeratotic keratinocytes. Dyskeratoses are most marked in the follicular epithelium. Sebaceous hyperplasia and a superficial dermal infiltrate of eosinophils, neutrophils, mast cells, histiocytes, and occasional melanophages are also typical.

Treatment and Prognosis

1. No specific therapy is known.
2. Any secondary bacterial or *Malassezia* skin infections should be treated with appropriate systemic medications for at least 3 to 4 weeks. Periodic retreatments are often needed because these cats are susceptible to recurring infection.
3. Alternatively, treatment with cyclosporine 5–7 mg/kg PO every 24 hours may be beneficial in some cats. Improvement should be seen within 4 to 6 weeks.
4. Treatments with prednisolone 1–3 mg/kg/day PO for 2 to 4 weeks, followed by 1–3 mg/kg PO every 48 hours, may partially control pruritus and symptoms in some cats. Adverse effects may be common and severe with long-term use.
5. The prognosis is guarded because most cats respond poorly to symptomatic therapy. Lesions may become refractory to ongoing therapy over time, especially if secondary bacterial or yeast infections are not identified and controlled. Affected cats should not be bred.

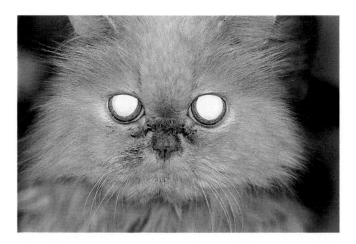

FIGURE 12-98 Facial Dermatitis of Persian Cats. Black, greasy exudate on the face of a young cat.

Facial Dermatitis of Persian Cats—*cont'd*

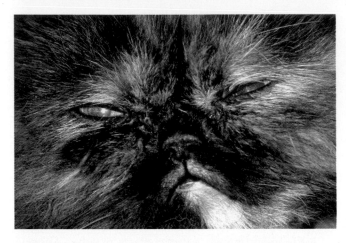

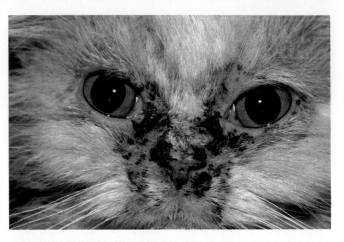

FIGURE 12-99 Facial Dermatitis of Persian Cats. Black, waxy exudate on the face of a young Persian cat. The normal coloration of this cat makes the lesions more difficult to visualize.

FIGURE 12-100 Facial Dermatitis of Persian Cats. Severe crusting and erosive dermatitis on the face and nasal planum of this young cat are typical of this syndrome but were caused by pemphigus foliaceus. Many conditions can mimic this syndrome, especially secondary *Malassezia* and bacterial infections.

CHAPTER 13

Diseases of Eyes, Claws, Anal Sacs, and Ear Canals

- Blepharitis
- Otitis Externa
- Aural Hematoma
- Melanoma
- Anal Sac Disease

- Perianal Fistulae (anal furunculosis)
- Bacterial Claw Infection
- Fungal Claw Infection (onychomycosis)
- Symmetrical Lupoid Onychodystrophy (idiopathic onychomadesis)

Blepharitis

Features

Blepharitis is inflammation of the eyelids that may be due to a primary bacterial infection or may be secondary to an underlying condition, such as a parasitic, allergic, autoimmune skin disease, or leishmaniasis. Eyelid involvement may occur alone or in conjunction with generalized skin disease. It is common in dogs and uncommon in cats.

Bacterial Blepharitis

The affected eyelids are mildly to markedly pruritic. They are often swollen or thickened, erythematous, and alopecic, with pustules, crusts, and sometimes cutaneous fistulae. One or more eyelid glands may be abscessed.

Insect Bite/Sting Hypersensitivity

Onset of eyelid erythema, with swelling (angioedema) or raised focal masses, is acute.

Contact Hypersensitivity (from topical ophthalmic medication)

This is characterized by acute onset of eyelid alopecia and depigmentation, with marked conjunctival injection. Secondary bacterial or yeast infections are common.

Allergy

Seasonal (atopy) or nonseasonal (atopy, food hypersensitivity) pruritus (eye rubbing) results in varying degrees of periocular erythema, alopecia, lichenification, and hyperpigmentation. Concurrent conjunctivitis and secondary bacterial blepharitis are common. Other skin involvement usually occurs.

Autoimmune Disease

This manifests as eyelid erythema, erosions, and crusting, which are not pruritic unless secondary bacterial infection is present. Similar lesions involving the dorsum or planum of the nose, lips, ears, footpads, or other mucocutaneous junctions, or generalized skin lesions, are present concurrently.

Leishmaniasis

Eyelid lesions may include periocular alopecia and dry seborrhea, ulcerated lid margins with moist dermatitis, diffuse blepharedema, and discrete nodular granulomas. Ophthalmic involvement is often characterized by anterior uveitis, conjunctivitis, or keratoconjunctivitis. Concurrent systemic signs such as malaise, weight loss, diarrhea, renal or liver failure, anemia, lameness, and skin lesions elsewhere on the body are common.

Blepharitis—*cont'd*

Top Differentials

Differentials include demodicosis, dermatophytosis, *Malassezia* dermatitis, juvenile cellulitis, autoimmune skin disease (pemphigus or lupus), and viral infection (rhinotracheitis, calicivirus).

Diagnosis

1. Usually based on history, clinical findings, and ruling out other differentials.
2. Cytology (pustule, abscess): suppurative inflammation and bacterial cocci, if primary or secondary bacterial blepharitis is present. *Malassezia* organisms, if secondary yeast dermatitis is present.
3. Bacterial culture (pustule, abscess): *Staphylococcus* is usually isolated, if primary or secondary bacterial blepharitis is present.
4. Dermatohistopathology: findings are variable, depending on the underlying cause.
5. Allergy workup: performed if atopy or food hypersensitivity is suspected.

Treatment and Prognosis

1. Any underlying cause should be identified and addressed.
2. Any topical medications should be discontinued, if contact dermatitis is suspected.
3. If pruritic, an Elizabethan collar should be used to prevent self-trauma.
4. Warm water compresses should be applied to affected areas two to three times daily to decrease swelling and remove exudate.
5. If bacterial infection is present, a topical antibiotic-glucocorticoid ophthalmic preparation should be applied to the affected eye every 8 to 12 hours for 2 to 3 weeks. Effective preparations include those containing the following:
   - Bacitracin-neomycin-polymyxin-hydrocortisone
   - Neomycin-prednisone
   - Gentamicin-betamethasone

   Do not use if contact dermatitis is suspected.
6. For bacterial blepharitis, appropriate systemic antibiotics should be administered for at least 3 weeks.
7. For autoimmune blepharitis, treatment with immunosuppressive medications should be provided (Tables 8-1 and 8-2).
8. Symptomatic treatment with topical ophthalmic preparations that contain glucocorticoids or antihistamines may be helpful in cases of allergic blepharitis.
9. The prognosis is good if the underlying cause can be identified and corrected or controlled.

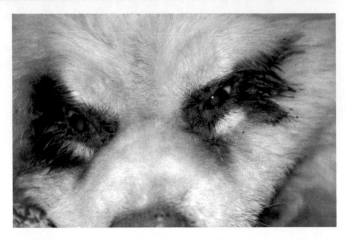

FIGURE 13-1 Blepharitis. Discoloration and matting of the hair around the eye in a dog with bilateral blepharitis.

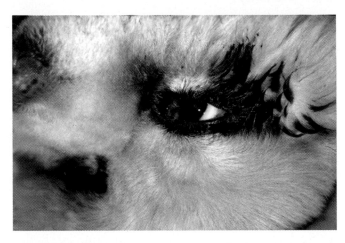

FIGURE 13-2 Blepharitis. Close-up of the dog in Figure 13-1. Discoloration and matting of the hair around the eye caused by the copious ocular discharge are apparent.

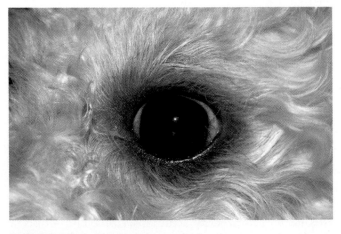

FIGURE 13-3 Blepharitis. Periocular alopecia and erythema associated with allergic dermatitis.

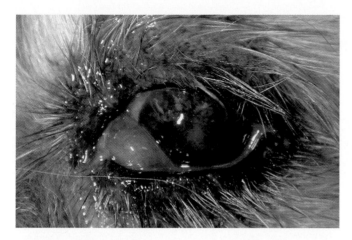

FIGURE 13-4 Blepharitis. Periocular alopecia and erythema associated with allergic dermatitis. The thick ocular exudate is caused by keratoconjunctivitis sicca (KCS) and the prolapsed third eyelid (cherry eye).

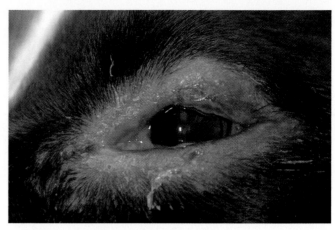

FIGURE 13-5 Blepharitis. "Marginal blepharitis" (immune-mediated syndrome) causing alopecic, papular, crusting periocular dermatitis.

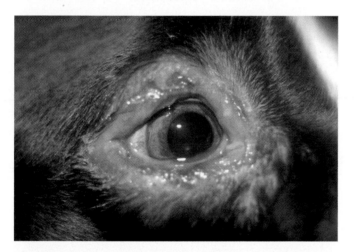

FIGURE 13-6 Blepharitis. Same dog as in Figure 13-5. The "marginal blepharitis" caused a bilateral, alopecic, papular dermatitis.

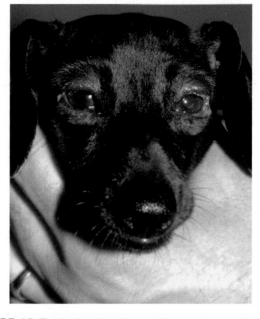

FIGURE 13-7 Blepharitis. The swollen, moist, erythematous dermatitis affecting both eyes was caused by a cutaneous bacterial infection. *(Courtesy S. McLaughlin.)*

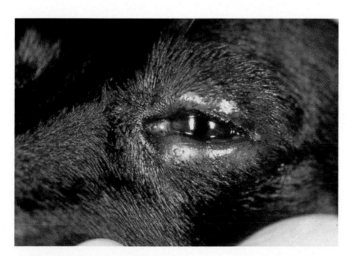

FIGURE 13-8 Blepharitis. Same dog as in Figure 13-7. Alopecia, erythema, and tissue swelling of the periocular skin. *(Courtesy S. McLaughlin.)*

Blepharitis—*cont'd*

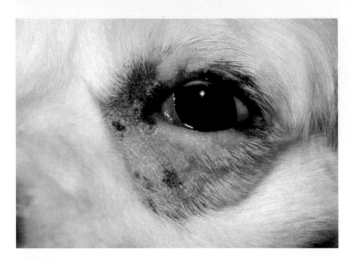

FIGURE 13-9 Blepharitis. Alopecia and erythema affecting the periocular skin caused by a secondary bacterial pyoderma. *(Courtesy E. Willis.)*

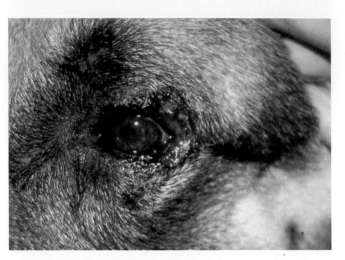

FIGURE 13-10 Blepharitis. Erosive lesions on the eyelids of this adult German shepherd were caused by a bacterial infection.

Otitis Externa

Features

Otitis externa is an acute or chronic inflammatory disease of the external ear canal. Its causes are numerous and almost always have an underlying primary disease (Table 13-1) that alters the normal structure and function of the canal, resulting in a secondary infection (Table 13-2). Otitis externa is common in cats and dogs, with Cocker spaniels especially at risk for developing severe and chronic disease.

TABLE 13-1 Primary Causes of Otitis Externa

Primary Factor	Characteristics	Comments
Parasites	*Otodectes cynotis*	Cause approximately 50% of otitis cases in cats and 5% to 10% of otitis in dogs. Dogs and cats can be asymptomatic carriers
	Demodicosis	Can cause a ceruminous otitis in dogs and cats
	Sarcoptes scabiei	Typically, the ear margin and ventral third of the outer ear pinna are affected. Otitis externa is not usually a feature of this disease
	Hard ticks, chiggers	May affect ear pinnae and external ear canal
	Spinous ear ticks	An uncommon cause of otitis externa in dogs and cats
Hypersensitivities	Atopy	Otitis externa is seen in 50% to 80% of atopic dogs. (In 3%–5% of them, otitis externa is the only symptom.) Usually, bilateral otitis
	Food hypersensitivity	Otitis externa is seen in up to 80% of dogs with food hypersensitivities. (In more than 20% of these dogs, otitis externa is the only symptom.)
	Contact dermatitis	Otic medication (e.g., neomycin, propylene glycol) can cause irritant reactions in the ear. Should be suspected any time ear disease worsens significantly while animal is undergoing topical treatment
Endocrine Disorders	Hypothyroidism	Bilateral ceruminous otitis externa. Most common in middle-aged to older dogs. Usually, skin involvement
		Usually, pinnae are more involved than ear canals, and other areas of the skin are affected. Lesions may include pustules, vesicles, scales, crusts, erosions, and ulcers
Foreign Bodies		Usually present as unilateral otitis externa. Look for plant material, dirt, small stones, impacted wax, loose hair, and dried medication. Often, the inciting foreign body is not identified because it becomes so coated with cerumen that, when removed during ear flushing, it is not recognizable
Keratinization Disorders	Canine primary seborrhea	Bilateral ceruminous otitis. Usually have other skin involvement, especially Cocker spaniels
	Facial dermatosis of Persians	Bilateral ceruminous otitis externa and seborrheic facial dermatitis. Secondary malasseziasis is common. Uncommon to rare in Persian cats
	Sebaceous adenitis	May cause dry, scaly ears and mild inflammation. Usually other skin involvement. Rare in dogs, with highest incidence in Standard Poodles, Akitas, and Samoyeds
Autoimmune/ Immune-Mediated Diseases	Juvenile cellulitis	Acute cellulitis of muzzle and periocular regions with marked submandibular and prescapular lymphadenomegaly. Exudative otitis externa, fever, and depression may also be present. Uncommon in puppies 3 weeks to 6 months old, with highest incidence in Golden retrievers, Labrador retrievers, Dachshunds, Pointers, and Lhasa apsos
Inflammatory Polyps (cats)		May present as recurrent, unilateral otitis externa. Polyps may originate from lining of tympanic cavity, auditory canal, or nasopharynx
Neoplasia	Cats	Ceruminous gland adenomas and adenocarcinomas, sebaceous gland adenomas and carcinomas, squamous cell carcinomas, papillomas
	Dogs	Ceruminous gland adenomas and adenocarcinomas, papillomas, basal cell carcinomas, squamous cell carcinomas
Conformation	Heavy, pendulous ears	May result in decreased air circulation, increased heat, and moisture
	Narrow ear canals Retention in the ear canal	Nidus for infection
	Hair in ear canals	
	Increased glandular tissue	

Otitis Externa—*cont'd*

TABLE 13-2 Secondary Causes of Otitis Externa

Secondary Factors	Comments
Bacterial infection	Include *Staphylococcus* spp., *Streptococcus*, *Pseudomonas* spp., *Proteus*, and *Escherichia coli*. Recurrent bacterial otitis is often associated with underlying allergies.
Yeast infection	*Malassezia pachydermatis*. Recurrent yeast otitis is often associated with underlying allergies.
Otitis media	Chronic otitis externa (2 months' duration or longer) often results in extension of the disease into the middle ear. The otitis media can then be a source for recurrent otitis externa.
Chronic pathologic changes	With chronic inflammation, the dermis and the subcutis become fibrotic, leading to permanent stenosis of the canal lumen. The auditory cartilage may become calcified and ossified. Secretions, desquamated cells, and proliferating microorganisms become entrapped. Calcified ear cartilage is a permanent change that cannot be resolved with medical therapy.

Otic pruritus or pain is a common symptom of otitis externa. Head rubbing, ear scratching, head shaking, aural hematomas, and a head tilt, with the affected ear tilted down, may be noted. An otic discharge that may be malodorous is often present. In acute cases, the inner ear pinna and the ear canal are usually erythematous and swollen. The ear canal may also be eroded or ulcerated. Pinnal alopecia, excoriations, and crusts are common. In chronic cases, pinnal hyperkeratosis, hyperpigmentation, and lichenification, as well as ear canal stenosis from fibrosis or ossification, are common. Decreased hearing may be noted. Concurrent otitis media should be suspected if otitis externa has been present for 2 months or longer, even if the tympanic membrane appears to be intact and no clinical signs of otitis media (drooping or inability to move ear or lip, drooling, decreased or absent palpebral reflex, exposure keratitis) are evident. Rarely, symptoms of otitis interna (head tilt, nystagmus, ataxia) may be present. Oral examination may reveal pain (severe otitis media), inflammation, or masses (especially polyps in cats). Depending on the underlying cause, concurrent skin disease may be seen.

Diagnosis

1. Based on history and clinical findings.
2. Otoscopic examination: assess degree of inflammation, ulceration, stenosis, and proliferative changes; amount and nature of debris and discharge; presence of foreign bodies, ectoparasites, and masses; and integrity of tympanic membrane.
3. Mineral oil prep (ear swab): look for otodectic and demodectic mites and ova.
4. Cytology (ear swab): look for bacteria, yeasts, fungal hyphae, cerumen, leukocytes, and neoplastic cells.
5. Bacterial culture (external or middle ear exudate): indicated when bacteria are found on cytology in spite of antibiotic therapy, or when otitis media is suspected.
6. Fungal culture: indicated when dermatophytic otitis is suspected, especially in long-haired cats that have ceruminous otitis.
7. Radiography (bulla series), computed tomography (CT), magnetic resonance imaging (MRI): evidence of bullous involvement (sclerosis, opacification) is seen in approximately 75% of otitis media cases.
8. Dermatohistopathology: may be indicated to identify primary cause (e.g., autoimmune disease, sebaceous adenitis, erythema multiforme), if neoplasia is suspected (ear canal mass), or if ear canal resection or ablation is performed because of end-stage otitis.

Treatment and Prognosis

1. Primary causes of the otitis should be identified and corrected, if possible (see Table 13-1).
2. **For swimmer's ear**, maceration of ear canals can be prevented by prophylactic instillation of a drying agent after the dog gets wet (swimming, bathing), or two to three times per week in very humid climates. Effective products are ear products that contain astringents/alcohol.
3. **For allergic otitis**, long-term management includes control of underlying allergies, resolution of any secondary bacterial and yeast otitis, and institution of ear cleaning and treatment every 3 to 7 days to prevent recurrence. In animals whose underlying allergies cannot be identified or completely controlled, judicious use of steroid-containing otic preparations as infrequently as needed may prevent otitis flare-ups.
4. **For mild/acute otitis**, at home, the owner should perform ear cleaning every 2 to 7 days with a ceruminolytic agent (that does not need to be flushed out) to prevent earwax and debris from accumulating. Lifelong ear cleaning every 3 to 7 days may be necessary to prevent relapses of otitis. The use of cotton swabs (which may damage the epithelium) is not recommended.
5. **For severe/chronic otitis**, in-hospital ear cleaning and flushing should be performed to remove accumulated exudate and debris from the vertical and horizontal ear canals (under sedation or anesthesia

if necessary). The procedure should be repeated every 2 to 7 days until all debris has been removed. Products that can be used for ear flushing include the following:

- Water or saline
- DSS diluted in warm water or saline

Non-ototoxic ear cleaning product

- Povidone-iodine 0.2% to 1% solution (may be ototoxic)
- Chlorhexidine 0.05% to 0.2% solution (may be ototoxic)
- Pretreatment (5 minutes before lavage) with a urea peroxide cleaning product is very effective at dissolving exudate, but the product MUST be flushed out of the canal (may be ototoxic).

6. **Systemic glucocorticoids** should be administered if the ear is painful or the canal is stenotic from tissue swelling or proliferation. For dogs, prednisone 0.25–0.5 mg/kg PO should be administered every 12 hours for 5 to 10 days. For cats, prednisolone 0.5–1.0 mg/kg PO should be administered every 12 hours for 7 to 14 days.

Individual Diseases

7. **For ear mites**, affected and all in-contact dogs and cats should be treated. When otic treatments are used, additional treatment to eliminate ectopic mites should be concurrently administered. Effective therapies for ear mites include the following:

- Otic miticide as per label directions (ivermectin and milbemycin products are safe and highly effective)
- Selemectin 6–12 mg/kg topically on skin twice 2 to 4 weeks apart (dogs)
- Tresaderm 0.125 to 0.25 mL AU q 12 hours for 2 to 3 weeks
- Ivermectin 0.3 mg/kg PO q 7 days for three to four treatments, or 0.3 mg/kg SC q 10–14 days for two to three treatments
- Fipronil 0.1 to 0.15 mL AU q 14 days for two to three treatments (based on anecdotal reports)

8. **For demodectic otitis**, effective therapies for ear mites include the following:

- Otic miticide as per label directions (ivermectin and milbemycin products are safe and highly effective)

  An alternative treatment is to use 1% injectable ivermectin solution 0.1 to 0.15 mL instilled AU every 24 hours, continuing at least 2 weeks past complete clinical resolution with no evidence of mites on follow-up ear smears.

9. **For yeast otitis**, antifungal-containing ear preparations should be repackaged into a bottle to provide more accurate dosing—dropper bottle, brown amber bottle, etc. Then, 0.2 to 0.5 mL ($\frac{1}{4}$–$\frac{1}{2}$ dropperful) should be instilled in the affected ear every 12 hours for at least 2 to 4 weeks. Treatment should be continued until follow-up ear smears are cytologically negative for microorganisms, the external canals are no longer edematous or inflamed, and the ear canal epithelium has normalized. Effective products include the following:

- Clotrimazole
- Ketoconazole
- Miconazole
- Thiabendazole
- Nystatin

10. **For severe refractory yeast otitis externa or otitis media**, in addition to topical antifungal treatment, systemic antifungal therapy may be helpful if administered for at least 3 to 4 weeks, then continued 1 to 2 weeks beyond complete clinical cure. Effective therapies include the following:

- Ketoconazole 5 mg/kg PO q 12 hours, or 10 mg/kg PO q 24 hours with food
- Fluconazole 5 mg/kg PO q 12 hours, or 10 mg/kg PO q 24 hours with food
- Itraconazole 5–10 mg/kg PO q 24 hours with food
- Pulse itraconazole 5–10 mg/kg PO q 24 hours with food on 2 consecutive days each week

11. **For bacterial otitis**, antibiotic-containing ear preparations should be repackaged into bottles to provide more accurate dosing—dropper bottle, brown amber bottle, etc. Then, 0.2 to 0.5 mL ($\frac{1}{4}$–$\frac{1}{2}$ dropperful) should be instilled in affected ears every 8 to 12 hours for at least 2 to 4 weeks. Treatment should be continued until follow-up ear smears are cytologically negative for microorganisms, the external canals are no longer edematous or inflamed, and the ear canal epithelium has normalized. Effective products include the following:

- Gentamicin
- Enrofloxacin
- Neomycin
- Polymyxin B
- Polymyxin E

12. **For bacterial otitis media**, systemic antibiotics may **not** achieve sufficient tissue concentrations to kill *Pseudomonas* and to prevent antibiotic resistance; the highest possible dose of antibiotic that is safe should be administered with concurrent high-concentration topical therapy of the same antibiotic. If topical treatment has been used aggressively and has been unsuccessful, systemic antibiotics may be indicated, based on culture and sensitivity results, for a minimum of 4 weeks, and continued 2 weeks beyond complete clinical cure.

Antibiotics include the following:

- Ormetoprim-sulfadimethoxine 27.5 mg/kg PO q 24 hours
- Trimethoprim-sulfa 22 mg/kg PO q 12 hours

Otitis Externa—cont'd

- Cephalexin, cephradine, or cefadroxil 22 mg/kg PO q 8 hours
- Ciprofloxacin 15 mg/kg PO q 12 hours *(may increase the risk of resistant bacteria)*
- Enrofloxacin 20 mg/kg PO q 24 hours *(may increase the risk of resistant bacteria)*
- Orbifloxacin 7.5 mg/kg PO q 24 hours *(may increase the risk of resistant bacteria)*
- Marbofloxacin 5.5 mg/kg PO q 24 hours *(may increase the risk of resistant bacteria)*

13. For Pseudomonas **otitis**, aggressive treatment should be provided for at least 2 to 4 weeks, then continued 2 weeks beyond complete clinical cure. All underlying/primary diseases should be identified and addressed. Currently, the most effective treatments include tris–ethylenediaminetetraacetic acid (EDTA) solutions with high concentrations of antibiotics instilled in high volumes (to ensure deep penetration and prevent dilution by exudate). Antibiotics should be selected according to culture and sensitivity results. Systemic antibiotics may **not** achieve sufficient tissue concentrations (mutation prevention concentration) to kill *Pseudomonas* and prevent antibiotic resistance. If systemic antibiotics are used, the highest possible dose that is safe should be administered, along with concurrent high-concentration topical therapy of the same antibiotic.

    - The EDTA solution should be combined with enrofloxacin to make a 10- to 20-mg/mL solution. The solution should be used q 12–24 hours to completely fill the ear canal. Even as the sole therapy, the surfactants in T8 Solution act to clean the ear while allowing the high concentration of enrofloxacin to penetrate into the deep canal. This treatment is 80% effective in chronic, recurrent otitis cases, even if the bacteria are reported to be resistant to enrofloxacin (because of the tris-EDTA and high concentration of antibiotic).

- Tris-EDTA solution (with/without enrofloxacin 10 mg/mL, gentamicin 3 mg/mL, or amikacin 9 mg/mL) 0.5 mL instilled q 8–12 hours
- Amikacin sulfate (Amiglyde V Injectable 50 mg/mL), undiluted, 0.1 to 0.2 mL instilled q 12 hours
- Silver sulfadiazine (Silvadene) 0.1% solution (mix 1.5 mL [⅓ tsp]) of Silvadene Cream with 13.5 mL distilled water, or mix 0.1 g silver sulfadiazine powder with 100 mL distilled water), and instill 0.5 mL q 12 hours
- Ticarcillin equine intrauterine infusion (Ticillin), undiluted, 0.2 to 0.3 mL q 8 hours
- Ticarcillin powder for injection (vial should be reconstituted as directed, then frozen in syringes as 1-mL aliquots). New syringe should be thawed each day and kept refrigerated. A dose of 0.2 to 0.3 mL should be instilled into affected ears q 8 hours.

For End-Stage Ears

14. **For chronic proliferative otitis,** aggressive medical therapy is needed. Weekly ear cleaning should be instituted. For bacterial/yeast otitis externa and media, long-term (minimum, 4 weeks) systemic and topical antibiotics or antifungal medications should be administered and continued beyond complete clinical resolution of the infection. To reduce tissue proliferation, prednisone 0.5 mg/kg PO should be administered every 12 hours for 2 weeks; then followed by 0.5 mg/kg PO every 48 hours for 2 weeks. These ears rarely return to complete normalcy, so long-term maintenance therapy with steroid-containing otic preparations, as described for allergic otitis, is almost always necessary.

15. **For end-stage ears, indications for surgery** include the following:
    - Traction-avulsion or surgical resection of inflammatory polyps/masses

---

Author's Note

The most important components for successful long-term treatment of otitis are the following:

1. Identify and control the underlying, primary disease; infectious otitis is secondary, and recurrence can be prevented only if the primary disease is treated.
2. Use sufficient volumes of otic medications to completely coat and penetrate the ear canal; most patients need a minimum of 0.25 mL to provide enough medication.
3. Don't treat and stop; treat and stop, but rather use frequent (every 3–7 days) cleaning or treatment to prevent otitis recurrence.

It is extremely important to base treatment decisions on cytology (initial and recheck) and clinical impressions together.

The most consistently successful and least ototoxic treatment for Pseudomonas otitis is a high-concentration enrofloxacin solution mixed into a tris-ethylenediaminetetraacetic acid (EDTA) (making a 10-mg/mL final solution). If the infection is not improving, consider a deep otic lavage and evaluation of the otic bullae. Systemic antibiotics do NOT seem to improve treatment efficacy beyond the topical solution alone.

- Lateral ear canal resection, which aids in ventilation and drainage and allows for easier application of medication but rarely results in cure because a large amount of diseased tissue is still present
- Vertical ear canal ablation, if proliferative changes are present in the vertical canal but the horizontal canal is not affected. Total ear canal ablation and lateral bulla osteotomy is usually indicated to alleviate chronic pain and discomfort when end-stage otitis externa and otitis media are no longer responsive to medical management.

16. The prognosis is variable, depending on whether the underlying cause can be identified and corrected, and on the chronicity and severity of the otitis externa. Because Cocker spaniels are especially at risk for chronic and severe otitis externa, early and aggressive management of primary otitis externa and secondary inflammation is warranted in this breed.

Text continued on page 410.

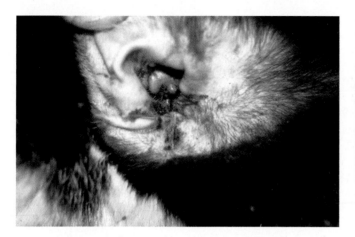

FIGURE 13-11 Otitis Externa. Brown, waxy exudate in a cat with otitis externa caused by a mixed bacterial and yeast infection.

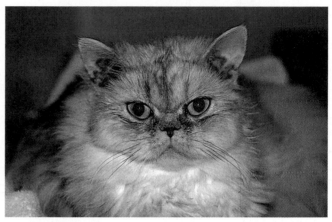

FIGURE 13-12 Otitis Externa. Bilateral otitis with brown, waxy exudate in a food-allergic cat.

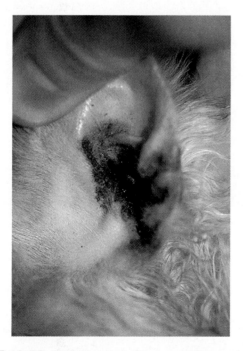

FIGURE 13-13 Otitis Externa. Close-up of the cat in Figure 13-12. The brown, waxy exudate was caused by a secondary yeast infection.

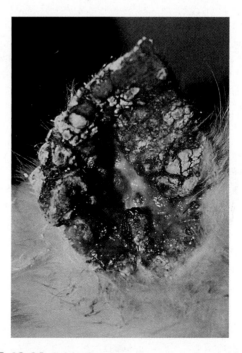

FIGURE 13-14 Otitis Externa. Severe erosive otitis with a crusting exudate and stenosis of the ear canal in a food-allergic cat. The gray adherent material is medicinal clay that the owner was using to pack the ears.

Otitis Externa—*cont'd*

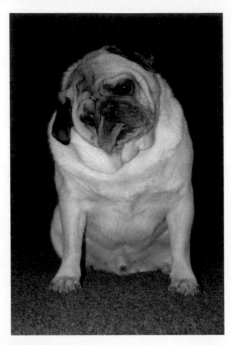

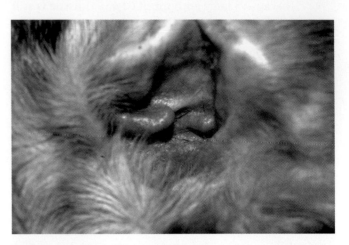

FIGURE 13-16 **Otitis Externa.** Erythema of the external ear canal and pinna in an allergic dog with noninfectious (sterile) allergic otitis.

FIGURE 13-15 **Otitis Externa.** Chronic otitis causing head tilt in a dog. Head tilts can be caused by the pain and discomfort of otitis externa or by vestibular symptoms associated with otitis media.

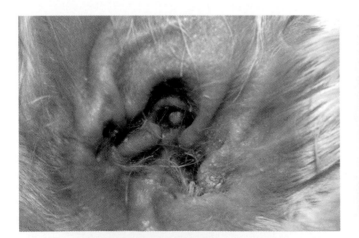

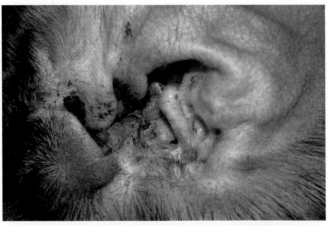

FIGURE 13-17 **Otitis Externa.** Erythema of the external ear canal and pinna with mild pale, waxy exudate caused by a secondary yeast infection associated with an underlying allergy.

FIGURE 13-18 **Otitis Externa.** Brown, waxy exudate with a secondary yeast infection associated with an underlying allergy.

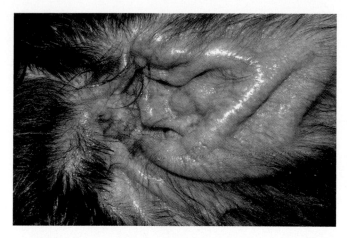

FIGURE 13-19 Otitis Externa. Erythema and lichenification of the ear canal and pinna in a dog with chronic allergic otitis. The lichenification is caused by chronic inflammation. Note the absence of apparent exudate and secondary infection (sterile allergic otitis).

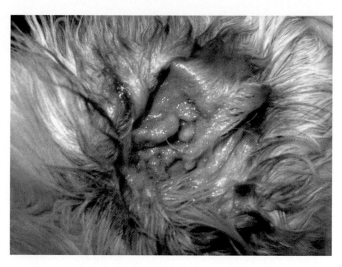

FIGURE 13-20 Otitis Externa. A purulent exudate in a dog with acute otitis. Note the absence of chronic inflammatory changes.

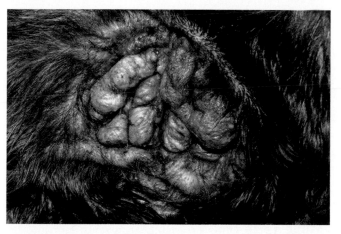

FIGURE 13-21 Otitis Externa. Severe swelling, lichenification, and stenosis in a dog with chronic recurrent otitis. The recurrent infections were secondary to underlying allergic dermatitis.

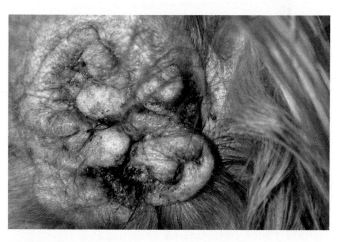

FIGURE 13-22 Otitis Externa. Severe swelling and lichenification causing complete stenosis of the ear canal in a dog with endocrine disease.

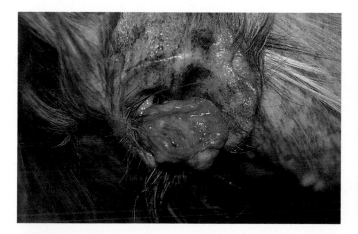

FIGURE 13-23 Otitis Externa. A ceruminous gland adenocarcinoma occluding the external ear canal.

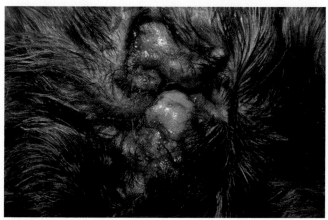

FIGURE 13-24 Otitis Externa. This ear tumor blocked the external ear canal and was a nidus for chronic, recurrent bacterial infection.

Otitis Externa—*cont'd*

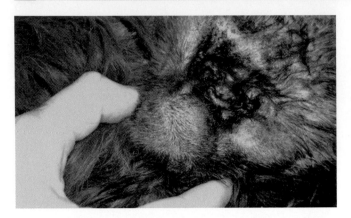

FIGURE 13-25 Otitis Externa. Calcification of the ear canal in a Cocker spaniel with chronic otitis. When palpated, the ear canal is firm and incompressible.

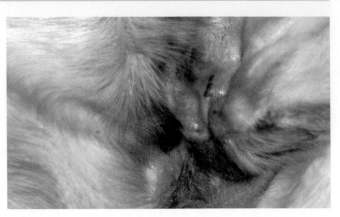

FIGURE 13-26 Otitis Externa. Erythema of the external ear canal and pinna in a Labrador that had previously undergone a lateral ear canal resection.

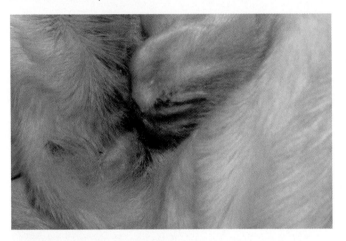

FIGURE 13-27 Otitis Externa. Same dog as in Figure 13-26. Despite the lateral ear canal resection, under normal circumstances (without traction), the ear canal would fold in on itself, thereby occluding the opening. This conformational abnormality caused recurrent infections.

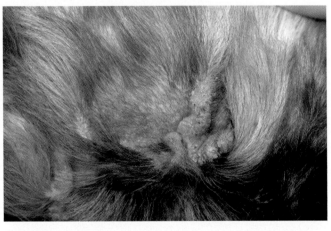

FIGURE 13-28 Otitis Externa. Erythematous dermatitis on the ear pinna of a dog that previously had a total ear canal resection. Persistent otitis (pinnal dermatitis) was caused by an underlying allergic disease that was never identified and controlled.

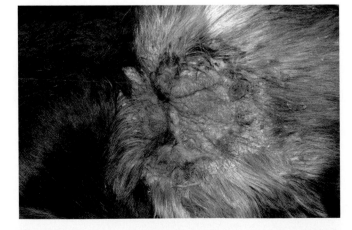

FIGURE 13-29 Otitis Externa. Severe otitis (pinnal dermatitis) with exudate in a dog that had a previous total ear canal resection. The underlying/primary disease was never identified and controlled, leading to recurrent otitis despite the surgery.

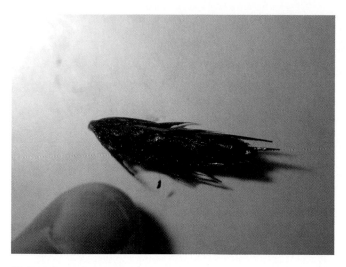

FIGURE 13-30 Otitis Externa. This grass awn was removed from the ear canal of a dog with chronic otitis. The otitis had persisted for several months before the foreign body was identified and removed.

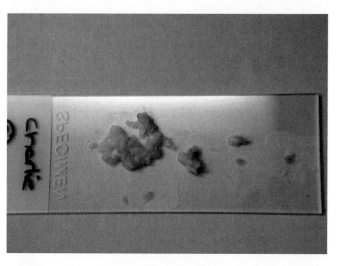

FIGURE 13-31 Otitis Externa. A large amount of inspissated pus and exudate that was flushed from the bulla of a dog with chronic otitis. This material, which remained in the bulla despite frequent ear cleaning, likely predisposed the animal to recurrent infection.

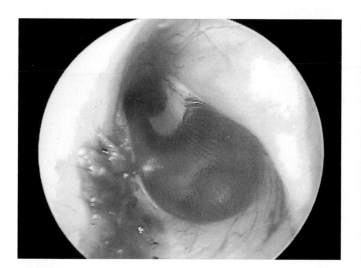

FIGURE 13-32 Otitis Externa. Otoscopic view of the normal eardrum. The tympanic membrane is translucent, and the hooked mallius is clearly visible. Minimal otic exudate is noted, with little inflammation.

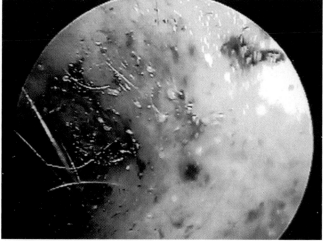

FIGURE 13-33 Otitis Externa. Dark black otic exudate within an inflamed external ear canal caused by *Otodectes*. The mites are visible as white specks along the ear canal.

Otitis Externa—*cont'd*

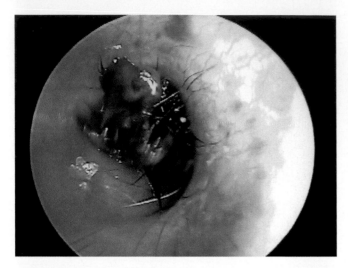

FIGURE 13-34 Otitis Externa. A wax plug sitting on top of the tympanic membrane within an inflamed ear canal. Note that the hairs in the deep canal can act as a nidus for recurrent infection.

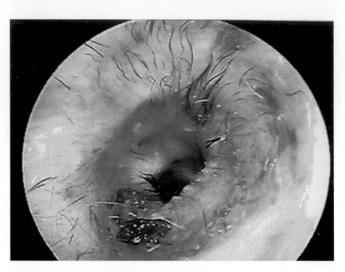

FIGURE 13-35 Otitis Externa. A moderately inflamed ear canal with purulent exudate. The tympanic membrane and mallius are barely visible but appear relatively normal.

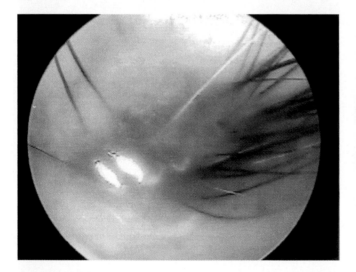

FIGURE 13-36 Otitis Externa. Visualization of the tympanic membrane was impossible because of pus filling the canal. Note the numerous hairs that can act as a nidus for recurrent infection.

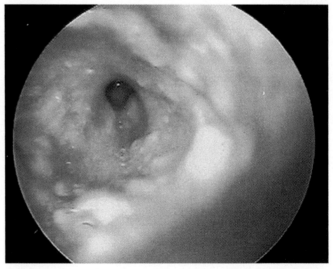

FIGURE 13-37 Otitis Externa. Severe otitis demonstrating a purulent exudate, glandular hypertrophy (cobblestone appearance of the canal wall), and stenosis of the deep canal. The tympanic membrane is covered with a purulent exudate.

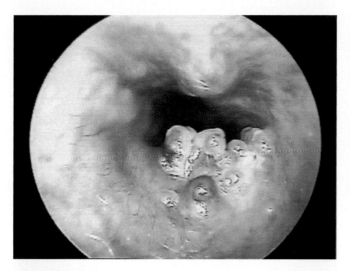

FIGURE 13-38 Otitis Externa. Numerous nodules in the external ear canal. Ceruminous gland hyperplasia/cysts may appear as bluish nodules. Without biopsy, it is impossible to rule out malignant tumors.

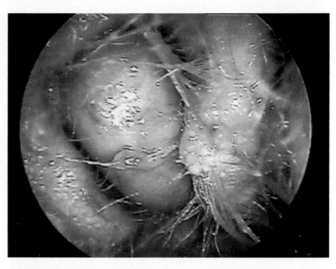

FIGURE 13-39 Otitis Externa. An otic tumor occluding the deep ear canal.

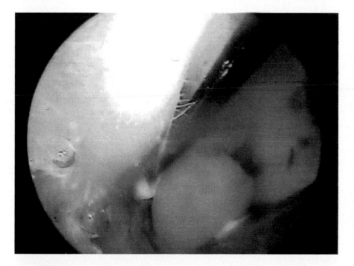

FIGURE 13-40 Otitis Externa. An otic polyp in a cat. Forceps can be seen extending into the deep canal in an attempt to grasp and remove the polyp.

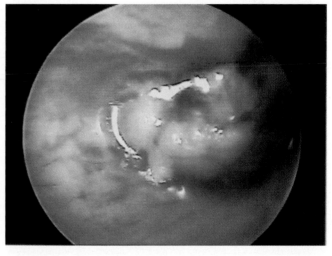

FIGURE 13-41 Otitis Externa. An otic tumor.

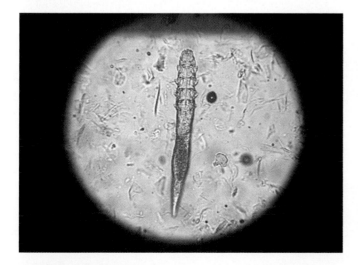

FIGURE 13-42 Otitis Externa. Microscopic image of a *Demodex* mite as seen with a 10× objective.

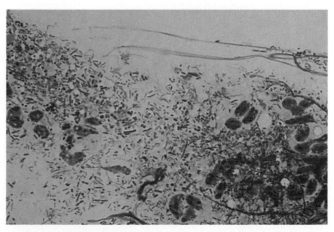

FIGURE 13-43 Otitis Externa. Microscopic image of a mixed bacterial infection from a dog with chronic, recurrent otitis as viewed with a 10× (oil) objective. Note the numerous species of bacteria that are present.

Otitis Externa—*cont'd*

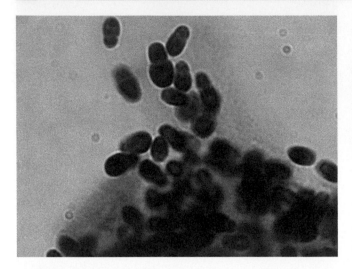

FIGURE 13-44 Otitis Externa. Microscopic image of *Malassezia* as viewed with a 100× (oil) objective.

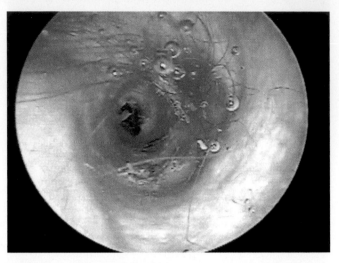

FIGURE 13-45 Otitis Externa. Inflammatory otitis externa with a ruptured tympanic membrane.

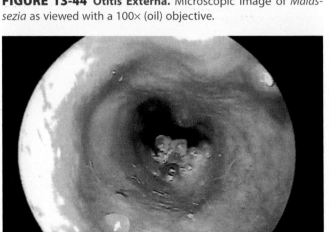

FIGURE 13-46 Otitis Externa. Numerous nodules in the external ear canal.

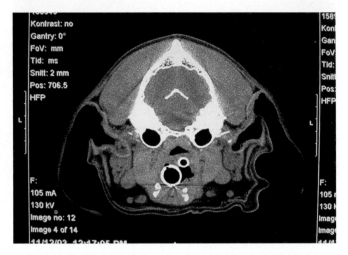

FIGURE 13-47 Otitis Externa. Computed tomographic image of a dog with chronic otitis. The bullae appear open, free of exudate, and without osteomyelitis. The left ear canal was occluded by a soft tissue mass. Radiology can help the clinician to identify calcification of the ear canal, tumors, and osteomyelitis of the bulla (which is a prognostic indicator).

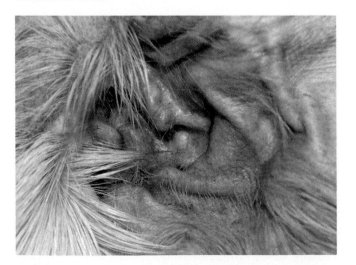

FIGURE 13-48 Otitis Externa. Generalized erythema affecting the external canal and pinna in an allergic dog without secondary infection; sterile allergic otitis.

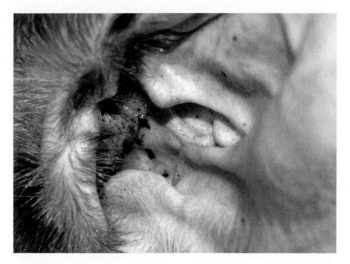

FIGURE 13-49 **Otitis Externa.** Sterile allergic otitis with mild otic exudate.

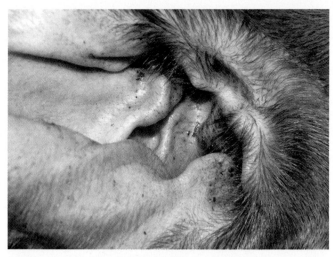

FIGURE 13-50 **Otitis Externa.** Sterile allergic otitis with mild waxy exudate without secondary infection.

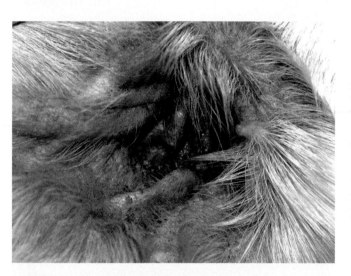

FIGURE 13-51 **Otitis Externa.** Severe erythema and waxy exudate in an allergic dog with a secondary mixed bacterial and yeast infection.

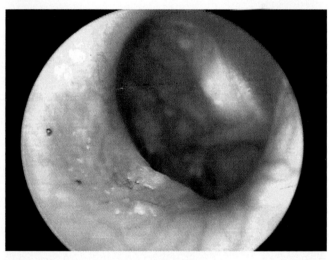

FIGURE 13-52 **Otitis Externa.** The shimmering tympanic membrane is being stretched over an expanding polyp in this cat. Note that the actual polyp is not recognizable.

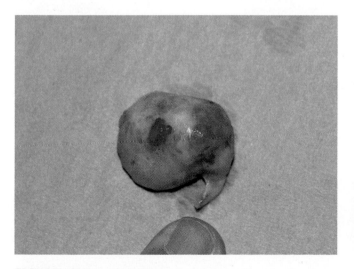

FIGURE 13-53 **Otitis Externa.** A feline otic polyp has been removed.

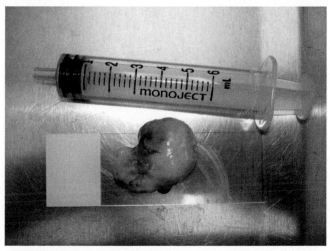

FIGURE 13-54 **Otitis Externa.** A feline otic polyp was removed and displayed.

Otitis Externa—*cont'd*

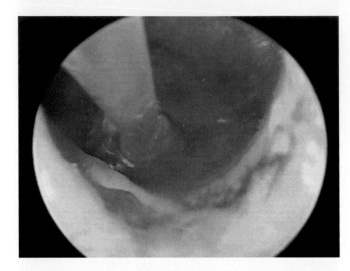

FIGURE 13-55 Otitis Externa. A myringotomy was performed with a Tom Cat catheter, and the bullae are being sampled and lavaged.

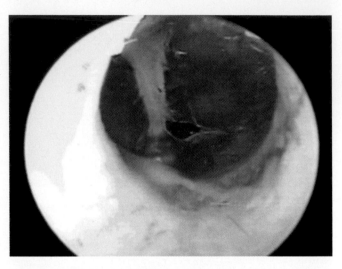

FIGURE 13-56 Otitis Externa. A myringotomy has been performed, and the opening is clearly visible just cranial to the mallius.

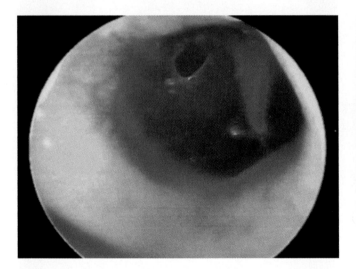

FIGURE 13-57 Otitis Externa. A myringotomy has been performed, and the opening is visible just caudal to the mallius.

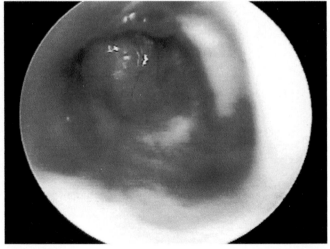

FIGURE 13-58 Otitis Externa. A tumor is visible almost completely obstructing the otic canal.

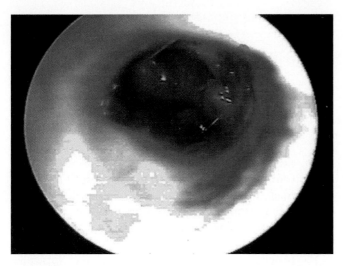

FIGURE 13-59 Otitis Externa. A tumor is visible at the end of the ear canal.

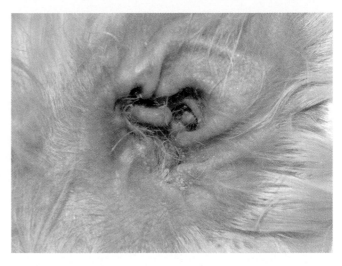

FIGURE 13-60 Otitis Externa. Erythema and a dry whitish otic exudate in an allergic dog with secondary yeast otitis.

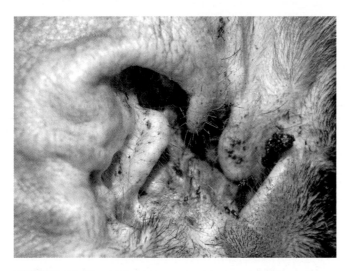

FIGURE 13-61 Otitis Externa. Moderate waxy otic exudate in a hypothyroid dog with a secondary bacterial otitis. Note that the exudate is of the character and quality that is usually associated with yeast, demonstrating the necessity of otic cytology.

Aural Hematoma

Features

This disease is caused by the traumatic rupture of vessels and capillaries within the ear pinnae. As the animal shakes its head severely, the centrifugal action and flopping of the pinnae cause the vessels to rupture. Blood then pools in the space between the skin and the cartilage, thereby creating a hematoma. The hematoma can be small, but persistent head shaking usually creates hematomas that extend the entire length of the ear pinnae. Hematomas are usually unilateral, but bilateral lesions may develop. Over time, the hematoma solidifies, becoming a firm mass. Concurrent otitis caused by ear mites, yeast, or bacteria is almost always present. This condition is uncommon in dogs and rare in cats.

Top Differentials

Differentials include neoplasia and cyst.

Diagnosis

1. Usually based on history and clinical signs.
2. Otoscopic examination of the ear canal identifying otitis externa.
3. Cytology of the ear canal reveals *Otodectes* mites, bacteria, or yeast.
4. Fine needle aspirate of the hematoma reveals blood.

Treatment and Prognosis

1. Otitis should be aggressively treated to decrease head shaking.
2. Oral prednisone 1 mg/kg administered every 12 to 24 hours for 5 days will help reduce the inflammation, intense pruritus, and discomfort that caused the head shaking.
3. Antibiotics should be administered to treat any secondary infection, until the ear has completely healed (see Table 2-1).
4. The hematoma should be drained as soon as possible. If the hematoma becomes organized, the surgical intervention is more difficult to perform, resulting in increased scar formation. Several techniques are commonly used to drain hematomas:
    - Surgical Technique: The ear pinna is incised over the length of the hematoma, and the contents are removed. The cavity is lavaged, and full-thickness sutures are placed at regular intervals (1 cm apart) to keep the tissue layers adhered. Some form of stent or suture-spacing device should be used to prevent sutures from becoming embedded in the skin, drain tubing, buttons, or pieces of x-ray film. Once the lesion has scarred, the sutures are removed (usually over several days to weeks). This technique is the most invasive and should be used for organized chronic hematomas that do not have a fluid center.
    - Cannula Technique: A small incision (0.5 mm) is made in the most dependent region of the hematoma. Blood is expressed and the cavity lavaged to remove any clots, and a bovine teat cannula is inserted into the incision and left unbandaged to provide drainage of the hematoma. Typically, drainage will diminish over several days. When the hematoma appears resolved and the tissue planes are adhered (several days to weeks), the teat cannula may be removed by gently wiggling it out of the incision. The remaining opening is left to heal.
    - Suction Drain Technique: Active suction drains can be inserted into the hematoma and bandaged onto the patient's head. These drains will maintain a constant negative pressure and will allow the tissue layers to adhere. One method involves modifying a butterfly catheter, removing the hub, and fenestrating the distal portion of the tubing. The tubing is then inserted into the hematoma through a small incision and is sutured into place. The butterfly needle is then bandaged onto the animal's head, and a Vacutainer tube is attached to the needle. The Vacutainer tube provides constant suction and allows the tissue layers to adhere. The Vacutainer tube should be replaced every 12 hours. When the exudate collected totals less than 2 mL/day, the apparatus can be removed (usually, 5–7 days).
    - Punch Biopsy Technique: A 6-mm punch biopsy is used to make one or several drainage holes that are left open to allow drainage while the tissue layers adhere. These biopsy holes are left to heal by second intention healing.
    - Laser Technique: A carbon dioxide (CO_2) laser is used to make several drainage holes over the hematoma. These open lesions provide drainage while the tissue layers adhere. The lesions created with the laser are allowed to heal through second intention. Simple removal of the blood through syringe aspiration results in immediate resolution, but the hematoma almost always recurs within several hours.
5. The prognosis is good, but recurrence is common, especially if the primary cause of the secondary otitis infection (allergies, endocrinopathies, polyps, neoplasia) is not controlled.

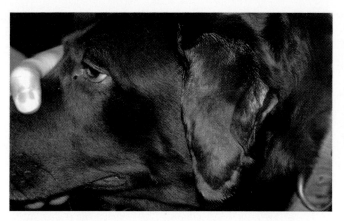

FIGURE 13-62 Aural Hematoma. An adult Labrador with a hematoma of the distal ear pinna. Swollen "ballooning" of the pinna is apparent.

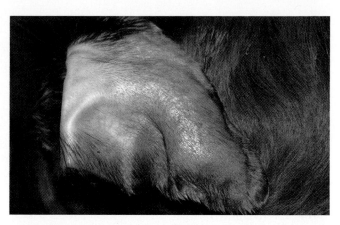

FIGURE 13-63 Aural Hematoma. Same dog as in Figure 13-62. The medial surface of the ear pinna clearly demonstrates ballooning caused by the accumulation of blood.

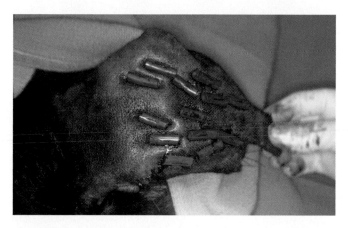

FIGURE 13-64 Aural Hematoma. The traditional suture technique used to treat aural hematomas is demonstrated. *(Courtesy D. J. Krahwinkel.)*

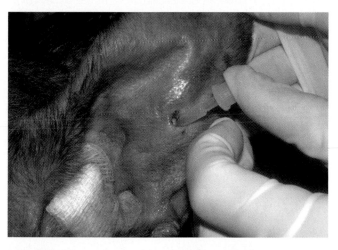

FIGURE 13-65 Aural Hematoma. A bovine teat cannula is being inserted into the dependent margin of the hematoma, which has been incised. Note that a gauze pad has been placed in the ear canal to prevent the introduction of blood and exudate.

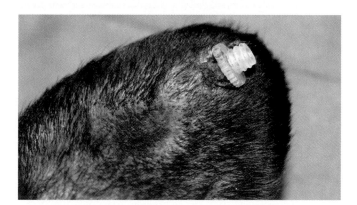

FIGURE 13-66 Aural Hematoma. A bovine teat cannula has been in place for approximately 7 days. Drainage has substantially decreased, and the tissue layers are adhered, which will prevent recurrence of the hematoma once the cannula has been removed.

Aural Hematoma—*cont'd*

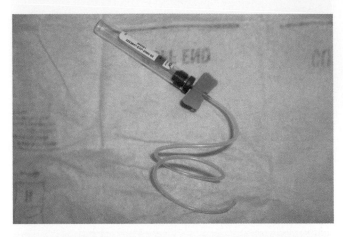

FIGURE 13-67 Aural Hematoma. A 22-gauge butterfly catheter has been modified by removing the syringe hub and cutting small openings in the tubing. This leaves the needle, which will be inserted into a Vacutainer tube to provide active suction.

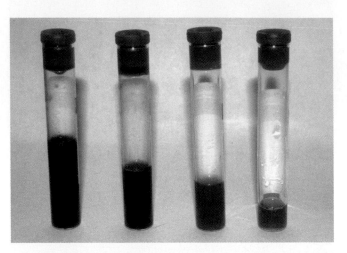

FIGURE 13-68 Aural Hematoma. Four Vacutainer tubes demonstrate a gradual decrease in collected drainage from the aural hematoma. Each Vacutainer tube was in place for 24 hours.

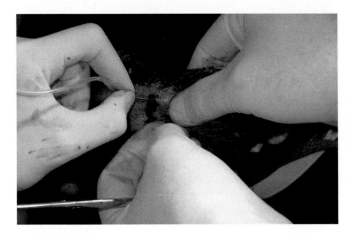

FIGURE 13-69 Aural Hematoma. An active drain has been placed with the use of a modified butterfly catheter and Vacutainer tubes. A small incision was made in the hematoma and the contents expressed before insertion of the tubing, which then was secured with suture.

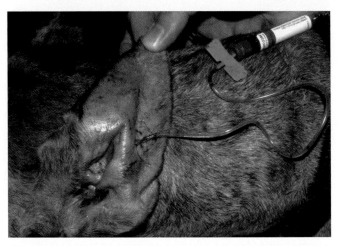

FIGURE 13-70 Aural Hematoma. The modified butterfly catheter has been inserted into the hematoma and sutured in place. The needle has been inserted into a Vacutainer tube.

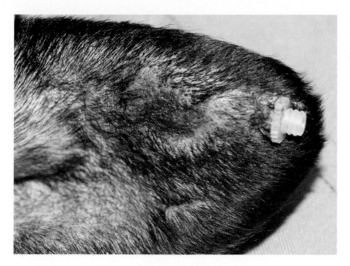

FIGURE 13-71 **Aural Hematoma.** A bovine teat cannula was placed into a small incision in the hematoma, providing several days of drainage while the tissues re-adhered.

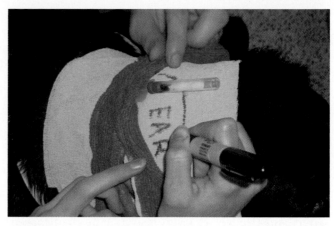

FIGURE 13-72 **Aural Hematoma.** The active suction device and the ear pinna are bandaged onto the top of the dog's head. Note that the bandage is clearly marked with the position of the ear pinna to prevent inadvertent trauma (cutting) during bandage removal.

Melanoma

Features

The tumor can be benign or malignant, but most melanomas involving the nail beds are malignant. In dogs, melanoma is the second most common digital neoplasm after squamous cell carcinoma. It is common in older dogs, with highest incidence noted in dogs with heavily pigmented skin, especially miniature Schnauzers, standard Schnauzers, and Scottish terriers. Irish setters and Golden retrievers also may be predisposed. It is rare in older cats.

Usually, melanoma appears as a solitary, well-circumscribed, dome-shaped, firm, brown to black, alopecic, pedunculated or wartlike growth ranging from 0.5 to 10 cm in diameter. Malignant melanomas can be pigmented or nonpigmented (amelanotic), may be ulcerated, and tend to be larger and more rapidly growing than benign melanomas. Secondary bacterial paronychia and deformed nails may also be present.

Top Differentials

Differentials include other neoplasms, bacterial claw infection/osteomyelitis, and fungal infection.

Diagnosis

1. Cytology: round, oval, stellate or spindle-shaped cells with a moderate amount of cytoplasm, containing granules of brown to green-black pigment. Malignant melanomas may have less pigment and show more pleomorphism, but malignancy cannot be reliably determined cytologically.
2. Dermatohistopathology: accumulation of neoplastic melanocytes, which may be spindle-shaped, epithelial, or round cell in appearance. Cells may be arranged in clusters, cords, or nervelike whorls and have variable degrees of pigmentation. Infiltration of pigment-laden macrophages is common. Benign neoplasms are circumscribed and have little nuclear variability and a low mitotic rate. Malignant melanomas may show more invasiveness, cellular pleomorphism, and mitotic figures (including atypical mitotic figures). Mitotic index is the most reliable way to predict biologic behavior; however, 10% of histologically benign melanomas behave in a malignant manner.
3. Radiography (affected digit): soft tissue swelling, bony proliferation, or bony lysis of P3 may be seen.
4. Affected animals should be screened for regional lymph node (aspirate/cytology, biopsy/histopathology) and internal metastasis (radiography, ultrasonography).

Treatment and Prognosis

1. The treatment of choice is radical surgical excision/P3 amputation because benign melanomas cannot be differentiated clinically from malignant ones.
2. Adjunct therapy with vaccine or chemotherapy may help prolong survival time in some dogs with malignant melanoma.
3. The prognosis is good for benign melanoma. The prognosis is poor for malignant melanoma because recurrence following surgery and metastasis are common.

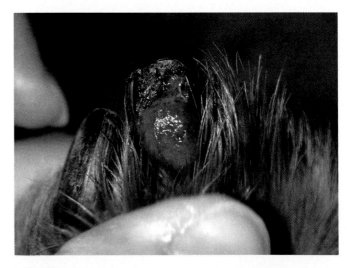

FIGURE 13-73 **Melanoma.** An amelanotic melanoma on the toe of a middle-aged rottweiler. *(Courtesy L. Frank.)*

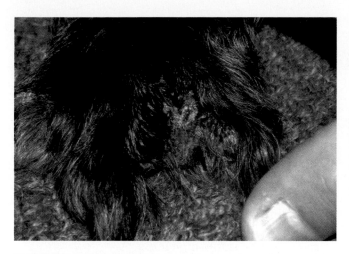

FIGURE 13-74 Melanoma. Recurrence of a malignant melanoma at the site of previous digital amputation. Malignant melanomas on the distal extremities are usually aggressive.

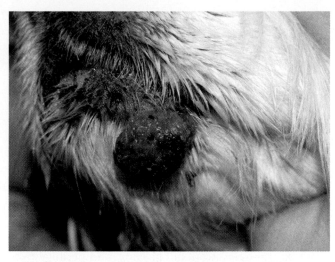

FIGURE 13-75 Melanoma. An amelanotic melanoma on the lip of an old Cocker spaniel. Note the similarity to more benign tumors that are more common in geriatric Cockers.

Anal Sac Disease

Features

Anal sac disease is a disease process that results in anal sac impaction, which may be followed by secondary infection (sacculitis) and abscess formation. Recurrent anal sac disease is often associated with underlying food hypersensitivity or atopy. It is common in dogs, with the highest incidence noted in small-breed dogs. It is rare in cats.

Scooting and perineal licking or biting are common symptoms of anal sac impaction and sacculitis. Tenesmus, painful defecation, tail chasing, and perineal pyotraumatic dermatitis may be seen. With abscessation, perianal erythema, swelling, an exudative draining tract (if abscess has ruptured), and fever may be present.

Top Differentials

Differentials include anal sac neoplasia, perianal fistulae, food allergy, and tapeworms.

Diagnosis

1. Digital palpation of distended, obstructed anal sacs.
2. Expression and examination of anal sac contents:
   ■ Normal anal sac: contains clear or pale yellow-brown fluid
   ■ Impacted anal sac: material is thick, brown, and pasty
   ■ Anal sacculitis: creamy yellow or thin yellow-green exudates
   ■ Anal sac abscess: usually contains a reddish-brown, purulent exudate

Treatment and Prognosis

1. Any underlying hypersensitivity should be identified and treated, especially food allergy.
2. For anal sac impaction, anal sacs should be expressed manually.
3. For anal sacculitis, anal sacs should be expressed manually and lavaged with 0.025% chlorhexidine or 0.4% povidone-iodine solution. Then, an antibiotic/glucocorticoid ointment (e.g., Panalog, Otomax) should be instilled into the anal sacs. Also, appropriate systemic, broad-spectrum antibiotics should be administered for 7 to 14 days.
4. For anal sac abscess, drainage should be established if the anal sac is not already ruptured. The anal sac should be cleansed and flushed with 0.25% chlorhexidine or 0.4% povidone-iodine solution, then an antibiotic/glucocorticoid ointment (e.g., Panalog, Otomax) instilled. Warm compresses applied to the affected area or hydrotherapy can be used every 12 to 24 hours to ensure drainage and promote healing. Topical antibiotic cream or ointment should be applied to the affected area every 12 hours, and appropriate systemic broad-spectrum antibiotics should be administered for 7 to 14 days.
5. For recurrent impactions, sacculitis, or abscesses, surgical excision of the affected anal sac is usually curative. However, temporary or permanent fecal incontinence is a possible postoperative complication, and draining fistulae will develop if the anal sacculectomy is incomplete.
6. The prognosis is variable. Routine manual anal sac expression may be useful in preventing recurrences.

Author's Note

- If patients have concurrent otitis, food allergy should be strongly considered as a possible underlying/primary cause of the anal sacculitis.
- Early and frequent expression of normal anal sacs may irritate the tissue and glands, increasing the need for even more frequent expression.

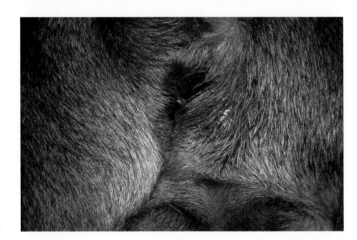

FIGURE 13-76 Anal Sac Disease. Alopecia and erythema over an inflamed, infected anal sac.

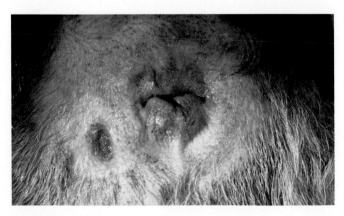

FIGURE 13-77 Anal Sac Disease. The infected anal sac abscess has ruptured, causing an ulcerative lesion.

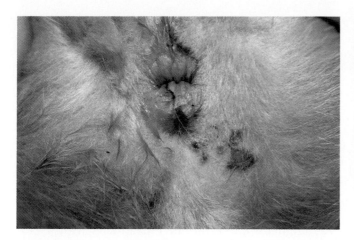

FIGURE 13-78 Anal Sac Disease. Alopecic, erosive dermatitis with crust formation in a cat with anal sacculitis.

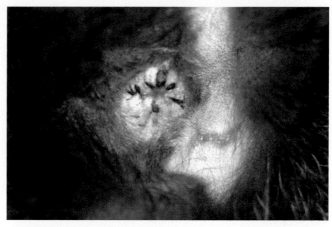

FIGURE 13-79 Anal Sac Disease. Alopecia and erythematous scar over a previously ruptured anal sac abscess in a cat.

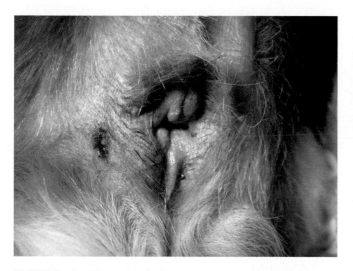

FIGURE 13-80 Anal Sac Disease. A ruptured anal sac abscess in a dog.

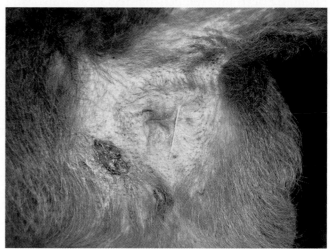

FIGURE 13-81 Anal Sac Disease. An alopecic, crusting lesion over the anal sac in a dog.

Perianal Fistulae (anal furunculosis)

Features

This is a chronic, progressive, often debilitating, inflammatory, ulcerative disease of perianal, anal, and perirectal tissues. The cause is unclear, but anatomic factors and a dysregulated immune response have been suspected. Food allergy is an incriminated but unproven cause. It is uncommon in dogs, with the highest incidence observed in middle-aged German shepherds.

Perianal lesions are usually painful and may be mild to severe, varying from small, pinpoint, draining sinuses, fistulous tracts, and erosions, to ulcerations, sometimes extending deep into the perianal region and involving the rectal tissue. Lesions usually are not associated with the anal sacs. On rectal palpation, the anus and rectum may be thickened and fibrotic. Associated symptoms may include frequent perianal licking, malodorous mucopurulent anorectal discharge, tenesmus, painful defecation, constipation, low tail carriage, increased frequency of defecation, pain on examination of the tail and perianal region, weight loss, and lethargy. Affected dogs may develop rectal strictures. Concurrent subclinical to clinical inflammatory bowel disease may be present.

Top Differentials

Differentials include neoplasia, ruptured anal sac abscess, and deep bacterial or fungal infection.

Diagnosis

1. Usually based on history, clinical findings, and ruling out other differentials.
2. Dermatohistopathology: inflammation with hidradenitis, epithelial necrosis at the follicular infundibulum, aggregates of eosinophils, and an intense inflammatory response, with plasma cells, lymphocytes, macrophages, and perivascular lymphoid nodules.
3. Histopathology (colon): mild to severe colitis may be present.

Treatment and Prognosis

1. Any underlying food hypersensitivity should be identified and treated.
2. Combining several treatments usually results in the most rapid and complete clinical resolution.
3. Topical hygiene (clipping of affected area, daily cleansing with 0.025% chlorhexidine rinses) should be provided.
4. Short-term (10–21 days) systemic antibiotics should be administered for secondary bacterial infection.
5. Topical nonalcohol steroid solutions applied q 12–24 hours may be beneficial.
6. Topical tacrolimus seems to be the most effective long-term therapy. It should be applied every 12 hours until lesions resolve, then tapered to every 24 to 72 hours to prevent relapse.
7. Long-term (3–5 months) treatment with cyclosporine (Atopica) is effective in many dogs; administer 5 mg/kg PO every 12 to 24 hours; this should be continued at least 4 weeks beyond complete resolution. Some dogs may require lifelong therapy with low-dose cyclosporine to maintain remission. The dosage and, therefore, the cost of cyclosporine may be reduced (30%–50%) if ketoconazole (5–10 mg/kg PO q 24 hours) is added to the treatment regimen (monitor liver function).
8. Long-term treatment with prednisone may be effective in some dogs. The clinician should administer 2 mg/kg PO every 24 hours for 2 weeks, followed by 1 mg/kg PO every 24 hours for 4 weeks, then 1 mg/kg PO every 48 hours for maintenance. The adverse effects of high dose, long-term steroid therapy may be severe.
9. Aggressive surgery to débride ulcers and remove fistulae may be effective in some dogs. Surgical procedures include excision, chemical cauterization, cryosurgery, deroofing and fulguration, and laser excision. However, multiple surgeries may be required, and postsurgical complications (e.g., recurrence of fistulae, anal stenosis, fecal incontinence) are common.
10. The prognosis is variable. To date, treatment with cyclosporine and surgical excision of residual lesions (if needed) seems to offer the best prognosis for cure. The recurrence rate is highest for dogs that have a long duration of disease before treatment is initiated.

Author's Note

- Most patients can be pushed into remission using systemic steroids with or without cyclosporine (Atopica) and then can be maintained on topical tacrolimus ointment alone without systemic therapy.
- Food allergy and neoplasia should be ruled out as underlying causes of the tissue destruction.

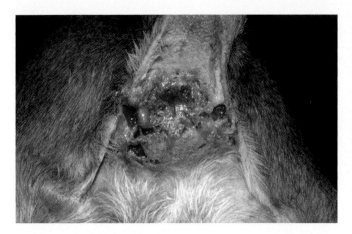

FIGURE 13-82 Perianal Fistulae. Multiple fistulae with severe destruction of the normal anal and perianal tissue. Note that the lesions are not limited to the anal sacs.

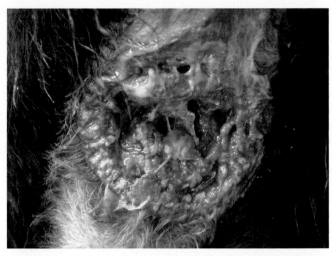

FIGURE 13-83 Perianal Fistulae. Severe ulcerative dermatitis of the entire perianal region with numerous deep fistulae. Note the purulent exudate.

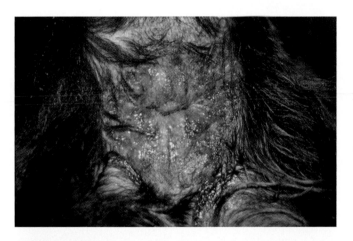

FIGURE 13-84 Perianal Fistulae. Numerous fistulae with a purulent exudate.

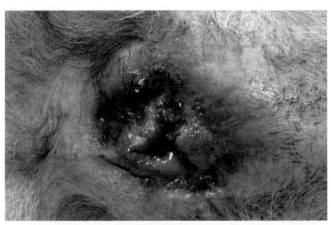

FIGURE 13-85 Perianal Fistulae. Deep fistula with swelling and inflammation. Note that the normal architecture of the anus is destroyed.

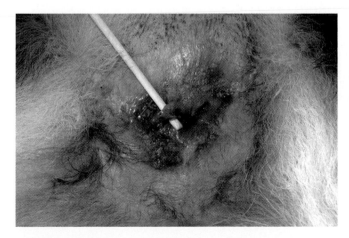

FIGURE 13-86 Perianal Fistulae. Numerous fistulae with redundant skin and tissue bridges.

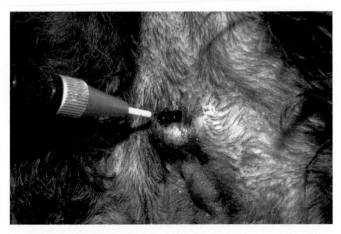

FIGURE 13-87 Perianal Fistulae. A laser was used to remove redundant tissue and to débride nonhealing fistulae. Treated tissue responds with a vigorous tissue-healing process.

Perianal Fistulae—cont'd

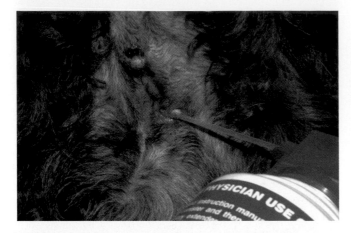

FIGURE 13-88 Perianal Fistulae. Canned cryosurgery solution was used to freeze a deep fistula. Treated tissue responds with a vigorous healing process.

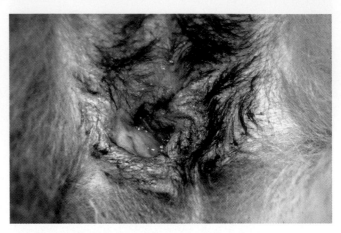

FIGURE 13-89 Perianal Fistulae. A deep perianal fistula.

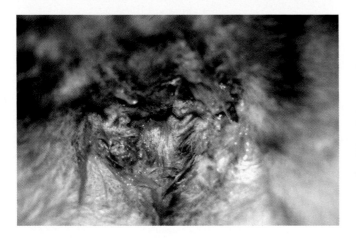

FIGURE 13-90 Perianal Fistulae. Perianal fistulae after immunosuppressive therapy has been instituted. Note the lack of active inflammation and the erythema.

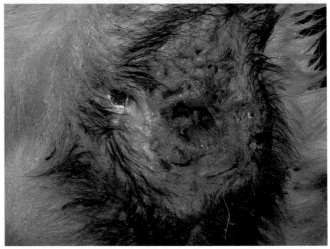

FIGURE 13-91 Perianal Fistulae. Multiple fistulae in a German shepherd. Note that the lesions are not limited to the anal sac areas.

Bacterial Claw Infection

Features

Bacterial claw infections are almost always secondary to an underlying cause. When one claw is affected, previous trauma should be suspected. When many claws are infected, underlying conditions to be ruled out include hypothyroidism, hyperadrenocorticism, allergies, autoimmune disorders, symmetrical lupoid onychodystrophy, and neoplasm.

Affected claws are often fractured and exudative, with associated paronychia, toe swelling, and pain. The nail may slough. Regional lymphadenomegaly may be seen. When multiple claws are involved, fever and depression may be noted. Osteomyelitis may develop as a sequela to chronic infection.

Top Differentials

Differentials include trauma, fungal infection, neoplasia, allergies, autoimmune skin disorders, symmetrical lupoid onychodystrophy, and neoplasm.

Diagnosis

1. Usually based on history, clinical findings, and ruling out other differentials.
2. Cytology (exudates from claw or claw fold): suppurative to (pyo)granulomatous inflammation with bacteria.
3. Bacterial culture (exudates from claw or claw fold, proximal portion of avulsed claw plate): *Staphylococcus* is usually isolated. Mixed bacterial infections are common.
4. Radiography (P3): evidence of osteomyelitis may be seen.

Treatment and Prognosis

1. The underlying cause should be identified and corrected.
2. Any loose claws or fractured portions of traumatized claws should be removed. In severe or refractory cases, the affected claw may need to be avulsed under general anesthesia.
3. Long-term (weeks to months) systemic antibiotics should be continued at least 2 weeks beyond complete clinical resolution. Antibiotic selection should be based on culture and sensitivity results. Pending these results, antibiotics that may be effective empirically include cephalosporins, clavulanated amoxicillin, and potentiated sulfonamides (see Table 2-1).
4. Topical foot scrubs with 2% to 4% chlorhexidine shampoo or foot soaks in 0.025% chlorhexidine solution every 8 to 12 hours for the first 7 to 10 days of antibiotic therapy may be helpful. Cleansing wipes (alcohol-free acne pads, chlorhexidine-containing pledgets, or other antimicrobial wipes) used every 12 to 72 hours work well.
5. In refractory cases with P3 osteomyelitis, P3 amputation may be necessary.
6. The prognosis for claw regrowth is good (unless P3 has been amputated).

Author's Note

- Fluoroquinolone antibiotics should be used only as a last resort because of possible increased risk for the development of methicillin-resistant Staph.
- Nails that regrow may never return to a completely normal condition; however, fragility and discomfort should resolve with treatment.

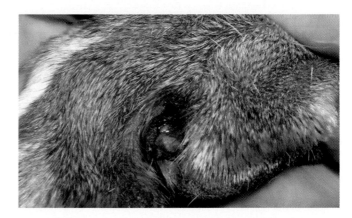

FIGURE 13-92 Bacterial Claw Infection. A dystrophic nail caused by a chronic bacterial infection.

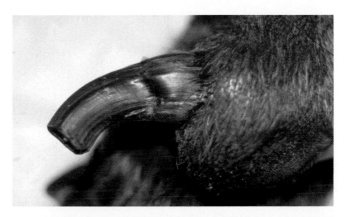

FIGURE 13-93 Bacterial Claw Infection. The base of this nail was split on the midline, and a purulent exudate was exuding from the fractured claw. A mixed bacterial population was cultured from the exudate.

Bacterial Claw Infection—*cont'd*

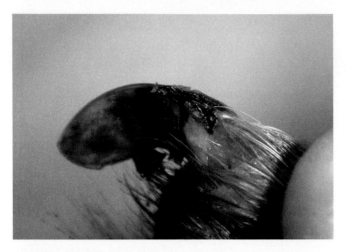

FIGURE 13-94 Bacterial Claw Infection. A fractured nail, demonstrating numerous cracks and fissures. The exudate contained numerous bacterial organisms.

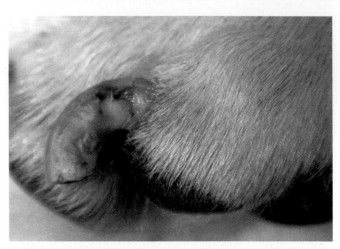

FIGURE 13-95 Bacterial Claw Infection. A fractured nail caused by trauma, with a secondary bacterial infection.

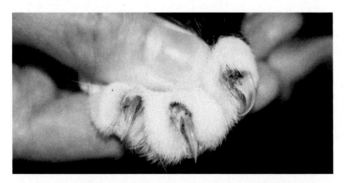

FIGURE 13-96 Bacterial Claw Infection. Paronychia (inflammation of the nail bed) caused by a bacterial infection in this cat. Note the similarity to *Pemphigus foliaceus*.

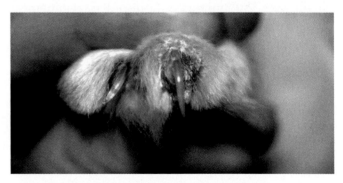

FIGURE 13-97 Bacterial Claw Infection. Paronychia and secondary bacterial infection in a cat with allergic dermatitis. Note the similarity to pemphigus in cats.

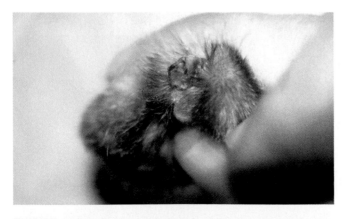

FIGURE 13-98 Bacterial Claw Infection. A stubby dystrophic nail caused by a chronic bacterial infection.

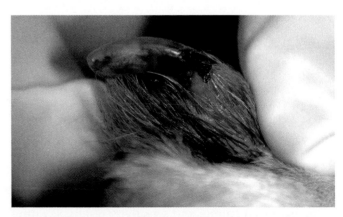

FIGURE 13-99 Bacterial Claw Infection. A fractured nail with a secondary infection.

Fungal Claw Infection (onychomycosis)

Features

Fungal claw infections are usually caused by dermatophytes, although isolated cases of nail infection from other fungi have been reported. Typically, only one or two claws are affected. These infections are rare in dogs and cats. Secondary yeast paronychia is common in allergic dogs.

Affected claws are often friable and misshapen. Associated paronychia is common. Generalized skin disease may be seen, especially if multiple claws are involved.

Top Differentials

Differentials include symmetrical lupoid onychodystrophy, trauma, bacterial infection, neoplasia, autoimmune skin disorders, and underlying allergies.

Diagnosis

1. Rule out other differentials.
2. Fungal culture (proximal claw shavings): *Trichophyton* spp. are most commonly isolated, but infection with *Microsporum* spp. and, more rarely, nondermatophytic fungi can occur (*Malassezia* spp.).

Treatment and Prognosis

1. Any loose or sloughing nails should be removed.
2. For true nail infections (soft, dystrophic nails), long-term (6 months or longer) systemic antifungal therapy should be administered at least 1 to 3 months beyond complete nail regrowth. Frequent nail trims should be performed to remove infected portions. Trimmings should be submitted for follow-up fungal cultures, and treatment continued until culture results are negative.
3. Antifungal drugs that may be effective include the following:
   - Ketoconazole 5–10 mg/kg PO q24 hours with food
   - Fluconazole 5–10 mg/kg PO q 24 hours with food
   - Terbinafine 15–30 mg/kg PO q 24 hours with food
   - Itraconazole 5–10 mg/kg PO q 24 hours with food
   - Historically, microsize griseofulvin 50–75 mg/kg PO q 12 hours with high-fat meal
4. Concurrent topical therapies that may be helpful include the following:
   - Clotrimazole-containing treatments applied q 12 hours
   - 0.2% enilconazole solution as a 5- to 10-minute foot soak q 24 hours
   - 0.025% chlorhexidine solution as a 5- to 10-minute foot soak q 12 hours
   - Thiabendazole-containing treatments, 1 drop on each claw q 8 hours (not as effective as other choices)
   - 0.4% povidone-iodine solution as a 5- to 10-minute foot soak q 6 hours (not as effective as other choices)
5. The prognosis is guarded to fair. Many dogs have incomplete resolution in spite of aggressive antifungal therapy. In these cases, P3 amputation or long-term, low-dose therapy with ketoconazole or itraconazole may be needed.

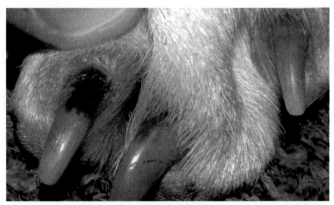

FIGURE 13-100 Fungal Claw Infection. Brown discoloration at the base of the nails was caused by a secondary *Malassezia* infection associated with allergic dermatitis. The brown exudate is tightly adhered to the claw and can be confused with normal pigmentation.

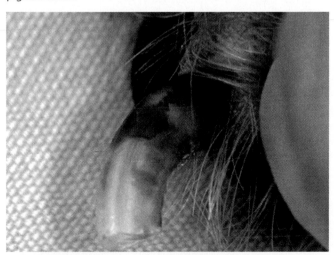

FIGURE 13-101 Fungal Claw Infection. Brown discoloration at the base of the claw is caused by a secondary *Malassezia* infection. This brown discoloration differs from normal pigmentation in that it does not extend the entire length of the nail.

Fungal Claw Infection—*cont'd*

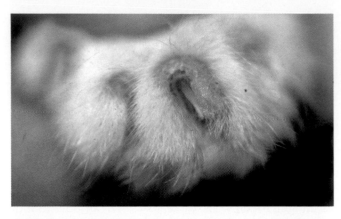

FIGURE 13-102 Fungal Claw Infection. Alopecia and erythema on the nail bed caused by a *Microsporum canis* infection.

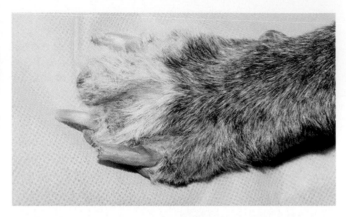

FIGURE 13-103 Fungal Claw Infection. Diffuse alopecia, erythema, and crusting on the foot caused by a *Trichophyton mentagrophytes* infection. Onychomycosis caused dystrophic nails that sloughed. *(Courtesy A. Yu.)*

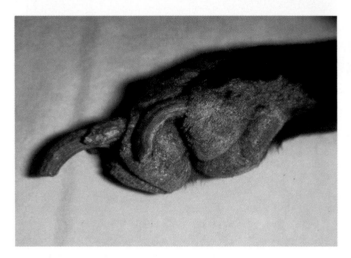

FIGURE 13-104 Fungal Claw Infection. Onychomycosis caused by a *Trichophyton mentagrophytes* infection. The nails are dystrophic, and there is an alopecic dermatitis. *(Courtesy D. Angarano.)*

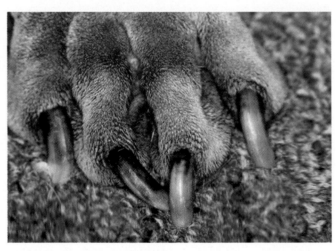

FIGURE 13-105 Fungal Claw Infection. Brown discoloration at the base of the nails was caused by a secondary *Malassezia* infection associated with allergic dermatitis.

Symmetrical Lupoid Onychodystrophy (idiopathic onychomadesis)

Features

This condition, which is suspected to be immune mediated, causes claw loss (onychomadesis). It is uncommon to rare in dogs, with the highest incidence reported in young adult to middle-aged dogs. German shepherds and rottweilers may be predisposed, but many breeds are affected.

Usually, an acute onset of nail loss occurs. Initially, one to two claws are lost, but over the course of a few weeks to several months, all claws slough. Replacement claws are misshapen, soft or brittle, discolored, and friable and usually slough again. Affected feet are often painful and pruritic. Paronychia is uncommon unless a secondary bacterial infection is present. Affected dogs have no other skin involvement and are otherwise healthy.

Top Differentials

Differentials include fungal and bacterial claw infection, autoimmune skin disorders, drug eruption, and vasculitis.

Diagnosis

1. Rule out other differentials.
2. Clinical symptoms and typical history.
3. Dermatohistopathology (P3 amputation) not recommended unless necessary to rule out neoplasia: basal cell hydropic degeneration, degeneration or apoptosis of individual keratinocytes in the basal cell layer, pigmentary incontinence, and a lichenoid interface dermatitis.

Treatment and Prognosis

1. Appropriate systemic antibiotics should be administered for at least 6 weeks, if secondary bacterial paronychia is present.
2. New nails should be trimmed frequently (approximately every 2 weeks) to prevent cracks.
3. Treatment with daily oral fatty acid supplementation administered 180 mg EPA/10 lb is often effective. Noticeable nail regrowth should be seen within 3 months of initiation of therapy.
4. If no improvement is seen with fatty acid supplementation, therapy with vitamin E 200 to 400 IU PO every 12 hours may be effective. Nail regrowth should be seen within 3 months of initiation of therapy.
5. Combined tetracycline and niacinamide therapy may also be effective. The clinician should give 250 mg of each drug (dogs <10 kg) or 500 mg of each drug (dogs >10 kg) PO every 8 hours until noticeable nail regrowth has occurred (approximately 3–6 months). Then, each drug should be administered every 12 hours for 2 months, followed by long-term maintenance therapy, with each drug administered every 24 hours. Alternatively, administering doxycycline 5–10 mg/kg (instead of tetracycline) every 12 to 24 hours may be effective.
6. Another treatment option is pentoxifylline 10–25 mg/kg PO administered every 8 to 12 hours.
7. Cyclosporine (Atopica) has demonstrated some benefit when administered at 10 mg/kg daily for 2 to 3 months, then tapered to the lowest possible dose that prevents relapse of the disease.
8. For severely painful cases refractory to medical management, therapeutic declawing may alleviate the discomfort.
9. In severe refractory cases, treatment as for autoimmune skin disease may be necessary; however, the adverse effects may make therapeutic declawing a better treatment option for long-term control without significant metabolic effects.
10. The prognosis for nail regrowth is good, although some nails may remain deformed or friable. In some dogs, therapy can be successfully discontinued after 6 months. In others, long-term maintenance therapy is necessary to maintain remission. In cases refractory to medical therapy, P3 amputation can be considered.

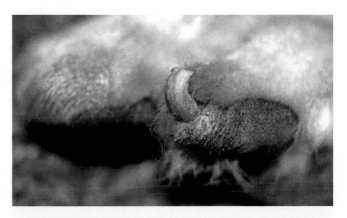

FIGURE 13-106 Symmetrical Lupoid Onychodystrophy. A dystrophic nail that is growing in the wrong direction. All nails were sloughed and replaced with deformed abnormal claws.

Symmetrical Lupoid Onychodystrophy—*cont'd*

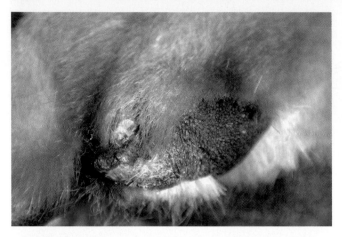

FIGURE 13-107 Symmetrical Lupoid Onychodystrophy. A dystrophic nail that is stubby and malformed. Abnormal nails are predisposed to fracture and traumatic avulsion.

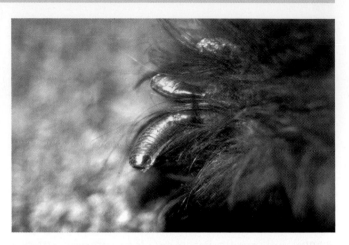

FIGURE 13-108 Symmetrical Lupoid Onychodystrophy. Numerous dystrophic nails growing in abnormal directions.

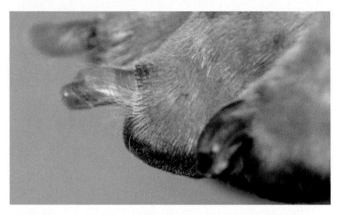

FIGURE 13-109 Symmetrical Lupoid Onychodystrophy. Multiple dystrophic nails on multiple feet are characteristic of this disorder. The skin was normal, except for iatrogenic changes associated with clipping.

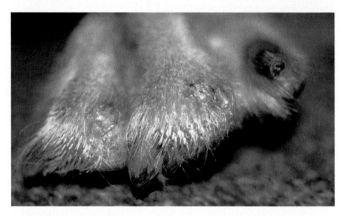

FIGURE 13-110 Symmetrical Lupoid Onychodystrophy. Multiple dystrophic nails.

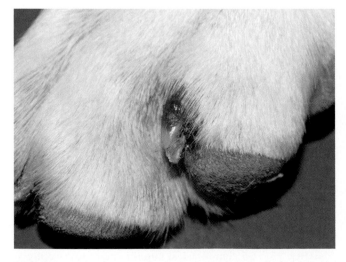

FIGURE 13-111 Symmetrical Lupoid Onychodystrophy. The nail is clearly severely affected while the surrounding nail bed lacks evidence of dermatitis.

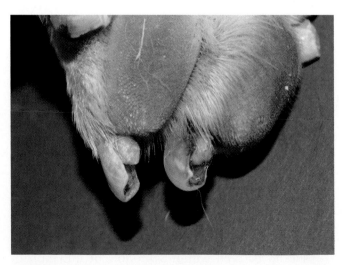

FIGURE 13-112 Symmetrical Lupoid Onychodystrophy. The keratin structure of the nail has separated from the underlying vascular tissue on multiple toes. These nails will eventually slough.

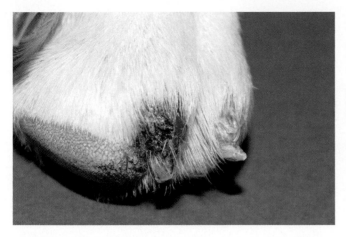

FIGURE 13-113 Symmetrical Lupoid Onychodystrophy. The nails have sloughed, leaving a painfully exposed vascular tissue. The nails will re-form but likely will never be completely normal.

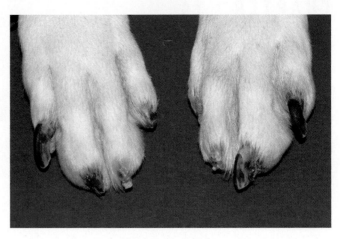

FIGURE 13-114 Symmetrical Lupoid Onychodystrophy. Lack of concurrent dermatitis with multiple nails sloughing is characteristic for this disease.

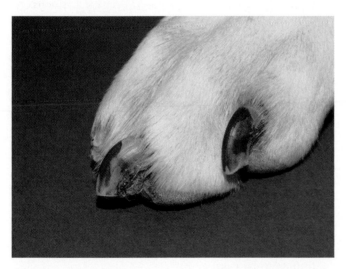

FIGURE 13-115 Symmetrical Lupoid Onychodystrophy. Multiple toes are affected without concurrent dermatitis.

CHAPTER 14

Neoplastic and Nonneoplastic Tumors

AMY LEBLANC*

- Intracutaneous Cornifying Epithelioma (keratoacanthoma, infundibular keratinizing acanthoma)
- Feline Solar Dermatosis
- Canine Solar Dermatosis
- Squamous Cell Carcinoma
- Bowen's Disease/Multifocal Squamous Cell Carcinoma In Situ
- Basal Cell Tumor/Carcinoma
- Hair Follicle Tumors
- Sebaceous Gland Tumors
- Perianal Gland Tumors
- Apocrine (epitrichial) Sweat Gland Cysts and Tumors
- Fibropruritic Nodule
- Fibroma
- Fibrosarcoma
- Nodular Dermatofibrosis
- Hemangioma
- Hemangiosarcoma
- Hemangiopericytoma
- Lipoma
- Liposarcoma
- Mast Cell Tumor
- Nonepitheliotropic Lymphoma (lymphosarcoma)
- Epitheliotropic Lymphoma (mycosis fungoides)
- Cutaneous Plasmacytoma
- Cutaneous Histiocytoma
- Cutaneous Histiocytosis
- Systemic Histiocytosis
- Malignant Histiocytosis
- Cutaneous Melanocytoma/Melanoma
- Transmissible Venereal Tumor (TVT)
- Collagenous Nevus
- Follicular Cyst–Epidermal Inclusion Cyst (infundibular cyst)
- Cutaneous Horns
- Skin Tags (fibrovascular papilloma)
- Calcinosis Circumscripta

Intracutaneous Cornifying Epithelioma (keratoacanthoma, infundibular keratinizing acanthoma)

Features

This is a benign neoplasm of hair follicle origin. It is uncommon in dogs. Solitary nodules can occur in any age or breed of dog; multicentric nodules occur most commonly in young male Norwegian elkhounds and Keeshonds.

This condition appears as single to multiple (as many as 40–50) firm to fluctuant, well-circumscribed, dermal or subcutaneous nodules ranging from 0.5 to 4 cm in diameter. Nodules may be partially alopecic, and most have a variably sized, dilated, central pore that opens directly to the skin surface; from this pore, gray-brown keratinaceous material can be expressed. Large pores may contain a hard, hornlike, keratin plug. Tumors deeply located in the dermis and subcutis may

*This chapter was originally written by K. S. Coyner.

not have pores. Lesions may appear anywhere on the body but are most commonly found on the dorsal neck, back, and tail.

Diagnosis

1. Cytology (usually nondiagnostic): amorphous cellular debris and mature cornified squamous epithelial cells with cholesterol crystals.
2. Dermatohistopathology: lamellated keratin-filled cavity (which may contain a pore to the skin surface) lined with stratified epithelial cells. Focal rupture may release keratin into the dermis, inciting a pyogranulomatous reaction in surrounding tissue.

Treatment and Prognosis

1. Surgical or laser excision is curative if lesions are solitary to few in number. Cryotherapy may also be effective.
2. For multiple lesions, treatment with acitretin 0.5–2 mg/kg/day or isotretinoin 1–3 mg/kg/day PO may be effective in some dogs. A good response should be seen after 3 months of treatment. Those that respond usually require lifelong therapy to maintain remission. Vitamin A (8000–10,000 IU/10 kg/day) may be a less potent alternative.
3. After surgical removal, the prognosis for cure is good for dogs with a solitary lesion, but dogs with more than one tumor are likely to develop new tumors at other sites. The prognosis for resolving multiple lesions is fair to good with medical treatment. These tumors are benign and do not metastasize.

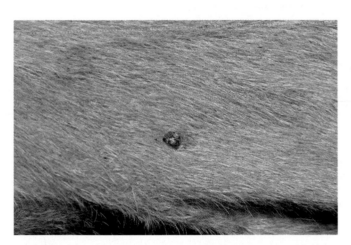

FIGURE 14-1 **Intracutaneous Cornifying Epithelioma.** A small keratin nodule associated with underlying tumor. The keratin nodule can easily be mistaken for a crust.

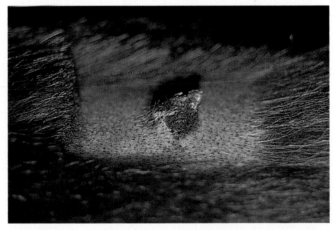

FIGURE 14-2 **Intracutaneous Cornifying Epithelioma.** An intracutaneous cornifying epithelioma and cutaneous horn on the lateral thorax of a young adult German shepherd.

Feline Solar Dermatosis

Features

This type of dermatosis is caused by actinic damage to white-haired skin. Initially, the skin becomes sunburned, but with repeated exposure to ultraviolet light, preneoplastic lesions (actinic keratoses, squamous cell carcinoma in situ) and squamous cell carcinoma may develop. The condition is common in older outdoor cats and indoor cats that like to sunbathe.

Initially, mild erythema, scaling, and alopecia of the white-haired skin may be observed. With continued exposure to sunlight, the skin becomes progressively erythematous and alopecic, crusted, ulcerated, and painful. The ear tips/margins are most commonly affected, but lesions may also occur on white-haired eyelids, nose/nasal planum, or lips.

Top Differentials

Differentials include dermatophytosis, trauma, autoimmune skin disease, vasculitis, hypersensitivity (flea, food, atopy), and squamous cell carcinoma.

Diagnosis

1. Usually based on signalment, history, and clinical findings.
2. Dermatohistopathology: in early lesions, epidermal hyperplasia and superficial perivascular dermatitis may be observed. Vacuolated epidermal cells, dyskeratotic keratinocytes, and basophilic degeneration

of elastin (solar elastosis) may be seen. In advanced lesions, the epidermis may be dysplastic, without invasion through the basement membrane (actinic keratosis), or the dermis may be invaded by nests of dysplastic epidermal cells (squamous cell carcinoma).

Treatment and Prognosis

1. Affected cats should be kept indoors and prevented from sunbathing between 9 AM and 4 PM.
2. If some sun exposure is unavoidable, a waterproof sunscreen (titanium dioxide) with a sun protection factor (SPF) of at least 30 can be applied twice daily to protect ears, but this is not recommended for use around the eyes, nose, or mouth in cats.
3. Treatment with β-carotene 30 mg/cat PO every 12 hours may be effective in resolving preneoplastic lesions. It is not effective if squamous cell carcinoma has developed.
4. Treatment with the synthetic retinoid, acitretin (5–10 mg/cat PO q 24 hours), may be effective in the treatment of nonneoplastic actinic lesions in some cats (monitor liver function). Vitamin A may be used as a less potent alternative.
5. Surgical excision, laser ablation, therapy for carcinoma in situ (see therapy for squamous cell carcinoma), or cryotherapy may be curative.
6. The prognosis is good if further sunlight exposure can be avoided before invasive squamous cell carcinomas develop.

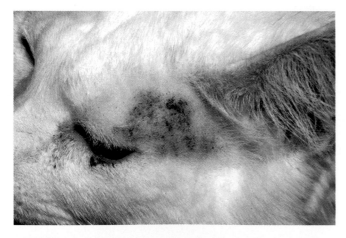

FIGURE 14-3 Feline Solar Dermatosis. Multifocal erythematous papular lesions on the preauricular region of the white cat are typical of actinic dermatitis. Note that the crusting obscures the actual dermatitis.

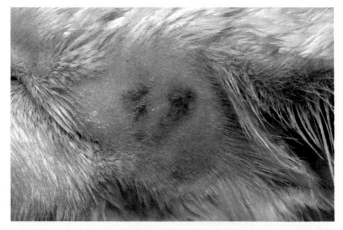

FIGURE 14-4 Feline Solar Dermatosis. Same cat as in Figure 14-3. The crusts have been removed, revealing the erythematous papular lesions.

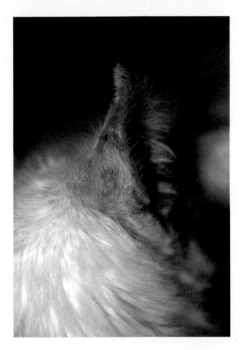

FIGURE 14-5 Feline Solar Dermatosis. Alopecia, erythema, erosions, and crusting on the ear pinna. As the disease progresses, papules will develop, with erosion and ulceration that suggest progression to squamous cell carcinoma.

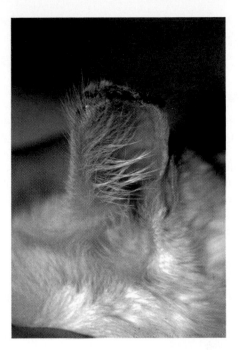

FIGURE 14-6 Feline Solar Dermatosis. The lesion on the distal ear margin of this cat has progressed to squamous cell carcinoma, destroying the normal ear architecture.

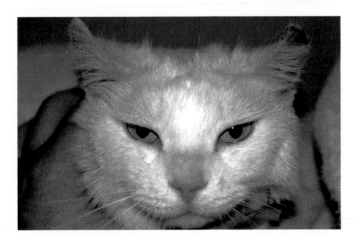

FIGURE 14-7 Feline Solar Dermatosis. Erythema and crust formation on the ear pinna of an aged cat.

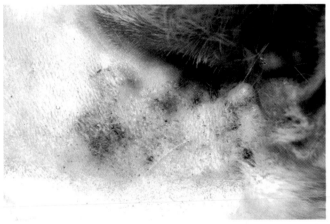

FIGURE 14-8 Feline Solar Dermatosis. Multiple erythematous papular lesions on the preauricular area of a white cat. Note that the focal area of erosion may have progressed to squamous cell carcinoma.

Canine Solar Dermatosis

Features

Canine solar dermatosis is caused by actinic damage to lightly pigmented or nonpigmented, sparsely haired skin on the nose or trunk. With repeated exposure to ultraviolet light, preneoplastic lesions (actinic keratoses, squamous cell carcinoma in situ) may develop. Nasal solar dermatosis is uncommon in dogs, with the greatest incidence in outdoor dogs. Truncal solar dermatosis is also uncommon in dogs, with the highest incidence noted in outdoor dogs that are avid sunbathers or are kept in unshaded areas. Predisposed breeds for truncal solar dermatosis include White Boxers and Bull terriers, American Staffordshire terriers, Beagles, Dalmatians, and German shorthaired pointers.

Nasal Lesions

Initially, the nose and adjacent nonpigmented, sparsely haired skin become erythematous and scaly (sunburned). Continued exposure to sunlight leads to alopecia, crusting, erosions, ulceration, and scarring.

Truncal Lesions

Initially, affected skin becomes erythematous and scaly (sunburned). With continued sun exposure, erythematous macules, papules, plaques, and nodules develop. These lesions may be crusted, eroded, and ulcerated. Palpable irregular thickenings of what appears to be visually normal skin may be detected. The ventral and lateral aspects of the abdomen and inner thighs are most frequently affected, but lesions may also develop on the flanks, tail tip, or distal extremities. Secondary pyoderma is common.

Top Differentials

Nasal Lesions

Differentials include nasal pyoderma, demodicosis, dermatophytosis, discoid lupus erythematosus, pemphigus erythematosus, and neoplasia (most common is squamous cell carcinoma).

Truncal Lesions

Differentials include demodicosis, dermatophytosis, pyoderma, drug reaction, and neoplasia.

Diagnosis

1. Usually based on history of prolonged sun exposure, clinical findings, and ruling out other differentials.
2. Dermatohistopathology: in early lesions, epidermal hyperplasia and superficial perivascular dermatitis are seen. Vacuolated epidermal cells, dyskeratotic keratinocytes, and basophilic degeneration of elastin (solar elastosis) may be noted. In advanced lesions, the epidermis may be hyperplastic and dysplastic, with no invasion through the basement membrane (actinic keratosis, carcinoma in situ).

Treatment and Prognosis

1. Further exposure to sunlight, especially between 9 AM and 4 PM, should be prevented.
2. If some sun exposure is unavoidable, sun block (zinc oxide) or sunscreen (titanium dioxide) should be applied to susceptible areas twice daily. For sunscreens, waterproof products with a sun protection factor (SPF) of at least 30 should be used.
3. If lesions are secondarily infected, appropriate systemic antibiotics should be administered for 2 to 3 weeks.
4. Treatment with vitamin A (8000–10,000 IU q 24 hours) or acitretin (0.5–1 mg/kg PO q 24 hours) may be effective in resolving lesions in some dogs with truncal solar dermatosis.
5. The prognosis is variable, depending on lesion chronicity. With sun avoidance, early cases of nasal solar dermatosis usually heal completely. However, chronic, ulcerative nasal lesions often heal by scarring, and with continued sun exposure, squamous cell carcinoma may develop. In early cases of truncal solar dermatosis, the prognosis is good if further exposure to sunlight is avoided. With continued exposure to sunlight, the likelihood of developing squamous cell carcinoma is high. Sun-damaged truncal skin is also predisposed to the development of hemangioma or hemangiosarcoma.

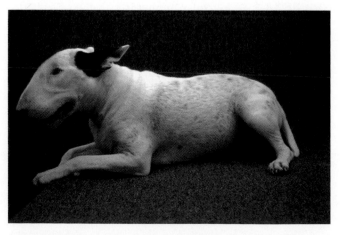

FIGURE 14-9 Canine Solar Dermatosis. Generalized alopecia and erythema covering the face and trunk of a Bull terrier.

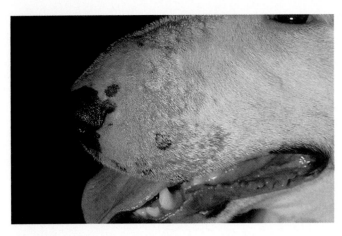

FIGURE 14-10 Canine Solar Dermatosis. Alopecia and erythema with papular dermatitis on the muzzle. *(Courtesy D. Angarano.)*

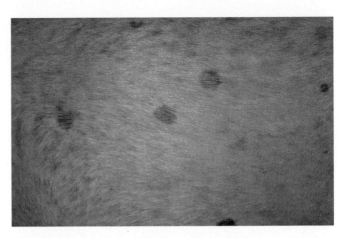

FIGURE 14-11 Canine Solar Dermatosis. Close-up of the lateral thorax of a dog with solar dermatitis. The skin is erythematous with moth-eaten alopecia. The pigmented areas may appear depressed or atrophied, which is an illusion caused by swelling of the surrounding unpigmented skin.

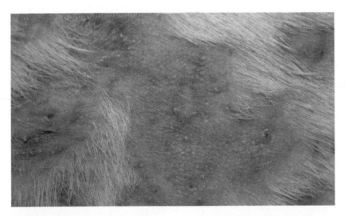

FIGURE 14-12 Canine Solar Dermatosis. A focal area of solar dermatitis demonstrating alopecic erythematous skin. Note that the hair follicles are partially occluded, forming comedones, which may become inflamed or secondarily infected.

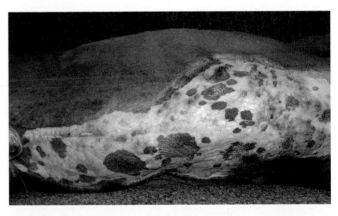

FIGURE 14-13 Canine Solar Dermatosis. Generalized solar dermatitis on the ventrum of a Boxer. The skin is erythematous and edematous with focal areas of scarring. Several ulcerated nodules, which may be squamous cell carcinoma, are apparent.

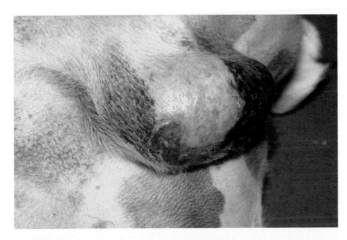

FIGURE 14-14 Canine Solar Dermatosis. This focal area of ulceration on the scrotum of a Boxer had progressed to squamous cell carcinoma.

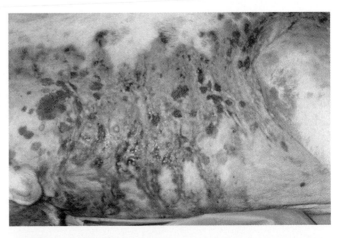

FIGURE 14-15 Canine Solar Dermatosis. This large, erythematous plaque on the abdomen was a combination of chronic solar dermatitis and squamous cell carcinoma. The pigmented areas of skin were protected and thus were not affected.

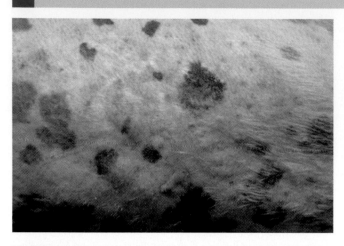

FIGURE 14-16 Canine Solar Dermatosis. Close-up of the abdomen of a dog with solar dermatitis. Note that the pigmented regions seem depressed or atrophied. This is an illusion caused by swelling of the unpigmented skin.

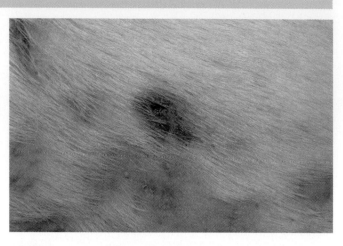

FIGURE 14-17 Canine Solar Dermatosis. A focal nodule with ulceration and drainage. This lesion had progressed to form a squamous cell carcinoma.

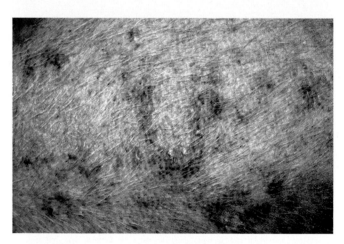

FIGURE 14-18 Canine Solar Dermatosis. Severe erythematous dermatitis with a coalescing papular rash caused by sun exposure.

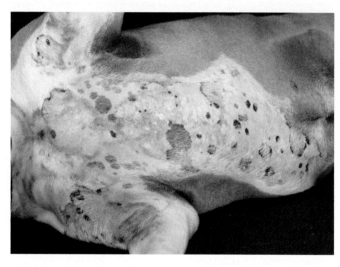

FIGURE 14-19 Canine Solar Dermatosis. Severe erythema affecting only the nonpigmented areas of skin on the ventrum of a Boxer.

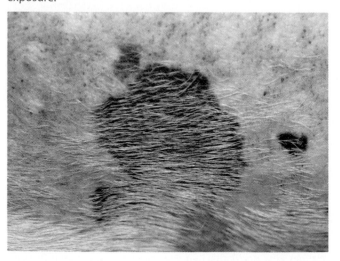

FIGURE 14-20 Canine Solar Dermatosis. Severe infiltrative dermatitis that only affects the nonpigmented skin. The pigmented areas often appear too thin, but it is actually the nonpigmented skin that is thickened by the abnormal cellular infiltrate.

Squamous Cell Carcinoma

Features

Squamous cell carcinoma is a malignant neoplasm of keratinocytes that accounts for 15% of cutaneous tumors in cats and 5% of cutaneous tumors in dogs. It most often occurs in thinly haired, nonpigmented, sun-damaged skin and may be preceded by actinic (solar) keratosis. Recently, papillomavirus infection has been implicated in tumor development in dogs, as papillomavirus antigen can be demonstrated in up to 50% of canine squamous cell carcinomas. Squamous cell carcinoma is common in dogs, with highest incidence in older dogs. Sunlight-induced tumors on the flank and ventrum occur most commonly in lightly pigmented dog breeds such as Dalmatians, Beagles, Whippets, and White English Bull terriers. The condition is common in cats, with highest incidence reported in older white cats. The incidence of solar-induced squamous cell carcinoma is highest in geographic areas with intense sunlight.

Dogs

Squamous cell carcinoma appears usually as single, but possibly multiple, proliferative or ulcerative lesions on the trunk, legs, digits, scrotum, nose, and lips. Proliferative tumors often have a cauliflower-like appearance, vary in size, and may ulcerate and bleed easily. Crater-like ulcerative lesions begin as crusted-over, shallow erosions that deepen. Nail bed tumors usually involve one digit, but multiple digits may be involved, especially in large, black-coated dogs such as black Labradors, German shepherds, and Standard Poodles. Affected digits are typically swollen and painful, and have a misshapen or absent nail.

Cats

Squamous cell carcinoma manifests as proliferative, crusting, or ulcerative lesions that may bleed easily. They most commonly involve nonpigmented ear pinnae, nose, and eyelids.

Diagnosis and Staging

1. Cytology (often nondiagnostic): cells may vary from poorly differentiated, small, round epithelial cells with basophilic cytoplasm to more mature, large, angular, nonkeratinized epithelial cells with abundant cytoplasm, retained nuclei, and perinuclear vacuolation.
2. Dermatohistopathology: irregular masses of atypical keratinocytes that proliferate downward and invade the dermis.
3. Regional lymph nodes and lungs should be screened carefully for tumor metastasis with lymph node cytology/biopsy and three-view thoracic radiographs, respectively.

Treatment and Prognosis

1. The treatment of choice is early, complete surgical excision that includes amputation of digital tumors. Excised tissues should be examined histopathologically for completeness of excision (margin assessment). Laser ablation may be appropriate for superficial lesions.
2. Cryotherapy or laser ablation may be appropriate for small, superficial lesions.
3. For nonresectable or partially resectable lesions, adjuvant radiotherapy (especially electron beam radiation) or strontium-90 (a form of superficial radiotherapy) may be effective.
4. Alternatively, for nonresectable lesions, intralesional chemotherapy (cisplatin, carboplatin, 5-fluorouracil), local hyperthermia, or photodynamic therapy may be effective in some cases. Systemic chemotherapy is less consistently effective for treatment of squamous cell carcinoma.
5. To prevent new solar-induced lesions from developing, future ultraviolet light exposure should be avoided. (See "Solar Dermatosis.")
6. The prognosis for dogs is variable, depending on the degree of differentiation and the site of the lesion. Most tumors are locally invasive and slow to metastasize, although squamous cell carcinoma of the digit tends to be more aggressive and may metastasize more readily. The prognosis in cats depends on the size and degree of differentiation, with smaller, well-differentiated tumors having a better prognosis than large or poorly differentiated ones.

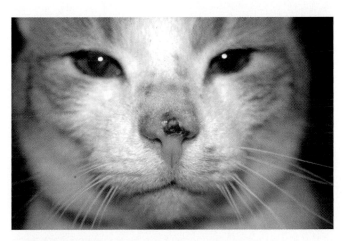

FIGURE 14-21 Squamous Cell Carcinoma. A small, ulcerated tumor on the nonpigmented nasal planum of a cat.

Squamous Cell Carcinoma—cont'd

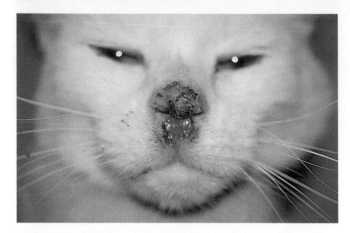

FIGURE 14-22 Squamous Cell Carcinoma. Erythema, ulceration, and crusting on the nose of an adult white cat. The initial lesions were typical of solar dermatosis.

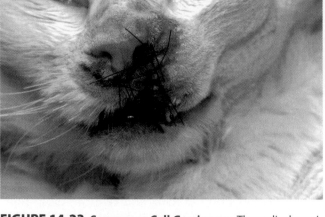

FIGURE 14-23 Squamous Cell Carcinoma. The radical surgical excision was necessary to remove the entire tumor. Surgical correction would have been much easier, if it had been performed earlier. *(Courtesy R. Seamen.)*

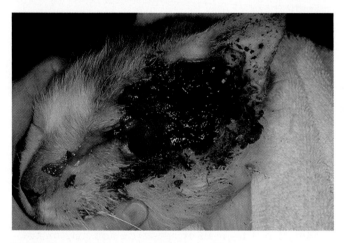

FIGURE 14-24 Squamous Cell Carcinoma. Severe tissue destruction and tumor proliferation on the face and periocular tissue of a cat. *(Courtesy S. McLaughlin.)*

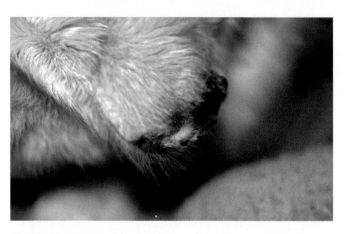

FIGURE 14-25 Squamous Cell Carcinoma. Necrosis and crusting of the distal ear margin of an adult white cat.

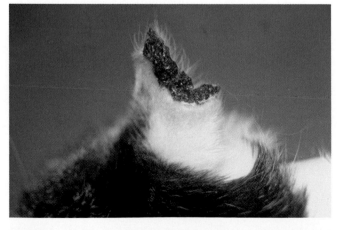

FIGURE 14-26 Squamous Cell Carcinoma. Severe tissue destruction of the entire distal ear pinna caused by progression of the squamous cell carcinoma. Early detection and therapeutic intervention provide better cosmetic outcomes.

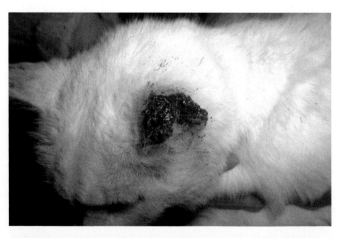

FIGURE 14-27 Squamous Cell Carcinoma. The squamous cell carcinoma has progressed beyond the ear pinna. Surgical resection of this tumor will be difficult and will require extreme reconstructive surgery.

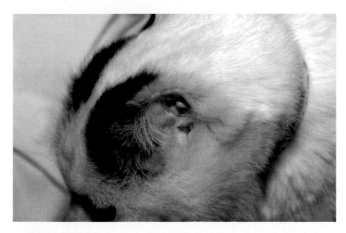

FIGURE 14-28 Squamous Cell Carcinoma. Amputation of this cat's ear pinna was performed to remove the tumor. Early detection and therapeutic intervention provide better cosmetic outcomes.

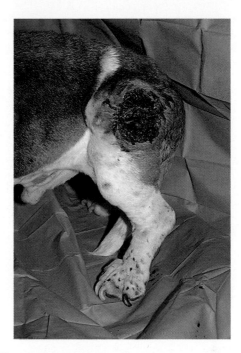

FIGURE 14-29 Squamous Cell Carcinoma. A large, ulcerated tumor on the hip of an aged Basset hound.

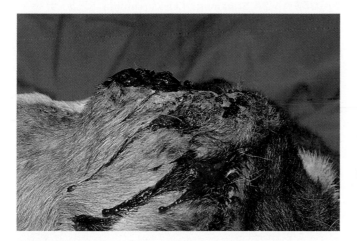

FIGURE 14-30 Squamous Cell Carcinoma. Close-up of the dog in Figure 14-29. This raised tumor has a deep ulcer, with tissue destruction forming a central crater.

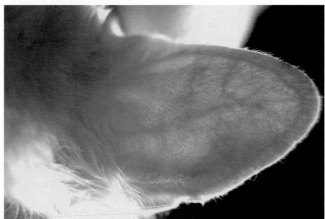

FIGURE 14-31 Squamous Cell Carcinoma. Focal area of carcinoma in situ on the ear pinna of a white cat. The ear pinnae have been illuminated from behind to demonstrate focal erythematous lesions.

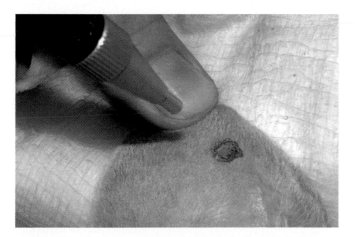

FIGURE 14-32 Squamous Cell Carcinoma. A carbon dioxide (CO_2) laser is used to ablate the focal neoplastic tissue. This technique allows for well-demarcated borders and minimal bystander tissue injury.

Squamous Cell Carcinoma—*cont'd*

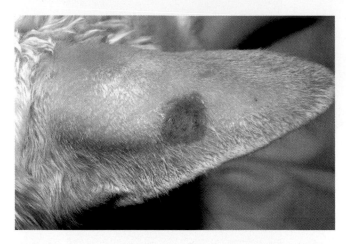

FIGURE 14-33 Squamous Cell Carcinoma. Same cat as in Figure 14-32. The tumor has been ablated, leaving a focal area of ulceration.

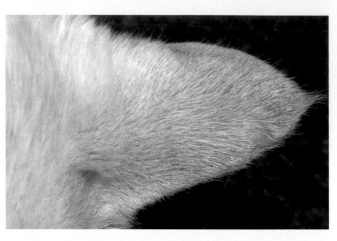

FIGURE 14-34 Squamous Cell Carcinoma. Same cat as in Figure 14-32. Three weeks after treatment, the focal area has healed and the hair is regrowing. Early detection and therapeutic intervention provide better cosmetic outcomes.

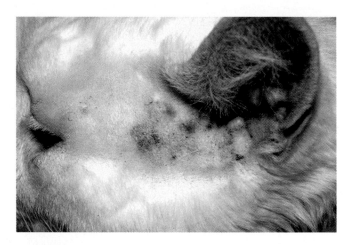

FIGURE 14-35 Squamous Cell Carcinoma. Multifocal squamous cell carcinoma on the preauricular area of a white cat.

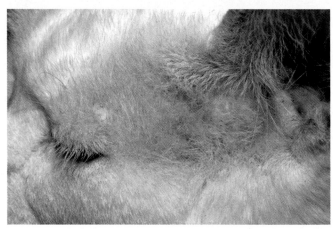

FIGURE 14-36 Squamous Cell Carcinoma. Same cat as in Figure 14-35. The tumors were ablated with a carbon dioxide (CO_2) laser and were allowed to heal. Early detection and therapeutic intervention provide better cosmetic outcomes.

Bowen's Disease/Multifocal Squamous Cell Carcinoma In Situ

Features

Bowen's disease is a syndrome of multifocal superficial neoplasms of keratinocytes. Lesions may occur in pigmented skin or skin that is not exposed to ultraviolet light. Bowen's disease occurs in older animals. It is uncommon in cats and rare in dogs. In cats, lesions are likely induced by papillomavirus infection.

Cats

Lesions are single to multiple crusting, often pigmented plaques 0.5 to 4 cm in diameter that are often alopecic, ulcerated, and painful, and bleed easily. They tend to be chronic (months to years) and may wax and wane. Lesions affect well-haired areas of the head, neck, shoulders, forelegs, and digits.

Dogs

Oral, genital, or nodular lesions may occur, in addition to lesions as described for cats. Progression of in situ lesions to invasive squamous cell carcinoma may occur but is unpredictable.

Diagnosis

Dermatohistopathology: irregular, superficial epithelial dysplasia with no disruption of the basement membrane. Hyperkeratosis and hypermelanosis are common,

and crusting with secondary infection and subsequent inflammation may occur. In cats, papillomatous changes may be evident at tumor margins, and 45% of lesions demonstrate papillomavirus antigen.

Treatment and Prognosis

1. For single to few lesions, surgical excision or laser ablation may be curative, but new lesions may arise elsewhere.
2. Lesions smaller than 2 to 4 mm in thickness may be treated with strontium-90 plesiotherapy.
3. In one report, a dog initially responded to topical 5-fluorouracil (frequency and duration of treatment not specified), which caused regression of skin lesions and controlled appearance of new lesions.
4. Acitretin 5–10 mg/cat PO every 24 hours may be effective in some cases.
5. 5% imiquimod cream (Aldara) applied topically to lesions may be helpful as immunomodulating therapy. It should be applied every 24 to 48 hours until response is noted (typically 2–3 weeks). (An Elizabethan collar can be used to prevent grooming during treatment.) Monitor liver function.
6. The prognosis for cure is guarded, as new lesions may continue to develop. Progression of in situ lesions to invasive squamous cell carcinoma may occur.

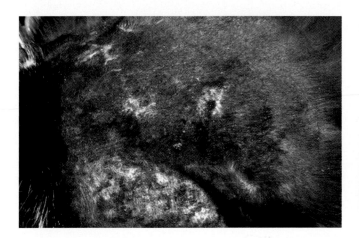

FIGURE 14-37 Bowen's Disease. Multifocal, crusting, papular lesions on the pigmented skin of an adult cat are typical of this syndrome.

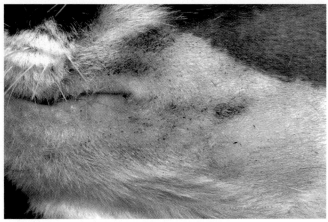

FIGURE 14-38 Bowen's Disease. Multifocal, crusting, papular lesions on the face. Note the mild, subtle nature of the lesions.

Bowen's Disease/Multifocal Squamous Cell Carcinoma In Situ—*cont'd*

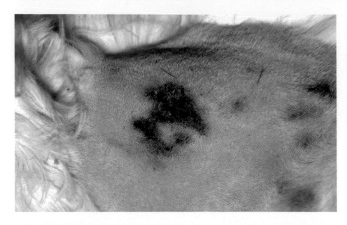

FIGURE 14-39 Bowen's Disease. Multifocal, pigmenting lesions. The extent of these lesions can be easily missed unless the hair is removed.

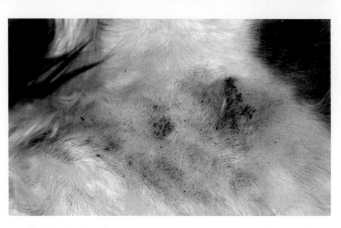

FIGURE 14-40 Bowen's Disease. Multifocal, crusting, papular lesions on the pigmented skin of an adult cat are typical of this syndrome.

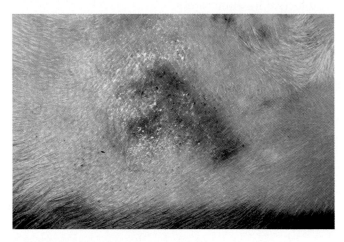

FIGURE 14-41 Bowen's Disease. Coalescing papules formed a plaque on the nonpigmented skin of this cat.

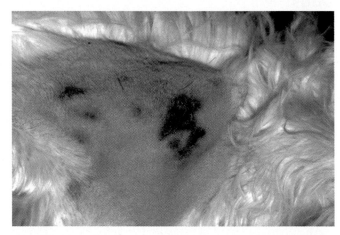

FIGURE 14-42 Bowen's Disease. Multifocal, pigmenting lesions.

Basal Cell Tumor/Carcinoma

Features

Basal cell tumor is a neoplasm originating from basal cells of the epidermis, hair follicles, sebaceous glands, or sweat glands that is usually behaviorally benign. It is uncommon in older dogs, with Cocker spaniels, Poodles, shelties, Kerry blue terriers, and Siberian huskies possibly predisposed. It is common in older cats (15%–26% of all feline skin tumors), with Siamese, Himalayan, and Persian cats possibly predisposed.

Usually, basal cell tumor manifests as solitary, well-circumscribed, raised, round, firm to fluctuant nodules that are 1 to 10 cm in diameter and may be pigmented, alopecic, or ulcerated. Lesions are most commonly found on the head, neck, thorax, or dorsal trunk.

Diagnosis

1. Cytology: basal cell tumors contain small, fairly uniform, round to cuboidal epithelial cells with scant basophilic cytoplasm that may be arranged in groups or ribbons. Basal cell carcinomas may show standard criteria for malignancy but can be difficult to differentiate cytologically from benign tumors.
2. Dermatohistopathology: nonencapsulated, often lobulated, intradermal to subcutaneous mass composed of cords or nests of neoplastic basal cells. Tumors may be pigmented or cystic, or may show central areas of squamous differentiation.

Treatment and Prognosis

1. The treatment of choice is complete surgical excision. Excised tissues should be examined histopathologically for completeness of excision (margin assessment).
2. Cryotherapy or laser ablation may be useful for smaller masses.
3. The prognosis is good. Basal cell tumors are benign, and basal cell carcinomas are of low-grade malignancy and very rarely metastasize.

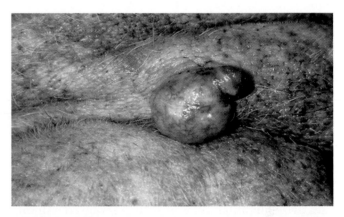

FIGURE 14-44 Basal Cell Tumors. A multilobulated nodule.

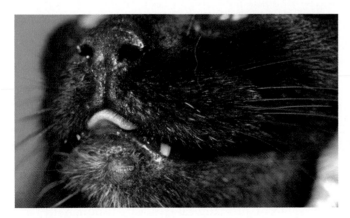

FIGURE 14-43 Basal Cell Tumors. A pigmented nodule on the chin of an adult cat.

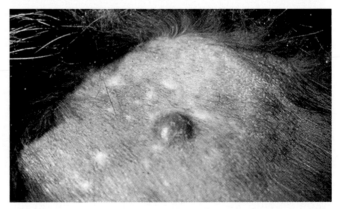

FIGURE 14-45 Basal Cell Tumors. This pigmented nodule on the trunk of an adult cat is typical of this tumor.

Hair Follicle Tumors

Features

Hair follicle tumors appear usually as benign neoplasms of germinal hair follicle cells that are classified according to the direction of adnexal differentiation. They are common in dogs and rare in cats. Trichoepitheliomas and pilomatrixomas are the most common follicular tumors.

Trichoepithelioma

Trichoepithelioma is a benign tumor of cells that differentiate toward hair follicles and shaft structures. It is common in dogs and uncommon in cats, with increased incidence reported in animals older than 5 years. Among dogs, Basset hounds, Golden retrievers, German shepherds, miniature Schnauzers, Standard Poodles, and spaniels may be predisposed. Among cats, Persians may be predisposed. Tumors usually occur as single (often multiple in Bassets), alopecic, firm, white to gray, multilobulated masses that may become ulcerated. Tumors range in size from 1 mm to 2 cm or larger. They are often located on the trunk and limbs in dogs, and on the head, tail, and limbs in cats.

Pilomatrixoma

This benign neoplasm arises from cells of the hair bulb/matrix. It is uncommon in dogs and very rare in cats, occurring in animals 5 to 10 years of age. Among dogs, Kerry blue terriers, Poodles, and Old English sheepdogs may be predisposed. Tumors are solitary, often alopecic, firm, sometimes ulcerated or calcified, well-circumscribed, dome-shaped to plaquelike, dermal or subcutaneous masses that may be cystic or pigmented and that range in size from 1 to 10 cm and occur most commonly on the trunk.

Trichoblastoma

This usually appears as a benign neoplasm of cells that originate from primitive hair germ epithelium. It is uncommon in middle-aged dogs and cats. Among dogs, Poodles and Cocker spaniels appear to be predisposed. Tumors range from 1 to 2 cm, and appear as solitary, firm, dome-shaped, alopecic nodules that occur most commonly on the head and neck in dogs and on the cranial half of the trunk in cats.

Tricholemmoma

This is a benign tumor of cells that differentiate toward the outer root sheath of the hair follicle. It is rare in dogs and cats, occurring in animals 5 to 13 years of age. Among dogs, Afghans may be predisposed. Tumors range from 1 to 7 cm, and appear as firm, circumscribed nodules, often on the head and neck.

Trichofolliculoma

This benign hair follicle tumor may actually be a follicular or pilosebaceous hamartoma, rather than a true neoplasm. It is rare in dogs and cats and has no known age, breed, or site predilection. Tumors occur as solitary, dome-shaped nodules that may have a central depression or opening that contains hair or sebaceous material.

Dilated Pore of Winer

This is a benign hair follicle tumor or cyst. It is uncommon in older cats and appears as a solitary firm mass or cyst (smaller than 1 cm) with a central keratin-filled opening. The keratin may occasionally appear to form a cutaneous horn. Nodules are most common on the trunk, head, and neck.

Diagnosis

1. Cytology (often nondiagnostic): hair follicle tumors are characterized by mature, cornified squamous epithelial cells and amorphous cellular debris. Small, uniform, basal-type epithelial cells occasionally can be seen.
2. Dermatohistopathology: hair follicle tumors are classified by the histologic pattern and appearance of basaloid tumor cells. Depending on tumor type, masses may be solid or cystic and may contain keratin.

Treatment and Prognosis

1. Observation without treatment is reasonable because these tumors are benign.
2. Surgical excision is curative.
3. The prognosis is good. Benign hair follicle tumors are not locally invasive, do not metastasize, and rarely recur after surgical removal. Although they are extremely rare, metastatic pilomatrixomas with neurologic complications have been reported in two dogs.

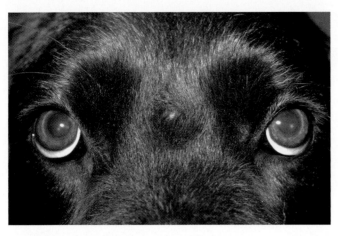

FIGURE 14-46 Hair Follicle Tumors. This small, nondraining nodule is typical of these tumors.

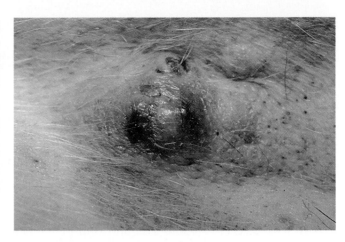

FIGURE 14-47 Hair Follicle Tumors. A small, pigmented nodule. Note the similarity to basal cell tumors, apocrine tumors, and melanoma.

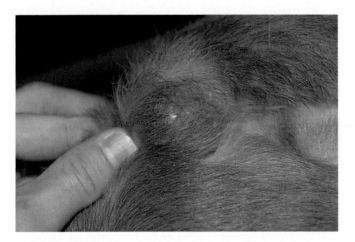

FIGURE 14-48 Hair Follicle Tumors. This large cyst on the ventral thorax of an aged hound mix was associated with a follicular tumor.

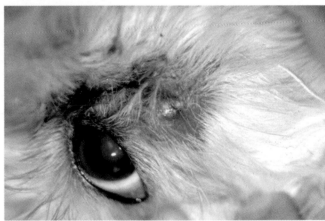

FIGURE 14-49 Hair Follicle Tumors. An alopecic, cystic nodule on the periocular skin.

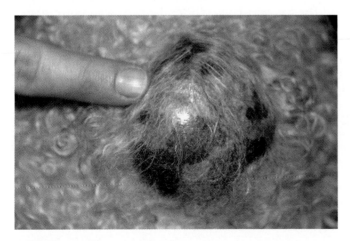

FIGURE 14-50 Hair Follicle Tumors. A large, alopecic, cystic tumor on the hip of a dog.

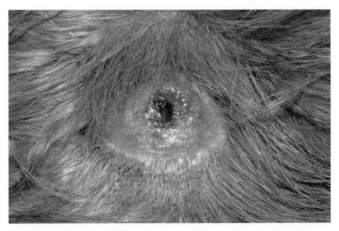

FIGURE 14-51 Hair Follicle Tumors. A focal, crusted, alopecic tumor.

Sebaceous Gland Tumors

Features

Nodular sebaceous hyperplasia, sebaceous epitheliomas, and sebaceous adenomas are benign tumors of sebocytes. They are common in older dogs, with highest incidence reported in Poodles, Cocker spaniels, miniature Schnauzers, and terriers (sebaceous adenomas/hyperplasia), and in Shih tzus, Lhasa apsos, Siberian huskies, and Irish setters (sebaceous epitheliomas). Benign sebaceous gland tumors are uncommon in older cats, with Persians possibly predisposed. Sebaceous gland adenocarcinomas are rare malignant tumors of older dogs and cats. Among dogs, Cocker spaniels are predisposed.

Benign sebaceous tumors are usually solitary, firm, elevated, wartlike or cauliflower-like growths that range from a few millimeters to several centimeters in diameter. Lesions may be yellowish or pigmented, alopecic, oily, or ulcerated. Nodules of sebaceous hyperplasia can be multiple. Sebaceous adenocarcinomas tend to appear as solitary, alopecic, ulcerated, or erythematous intradermal nodules smaller than 4 cm that invade into the subcutis. Sebaceous gland tumors occur most commonly on the trunk, legs, head, and eyelids in dogs, and on the head in cats.

Diagnosis

1. Distinctive wartlike, cauliflower growths.
2. Cytology:
   - *Sebaceous hyperplasia/adenoma:* cells exfoliate in groups and appear similar to normal sebaceous cells, with foamy pale blue cytoplasm and small dark nuclei.
   - *Sebaceous epithelioma:* small, fairly uniform, sometimes melanotic epithelial cells with low numbers of sebaceous cells
   - *Sebaceous carcinoma:* extremely basophilic basal-type cells with nuclear and cellular pleomorphism

3. Dermatohistopathology:
   - *Sebaceous hyperplasia:* multiple enlarged mature sebaceous lobules with a single peripheral layer of basaloid germinal cells and a central duct. No mitotic figures are seen.
   - *Sebaceous adenoma:* similar to hyperplasia but with increased numbers of basaloid germinal cells and immature sebocytes. Low mitotic activity and loss of organization are noted around the central duct.
   - *Sebaceous epithelioma:* multiple lobules of basaloid epithelial cells interspersed with reactive collagenous tissue and secondary inflammation. Fairly high mitotic activity has been demonstrated. Scattered areas of sebaceous differentiation, squamous metaplasia, or melanization may be observed.
   - *Sebaceous gland adenocarcinoma:* poorly defined lobules of large epithelial cells with varying degrees of sebaceous differentiation and cytoplasmic vacuolation. Nuclei are large, and mitotic activity is moderately high.

Treatment and Prognosis

1. For benign sebaceous gland tumors, observation without treatment is reasonable.
2. Surgical excision (laser ablation or cryosurgery) of benign sebaceous gland tumors is usually curative for cosmetically unacceptable lesions or for lesions that bother the dog.
3. For sebaceous gland adenocarcinomas, complete surgical excision is recommended.
4. The prognosis is good. Benign sebaceous gland tumors are not locally invasive, do not metastasize, and rarely recur after surgical removal. Sebaceous gland adenocarcinomas are locally infiltrative and occasionally involve regional lymph nodes, but distant metastases are uncommon.

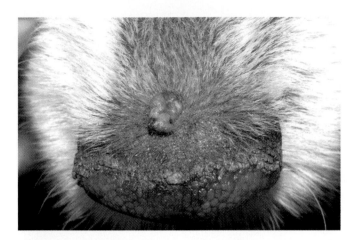

FIGURE 14-52 Sebaceous Gland Tumors. This sebaceous adenoma on the nasal planum demonstrates the characteristic cauliflower appearance.

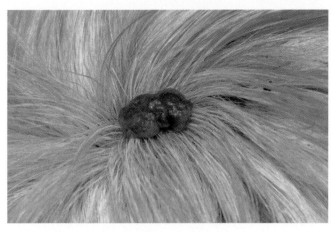

FIGURE 14-53 Sebaceous Gland Tumors. This sebaceous adenoma had persisted for several years with little progression.

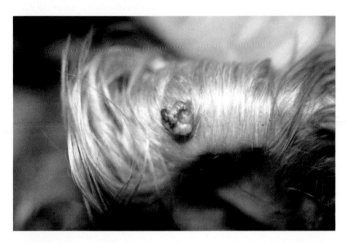

FIGURE 14-54 Sebaceous Gland Tumors. This sebaceous adenoma on the ear pinna demonstrates the characteristic size and shape of these tumors.

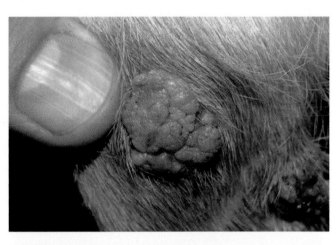

FIGURE 14-55 Sebaceous Gland Tumors. Sebaceous adenomas are usually small (the size of a pencil eraser) but may progress into larger lesions.

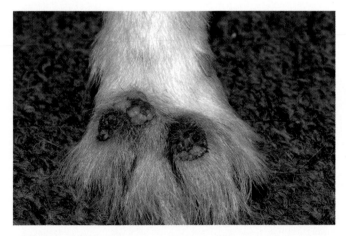

FIGURE 14-56 Sebaceous Gland Tumors. Multiple sebaceous adenomas on the foot. Some dogs develop multiple tumors distributed over their entire body.

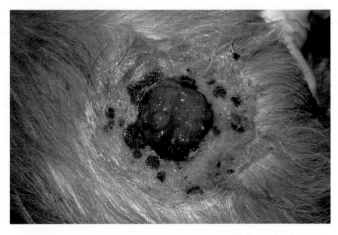

FIGURE 14-57 Sebaceous Gland Tumors. An aggressive, infiltrative sebaceous tumor.

Sebaceous Gland Tumors—*cont'd*

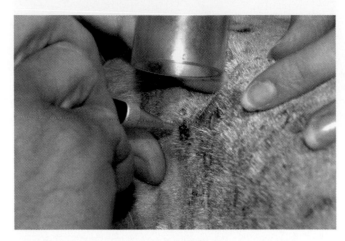

FIGURE 14-58 Sebaceous Gland Tumors. Carbon dioxide (CO_2) laser ablation provides a good method of treating patients with numerous sebaceous adenomas.

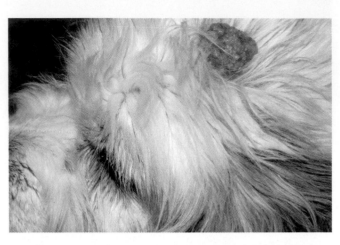

FIGURE 14-59 Sebaceous Gland Tumors. A large tumor on the head of a geriatric Cocker spaniel demonstrates the classic cauliflower shape of this tumor type.

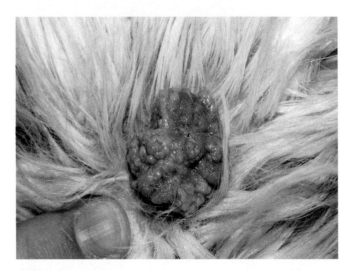

FIGURE 14-60 Sebaceous Gland Tumors. The cauliflower shape is characteristic for this type of tumor.

Perianal Gland Tumors

Features

These are usually benign growths that arise from the circumanal (hepatoid) glands, possibly secondary to androgenic stimulation. Perianal adenomas are common in older intact male dogs, and they are uncommon in female and neutered male dogs. Perianal gland adenocarcinomas are uncommon and occur with equal frequency in older male and female dogs, regardless of neuter status.

Adenomas are solitary or multiple slow-growing, firm, round to lobular, dermal nodules of variable size that may ulcerate. Tumors usually occur adjacent to the anus but may also occur on the tail, tail head, perineum, or prepuce, or can appear as a diffuse, bulging ring of tissue around the anus. Perianal adenocarcinomas appear similar to adenomas but tend to grow and ulcerate more rapidly.

Diagnosis

1. Cytology: clumps of large, round to polyhedral, hepatoid epithelial cells that contain abundant pale blue cytoplasm, round to oval nuclei, and one to two nucleoli. A second population of smaller epithelial "reserve cells" is also commonly present. Adenocarcinomas cannot be reliably differentiated cytologically from adenomas.
2. Dermatohistopathology: lobules of polygonal cells resembling hepatocytes with abundant, finely vacuolated eosinophilic cytoplasm and central round nuclei. A rim of basal reserve cells surrounds each lobule. Squamous metaplasia may occur. Mitotic figures are rarely seen in adenomas. Adenocarcinomas appear similar to adenomas but have increased anisocytosis/anisokaryosis and frequent mitotic figures.

Treatment and Prognosis

1. For intact male dogs, castration and tumor removal is the treatment of choice for most perianal adenomas.
2. For large or diffuse benign lesions, neutering first and waiting several months will allow reduction in tumor volume to facilitate safer and easier mass removal.
3. Surgical excision is also indicated for adenomas occurring in female or neutered male dogs.
4. Cryotherapy or laser ablation may be useful for adenomas smaller than 1 to 2 cm in diameter.
5. Estrogen therapy may reduce adenoma size but can cause fatal bone marrow suppression and therefore is not recommended.
6. Perianal adenocarcinomas will not regress after castration, and complete surgical excision is the treatment of choice. Radiation or chemotherapy may slow disease progression in incompletely excised tumors.
7. Recurrence of adenomas after castration or resection warrants investigation of possible underlying hyperadrenocorticism.
8. The prognosis for perianal adenoma is good, as tumors are benign and do not usually recur after castration. The prognosis for perianal adenocarcinomas is fair to guarded, as recurrence with local invasion after surgery or metastasis may occur, most commonly to regional (sublumbar/pelvic) lymph nodes, liver, and lung.. Dogs with adenocarcinomas larger than 5 cm and those with metastasis present at the time of diagnosis have the poorest prognosis and may live for only a few months.

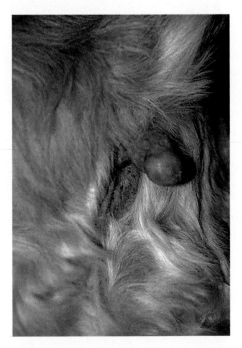

FIGURE 14-61 Perianal Gland Tumors. An elongated, pedunculated tumor on the perianal tissue of an aged Cocker spaniel.

Perianal Gland Tumors—*cont'd*

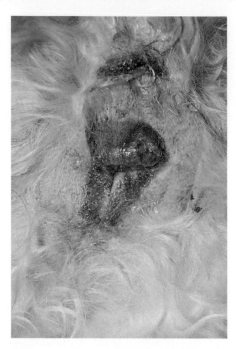

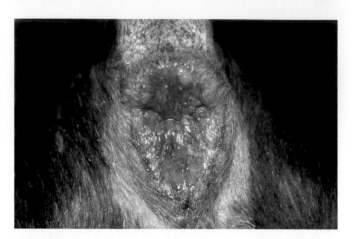

FIGURE 14-63 **Perianal Gland Tumors.** Severe tissue proliferation surrounding the anal mucosa.

FIGURE 14-62 **Perianal Gland Tumors.** An ulcerated nodule on the perianal tissue of an aged Cocker spaniel.

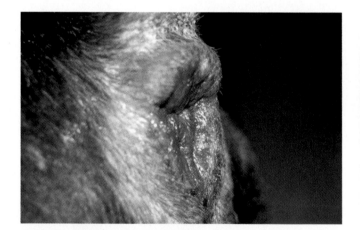

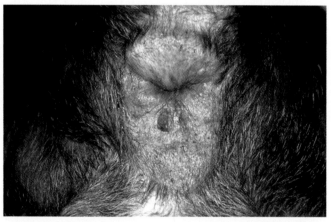

FIGURE 14-64 **Perianal Gland Tumors.** Same dog as in Figure 14-63. Swollen tissue protrudes beyond the normal anal architecture.

FIGURE 14-65 **Perianal Gland Tumors.** Swollen anal tissue with a focal nodule.

Apocrine (epitrichial) Sweat Gland Cysts and Tumors

Features

Cysts of apocrine sweat glands are benign tumor-like lesions. Apocrine sweat gland adenomas and adenocarcinomas can arise from apocrine gland or apocrine duct cells. Lesions are uncommon in dogs and cats, with highest incidence reported in older animals. Among dogs, German shepherds and Golden retrievers may be predisposed to apocrine tumors. Siamese cats may be predisposed to carcinomas.

Dogs

Apocrine cysts appear as raised, round, fluctuant intradermal nodules that measure 0.5 to 3.0 cm and contain a clear fluid. Cysts occur most commonly on the head. Apocrine sweat gland adenomas are usually solitary, raised, alopecic, circumscribed, dermal or subcutaneous tumors that may have a bluish tint. Tumors may be firm, cystic, or ulcerated and range in size from 0.5 to 4 cm in diameter. Apocrine sweat gland carcinomas are usually solitary growths that may appear clinically similar to an adenoma. Sweat gland tumors are most common on the head, neck, trunk, and legs.

Cats

Multiple apocrine cysts measuring 2 to 10 mm have been described on the eyelids of Persian and Himalayan cats. Apocrine adenomas and adenocarcinomas may be clinically indistinguishable from each other; however, adenocarcinomas tend to be more ulcerative, firm, and inflamed. Tumors are usually solitary, well-circumscribed, raised, firm, or cystic lesions ranging from a few millimeters to a few centimeters in diameter. Nodules may have a bluish tinge and may be ulcerated. Adenomas occur most commonly on the head in cats; adenocarcinomas may occur anywhere on the body.

Diagnosis

1. Cytology (often nondiagnostic):
   - *Apocrine cyst:* usually acellular fluid with occasional macrophages
   - *Apocrine adenoma:* few medium, round or oval cells with eccentric nuclei and large intracytoplasmic droplets of secretory product
   - *Apocrine adenocarcinoma:* groups of small, basophilic, epithelial cells with scant blue cytoplasm. Most cells may appear fairly uniform with a subpopulation of larger, more pleomorphic cells.
2. Dermatohistopathology:
   - *Apocrine cyst:* variably sized, single to multiple, dilated epitrichial gland cysts lined by one or two layers of normal to attenuated columnar secretory epithelium
   - *Apocrine adenoma:* circumscribed dermal nodule comprising multiple cysts, lined by often proliferative columnar epithelium and containing clear or eosinophilic fluid. Mitotic activity is low.
   - *Apocrine adenocarcinoma:* architecturally similar to adenoma. However, nuclear pleomorphism and increased mitotic activity are present, and neoplastic cells may be locally invasive.

Treatment and Prognosis

1. The treatment of choice is complete surgical excision.
2. Observation without treatment is also an option for apocrine cysts and adenomas, as these lesions are benign.
3. The prognosis for apocrine cysts and adenomas is good, as surgical removal is curative. The prognosis for apocrine gland adenocarcinomas is variable. Tumors may be locally invasive and may recur after surgery; up to 20% of cases have lymphatic involvement or distant metastasis.

Apocrine (epitrichial) Sweat Gland Cysts and Tumors—*cont'd*

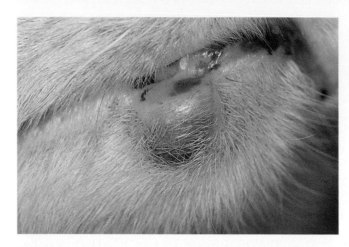

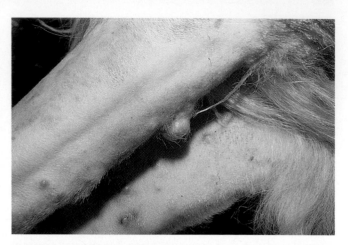

FIGURE 14-66 **Apocrine Gland Tumor.** The blue nodule on the lower lip of this adult cat is typical of an apocrine tumor. Note the similarity to basal cell tumors, melanomas, and follicular tumors.

FIGURE 14-67 **Apocrine Gland Tumor.** An apocrine gland cyst on the leg of an adult dog.

Fibropruritic Nodule

Features

Although the pathogenesis is unknown, fibropruritic nodules occur only in dogs with chronic flea bite hypersensitivity. They are uncommon in dogs, with highest incidence in older dogs, especially purebred and mixed-breed German shepherd dogs.

Fibropruritic nodules are multiple, alopecic, firm, sessile or pedunculated nodules measuring 0.5 to 2 cm in diameter that may be erythematous or hyperpigmented. Lesions may be smooth or hyperkeratotic, and they occasionally ulcerate. These lesions are found along the dorsal lumbosacral area in dogs with chronic flea bite hypersensitivity.

Diagnosis

1. Usually based on history and clinical findings.
2. Dermatohistopathology: severely hyperplastic, sometimes ulcerated, epidermis overlying dermal fibrosis, and inflammation that may obscure adnexal structures.

Treatment and Prognosis

1. Underlying flea bite hypersensitivity should be treated.
2. Cosmetically unacceptable lesions can be surgically excised.
3. The prognosis is good. Although fibropruritic nodules rarely resolve spontaneously, they are benign lesions that do not affect the dog's quality of life. Flea control should prevent development of additional lesions.

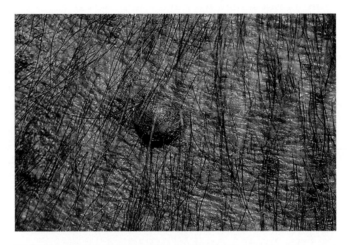

FIGURE 14-68 Fibropruritic Nodule. This small, pigmented nodule developed on the lumbar region of an adult Schnauzer with severe flea allergy dermatitis.

Fibroma

Features

A fibroma is a benign neoplasm of dermal or subcutaneous fibroblasts. It is uncommon in middle-aged to older cats and dogs, with highest incidence in Boxers, Golden retrievers, and Dobermann pinschers.

Usually, fibroma manifests as a solitary, well-circumscribed, firm, dome-shaped or pedunculated, dermal or subcutaneous mass that ranges from 1 to 5 cm in diameter. The overlying epidermis may be alopecic and atrophic. Lesions can occur anywhere on the body, most commonly on the limbs and flanks.

Diagnosis

1. Cytology (often nondiagnostic as mesenchymal tumors are poorly exfoliative): few uniform spindle cells with round or oval dark nuclei containing one to two small nucleoli.
2. Dermatohistopathology: well-circumscribed dermal or subcutaneous nodule of mature fibroblasts with abundant collagen production that displaces normal dermal adnexal structures. Mitotic figures are very rare.

Treatment and Prognosis

1. Observation without treatment is reasonable because these tumors are benign.

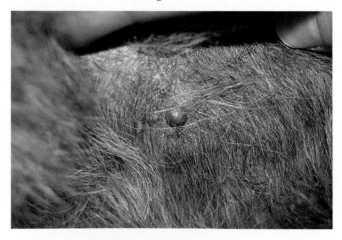

FIGURE 14-69 Fibroma. A small, nonpigmented nodule on the lateral thorax of an aged Schnauzer.

2. Complete surgical excision is curative for cosmetically unacceptable tumors.
3. The prognosis is good. Fibromas are benign, noninvasive, and nonmetastatic.

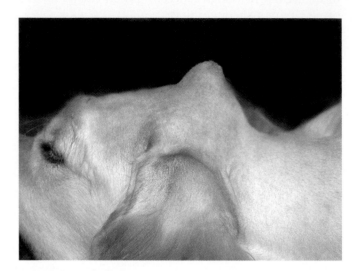

FIGURE 14-70 Fibroma. A large tumor on the head of a young Golden retriever. The hair has been clipped in preparation for surgical removal.

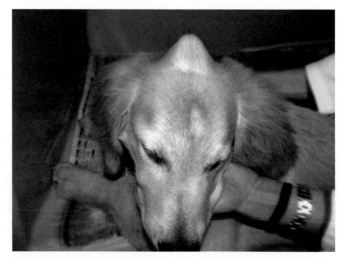

FIGURE 14-71 Fibroma. Same dog as in Figure 14-70. A large tumor on the head of a young Golden retriever.

Fibrosarcoma

Features

A fibrosarcoma is a malignant neoplasm that arises from dermal or subcutaneous fibroblasts. In dogs, it occurs spontaneously. In cats, it may arise spontaneously, may be induced by feline sarcoma virus (FeSV), or may be vaccine induced, especially by feline leukemia, rabies, or adjuvant vaccines. Fibrosarcoma is uncommon in dogs, with highest reported incidence in older dogs, especially Golden retrievers and Dobermanns. It is common in cats, with highest incidence of FeSV-induced lesions in cats younger than 5 years old, and highest incidence in older cats of tumors not associated with FeSV or vaccinations.

Dogs

Usually, fibrosarcoma appears as a solitary, firm subcutaneous mass that is poorly circumscribed and nodular to irregular in shape, and ranges from 1 to 15 cm in diameter. The surface may be alopecic and ulcerated. Tumors often arise on the head and proximal limbs and may be fixed to underlying tissue.

Cats

Fibrosarcomas manifest as rapidly infiltrating dermal or subcutaneous masses that are firm, poorly circumscribed, and nodular to irregular in shape, and range from 0.5 to 15 cm in diameter. Lesions may be alopecic and ulcerated. FeSV-associated fibrosarcomas are usually multicentric, whereas those not caused by FeSV are usually solitary. Tumors most commonly involve the trunk, distal limbs, and ear pinnae. Postvaccination fibrosarcomas arise subcutaneously at previous vaccination sites 1 month to 4 years post vaccination, and are larger and more rapidly growing than non–vaccine-induced lesions.

Diagnosis

1. Feline leukemia test: positive for cats with FeSV-induced tumors.
2. Cytology (often nondiagnostic): cells may be fusiform, oval, or stellate and may contain multiple nuclei. Cellular pleomorphism, nuclear size, and cytoplasmic basophilia vary with degree of tumor differentiation.
3. Dermatohistopathology: haphazardly interlacing bundles of plump spindle cells that are infiltrative and nonencapsulated. Mitotic activity, multinucleated cells, and collagen production are variable. In vaccination-induced lesions, peripheral lymphoid and granulomatous inflammation may be observed, along with epithelioid macrophages and multinucleated histiocytic giant cells that contain an intracytoplasmic, amorphous basophilic material (presumed to be adjuvant). Vaccine-induced tumors in cats tend to have more extensive necrosis, greater pleomorphism, and an increased mitotic index compared with non–vaccine-induced lesions.

Treatment and Prognosis

1. The treatment of choice for single tumors is wide surgical excision or amputation of the affected limb. Surgical excision should be carried out with preoperative cross-sectional imaging (computed tomography [CT] or magnetic resonance image [MRI] scanning).
2. Radiation therapy is often used preoperatively or postoperatively in cases in which complete excision is difficult, and is especially important in conjunction with surgery in treatment of feline vaccine–associated sarcomas.
3. Chemotherapy (doxorubicin hydrochloride [Adriamycin], mitoxantrone) may be effective for palliation of nonresectable tumors.
4. The prognosis for solitary tumors is variable. Factors that influence prognosis include tumor size, completeness of excision, histologic grade, location, and depth of invasion. Small, superficial, low-grade tumors or tumors on extremities treated with amputation have a better prognosis, whereas large, deep, truncal, vaccine-induced, or high-grade tumors have a poor prognosis and usually recur locally after surgery. The median disease-free interval for cats treated with surgery in a private practice setting (2 months) is significantly shorter than if the surgery is carried out by a board-certified veterinary surgeon (9 months). Distant metastasis is generally uncommon but can occur in up to 24% of cats with vaccine-induced tumors.
5. The prognosis for multiple FeSV-induced tumors is poor. Surgery is ineffective for cats with tumors induced by FeSV because of the multicentric nature of the disease.

Fibrosarcoma—cont'd

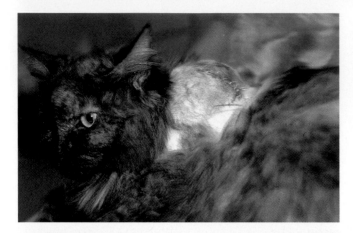

FIGURE 14-72 **Fibrosarcoma.** A large vaccine-induced fibrosarcoma on the dorsum of a cat.

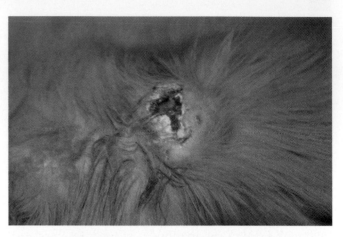

FIGURE 14-73 **Fibrosarcoma.** A large tumor with an ulcerated cutaneous surface.

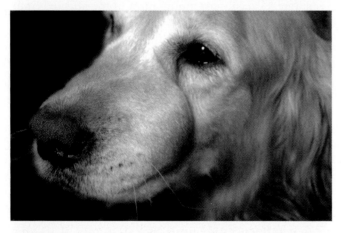

FIGURE 14-74 **Fibrosarcoma.** This rapidly progressive tumor caused asymmetrical swelling on the face of this Golden retriever.

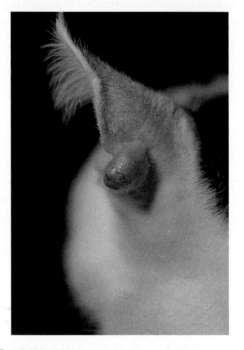

FIGURE 14-76 **Fibrosarcoma.** A small fibrosarcoma on the ear pinna of an adult cat.

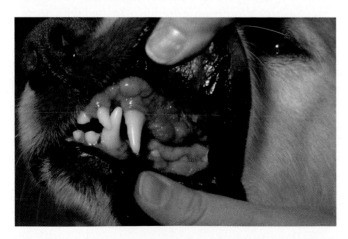

FIGURE 14-75 **Fibrosarcoma.** Same dog as in Figure 14-74. Multiple neoplastic nodules are apparent on the gingiva.

Nodular Dermatofibrosis

Features

Nodular dermatofibrosis is a syndrome in which the appearance of dermal fibrotic nodules is associated with concurrent renal cystic disease and, in intact females, uterine leiomyomas. Although the exact pathogenesis is unknown, an autosomal dominant mode of inheritance has been postulated in affected German shepherd dogs. The condition is rare in dogs, with the highest incidence in middle-aged to older German shepherds.

The disease is characterized by the sudden appearance of multiple cutaneous nodules. Nodules are firm, well circumscribed, and dermal to subcutaneous, and range from several millimeters to 4 cm in diameter. The skin overlying the nodules may be thickened, hyperpigmented, alopecic, or ulcerated. Lesions occur most commonly on the limbs, head, and ears. Concurrent unilateral or bilateral renal epithelial cysts, cystadenomas or cystadenocarcinomas, or uterine leiomyomas are present. Skin lesions often precede clinical signs of underlying disease by months to years.

Diagnosis

1. Dermatohistopathology: circumscribed dermal or subcutaneous mass composed of structurally normal collagenous bundles.
2. Radiography, ultrasonography, or exploratory laparotomy: renal cystic or neoplastic disease or uterine neoplastic disease.

Treatment and Prognosis

1. The treatment of choice is nephrectomy if only one kidney is involved, and ovariohysterectomy for uterine leiomyomas. Unfortunately, the renal disease is usually bilateral.
2. Skin lesions are removed only for cosmetic reasons, or if they interfere with function.
3. The long-term prognosis is poor, as the underlying renal cystic or neoplastic disease is invariably fatal. However, in one large compilation of cases, the mean age of diagnosis of skin lesions preceded mean animal death by 3 years. Affected dogs should not be bred.

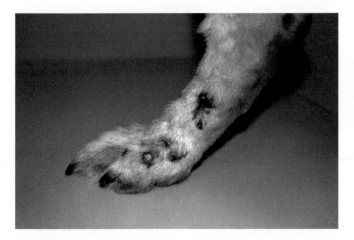

FIGURE 14-77 Nodular Dermatofibrosis. Multiple, alopecic, hyperpigmented nodules on the leg of a German shepherd are characteristic of this syndrome.

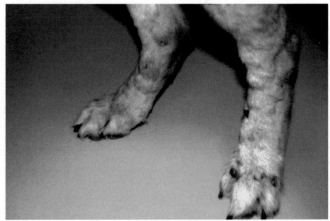

FIGURE 14-78 Nodular Dermatofibrosis. Same dog as in Figure 14-77. Alopecic, hyperpigmented nodules cover the legs.

Hemangioma

Features

A hemangioma is a benign tumor of blood vessel endothelial cells. It is uncommon in dogs, with highest incidence reported in older dogs, especially those with lightly pigmented and sparsely haired ventrums (e.g., Pit Bulls, Dalmatians, Beagles, Greyhounds, Whippets, Italian Greyhounds), suggesting ultraviolet light exposure as a causal factor. Predisposed breeds for non–sunlight-induced lesions include Airedales, Boxers, Springer spaniels, German shepherds, and Golden retrievers. Hemangioma is rare in cats, with highest incidence in older male cats.

Hemangioma usually appears as a solitary, rounded, well-circumscribed, firm to fluctuant, raised, bluish to reddish black, dermal or subcutaneous growth ranging from 0.5 to 4 cm in diameter. Hemangiomas of the glabrous skin can appear as clusters or plaquelike aggregates of blood vessels. Tumors are more common on the trunk and limbs of dogs and on the head and limbs of cats.

Diagnosis

1. Cytology (often nondiagnostic): mostly blood with a few normal-appearing endothelial cells, which may be oval, stellate or spindle cells with moderate blue cytoplasm and a medium, round nucleus with one to two small nucleoli.
2. Dermatohistopathology: well-circumscribed dermal or subcutaneous nodule formed by dilated blood-filled spaces lined by relatively normal-appearing flattened endothelial cells. No mitotic figures are seen. Solar-induced lesions may have accompanying solar dermatitis and elastosis.

Treatment and Prognosis

1. Complete surgical excision is curative. Cryotherapy can also be used in conjunction with surgery for small dermal lesions.
2. If surgery is otherwise contraindicated, benign neglect and observation without treatment may be reasonable because these tumors are benign.
3. To prevent new solar-induced lesions from developing, future ultraviolet light exposure should be avoided.
4. The prognosis is good. Hemangiomas are benign and not invasive and do not recur after surgical excision; however, malignant transformation of solar-induced lesions may occasionally occur.

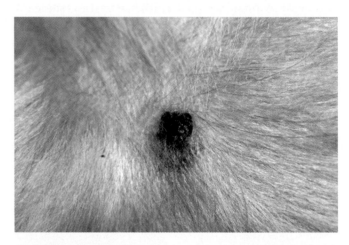

FIGURE 14-79 Hemangioma. A focal vascular proliferation typical of this neoplasm. Note the "bruised" coloration of the nodule.

Hemangiosarcoma

Features

A hemangiosarcoma is a malignant neoplasm of blood vessel endothelial cells that can involve the skin as a primary or metastatic site. Solar damage may be involved in the development of tumors on the ventral glabrous skin in short-coated, lightly pigmented dogs (especially Whippets, Italian Greyhounds, Beagles, Great Danes, and English bulldogs), and on the head and ears in white cats. Hemangiosarcoma is uncommon in older dogs and cats. Among dogs, German shepherds and Golden retrievers may be predisposed to non–sunlight-induced lesions.

Tumors can occur in the dermis (especially of the ventral glabrous skin) or subcutaneous tissue. Tumors may appear clinically similar to hemangioma (bluish to reddish-black plaques or nodules <4 cm), or they can present as poorly defined, subcutaneous, spongy, dark red to black masses that measure up to 10 cm in diameter. Alopecia, bleeding, and ulceration are common. Hemostatic abnormalities such as thrombocytopenia and disseminated intravascular coagulation (DIC) may occur. Lesions occur most commonly on the limbs and trunk in dogs, and on the head, ears, ventral trunk, and distal limbs in cats.

Diagnosis

1. Cytology (may be nondiagnostic): mostly blood with neoplastic endothelial cells that vary in appearance from normal to large, pleomorphic cells with basophilic cytoplasm and prominent nucleoli.
2. Dermatohistopathology: dermal or subcutaneous infiltrative mass of atypical pleomorphic hyperchromatic spindle cells with a tendency to form vascular channels. Mitotic rate is variable.
3. Affected animals should be screened for internal neoplasia and other sites of metastasis (thoracic radiography/abdominal ultrasound).

Treatment and Prognosis

1. Radical surgical excision alone is adequate for dermal tumors.
2. Surgical excision and adjunctive chemotherapy (doxorubicin hydrochloride [Adriamycin], cyclophosphamide [Cytoxan]) are indicated in cases that involve structures deeper than the dermis.
3. The prognosis for strictly dermal tumors is good after complete surgical excision. The prognosis for subcutaneous tumors is poor because of the high incidence of local recurrence or metastasis.

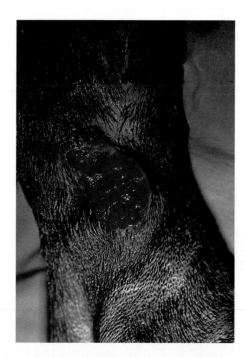

FIGURE 14-80 Hemangiosarcoma. An ulcerated, proliferative tumor on the distal limb of a dog. *(Courtesy L. Schmeitzel.)*

Hemangiopericytoma

Features

A hemangiopericytoma is a neoplasm that arises from vascular pericytes belonging to the diverse family of soft tissue sarcomas. It is common in older dogs, with highest incidence reported in large breeds, especially German shepherds, Irish setters, and Siberian huskies. It is rare in cats.

Usually, hemangiopericytoma manifests as a solitary, well-circumscribed, soft to firm, multinodular, dermal to subcutaneous tumor that ranges from 2 to 25 cm in diameter. Tumor may be fixed to underlying tissue. Lesions may be hyperpigmented, alopecic, or ulcerated and are most commonly found on the limbs, thorax, and flank.

Diagnosis

1. Cytology (these tumors, although mesenchymal in origin, often exfoliate well, resulting in highly cellular samples): tumor cell morphology varies from spindle-shaped to stellate, with wispy light to medium blue cytoplasm and a round or oval nucleus with uniformly stippled chromatin and one to two prominent nucleoli.
2. Dermatohistopathology: multilobular nonencapsulated subcutaneous or dermal mass consisting of small spindle and polygonal cells with few mitotic figures arranged in sheets and concentric whorls around a central vascular lumen. Tumor cells that are not in whorls may appear as plump epithelioid cells with abundant eosinophilic cytoplasm.

Treatment and Prognosis

1. The treatment of choice is radical surgical excision of tumor (2–3 cm lateral margins with inclusion of one deep facial plane) or amputation of the affected limb, if complete excision is not possible.
2. Adjunctive radiation therapy will significantly prolong the disease-free interval for animals with incompletely excised tumors.
3. The prognosis is variable. Tumors may recur locally postsurgically, but metastasis is rare. The tumor's histologic grade, based on mitotic index, degree of histologic differentiation, and percentage of necrosis, will predict the metastatic potential. Tumors present longer than 2 months before surgery and tumors with increased necrosis histologically may have a higher rate of recurrence. Similarly, tumors with a histologically epithelioid pattern and noncutaneous location may present an increased risk for recurrence or metastasis.

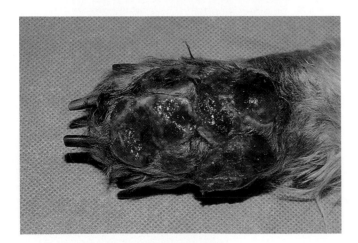

FIGURE 14-81 Hemangiopericytoma. This alopecic, ulcerated tumor on the dorsal surface of the paw is typical of hemangiopericytoma.

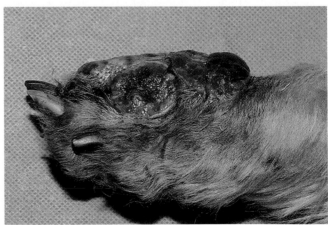

FIGURE 14-82 Hemangiopericytoma. Close-up of the dog in Figure 14-81. This ulcerated, proliferative tumor extends above the foot.

Lipoma

Features

A lipoma is a benign neoplasm of subcutaneous (occasionally dermal) lipocytes. It is common in middle-aged to older dogs, especially Dobermanns, Labradors, and miniature Schnauzers. It is uncommon in older cats, with Siamese cats possibly predisposed.

Lipoma manifests as single to multiple movable, well-circumscribed, dome-shaped to multilobulated, soft to firm, subcutaneous masses that range from 1 to 30 cm in diameter. Less commonly, tumors may be large, soft, poorly circumscribed masses that infiltrate underlying muscle, tendons, and fascia (infiltrative lipoma). Lesions most often occur on the thorax, abdomen, and limbs.

Diagnosis

1. Cytology: aspirates have an oily appearance grossly and often are dissolved in alcohol-containing stains, leaving clear areas with variable numbers of lipocytes containing pyknotic nuclei, which are compressed to the cell membrane by intracellular fat globules.
2. Dermatohistopathology: well-circumscribed nodules composed of solid sheets of mature lipocytes that may have a capsule of mature fibrous tissue. Mitotic figures are not present. Infiltrative lipomas are composed of sheets of mature lipocytes, which spread along fascial planes into muscle bundles and connective tissue.

Treatment and Prognosis

1. For small, well-circumscribed tumors, observation without treatment is reasonable.
2. Surgical excision is the treatment of choice for cosmetically unacceptable or rapidly enlarging tumors.
3. Infiltrative lipomas should be treated with early aggressive surgery, which can be followed by adjunctive radiation, if excision is incomplete.
4. The prognosis is good for well-encapsulated lipomas. The prognosis is guarded for infiltrative lipomas, which often recur postsurgically. Infiltrative lipomas cause destruction of muscle and connective tissue but are not metastatic.

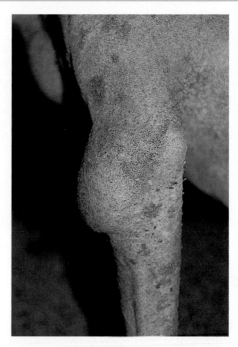

FIGURE 14-83 Lipoma. This soft tumor developed over several years on the forearm of this aged dog.

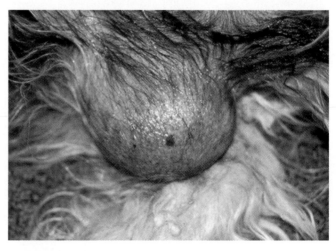

FIGURE 14-84 Lipoma. A large lipoma on the ventral chest of an aged Schnauzer.

Lipoma—*cont'd*

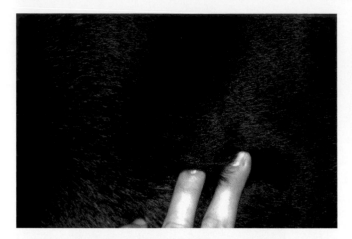

FIGURE 14-85 Lipoma. The lipoma on the lateral thorax of this aged Labrador mix breed was difficult to visualize but was easily palpated.

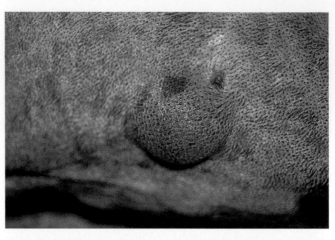

FIGURE 14-86 Lipoma. Close-up of the dog in Figure 14-84. The clipped fur coat allows the tumor to be visualized more easily.

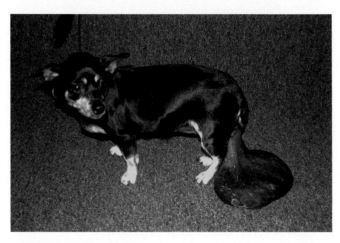

FIGURE 14-87 Lipoma. A huge, pendulous lipoma, originating from the perianal tissue.

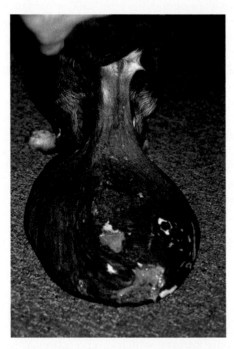

FIGURE 14-88 Lipoma. Same dog as in Figure 14-87. The pendulous nature of this huge lipoma is apparent.

Liposarcoma

Features

A liposarcoma is a malignant tumor of subcutaneous lipoblasts. Liposarcomas are locally invasive and may metastasize to lungs, liver, spleen, or bone. They are rare in dogs and cats. Older animals are predisposed.

Liposarcomas are solitary, poorly circumscribed, soft to firm masses that range from 0.5 to 20 cm in diameter. These tumors are more common in the deep subcutaneous tissue of the chest, ventral abdomen, trunk, and proximal legs.

Diagnosis

1. Liposarcomas are often clinically and cytologically indistinguishable from lipomas, so biopsy is needed for definitive diagnosis.

2. Dermatohistopathology: variably differentiated, stellate, spindle-shaped or round neoplastic lipoblasts with finely vacuolated eosinophilic cytoplasm that stains positively for fat.

Treatment and Prognosis

1. Aggressive surgical excision is the treatment of choice, as tumors are locally invasive.
2. External beam radiation therapy may be useful adjunctive therapy for incompletely resectable masses.
3. The prognosis for cure is guarded because of the invasive nature of this tumor, although postsurgery survival time is often significantly prolonged.

Mast Cell Tumor

Features

A mast cell tumor is a malignant tumor that arises from dermal tissue mast cells. It is the most common cutaneous tumor of the dog (16%–21% of reported tumors) and the second most common tumor of the cat (20% of reported tumors), with highest incidence in older animals. Among dogs, predisposed breeds include Boxers, Pugs, Boston terriers, Labradors, Weimaraners, Beagles, Chinese Shar peis, and Golden retrievers. Among cats, Siamese cats are predisposed.

Dogs

Lesions are variable and may include dermal or subcutaneous edema, papules, nodules, or pedunculated masses that range from a few millimeters to several centimeters in diameter. Lesions may be poorly or well circumscribed, soft or firm, alopecic or ulcerated, and erythematous, hyperpigmented, or flesh colored. Tumors are usually solitary but may be multiple and are most commonly found on the trunk, perineum, and limbs. Concurrent gastric or duodenal ulcers or blood coagulopathy may be seen secondary to release of mast cell granule products (e.g., histamine, heparin).

Cats

Usually, mast cell tumor appears as a solitary intradermal nodule that may be erythematous and alopecic or ulcerated, and that ranges in size from 0.2 to 3 cm. Diffusely swollen infiltrative lesions may occur. Multiple clusters of subcutaneous nodules ranging in size from 0.5 to 1 cm may be found in young (<4 years of age) cats (histiocytic subtype); these tumors may spontaneously regress. Siamese cats appear to be predisposed to both types of mast cell tumors. Tumors are most commonly found on the head and neck. Most cutaneous mast cell tumors in cats are well differentiated and are considered behaviorally benign. Affected cats rarely have systemic abnormalities, although intermittent pruritus and self-trauma are common. Uncommonly, histopathologically anaplastic and behaviorally malignant cutaneous tumors may occur in cats, and metastasis to the skin from a primary visceral mast cell tumor, typically involving the spleen, has been reported.

Diagnosis

1. Cytology: many round cells with round nuclei and basophilic intracytoplasmic granules that stain variably depending on degree of tumor differentiation. Eosinophils may also be seen in association with tumor cells.

2. Dermatohistopathology: nonencapsulated, infiltrative sheets or densely packed cords of round cells with central nuclei and abundant cytoplasm with variably basophilic granules. Eosinophils may be numerous. Histiocytic mast cell tumors of young cats are poorly granulated and contain lymphoid aggregates.

3. Animals with poorly differentiated or incompletely excised tumors or that have signs of systemic disease should be screened for metastasis (regional lymph node aspirate, radiography, ultrasound, ± liver/spleen or bone marrow aspirate).

Treatment and Prognosis

1. For solitary tumors with no metastasis, wide surgical excision (minimum 3-cm margins) is the treatment of choice and is often curative for Grade I (well-differentiated) and Grade II (intermediately differentiated) tumors. Postoperatively, routine follow-up should be performed every 2 to 3 months for reexamination of the surgery site and regional lymph nodes.

2. Radiation therapy prolongs the disease-free interval of incompletely excised tumors.

3. Intralesional triamcinolone has been used in selected cases of incompletely resected or nonresectable tumors, with variable results.

4. For disseminated lesions, treatment with oral prednisone 2 mg/kg/day for 2 weeks, then 1 mg/kg/day for 2 weeks, then 1 mg/kg every 48 hours indefinitely may induce temporary remission/palliation.

5. Additional palliative therapies for metastatic disease include the use of H_1 blockers (e.g., diphenhydramine), H_2 blockers (e.g., cimetidine, famotidine, ranitidine), or the proton pump blocker omeprazole to decrease gastrointestinal effects from hyperhistaminemia. For cases with active gastrointestinal ulceration, sucralfate and misoprostol may be helpful.

6. Chemotherapy in general is of limited value in disseminated disease; however, lomustine (CCNU), vinblastine, or toceranib (Palladia, Pfizer Animal Health) may be effective.

7. The prognosis in dogs is variable and is highly dependent on tumor grade, disease stage, and type of therapy employed. The most important prognostic factor is histologic grade of the tumor; complete excision of Grade I (well-differentiated) tumor is usually curative (<10% metastasis), whereas dogs with Grade III tumors (poorly differentiated) often succumb to local recurrence or metastasis within months (55%–96% metastasis). Increases in cell proliferation markers such as mitotic index >5

(number of mitoses per 10 high power fields), argyrophilic nucleolar staining organizing regions (AgNOR), and Ki-67 confer a poorer prognosis. Tumor location is also prognostically important; tumors in the inguinal, perineal, and subungual regions, on the muzzle, and in the oral or nasal cavity frequently metastasize, whereas appendicular tumors tend to have a better prognosis. Breed can also be prognostic; Boxers tend to have more well-differentiated tumors, and Shar peis tend to have poorly differentiated tumors that are behaviorally aggressive. Multifocal mast cell disease is common in weimaraners, Pugs, Boxers, and Boston terriers. The prognosis for primary cutaneous mast cell tumors in cats is good. Primary cutaneous mast cell tumors in cats are usually benign, and excision is curative. Histiocytic mast cell tumors in young cats usually regress spontaneously over 4 to 24 months.

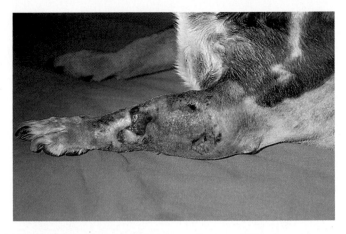

FIGURE 14-91 **Mast Cell Tumor.** Close-up of the dog in Figure 14-90. The forelimb is swollen because of angioedema caused by the histamine that was released. *(Courtesy D. Angarano.)*

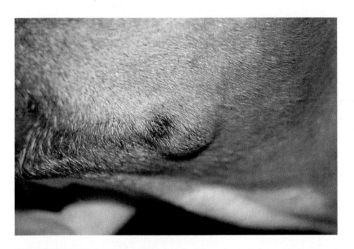

FIGURE 14-89 **Mast Cell Tumor.** A large nodule on the ventral mandible of an adult Boxer.

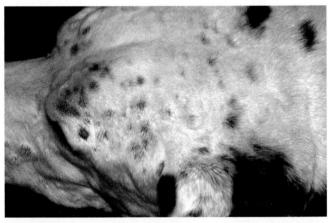

FIGURE 14-92 **Mast Cell Tumor.** Multiple alopecic, erythematous tumors on the head and ear pinna of a Dalmatian.

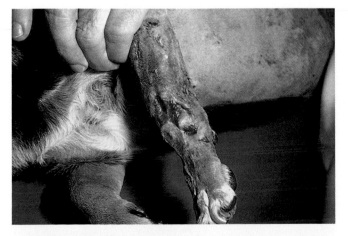

FIGURE 14-90 **Mast Cell Tumor.** Multiple nodules and ulcerations on the distal limb. Just after this picture was taken, the limb began to swell from histamine release that occurred during diagnostic palpation of the tumor. *(Courtesy D. Angarano.)*

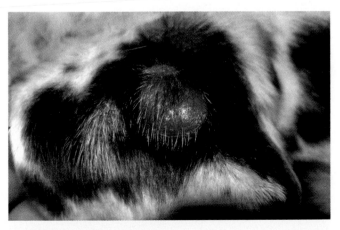

FIGURE 14-93 **Mast Cell Tumor.** Same dog as in Figure 14-92. The alopecic, erythematous nodule on the ear pinna is characteristic of this tumor type.

Mast Cell Tumor—cont'd

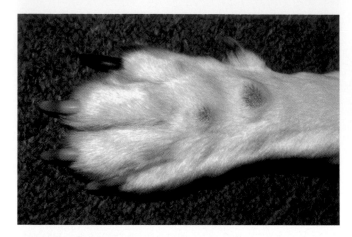

FIGURE 14-94 **Mast Cell Tumor.** Multiple alopecic, erythematous tumors on the foot.

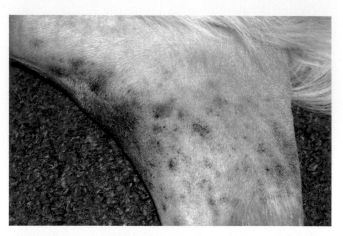

FIGURE 14-95 **Mast Cell Tumor.** Multiple, papular, erythematous lesions on the inner rear leg of an older Golden retriever. Note the similarity to lesions caused by folliculitis (pyoderma, *Demodex*, dermatophytosis).

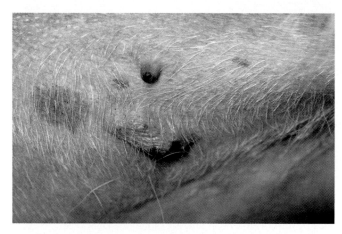

FIGURE 14-96 **Mast Cell Tumor.** A focal mast cell tumor. Note the unusual appearance (droopy skin and absence of a solid nodule, alopecia, or erythema).

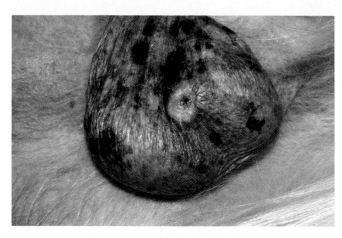

FIGURE 14-97 **Mast Cell Tumor.** A focal, ulcerated mast cell tumor on the scrotum. Note similarity to squamous cell carcinoma.

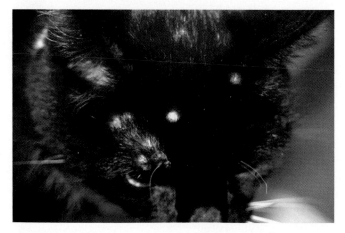

FIGURE 14-98 **Mast Cell Tumor.** Multiple alopecic nodules on the head of an adult cat are typical of this tumor in felines.

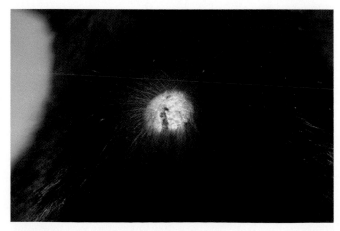

FIGURE 14-99 **Mast Cell Tumor.** Focal alopecia at the nodule on the dorsum of an adult cat.

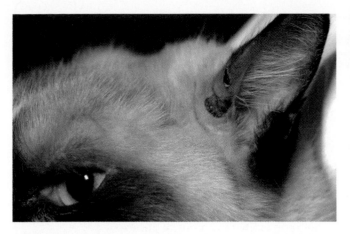

FIGURE 14-100 **Mast Cell Tumor.** An erythematous, alopecic nodule at the base of the ear pinna on an adult Siamese cat. *(Courtesy R. Seamen.)*

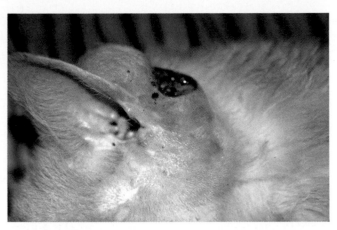

FIGURE 14-101 **Mast Cell Tumor.** A large, ulcerated tumor at the base of a cat's ear pinna.

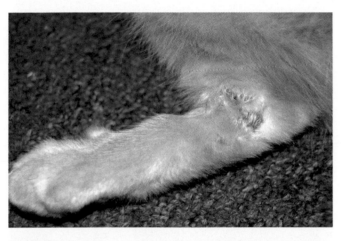

FIGURE 14-102 **Mast Cell Tumor.** Same cat as in Figure 14-101. Multiple nodular tumors on the distal extremity of a cat with metastatic mast cell tumors.

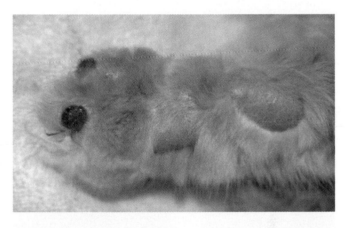

FIGURE 14-103 **Mast Cell Tumor.** Multiple alopecic nodules on the distal extremity of an adult cat. Note the variation in tumor characteristics, with some lesions being erythematous and ulcerated.

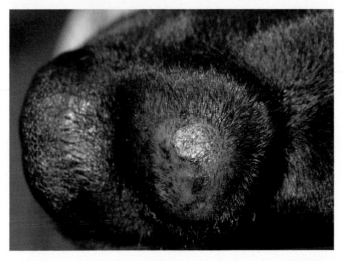

FIGURE 14-104 **Mast Cell Tumor.** This focal infiltrated lesion with alopecia and erosion of the skin surface is typical for mast cell tumors. Note the similarity to a fungal kerion.

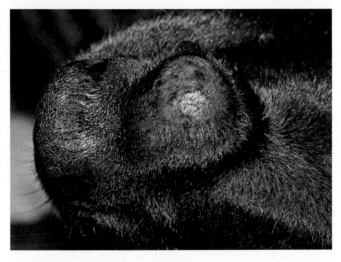

FIGURE 14-105 **Mast Cell Tumor.** A focal tumor on the nose of a middle-aged dog demonstrating alopecia and cutaneous erosion. Note the similarity to a fungal kerion.

Nonepitheliotropic Lymphoma (lymphosarcoma)

Features

Nonepitheliotropic lymphoma is a malignant neoplasm that may arise from B or T lymphocytes. It is uncommon in dogs and cats, with highest incidence in older animals.

Usually, nonepitheliotropic lymphoma appears as multiple, firm, dermal to subcutaneous nodules that may be alopecic and frequently ulcerated. Tumors may occur in arciform or serpiginous shapes. Lesions occur most frequently on the trunk, head, and extremities. Pruritus and oral mucosal involvement are rare. Concurrent signs of systemic involvement are common.

Diagnosis

1. Cytology: numerous neoplastic lymphocytes.
2. Dermatohistopathology: nodular to diffuse infiltration of dermis ± subcutis by sheets of homogenous neoplastic lymphocytes that do not involve glands or hair follicles.
3. Affected animals should be screened for internal organ and lymph node involvement.

Treatment and Prognosis

1. For solitary lesions, surgical excision or radiation therapy is the treatment of choice.
2. For disseminated disease, combination chemotherapy (prednisone with cytotoxic drugs such as cyclophosphamide, vincristine, L-asparaginase, and doxorubicin) may induce a durable remission, especially in non–T-cell lymphoma.
3. The prognosis is poor. Tumors are highly malignant and typically involve multiple organs and other body systems.

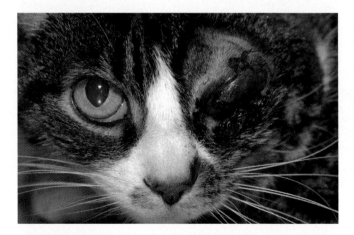

FIGURE 14-106 Nonepitheliotropic Lymphoma. A large, erosive tumor originating from the conjunctival tissue of an adult cat. *(Courtesy R. Seamen.)*

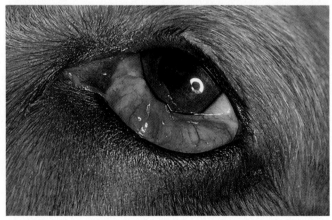

FIGURE 14-107 Nonepitheliotropic Lymphoma. Conjunctival tissue was infiltrated with neoplastic lymphocytes. *(Courtesy J. MacDonald.)*

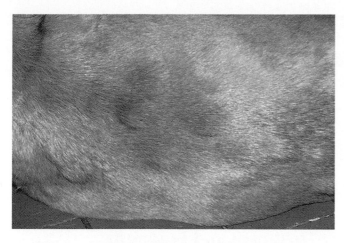

FIGURE 14-108 Nonepitheliotropic Lymphoma. Multiple nodules on the dorsum of an aged Labrador. *(Courtesy J. MacDonald.)*

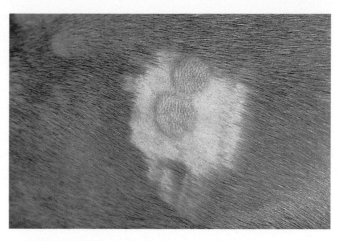

FIGURE 14-109 Nonepitheliotropic Lymphoma. Close-up of the dog in Figure 14-108. The area has been clipped to provide better visualization of the tumors. *(Courtesy J. MacDonald.)*

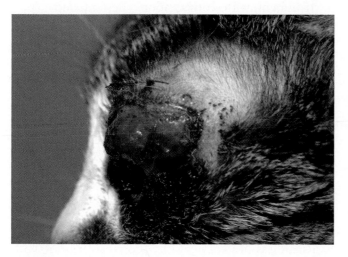

FIGURE 14-110 Nonepitheliotropic Lymphoma. The large, eroded, conjunctival tumor protrudes from the cat's eye. *(Courtesy R. Seamen.)*

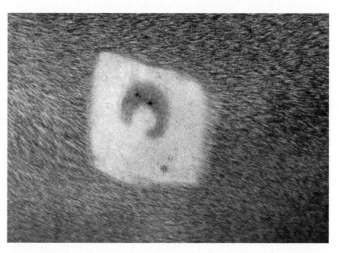

FIGURE 14-111 Nonepitheliotropic Lymphoma. A C-shaped tumor on the trunk of an aged dog. *(Courtesy D. Angarano.)*

Epitheliotropic Lymphoma (mycosis fungoides)

Features

Epitheliotropic lymphoma is a malignant neoplasm that arises from T lymphocytes. It is uncommon in dogs and cats, with highest incidence in older animals. Among dogs, Scottish terriers, Boxers, and Golden retrievers are predisposed.

Dogs

Cutaneous symptoms may include single to multiple plaques or nodules that range from a few millimeters to several centimeters in diameter. Mucocutaneous depigmentation and ulceration or generalized erythema, alopecia, scaling, and pruritus may occur. Footpads may be hyperkeratotic, ulcerated, or depigmented. Ulcerative stomatitis may be present. Most cases occur as a slowly progressive disease; chronicity, peripheral lymphadenomegaly, and signs of systemic involvement are commonly seen.

Cats

Cutaneous symptoms include pruritic exfoliative erythroderma with alopecia and crusting. Erythematous plaques or nodules may occur, especially on the head and neck. Oral and mucocutaneous involvement is less common than in the dog.

Diagnosis

1. Cytology: abundant round neoplastic lymphoid cells that are often histiocytic, with basophilic cytoplasm and pleomorphic, indented to lobular nuclei.

2. Dermatohistopathology: lichenoid band of pleomorphic neoplastic lymphocytes that infiltrate the superficial dermis and the surface of follicular and sweat gland epithelia. Neoplastic cells may occur within small intraepidermal vesicles (Pautrier's microabscesses).

3. Affected animals should be screened for internal organ and lymph node involvement.

Treatment and Prognosis

1. For solitary lesions, surgical excision or radiation therapy (especially, electron beam therapy) is the treatment of choice.

2. Treatment with combination chemotherapy (prednisone and cytotoxic drugs) is only minimally effective. Anecdotally, lomustine (CCNU), pegasparaginase, or pegylated liposomal doxorubicin (Doxil) may be more effective than other drugs.

3. Treatment with isotretinoin 3–4 mg/kg/day (dogs) or 10 mg/cat every 24 hours (cats) PO may improve clinical signs in some affected animals.

4. Anecdotally, interferon (Roferon-A, Hoffmann-LaRoche) 1–1.5 million U/m² administered SC three times weekly may be effective in some dogs.

5. Supplementation with safflower oil (which contains high levels of linoleic acid) 3 mL/kg PO mixed with food twice weekly may improve clinical signs in some animals.

6. Regardless of treatment, the prognosis is poor, with most animals surviving less than 6 months after diagnosis.

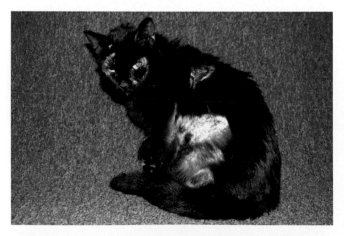

FIGURE 14-112 Epitheliotropic Lymphoma. Multiple alopecic, crusting, ulcerated tumors covering the entire body of an adult cat. The cat had been previously treated for allergic dermatitis without response.

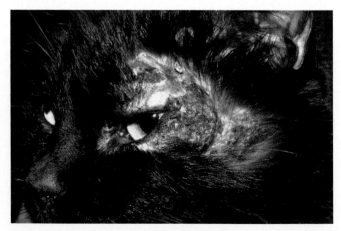

FIGURE 14-113 Epitheliotropic Lymphoma. Same cat as in Figure 14-112. Alopecic, crusting, ulcerated lesions surround the eye.

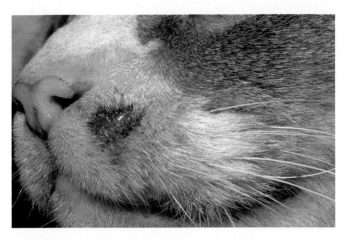

FIGURE 14-114 Epitheliotropic Lymphoma. Focal, alopecic, ulcerated lesions on a cat's lip. Note that the entire lip is swollen, which is caused by the infiltrating neoplastic cells.

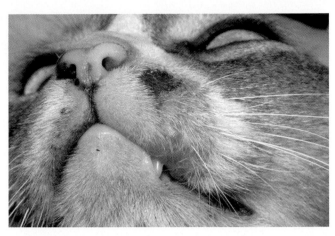

FIGURE 14-115 Epitheliotropic Lymphoma. Same cat as in Figure 14-114. The ulcerated lesion and a symmetrical swollen lip are apparent.

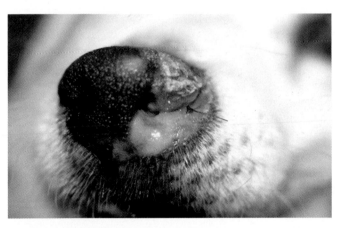

FIGURE 14-116 Epitheliotropic Lymphoma. Unilateral depigmentation, ulceration, and tissue destruction on the nasal planum of a dog. Note the similarity to autoimmune skin disease, vasculitis, and drug reaction.

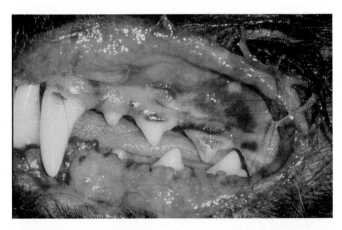

FIGURE 14-117 Epitheliotropic Lymphoma. Severe swelling and exudation of the oral mucosa caused by tumor infiltration. Note the similarity to autoimmune skin disease, vasculitis, and drug reaction.

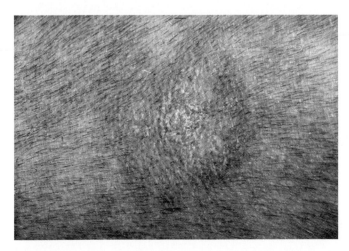

FIGURE 14-118 Epitheliotropic Lymphoma. This erythematous, scaling plaque is typical of mild tumor lesions.

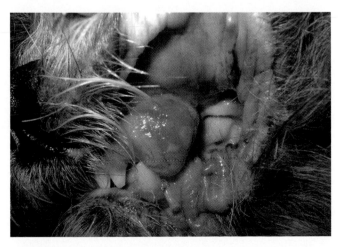

FIGURE 14-119 Epitheliotropic Lymphoma. Focal mass on the gingiva.

Epitheliotropic Lymphoma—*cont'd*

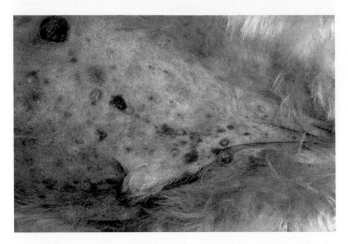

FIGURE 14-120 Epitheliotropic Lymphoma. Multiple erythematous papules and nodules on the abdomen. Note the similarity to lesions caused by folliculitis (pyoderma, *Demodex*, dermatophytosis).

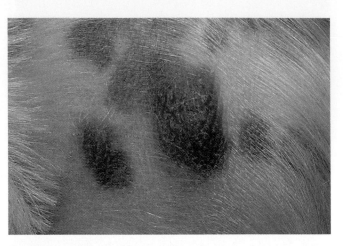

FIGURE 14-121 Epitheliotropic Lymphoma. Erythematous nodules on the trunk.

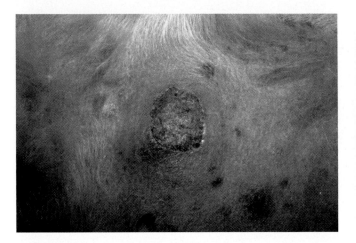

FIGURE 14-122 Epitheliotropic Lymphoma. A large, crusting, ulcerative lesion on the abdomen. Note the surrounding erythematous papular lesions, which could easily be confused with folliculitis.

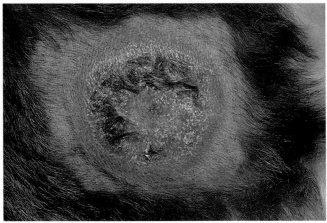

FIGURE 14-123 Epitheliotropic Lymphoma. This large, erythematous, alopecic tumor has a central crater-like depression.

Cutaneous Plasmacytoma

Features

Cutaneous plasmacytoma is a neoplasm of plasma cell origin. It is uncommon in dogs, with highest incidence in older animals. Cocker spaniels may be predisposed. The condition is very rare in cats.

Usually, cutaneous plasmacytoma appears as a solitary, well-circumscribed, soft or firm, occasionally pedunculated or ulcerated, erythematous, dermal nodule that ranges from a few millimeters to several centimeters (usually 1–2 cm) in diameter. Lesions most often are found in the external ear canal, or on the lips, trunk, or digits. Digital lesions may be ulcerated and may bleed easily. Concurrent multiple myeloma is rare in dogs but may be more common in cats, especially with plasmacytomas localized to the hock region.

Diagnosis

1. Cytology: many round cells that may appear like typical plasma cells with perinuclear halos or that may be less plasmacytoid with a moderate amount of dark blue cytoplasm and round eccentric nuclei with stippled chromatin. Binucleate and multinucleate cells are common.
2. Dermatohistopathology: well-circumscribed round cell tumor with cells arranged in small solid lobules separated by a delicate stroma. Marked cellular pleomorphism, occasional binucleate cells, and moderate to marked mitotic index are present. Recognizable plasma cells with perinuclear halos are visible, mostly on the periphery.

Treatment and Prognosis

1. The treatment of choice is complete surgical excision.
2. The prognosis is good in dogs. Local recurrence and metastasis are rare. In cats, the prognosis is guarded, with systemic disease or metastasis to regional lymph nodes likely.

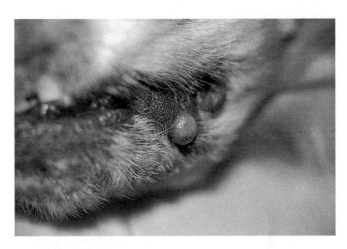

FIGURE 14-125 Cutaneous Plasmacytoma. Small alopecic nodule on the lower lip of an adult mixed breed.

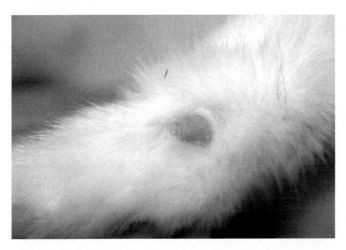

FIGURE 14-124 Cutaneous Plasmacytoma. Focal, alopecic nodule on the distal leg.

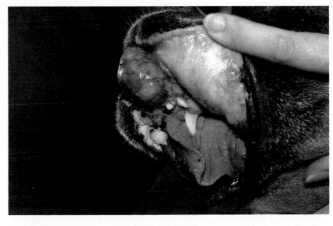

FIGURE 14-126 Cutaneous Plasmacytoma. Large proliferative tumor on the gingiva.

Cutaneous Histiocytoma

Features

Cutaneous histiocytoma is a benign neoplasm of mononuclear cells derived from epidermal Langerhans' cells. It is common in dogs, with highest incidence in young adults younger than 4 years old. It is rare in cats.

Usually, this condition manifests as a solitary, rapidly growing, firm, well-circumscribed, erythematous, raised, alopecic dermal nodule that ranges from 0.5 to 4 cm in diameter. Lesions may be ulcerated and occur most commonly on the head, ear pinnae, and legs.

Diagnosis

1. Cytology: large, round cells with a moderate amount of pale blue, finely granular cytoplasm and round or kidney bean–shaped nuclei with lacy chromatin, multiple indistinct nucleoli, and occasional to many mitotic figures. Aspirates from regressing lesions also contain lymphocytes.
2. Dermatohistopathology: circumscribed, dense dermal infiltrative sheets of homogenous to pleomorphic histiocytes that may extend to the epithelium. Mitotic figures may be seen, and lymphocytic infiltration is common. Older lesions often contain multifocal areas of necrosis.

Treatment and Prognosis

1. Observation without treatment is reasonable because most lesions regress spontaneously within 3 months.
2. Surgical excision or cryotherapy is curative for lesions that do not regress spontaneously.
3. The prognosis is good.

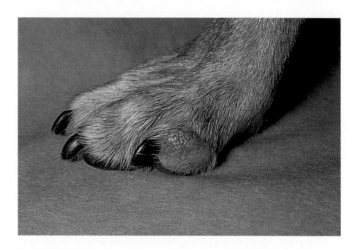

FIGURE 14-128 Cutaneous Histiocytoma. The alopecic, erythematous tumor on the foot of this young dog is typical of cutaneous histiocytoma. *(Courtesy D. Angarano.)*

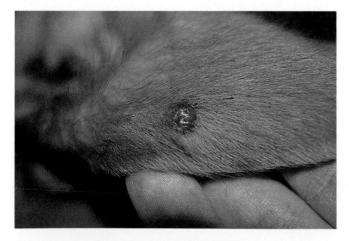

FIGURE 14-127 Cutaneous Histiocytoma. Small, alopecic, erythematous nodule on the ear pinna of a young adult dog.

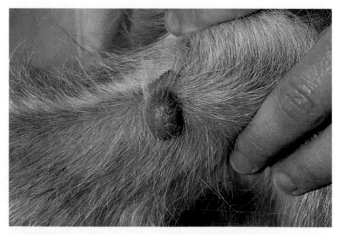

FIGURE 14-129 Cutaneous Histiocytoma. An alopecic, erythematous tumor on the distal limb of a young dog is typical of this neoplasia. *(Courtesy D. Angarano.)*

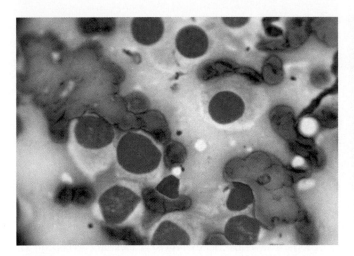

FIGURE 14-130 Cutaneous Histiocytoma. Microscopic image of typical round cells from a fine needle aspirate of a histiocytoma as seen with a 100× (oil) objective.

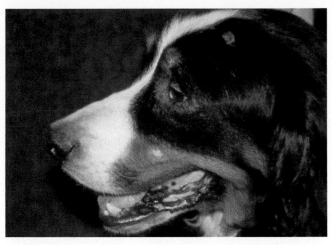

FIGURE 14-131 Cutaneous Histiocytoma. Multiple alopecic nodules on the head of an adult Bernese mountain Dog.

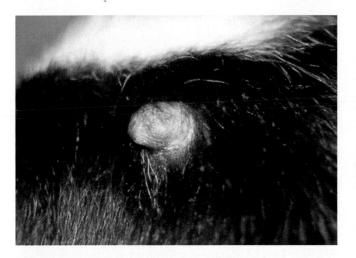

FIGURE 14-132 Cutaneous Histiocytoma. Close-up of the dog in Figure 14-131. The alopecic nodule on the head is apparent.

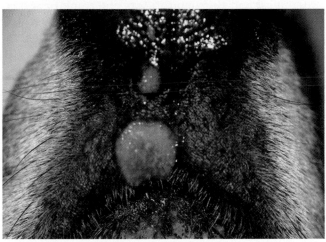

FIGURE 14-133 Cutaneous Histiocytoma. A focal lesion on the muzzle of a young dog demonstrating the thickened infiltrative nature of the lesion.

Cutaneous Histiocytosis

Features

Cutaneous histiocytosis is a rare, benign, histiocytic, proliferative disorder in dogs that involves cutaneous structures only and is thought to represent a reactive, not a neoplastic, process. Affected dogs range in age from 2 to 13 years. Golden Retrievers, Shelties, and collies may be predisposed.

Multiple dermal (rarely subcutaneous) erythematous nodules or plaques may be alopecic or ulcerated and range in size from 1 to 5 cm. Nodules are not painful or pruritic unless they become secondarily infected. The number of lesions is variable and can range from a few to more than 50. Lesions occur most frequently on the head, neck, perineum, scrotum, and extremities, and they tend to wax and wane or regress and appear at new areas. Nasal mucosal involvement may occur, but systemic and lymph node involvement does not occur.

Diagnosis

1. Cytology: numerous large, pale, round to oval histiocytes.
2. Dermatohistopathology: diffuse, often periadnexal or perivascular accumulations of a mixture of lymphocytes, plasma cells, neutrophils, and large histiocytes, with large vesicular and often indented nuclei. Mitotic figures are numerous, and vascular involvement or thrombosis may occur. Special stains are required to rule out infectious causes of histiocytic inflammation.

Treatment and Prognosis

1. Approximately 50% of cases respond to immunosuppressive doses of glucocorticosteroids. Addition of cytotoxic drugs to the treatment regimen may improve response.
2. Cyclosporine (Atopica) A or leflunomide is useful in cases that respond poorly to corticosteroids.
3. Surgical excision is successful in a minority of cases.
4. The prognosis is guarded. Although systemic involvement does not occur, most cases are episodic or continually progressive and need long-term immunosuppressive therapy for control.

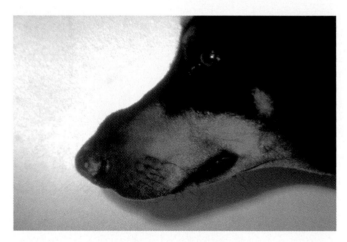

FIGURE 14-134 Cutaneous Histiocytosis. Multiple nodules on the face of an adult dog. *(Courtesy L. Frank.)*

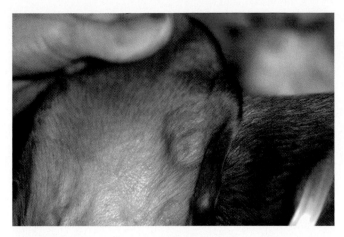

FIGURE 14-135 Cutaneous Histiocytosis. Same dog as in Figure 14-134. Multiple nodules on the ear pinna. *(Courtesy L. Frank.)*

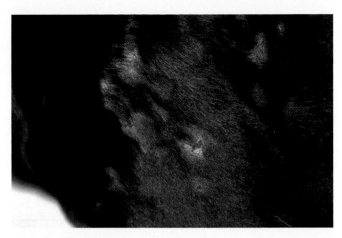

FIGURE 14-136 Cutaneous Histiocytosis. Same dog as in Figure 14-134. Note multiple nodules on the body. *(Courtesy L. Frank.)*

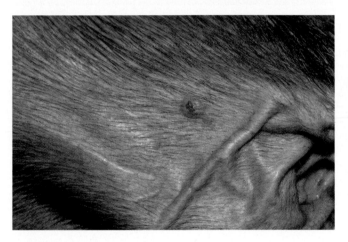

FIGURE 14-137 Cutaneous Histiocytosis. A focal lesion on the ear pinna of an infected dog.

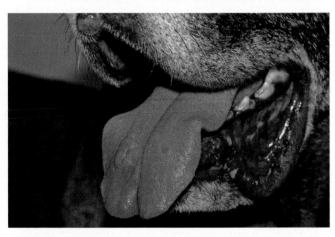

FIGURE 14-138 Cutaneous Histiocytosis. A focal infiltrative lesion on the tongue of an infected dog. This patient developed multiple focal lesions caused by the infection.

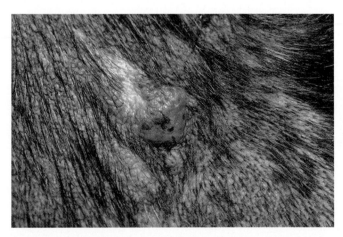

FIGURE 14-139 Cutaneous Histiocytosis. A focal lesion without purulent drainage, which is typical of other deep infections.

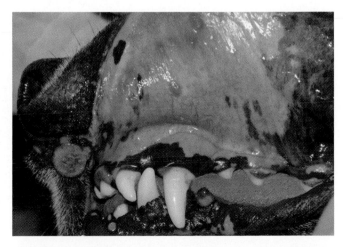

FIGURE 14-140 Cutaneous Histiocytosis. Focal infiltrative lesion on the lips and nasal planum caused by the infection.

Cutaneous Histiocytosis—*cont'd*

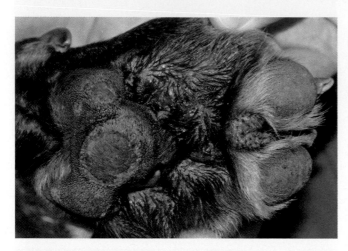

FIGURE 14-141 Cutaneous Histiocytosis. Deep ulceration of the footpads caused by the deep infection. Note the similarity to autoimmune skin disease. A biopsy and culture would differentiate the two diseases.

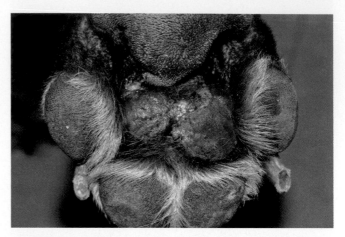

FIGURE 14-142 Cutaneous Histiocytosis. Same dog as in Figure 14-141. Multiple footpads have ulcerated as a result of the deep infection.

Systemic Histiocytosis

Features

Systemic histiocytosis is a proliferative disorder of histiocytes that involves the skin and internal organs. It is rare in dogs, with highest incidence in young adult to middle-aged male Bernese mountain dogs.

Multifocal haired or alopecic papules, plaques, and nodules may be alopecic or ulcerated. Lesions affect eyelids, muzzle, planum nasale, extremities, and scrotum most severely. Nodules measure up to 4 cm in diameter, may extend into the subcutis, and are not painful or pruritic. Generalized lymphadenomegaly may occur. Lesions may also develop in the lung, spleen, liver, bone marrow, and nasal cavity, causing noncutaneous signs of anorexia, weight loss, and respiratory stertor; in these cases, the disease more closely resembles malignant histiocytosis (see below). In some dogs, the disease is rapidly progressive, whereas in others, the course is more prolonged with alternating episodes of exacerbation and remission.

Diagnosis

1. Cytology: numerous large, pale, round to oval histiocytes.
2. Dermatohistopathology of skin/affected internal organs: diffuse, often periadnexal or perivascular accumulations of a mixture of lymphocytes, plasma cells, neutrophils, and large histiocytes with large vesicular and often indented nuclei. Mitotic figures are numerous, and vascular involvement or thrombosis is common. Special stains are required to rule out infectious causes of histiocytic inflammation.

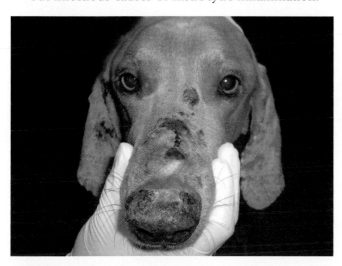

FIGURE 14-143 Systemic Histiocytosis. Multiple ulcerated nodules on the face and nasal planum of an adult Weimaraner. Note the similarity of the lesions on the nasal planum to autoimmune skin disease and epitheliotropic lymphoma.

Treatment and Prognosis

1. Immunosuppressive doses of glucocorticosteroids are usually ineffective.
2. Cyclosporine (Atopica) A or leflunomide has been used successfully in some cases. Although some dogs may remain asymptomatic for an indefinite time after cessation of therapy, others need continuous therapy to maintain remission.
3. The prognosis is guarded to poor. Most cases are episodic or continually progressive and require long-term immunosuppressive therapy.

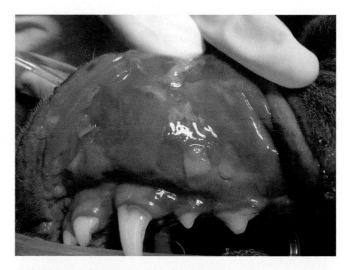

FIGURE 14-144 Systemic Histiocytosis. Same dog as in Figure 14-143. Erosions on the oral mucosa.

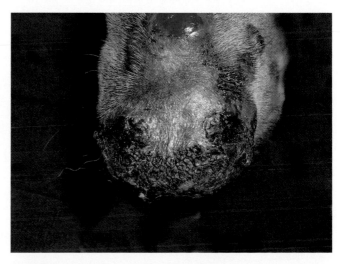

FIGURE 14-145 Systemic Histiocytosis. Same dog as in Figure 14-143. Multiple ulcerated nodules on the face and nasal planum of an adult Weimaraner. Note the similarity of the lesions on the nasal planum to autoimmune skin disease and epitheliotropic lymphoma.

Systemic Histiocytosis—*cont'd*

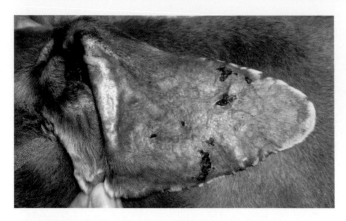

FIGURE 14-146 Systemic Histiocytosis. Same dog as in Figure 14-143. Multiple nodules on the ear pinna.

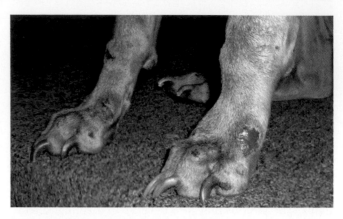

FIGURE 14-147 Systemic Histiocytosis. Same dog as in Figure 14-143. Multiple ulcerated nodules on the legs and feet of an adult Weimaraner.

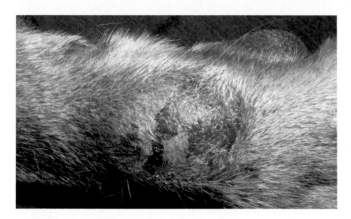

FIGURE 14-148 Systemic Histiocytosis. Same dog as in Figure 14-143. Alopecic eroded nodule on the leg.

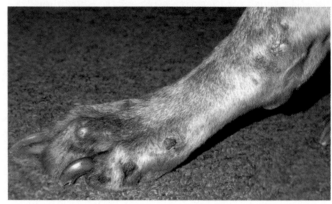

FIGURE 14-149 Systemic Histiocytosis. Same dog as in Figure 14-143. Multiple ulcerated nodules on the legs and feet of an adult Weimaraner.

Malignant Histiocytosis

Features

Malignant histiocytosis is a malignant neoplasm of histiocytes. It is rare in dogs, with highest incidence in middle-aged to older dogs and in Bernese mountain dogs. Other predisposed breeds include Labradors, Rottweilers, Golden retrievers, and Flat coated retrievers.

Cutaneous lesions are uncommon, but if present, they are characterized by multiple, firm, dermal to subcutaneous nodules that may be alopecic or ulcerated. Lesions may appear anywhere on the body. The spleen, lymph nodes, lung, and bone marrow are primarily affected, and animals with widespread disease may have lesions in other organs, such as the liver, bone, central nervous system (CNS), and kidneys. Common clinical symptoms include lethargy, weight loss, lymphadenomegaly, hepatosplenomegaly, pancytopenia, respiratory signs, and CNS disease.

Diagnosis

1. Cytology (may be nondiagnostic): large pleomorphic, atypical histiocytes with abundant finely granulated or vacuolated cytoplasm and single or multiple oval to reniform nuclei. Phagocytosis of erythrocytes and leukocytes by multinucleated tumor cells is commonly seen.
2. Dermatohistopathology (skin or affected internal organs): nonencapsulated, poorly demarcated proliferation of pleomorphic anaplastic histiocytes that may be round or spindle-shaped. Multinucleated giant cells, cells with abnormal nuclei, and bizarre mitotic figures are common.

Treatment and Prognosis

Although chemotherapy may prolong survival in some cases, the prognosis is poor. Malignant histiocytosis is a highly malignant, rapidly progressive, and fatal disease.

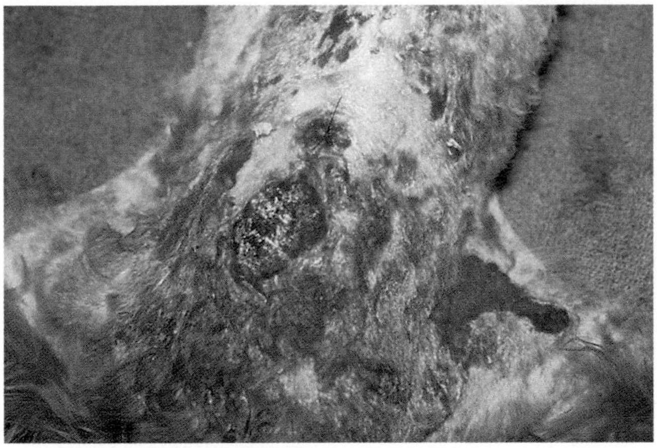

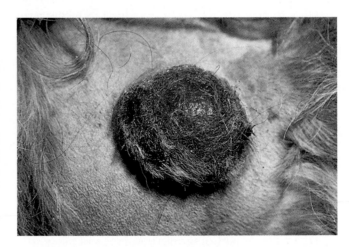

FIGURE 14-150 Malignant Histiocytosis. Generalized areas of alopecia, erythema, erosions, and crusting. *(Courtesy D. Angarano.)*

FIGURE 14-151 Malignant Histiocytosis. Close-up of the dog in Figure 14-150. Alopecia, erythema, and erosions on the scrotum. *(Courtesy D. Angarano.)*

Cutaneous Melanocytoma/Melanoma

Features

This condition is characterized by a benign (melanocytoma) or malignant (melanoma) proliferation of melanocytes. Most cases (85%) are benign. Because in dogs melanocytomas/melanomas arise from the haired skin or oral cavity, sun exposure does not appear to be a causative factor. Breed and familial clustering in domestic animals suggests that genetic susceptibility may be a factor. Alterations in oncogenes, tumor suppressor genes, and immune surveillance are also involved. These tumors are common in older dogs and are rare in older cats. Among dogs, predisposed breeds include Scottish terriers, Airedales, Dobermann pinschers, Cocker spaniels, Poodles, Irish setters, and Schnauzers.

Melanocytomas are usually solitary, well-circumscribed, dome-shaped, firm, brown to black, alopecic, pedunculated or wartlike growths that range from 0.5 to 10 cm in diameter. Plaquelike tumors can also occur. Malignant melanomas may be pigmented or nonpigmented (amelanotic), may be ulcerated, and tend to be larger and more rapidly growing than benign melanocytomas. Malignant tumors tend to metastasize first to regional lymph nodes, then to the lungs. Lesions may appear anywhere on the body, but in dogs, they occur most commonly on the head, trunk, and digits. In cats, lesions are found most commonly on the head.

Diagnosis

1. Cytology: round, oval, stellate or spindle-shaped cells with a moderate amount of cytoplasm, containing granules of brown to green-black pigment. Malignant melanomas may have less pigment and show greater pleomorphism, but malignancy cannot be reliably determined cytologically.
2. Dermatohistopathology: accumulation of neoplastic melanocytes that may be spindle, epithelial, or round cell in appearance with variable degrees of pigmentation. Cells may be arranged in clusters, cords, or nervelike whorls. Infiltration of pigment-laden macrophages is common. Benign neoplasms are circumscribed and have low nuclear variability and a low mitotic rate. Malignant melanomas may show greater invasiveness, more extensive cellular pleomorphism, and increased mitotic figures (including atypical mitotic figures). Mitotic index is the most reliable way to predict biologic behavior (a mitotic rate of <3 mitoses/10 high power fields is usually associated with benign behavior); however, 10% of histologically benign melanocytomas behave in a malignant manner.
3. Animals with malignant melanomas should be screened for regional lymph node and internal metastasis to the thorax and abdomen.

Treatment and Prognosis

1. The treatment of choice is radical surgical excision because benign melanocytomas cannot be clinically differentiated from malignant melanomas.
2. If surgical excision is incomplete, adjunctive treatment options include radiation therapy and local hyperthermia.
3. Chemotherapy (carboplatin, doxorubicin, piroxicam, and dacarbazine) may prolong survival in some cases of malignant disease, but in general, response rates to chemotherapy are low.
4. Although it was evaluated primarily in canine oral malignant melanoma, the Merial melanoma xenogenic DNA vaccine may be useful to combat systemic metastasis in malignant cutaneous melanocytomas.
5. The prognosis is good for benign melanocytomas. The prognosis is poor for malignant melanomas, especially if the tumor is large, with recurrence following surgery and metastasis common. Tumor location is prognostic: most oral and mucocutaneous melanomas (except the eyelid) and 50% of melanomas involving the nail beds are malignant. Breed is also prognostic: >75% of melanocytic neoplasms in Dobermanns and miniature Schnauzers are behaviorally benign, and 85% of those in miniature Poodles are behaviorally malignant.

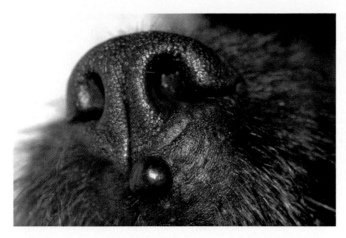

FIGURE 14-152 Cutaneous Melanocytoma/Melanoma. A pigmented nodule in close proximity to the nasal planum of an adult dog.

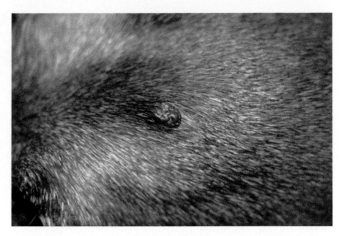

FIGURE 14-153 Cutaneous Melanocytoma/Melanoma. A focal pigmented nodule on the head of an adult dog.

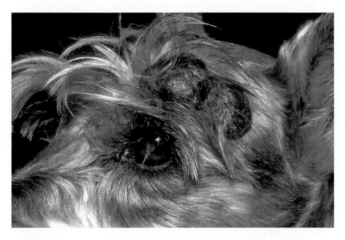

FIGURE 14-154 Cutaneous Melanocytoma/Melanoma. A multilobulated, alopecic, hyperpigmented melanoma on the head of an adult Schnauzer.

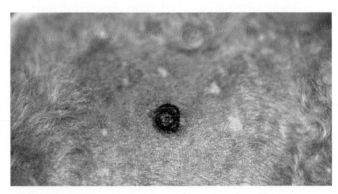

FIGURE 14-155 Cutaneous Melanocytoma/Melanoma. A focal pigmented nodule.

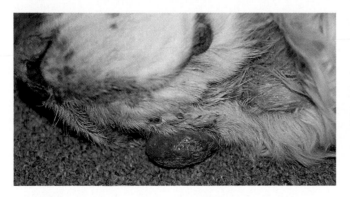

FIGURE 14-156 Cutaneous Melanocytoma/Melanoma. An ulcerated, amelanotic melanoma on the ventral neck of an aged Cocker spaniel.

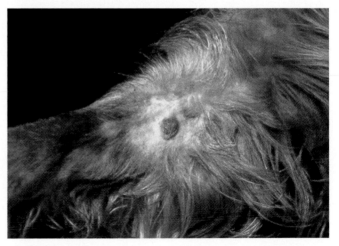

FIGURE 14-157 Cutaneous Melanocytoma/Melanoma. A small, pigmented nodule on the distal limb of an adult Golden retriever.

Transmissible Venereal Tumor (TVT)

Features

Transmissible venereal tumor (TVT) is a benign to malignant neoplasm of unknown cell origin that may be virally induced. Most TVT tumor cells have 59 chromosomes, in contrast to normal dog cells, which have 78. The expression of major histocompatibility class (MHC) II antigen by canine TVT cells has suggested a reticuloendothelial origin. Neoplastic cells also express lysozyme and α_1-antitrypsin immunoreactivity, along with a canine macrophage marker, supporting a monocyte/macrophage lineage histogenesis of TVT. Viable neoplastic cells are most often transplanted during coitus but can be inoculated into multiple sites by licking, sniffing, or scratching. Naturally infected dogs may develop an antitumor immunologic response, which induces spontaneous resolution of disease. This condition is uncommon in dogs, with highest incidence reported in sexually active female dogs in the tropics and subtropics.

Single to multiple, firm to friable, red to flesh-colored, often hemorrhagic, dermal or subcutaneous, nodular or wartlike masses range from 1 to 20 cm in diameter. Lesions most commonly involve external genitalia but may also occur elsewhere on the body, especially on the face and limbs. Ulceration and secondary bacterial infection may occur. Metastasis (to lymph nodes, skin, eye, liver, or brain) is rare but can occur, especially in immunosuppressed animals and puppies.

Diagnosis

1. Cytology: large, pleomorphic, round cells with a moderate amount of medium blue, distinctly vacuolated cytoplasm, and round nuclei with coarse chromatin and one to two large nucleoli. Mitotic figures and low numbers of lymphocytes, plasma cells, and histiocytes may be seen.
2. Dermatohistopathology: sheets of uniform round cells interspersed with a delicate collagenous stroma. Nuclei are large and hyperchromatic, and cells contain abundant light blue vacuolated cytoplasm. The mitotic index is high. Necrosis or lymphocytic infiltration may be present.

Treatment and Prognosis

1. The treatment of choice is vincristine 0.5–0.7 mg/m^2 IV every 7 days until complete clinical remission occurs (approximately 4–6 weeks).
2. Alternatively, treatment with external beam radiation therapy may be effective in vincristine-resistant cases.
3. Although surgical removal may be considered for small, localized lesions, the postsurgical recurrence rate is 20% to 60%.
4. The prognosis is generally good. Although tumors may spontaneously regress, treatment is recommended to prevent metastasis.

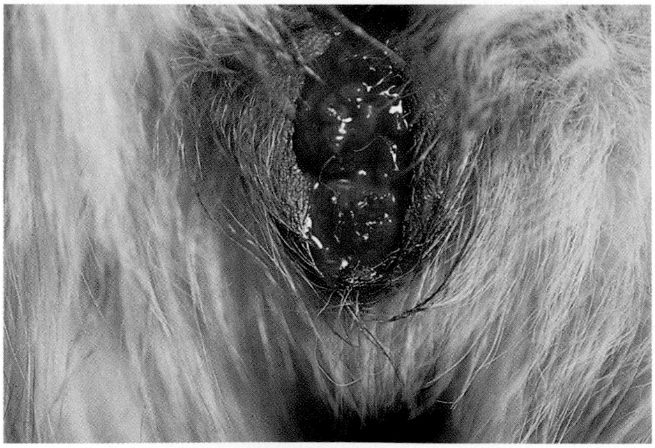

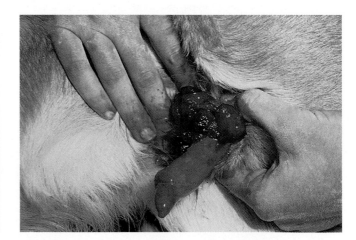

FIGURE 14-158 Transmissible Venereal Tumor. A multilobulated tumor on the vaginal mucosa of an adult dog. The cauliflower-shaped mass is typical of transmissible venereal tumor.

FIGURE 14-159 Transmissible Venereal Tumor. A large, multilobulated mass on the base of the penis of an adult dog. The hemorrhage was caused by prepuce that traumatized the tumor. *(Courtesy C. Calvert.)*

Collagenous Nevus

Features

Collagenous nevus is a developmental defect of the skin that may or may not be congenital, and is characterized by collagenous hyperplasia. The condition is uncommon in dogs.

Usually, collagenous nevus appears as single, firm, well-circumscribed, flat to dome-shaped dermal nodules 0.5 to 5 cm in diameter (usually <1 cm). Lesions may have pitted surfaces and may be alopecic or hyperpigmented. Lesions may appear anywhere on the body but are most common on the head, neck, and legs.

Diagnosis

Dermatohistopathology: poorly cellular mass of mature collagen that does not usually displace adnexal structures.

Treatment and Prognosis

1. Observation without treatment is reasonable because these are benign lesions.
2. For cosmetically unacceptable lesions, surgical excision is curative.
3. The prognosis is good, as tumors are not neoplastic.

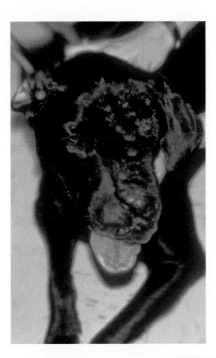

FIGURE 14-160 Collagenous Nevus. Multiple nodules and tumors on the head of an adult Labrador. *(Courtesy University of Florida, case material.)*

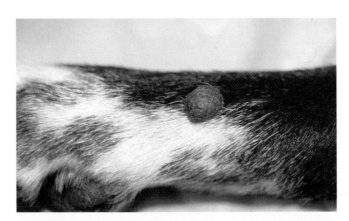

FIGURE 14-161 Collagenous Nevus. This solitary alopecic, hyperpigmented nodule is typical of this tumor.

Follicular Cyst–Epidermal Inclusion Cyst (infundibular cyst)

Features

This is a nonneoplastic cystic structure that contains an epithelial lining. It is common in dogs and uncommon in cats, with highest incidence reported in middle-aged animals. In dogs, predisposed breeds may include Boxers, Shih tzus, Schnauzers, and Basset hounds.

Usually, a solitary, well-circumscribed, firm to fluctuant, intradermal swelling that measures 0.5 to 5 cm (usually <2 cm) in diameter may be alopecic. The lesion may become inflamed, secondarily infected, painful, or pruritic, or may rupture and discharge a thick gray to yellow-brown caseous material. Lesions are most commonly found on the head, trunk, or proximal limb in dogs, and on the head, neck, and trunk in cats.

Diagnosis

1. Cytology (may be nondiagnostic): amorphous cellular debris and mature keratinized epithelial cells with cholesterol crystals.
2. Dermatohistopathology: a cystic structure filled with lamellated keratin and lined by normal stratified squamous epithelium. Rupture of cyst contents may incite a surrounding pyogranulomatous inflammatory response.

Treatment and Prognosis

1. Observation without treatment is reasonable because lesions are benign.

2. Surgical excision is curative for cosmetically unacceptable lesions.
3. Cyst contents should not be manually expressed because if the cyst wall ruptures through the dermis, a foreign body reaction and infection may develop.
4. The prognosis is good as cysts are not neoplastic.

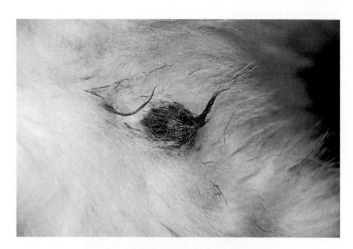

FIGURE 14-163 Follicular-Epidermal Inclusion Cyst. Close-up of the dog in Figure 14-162. The follicular cyst ruptured upon palpation.

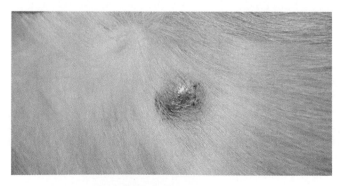

FIGURE 14-162 Follicular-Epidermal Inclusion Cyst. This alopecic, erythematous nodule is typical of small follicular cysts. When the cyst was palpated, it ruptured.

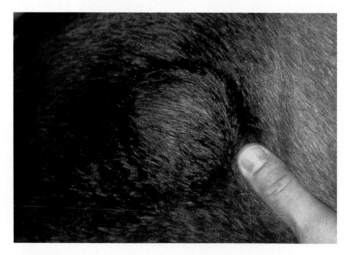

FIGURE 14-164 Follicular-Epidermal Inclusion Cyst. This large follicular cyst was associated with a primary follicular tumor.

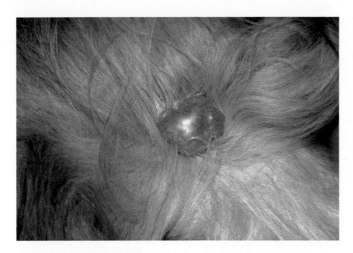

FIGURE 14-165 **Follicular-Epidermal Inclusion Cyst.** A large follicular cyst. The fluid-filled vesicle is apparent.

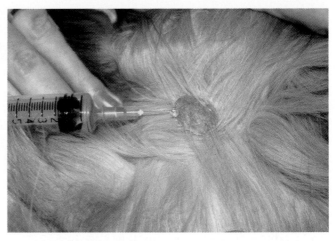

FIGURE 14-166 **Follicular-Epidermal Inclusion Cyst.** Same dog as in Figure 14-165. The fluid is being drained from the cyst.

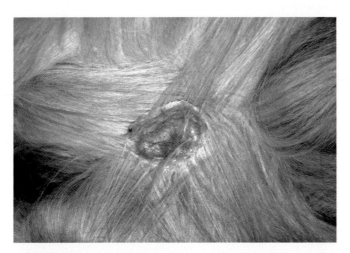

FIGURE 14-167 **Follicular-Epidermal Inclusion Cyst.** Same dog as in Figure 14-165. The fluid has been removed, and the cyst has deflated.

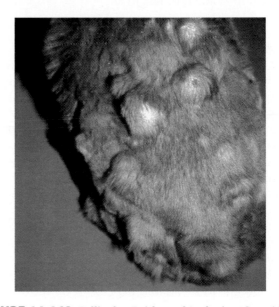

FIGURE 14-168 **Follicular-Epidermal Inclusion Cyst.** Multiple follicular cysts on the body of an adult cat. *(Courtesy D. Angarano.)*

Cutaneous Horns

Features

A cutaneous horn is a circumscribed, conical or cylindrical mass of keratin that may originate from underlying actinic keratosis, squamous cell carcinoma, papilloma, a dilated pore, or infundibular keratinizing acanthoma. It also may be seen as a unique entity on the footpads of cats infected with feline leukemia virus. Multiple cutaneous horns arising from under the claws have also been described in feline leukemia virus–negative cats. The condition is uncommon in dogs and cats.

Single or multiple conical to cylindrical hornlike masses of firm keratin are several millimeters in diameter and up to 2 cm in length.

Diagnosis

1. Dermatohistopathology: a well-demarcated area of papillomatous epidermal hyperplasia from which a compact column of keratin protrudes, resembling a toenail. The epidermis of feline leukemia–associated cutaneous horns may show dyskeratotic or multinucleate keratinocytes.
2. Cats with footpad lesions should be screened for feline leukemia virus infection.

Treatment and Prognosis

1. The treatment of choice is complete surgical excision.
2. Although cutaneous horns themselves are benign, the prognosis is variable, depending on the underlying cause.

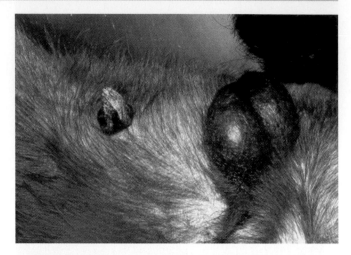

FIGURE 14-170 Cutaneous Horn. A cutaneous horn on the caudal thigh of an adult mixed-breed dog.

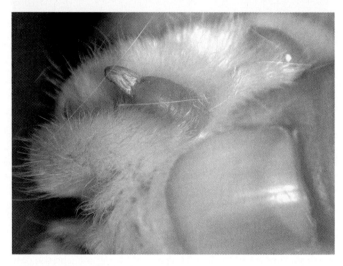

FIGURE 14-171 Cutaneous Horn. A small, cutaneous horn originating from the digital footpad of an adult cat.

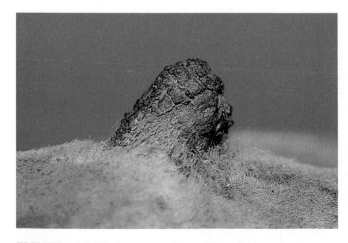

FIGURE 14-169 Cutaneous Horn. The solid keratin structure of this cutaneous horn is apparent.

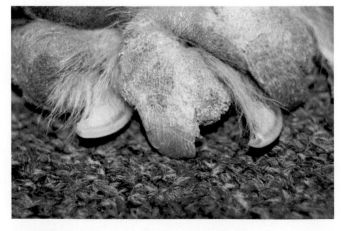

FIGURE 14-172 Cutaneous Horn. A cutaneous horn originating from the digital footpad of a dog with primary seborrhea.

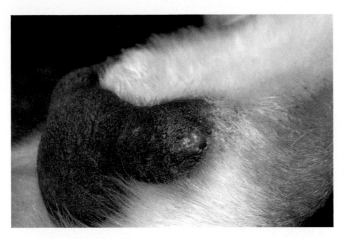

FIGURE 14-173 Cutaneous Horn. A focal hyperkeratotic lesion ("corn") on the central footpad of an adult Greyhound.

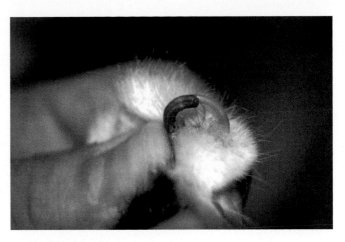

FIGURE 14-174 Cutaneous Horn. A cutaneous horn originating from the digital footpad of an adult cat.

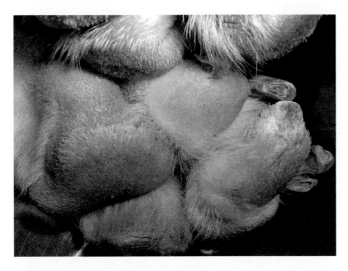

FIGURE 14-175 Cutaneous Horn. A hyperkeratotic lesion originating from the digital footpad of an adult dog.

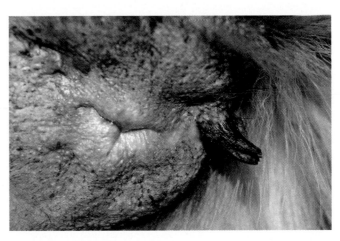

FIGURE 14-176 Cutaneous Horn. This cutaneous horn developed on the perianal tissue of a dog.

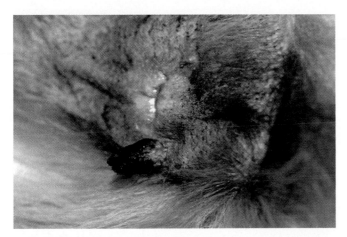

FIGURE 14-177 Cutaneous Horn. Same dog as in Figure 14-176. The abnormal keratin production actually appears like a toenail originating from perianal tissue.

Skin Tags (fibrovascular papilloma)

Features

A skin tag is a benign growth of fibrovascular origin that may be a hyperplastic skin response to repetitive trauma. It is uncommon in dogs, with highest incidence in middle-aged to older large and giant breeds. The condition is rare in cats.

Firm, pedunculated growths measure between 1 and 2 cm long and a few millimeters in diameter. Larger lesions may become ulcerated. Lesions are most common on the sternum, bony prominences, and trunk.

Diagnosis

Dermatohistopathology: hyperplastic epidermis overlying a core of vascularized collagenous connective tissue. Adnexa are absent.

Treatment and Prognosis

1. Observation without treatment is reasonable because these lesions are benign.
2. Surgical excision, laser ablation, or cryosurgery is curative for cosmetically unacceptable lesions.
3. The prognosis is good because growths are not neoplastic.

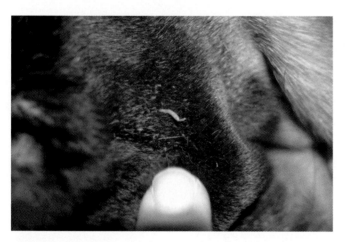

FIGURE 14-178 Skin Tag. A small, focal cutaneous tag on the face of an adult dog.

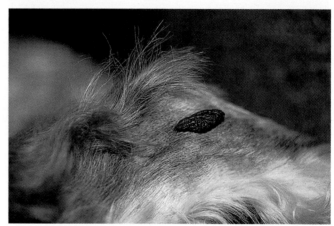

FIGURE 14-180 Skin Tag. A pigmented skin tag on the trunk of an adult Schnauzer.

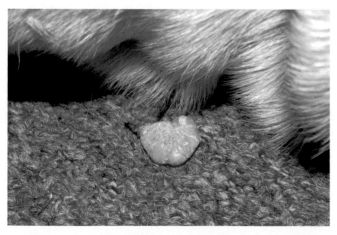

FIGURE 14-179 Skin Tag. A skin tag on the neck of an adult dog.

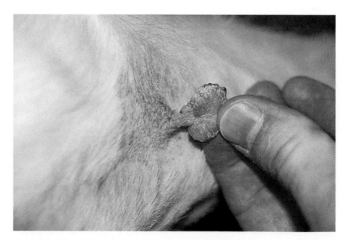

FIGURE 14-181 Skin Tag. Close-up of the dog in Figure 14-179. The small pedicle that attaches the skin tag to the body is visible.

Calcinosis Circumscripta

Features

Calcinosis circumscripta is seen as a focal area of dystrophic calcification that occurs at sites of repetitive or previous trauma, such as pressure points, footpads, ear cropping sites, or injection or injury sites (e.g., bite wounds, repetitive choke chain trauma). Multiple nodules have been described in association with canine hypertrophic osteodystrophy (HOD) and polyarthritis. The condition is uncommon in dogs, with highest incidence in young (<2 years old) large breeds (especially German shepherds). It is very rare in cats.

Usually, calcinosis circumscripta manifests as a single, firm, haired or alopecic, dome-shaped, subcutaneous or deep dermal mass that may ulcerate and discharge a white gritty substance. Nodules range from 0.5 to 7 cm in diameter. Lesions are most frequently seen over bony prominences, such as the elbow and lateral metatarsal and phalangeal areas of the rear leg. Rarely, lesions may occur on the dorsal neck, tongue, cheek, or base of the pinna.

Diagnosis

1. Cytology (may be nondiagnostic): amorphous, gritty white material that becomes basophilic when stained.
2. Dermatohistopathology: multifocal accumulations of finely or coarsely granular amorphous basophilic debris in the deep dermal or subcutaneous tissue, surrounded by granulomatous inflammation.

Treatment and Prognosis

1. Complete surgical excision is curative.
2. Multiple lesions associated with HOD or polyarthritis may spontaneously resolve with resolution of associated disease.
3. The prognosis is good in that growths are not neoplastic.

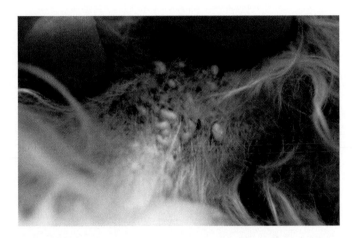

FIGURE 14-183 Calcinosis Circumscripta. Same dog as in Figure 14-182. Multiple white papules.

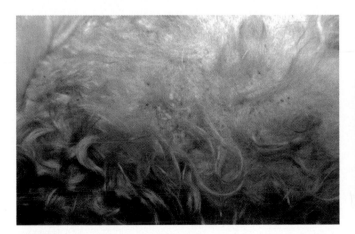

FIGURE 14-182 Calcinosis Circumscripta. Multiple white papules. Note the similarity with milia, which is typically seen in alopecic breeds or with follicular dysplasia.

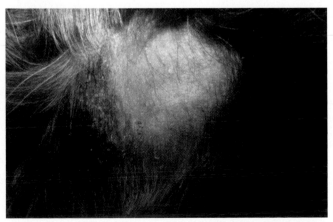

FIGURE 14-184 Calcinosis Circumscripta. Alopecia allows visualization of the calcified material within the skin. *(Courtesy M. Austel.)*

CHAPTER | 15

Avian and Exotic Animal Dermatology

CHERYL GREENACRE

PARASITIC
- Acariasis
- Pediculosis
- Subcutaneous Parasites
- Myiasis, Flea or Tick Infestation

BACTERIAL
- Rabbit Syphilis (*Treponema cuniculi*)
- Ulcerative Pododermatitis—rabbit (sore hock), bird (bumblefoot)
- Mycobacteriosis—bird
- Bacterial Dermatitis—bird, ferret
- Sepsis in Reptiles versus Shedding
- Aural (Ear) Abscess—turtle

VIRAL
- Psittacine Beak and Feather Disease—bird
- Papillomavirus—ferret (toe), rabbit (oral/rectal), rabbit (facial)
- Papillomatous Cloacal/Oral Masses—bird
- Inclusion Body Disease (IBD)—snake

FUNGAL
- Fungal Dermatitis (ringworm)—chinchilla
- Fungal Dermatitis (*Chrysosporium* spp.)—reptile

NEOPLASIA
- Mast Cell Tumor—ferret
- Adrenal Cortical Tumor—ferret
- Mammary Fibroadenoma—rat, mouse
- Hamster Cheek Pouch

- Tumor of Ventral Scent Gland—gerbil
- Squamous Cell Carcinoma—bird, turtle
- Lipoma—bird
- Xanthoma—bird
- Brown Hypertrophy of the Cere—budgerigar (parakeet)

TRAUMA
- Bruise—bird
- Necrosis From Injectable Enrofloxacin
- Air Sac Rupture—bird
- Constricted Toe Syndrome—bird
- Hernia—bird
- Cloacal Prolapse—bird
- Bite Trauma—snake, iguana
- Shell Repair—turtle, tortoise

METABOLIC/NUTRITIONAL/ENDOCRINE-RELATED
- Vitamin A Deficiency—bird, turtle
- Cystic Ovary—guinea pig

OTHER DISEASES
- Feather Picking/Chewing/Self-Mutilation—bird
- Feather Cyst—bird
- Excess Keratin—guinea pig foot
- Porphyrin Tears—rat
- Improper Vaccine Delivery—bird
- Hairless Varieties
- Tattoo—ferret, rabbit, bird

PARASITIC

Acariasis

Features

Common mites of avian and exotic animal pet species are generally species specific (Table 15-1). Fur mites generally cause dandruff and patchy alopecia with little associated pruritus. The rabbit fur mite (*Cheyletiella parasitovorax*) is considered zoonotic, causing mild hyperemia and pruritus in humans. The ear mite, *Otodectes cynotis*, is commonly found in ferrets and can spread between cats and ferrets; therefore it is important to treat all susceptible pets in the household. The presence of black earwax in ferrets does not necessarily denote ear mite infestation. The rabbit ear mite, *Psoroptes cuniculi*, can cause such an accumulation of dry crusts that an upright ear can be weighted down into the lop-ear position. *Demodex* spp. are commonly demonstrated in hamsters greater than 2 years of age with concomitant Cushing's disease. Hamsters are generally exposed to the mites when young but do not exhibit clinical signs until immunocompromised. Rabbits and guinea pigs with intense pruritus should be checked for their respective mites because this would be the most common differential. Birds, typically budgerigars and canaries, infected with *Knemidokoptes* generally show pitting of the beak and facial skin (budgerigars), or pitting of the skin of the legs (canaries). Snake mites (*Oophyionysus* spp.) can be found anywhere on the snake's body, but typically they can be found around the eye or between the cleft of skin under the chin. Severe infestations in snakes can cause significant anemia. African hedgehogs kept as pets in the United States can present with *Chorioptes* spp. mites, resulting in quill loss and skin crusting and flaking.

Top Differentials

Differentials include superficial pyoderma, dermatophytosis, and trauma. Rabbit syphilis (*Treponema cuniculi*) is a differential in rabbits.

Diagnosis

Microscopy of skin scrapes (deep if suspecting *Sarcoptes scabiei*) or tape preparations for fur mites, demonstrating the parasite or ova.

TABLE 15-1 Common Mites of Avian and Exotic Animal Pets

Mite	Characteristics
Fur Mites	
Mouse	
Myobia musculi	Found over head, neck, and shoulder area
Radfordia affinis	
Myocoptes musculinus	Found over entire body
Rat	
Radfordia ensifera	
Rabbit	
Cheyletiella parasitovorax	"Walking dandruff mite," zoonotic
Listrophus gibbus	
Ear Mites	
Rat	
Notoedres muris	
Rabbit	
Psoroptes cuniculi	Dry crusts in ear canal and pinna
Ferret	
Otodectes cynotis	Dark, waxy discharge in ears
Hamster	
Notoedres notedres	Found over ears, nose, feet, and anus
Skin	
Hamster	Common secondary to Cushing's disease
Demodex criceti	Found in epidermis
Demodex aurati	Found deep (hair follicles, sebaceous glands)
Guinea Pig	
Trixacarus caviae	Marked purities: neck, shoulder, inguinal
Chirodiscoides caviae	Nonpruritic: lumbar, lateral rear limbs
Rabbit	
Sarcoptes scabiei	Intense pruritus, self-mutilation
Budgerigars and Canaries	
Knemidokoptes pili	"Scaly leg and face mite," pitting beak, skin
Snake	
Ophionyssus natricis	Check crypts around eye and cleft under chin
Hedgehog	
Chorioptes spp.	Quill loss; skin crusting and flaking

Acariasis—*cont'd*

Treatment and Prognosis

In general, the treatment for mites in most species is ivermectin at 0.2 mg/kg PO, SC, or preferably topically repeated in 10 to 14 days, with some important exceptions: never use ivermectin in turtles or tortoises—it can cause paralysis, coma, death as a result of their permeable blood-brain barrier; never inject ivermectin into birds, especially small birds, as the propylene glycol base can cause an anaphylactic reaction and death.

- Do not hang mite treatments, such as those that contain paradichlorobenzene, on the side of the cage, as they may be toxic to birds and they do not rid the bird of mites.

- In rabbits, selamectin has been shown to clear infection of ear mites with one dose. When treating rabbits for ear mites, it is important to not remove the crusts, as they will fall out within 1 week after treatment with very little trauma.

- Hamsters with concurrent adrenal hyperplasia may respond to op'DDD.

- Because snake mites spend time off the host, any porous material in the enclosure should be discarded, and nonporous surfaces can be sprayed with a well-shaken mixture of ivermectin at 5 mg/L water. The propylene glycol base does not mix well with water.

- Consult *Carpenter's Exotic Animal Formulary* for further drug information.

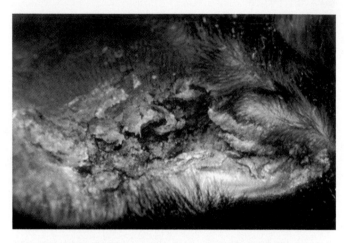

FIGURE 15-2 Acariasis. Rabbit with a typical mild case of ear mites due to *Psoroptes cuniculi.*

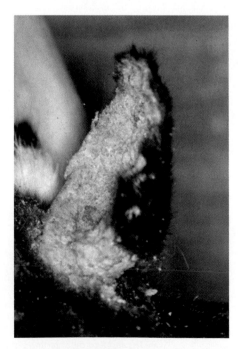

FIGURE 15-1 Acariasis. Rabbit with a severe case of ear mites due to *Psoroptes cuniculi.*

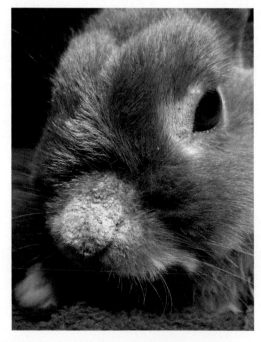

FIGURE 15-3 Acariasis. Rabbit with scabies due to a *Sarcoptes* spp. mite. This rabbit had intense pruritus.

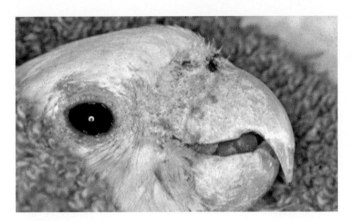

FIGURE 15-4 Acariasis. Cockatiel with *Knemidokoptes pili* mite infestation, known as the *scaly leg and face mite (side view).*

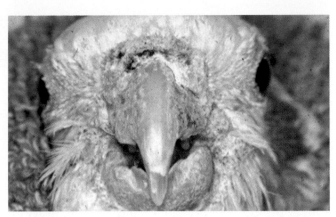

FIGURE 15-5 Acariasis. Cockatiel with *Knemidokoptes pili* mite infestation, known as the *scaly leg and face mite (front view).*

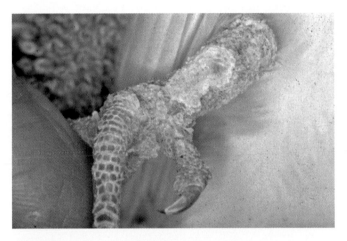

FIGURE 15-6 Acariasis. Cockatiel with *Knemidokoptes pili* mite infestation, known as the *scaly leg and face mite (view of plantar surface of foot).*

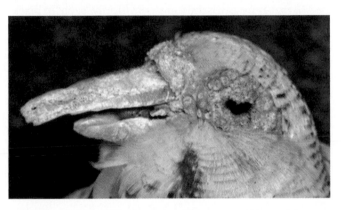

FIGURE 15-7 Acariasis. Budgerigar with severe case of *Knemidokoptes pili* mite infestation, known as the *scaly leg and face mite,* which has caused deformation of the beak.

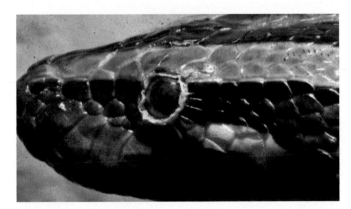

FIGURE 15-8 Acariasis. Ball python with retained spectacle over the eye due to *Oophinysus* spp. mite infestation. The mites live in the crypt around the eye and interfere with normal shed in this area.

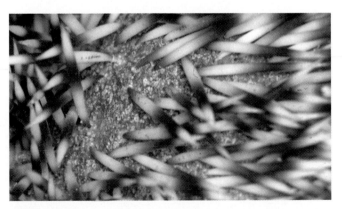

FIGURE 15-9 Acariasis. African hedgehog with *Chorioptes* spp. mite infestation. Loss of quills and dry, flaky skin are typical, as is pruritus.

Pediculosis

Features

The mouse louse *(Polyplax serrata)* is common in wild mice, causing anemia, debilitation, and intense pruritus. If it is found in pet mice, there is usually exposure to wild mice. The spined rat louse *(Polyplax spinulosa)* is rare but can cause pruritus, irritability, and anemia. The lice of guinea pigs *(Gliricola porcelli, Gyropus ovalis)* are commonly seen in pet guinea pigs, and if heavy in number can cause pruritus, rough hair coat, and alopecia. Typically, infestation with *Gyropus* spp. is associated with intense pruritus. Bird lice are uncommonly seen in pet parrot-type birds but are commonly seen in backyard poultry and peafowl. The chicken head louse *(Cuclotogaster heterographus)* is found about the head of chickens and peafowl. The chicken body louse *(Menacanthus stramineus)* is found near the vent of a variety of domestic fowl, including chickens, peafowl, guinea fowl, quail, pheasant, ducks, and geese.

Top Differentials

Differentials include other ectoparasites.

Diagnosis

Microscopy of tape preparation or plucked hair demonstrates the parasite or the ova (nits).

Treatment and Prognosis

In general, the treatment for lice is ivermectin at 0.2 mg/kg PO, SC, or topical, except for these important exceptions: never use ivermectin in turtles or tortoises—it may cause paralysis, coma, or death because of their permeable blood-brain barrier; never inject ivermectin IM into birds, especially small birds, as the propylene glycol base can cause an anaphylactic reaction and death. Other susceptable animals in the group should be treated as well as the environment.

Consult *Carpenter's Exotic Animal Formulary* for further drug information.

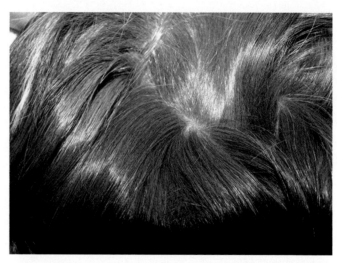

FIGURE 15-11 Pediculosis. Guinea pig infested with unidentified lice, but probably *Gliricola* spp. because this animal was not pruritic. Lice and nits were visible with the naked eye over the rump area.

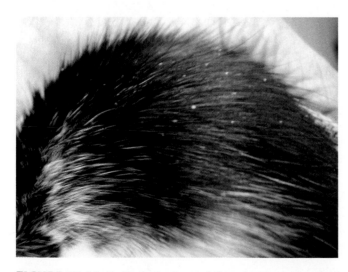

FIGURE 15-10 Pediculosis. Pet rat infested with unidentified lice. Lice and nits were visible with the naked eye over the entire dorsum.

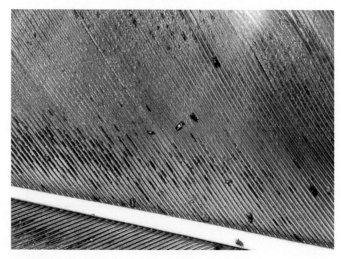

FIGURE 15-12 Pediculosis. Chicken with unidentified louse on feathers.

Subcutaneous Parasites

Features

Recently imported parrots may occasionally have a subcutaneous mass of adult *Pelicitus* spp. nematodes. Recently imported reptiles, including day geckos, may have a coelomic or SC mass of adult *Thamagadia* or *Magnathamagadia* spp. Rabbits that graze outside or are fed fresh-cut grass from outside can get *Cuterebra* spp. bot larva subcutaneously. The *Cuterebra* is ingested and migrates out of the oral cavity or esophagus to a subcutaneous site and is distinguished by the presence of a breathing hole in the skin.

Top Differentials

Differentials include neoplasia, abscess, or other granuloma.

Diagnosis

In reptiles and birds, the roughly 1 × 1-cm SC mass may have a vermiform shape. In rabbits, the roughly 4 × 2-cm SC mass will have a tell-tale breathing hole, and sometimes movement can be observed through the breathing hole under the skin.

Treatment and Prognosis

Surgical removal is best.
- For rabbits, remove the parasite under general anesthesia by surgically incising the skin in each direction from the breathing hole, taking care not to traumatize the parasite to prevent release of parasite antigen. Clean and débride the wound and leave open to heal by second intention, with daily cleansing.
- For birds and reptiles, surgical removal, cleansing, and primary closure is usually best.

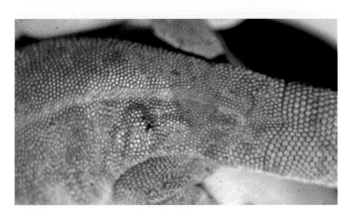

FIGURE 15-13 Subcutaneous Parasites. A day gecko with *Magnathamagadia* or *Thamagadia* spp. nematode SC. These were easily surgically removed. Later, the same nematode was found in the coelomic area.

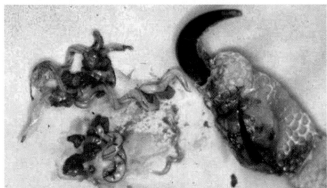

FIGURE 15-14 Subcutaneous Parasites. A recently imported parrot with *Pelicitus* spp. nematodes SC. These were easily surgically removed. Diagnosis was made in this case by visualization of nematode ova on cytological examination of an aspirate of the mass.

Myiasis, Flea or Tick Infestation

Features

Maggots are seen most commonly in the perineal area of rabbits housed outdoors and wild bird patients after trauma. A variety of ticks can infest domestic rabbits housed outdoors or wild rabbits. Fleas are occasionally seen in rabbits and ferrets, with ferrets seeming particularly susceptible to heavy infestations and subsequent fatal anemia. Pruritus is generally mild.

Diagnosis

Direct visualization of maggots, fleas, or ticks on skin.

Treatment and Prognosis

■ Maggots: Direct removal, or can use Capstar PO (nitenpyram 1 mg/kg PO).
■ Fleas: In general, the treatment for fleas in ferrets is similar to that for cats. Rabbits on the other hand should never be given fipronil (Frontline) as it causes seizures and/or death in rabbits. Rabbits can be given imidocloprid (Advantage) or pyrethrin products.
■ Ticks: Direct removal. Recently imported animals with ticks should have the ticks submitted for identification to be sure they are not foreign. Always save parasite specimens in 70% alcohol, never formalin, as formalin renders physically indentifying structures on the parasite unusable.

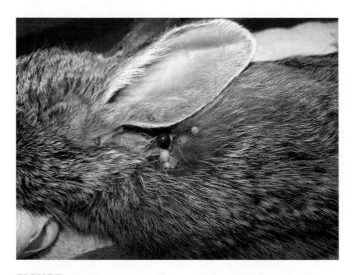

FIGURE 15-15 Myiasis, Flea or Tick Infestation. Wild cottontail rabbit infested with unidentified tick species.

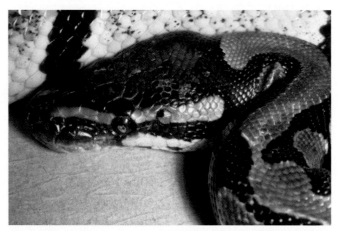

FIGURE 15-16 Myiasis, Flea or Tick Infestation. Recently imported ball python with a flat-bodied snake tick. This tick was submitted for identification and was found not to be a species that could bring heartwater disease into this country from Africa.

BACTERIAL

Rabbit Syphilis *(Treponema cuniculi)*

Features

This sexually transmitted disease of rabbits causes crusting and erosive lesions of the skin and mucocutaneous junctions of the perineum, periocular and perioral areas, and sometimes the base of the ear. This disease is NOT zoonotic; human syphilis is caused by *T. pallidum*. The incubation period is long, approximately 3 to 6 weeks. Males without obvious signs can transmit the disease.

Top Differentials

Differentials include acariasis (see Figure 15-3) and papillomavirus, (see Figure 15-45), which typically involve other areas of the body than the mucocutaneous junctions.

Diagnosis

Diagnosis is often based on typical clinical signs and response to treatment, but a definitive diagnosis can be obtained by identifying the organism on biopsy or via direct microscopic examination of the fluid obtained after removing superficial crusts and squeezing the skin. After a few drops of saline are added and the condenser is turned down on the microscope, the motile bacteria can be seen.

Treatment and Prognosis

Sometimes this is a self-limiting disease. If the rabbit is to be bred or the lesions are troublesome, then treatment is recommended with procaine penicillin G with benzathine given subcutaneously ONLY every 7 days for 3 treatments. Remember never to give rabbits oral penicillin as this may cause fatal enteritis.

Consult *Carpenter's Exotic Animal Formulary* for further drug information.

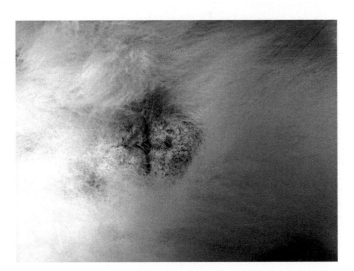

FIGURE 15-17 Rabbit Syphilis. Perineal region of the same rabbit as in Figure 15-18, with typical mild to moderate case of rabbit syphilis caused by *Treponema cuniculi*. Lesions are near mucocutaneous junctions.

Rabbit Syphilis—*cont'd*

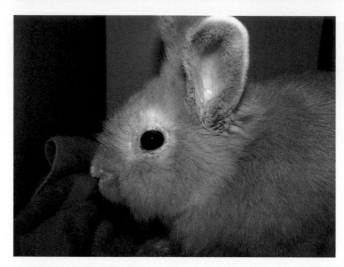

FIGURE 15-18 Rabbit Syphilis. Young adult, female rabbit with typical mild to moderate case of rabbit syphilis caused by *Treponema cuniculi*. Lesions are near mucocutaneous junctions.

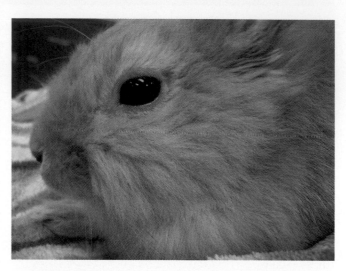

FIGURE 15-19 Rabbit Syphilis. Rabbit syphilis after treatment. Same rabbit as in Figure 15-18, after 3 weeks of treatment with subcutaneous procaine benzathine penicillin every 7 days.

Ulcerative Pododermatitis—rabbit (sore hock), bird (bumblefoot)

Features

The causes of ulcerative pododermatitis in rabbits include obesity, genetically sparse hair cover over the plantar surface of the "hock" (actually the plantar surface of the proximal metatarsus), and trauma from wire-only substrate or carpet, causing shearing forces on the hair. The hair provides the cushion for the plantar surface. Mild pododermatitis includes alopecia and hyperemia of the intact skin. Moderate pododermatitis involves breakdown of the skin with erosions, scabs, proliferative tissue, and swelling or infection of skin. Severe pododermatitis with osteomyelitis can easily occur because there is very little soft tissue coverage in this area. Guinea pigs present with this same disease, but the cause is usually unsanitary conditions past or present, and it is very difficult to treat.

Captive raptors commonly present with pododermatitis because they stand most of the day. It has been shown that during flight, the temperature and blood supply to a raptor foot increase dramatically. The plantar surfaces of the digits and tarsometatarsal area are more commonly affected in raptors, passerines and small psittacines, whereas parrots are usually affected on the plantar surface of the tarsometatarsus. Small or uniform-size perches, hypovitaminosis A, obesity, and "sitting back on the hocks" are usual causes in pet parrots.

Top Differentials

Perhaps a tumor, such as a fibrosarcoma, could form a mass in this area on a rabbit that may look like podo-dermatitis or trauma from other causes.

Diagnosis

Diagnosis is based on direct visualization. A radiograph can determine if there is osteomyelitis.

Treatment and Prognosis

Rabbits

Mild pododermatitis of rabbits can be improved with changes in husbandry, such as providing a flat place to stand (kitchen cutting boards work well), removing wire substrate, limiting or eliminating time on carpet, providing towels or hay, or making a "bunny bootie" to bandage or somehow cover and protect the proximal metatarsus. The prognosis is good for mild pododermatitis. Moderate to severe cases may require surgery to remove abscessed areas, multiple days of flushing an infected joint, and antibiotics (based on aerobic and anaerobic culture). The prognosis is guarded to grave for moderate and severe pododermatitis, respectively. Enrofloxacin is a safer antibiotic for use in rabbits; it provides good bone penetration but is not effective against anaerobic bacteria. Metronidazole is typically used in rabbits if *Fusobacterium necrophorum* or a similar organism is cultured. If anaerobic bacteria is cultured, such as *Fusobacterium necrophorum*, then metronidazole is typically used in rabbits, or subcutaneous Procain Pen G. Remember, do **not** give penicillins orally to rabbits as it can be fatal.

Guinea Pigs

The very chronic form of pododermatitis in Guinea pigs requires improved substrate, soaking feet in warm water to increase circulation, frequent cleaning and moisturizing of feet, and long-term antibiotics.

Birds

Birds with mild pododermatitis may improve with husbandry changes such as a wider perch, a perch with varying diameters, a padded perch, improved diet with less fat or fewer calories or with needed vitamin A, and, most important, increased exercise. If infection is present, then surgery or long-term antibiotics based on culture (both aerobic and anaerobic) and bandaging may be necessary. A variety of bandages have been described, such as "ball," where the foot is bandaged into a ball; "snowshoe," where the bandage is flat-bottomed to disperse the weight over a larger surface area; or a bandage that puts no weight on the bottom of the foot because a U-shaped bar is strapped to the leg. The prognosis is guarded to grave for moderate and severe pododermatitis, respectively.

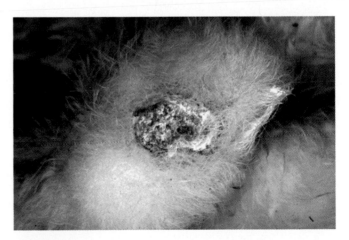

FIGURE 15-20 Ulcerative Pododermatitis. Rabbit with moderate case of ulcerative pododermatitis that has eroded through the skin and developed a scab with inflammation on the plantar surface of the foot.

Ulcerative Pododermatitis—rabbit, bird—*cont'd*

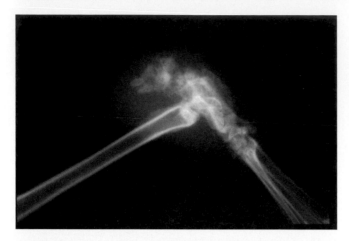

FIGURE 15-21 Ulcerative Pododermatitis. Radiograph of a rabbit with a severe case of ulcerative pododermatitis that includes osteomyelitis of the tarsus and tibiotarsal joint.

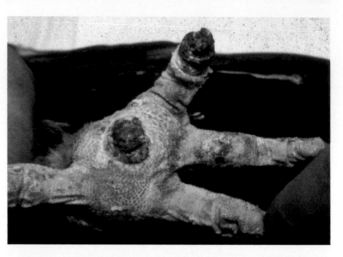

FIGURE 15-22 Ulcerative Pododermatitis. Raptor under anesthesia with a severe case of ulcerative pododermatitis (bumblefoot) on the plantar surface of the foot. The affected area of the foot is typical for raptors.

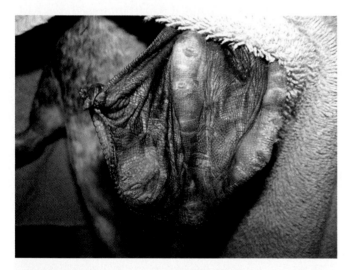

FIGURE 15-23 Ulcerative Pododermatitis. Duck with a moderate to severe case of ulcerative pododermatitis (bumblefoot) on the plantar surface of the foot. The affected area of the foot is typical for Anseriformes (ducks, geese, swans).

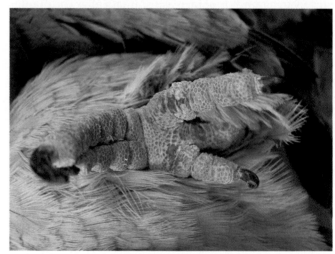

FIGURE 15-24 Ulcerative Pododermatitis. Amazon parrot with a mild case of ulcerative pododermatitis. This case started as hypovitaminosis A from an all-seed diet, causing unhealthy, thin skin predisposing to plantar erosions.

Mycobacteriosis—bird

Features

Mycobacteriosis caused by *Mycobacterium avium, Mycobacterium genovense,* and other species has been described periodically in parrots. A rare cutaneous form has been described and presents as nonhealing raised lesions over the legs that do not heal or respond to typical antibiotics. The typical form of mycobacteriosis in birds generally affects the hepatic and gastrointestinal (GI) systems.

Top Differentials

A slow-healing secondarily infected traumatic wound may resemble this lesion.

Diagnosis

A histopathologic diagnosis of a chronic granulomatous lesion with no obvious organisms should be suspicious of mycobacteriosis and further testing should be pursued. *Mycobacteria* spp. can be detected on special stains of a biopsy sample. Specifically, a Fite's modified acid-fast stain should be requested because a regular acid-fast stain may destroy the delicate types of mycobacterial species that infect birds. A PCR test can also be performed on tissues.

Treatment and Prognosis

Euthanasia, not treatment, is recommended because of the zoonotic potential of this disease, which is historically difficult to treat in people and can be fatal. Nevertheless, treatments have been attempted with three to five medications, including ethambutol, given daily or twice daily for a year or longer, with documented recurrence after medication is stopped. Check with your local health department regarding the legal implications of treating an animal in your area.

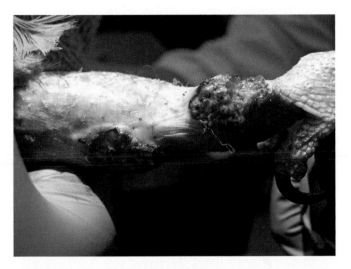

FIGURE 15-25 Mycobacteriosis. Amazon parrot with chronic nonhealing wounds on the leg caused by *Mycobacterium kansasii*. The parrot was euthanized after confirmatory diagnosis with a Fite's modified acid-fast stain and polymerase chain reaction (PCR) performed at washington State Diagnostic Laboratory.

Bacterial Dermatitis—bird, ferret

Features

It is not common for birds to present with a bacterial dermatitis unless it is involving the plantar surface of the foot, as described under ulcerative pododermatitis, or there is underlying trauma that allowed the infection to start; if present, this generally involves gram-negative bacteria. A ferret developed suspected allergy and secondary *Pseudomonas* spp. dermatitis after the owner built it a cage made of redwood. After removal of the new homemade cage and appropriate antibiotic treatment, the ferret made a complete recovery.

Top Differentials

Fungal infection or neoplasia.

Diagnosis

Diagnosis usually involves aerobic and anaerobic culture and sensitivity, but may also include cytology, biopsy, or fungal culture. No allergy testing has been reported in ferrets. In this case, suspicion was high because the disease occurred after exposure to the new cage.

Treatment and Prognosis

Clean and débride the wound; this is sometimes repeated over the course of days. Primary closure is performed once infection is controlled. Birds' heterophils lack myeloperoxidase, an enzyme that liquefies pus; therefore do not place drains in the wound. Contaminated wounds are treated as in other animals. Antibiotic is based on culture.

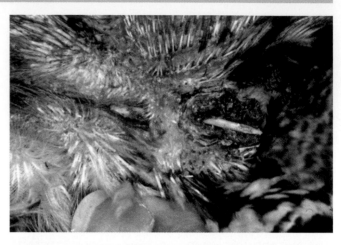

FIGURE 15-27 Bacterial Dermatitis. Close-up of owl in Figure 15-26.

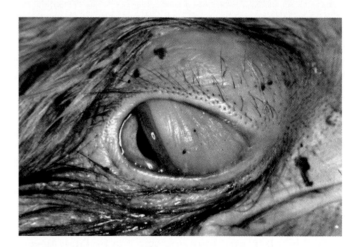

FIGURE 15-28 Bacterial Dermatitis. Captive adult bald eagle with a supraorbital SC abscess.

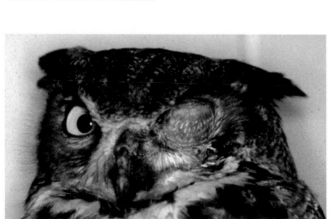

FIGURE 15-26 Bacterial Dermatitis. Wild great horned owl with a porcupine quill through the skin under the left eye. The quill was removed under anesthesia and the wound cleaned to heal by second intention healing.

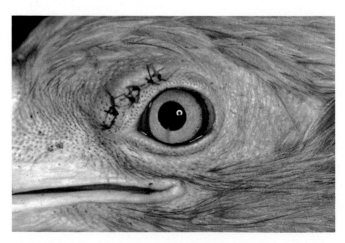

FIGURE 15-29 Bacterial Dermatitis. Same captive adult bald eagle with a supraorbital SC abscess after surgical removal.

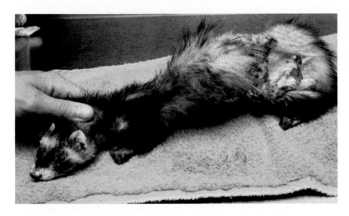

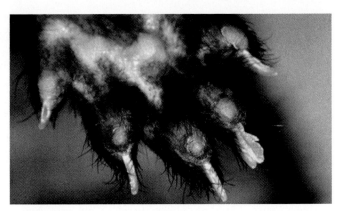

FIGURE 15-30 Bacterial Dermatitis. Young adult ferret with severe bacterial dermatitis due to *Pseudomonas aeruginosa*. The owner had recently hand-made an enclosure of redwood for the ferret, and although this was not proved, it was suspected that the ferret was allergic to the redwood. The ferret responded well to appropriate antibiotic therapy based on culture.

FIGURE 15-31 Bacterial Dermatitis. Same ferret as in Figure 15-30, with bacterial dermatitis showing plantar surface of foot.

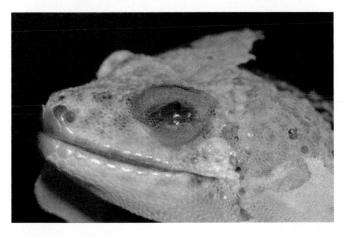

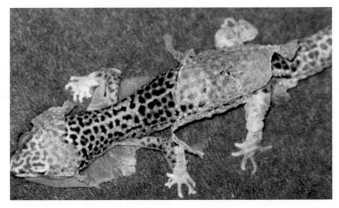

FIGURE 15-32 Bacterial Dermatitis. Adult leopard gecko with severe case of dysecdysis (abnormal shedding) with two or three successive sheds still in place. A culture of the green ocular discharge grew *Pseudomonas aeruginosa*.

FIGURE 15-33 Bacterial Dermatitis. Same gecko as in Figure 15-32 showing dysecdysis (abnormal shedding of the entire body). Retained sheds on toes have a constricted blood supply and cause necrosis of the toes. This gecko ended up responding to appropriate antibiotic therapy based on culture and multiple warm water soaks but lost almost all its toes.

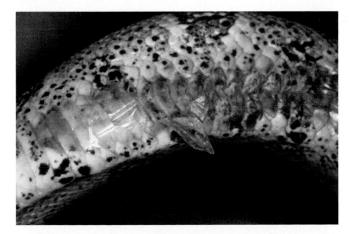

FIGURE 15-34 Bacterial Dermatitis. Ventral surface of snake (boa) with bacterial dermatitis secondary to a burn.

Sepsis in Reptiles versus Shedding

Features

Bacterial sepsis in reptiles can manifest as hyperemia of the ventrum in turtles or snakes, and as hyperemic conjunctiva in lizards. Historically, *Pseudomonas* and *Aeromonas* are the most common bacterial isolates from reptiles. Occasionally, boa-type snakes can also develop a cellulitis at the site of infection, which causes tremendous swelling. Snakes normally shed in one piece, whereas lizards shed in a piecemeal fashion from head to toe. Snakes will shed the spectacle over the eye first, turning the bluish color of the eye clear, which marks the beginning of a shed. Then, the snake sheds (ecdysis) the entire skin in one everted piece. Dysecdysis is an abnormal shed and is usually due to low humidity in the environment. During the week before and after a shed, a snake can mimic respiratory disease because of partial occlusion of the nares, and they may also develop a hyperemic ventrum.

Top Differentials

Localized skin or shell infection on the ventrum can also present with hyperemia, but it is usually localized—not generalized. Days to weeks before a normal shed, a snake can mimic sepsis, showing a hyperemic ventrum and even increased respiratory sounds. A haziness to the skin and a "bluing" of the spectacle (scale over the eye) occurs just before a shed due to increase in lymph fluid under the spectacle. Inclusion body disease caused by a retrovirus-like agent can cause an abnormal shed, as well as neurologic signs. Sepsis can also cause a hyperemic ventrum. Respiratory disease can cause wet crackles.

Diagnosis

If the skin blanches with digital pressure, it is hyperemia, and not the pigmentation of the animal.

Treatment and Prognosis

Find the source of infection, obtain a culture or blood culture, and treat with appropriate antibiotics. Antibiotic treatment in reptiles is routinely given for 6 to 10 weeks. To encourage a shed, the reptile should be soaked in warm water. Never pull off the shed, especially the spectacle over the eye, as skin or corneal damage may occur. The old shed can be gently rubbed off in the water. Increase humidity in the habitat by adding a wide, shallow dish of water big enough for the reptile to soak on its own.

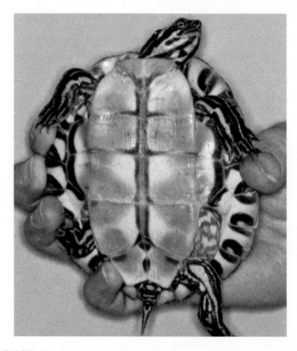

FIGURE 15-35 Sepsis. Ventral hyperemia of the plastron of a red-eared slider turtle secondary to sepsis from bacterial pneumonia.

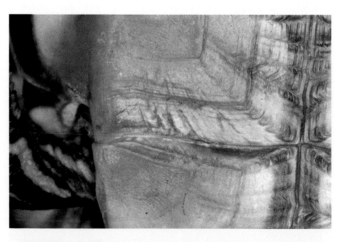

FIGURE 15-36 Sepsis. Close-up of turtle in Figure 15-35.

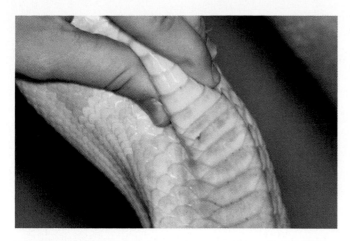

FIGURE 15-37 **Sepsis.** Ventral hyperemia of the scutes (scales) of an amelanistic snake secondary to sepsis from a bacterial pneumonia.

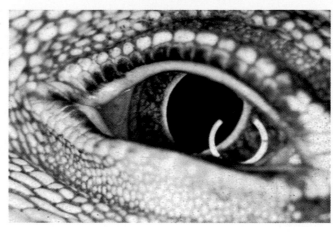

FIGURE 15-38 **Sepsis.** Hyperemia of the conjunctiva of a green iguana secondary to sepsis from a bacterial pneumonia.

Aural (Ear) Abscess—turtle

Features

A caseous abscess, presenting as a swelling, often large, under the external tympanic membrane on the side of the head. It can occur bilaterally and is often seen in wild box turtles or pet red-eared slider turtles. There is some evidence that it may be due to hypovitaminosis A, and its occurrence in wild turtles may be linked to exposure to organophosphates. This disease is very common.

Top Differentials

Differentials include neoplasia or other granuloma.

Diagnosis

By clinical appearance.

Treatment and Prognosis

■ Surgical removal of caseated pus after lancing the tympanic membrane (myringotomy). It is important to remove about 50% of the tympanum to leave a wide hole for flushing with warm saline for as many days as possible after surgery (try for 3 days). In other words, leave it open to heal by second intention healing for as long as possible.

■ Often the caseated plug can be removed in one piece, like a casting of the inner ear.

■ Dry dock water turtles until the surgery site is healed.

■ Do not instill products into the ear that may be ototoxic (amikacin, enrofloxacin, chlorhexidine, or iodine solutions).

■ Systemic antibiotics are often administered, including enrofloxacin, cephazolin, and long-acting ceftriofun (see Carpenter's formulary), or other. Ideally, antibiotic therapy should be based on culture sensitivity.

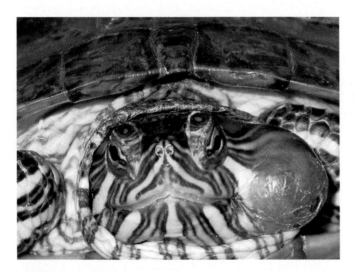

FIGURE 15-39 Aural Abscess. A captive red-eared slider turtle with an aural abscess of the left ear. The skin over the abscess is the tympanic membrane. Surgery under anesthesia to lance, remove the abscess, and flush the cavity resolved the disease.

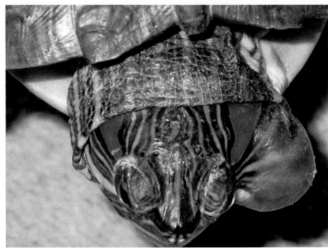

FIGURE 15-40 Aural Abscess. Different view of turtle in Figure 15-39 with an aural abscess.

VIRAL

Psittacine Beak and Feather Disease—bird

Features

The psittacine beak and feather disease (PBFD) virus most commonly causes clinical signs in captive and free-ranging Old World (Australian and African) psittacine birds such as cockatoos, lovebirds, African gray parrots, and cockatiels. The PBFD virus is endemic in many free-ranging flocks of psittacines in Australia. A few cases of clinical PBFD have been documented in New World species, including Scarlet macaws, red-lored and blue-fronted Amazon parrots, and Jenday conures. PBFD virus is shed in feces, feather dander, and various excretions and secretions. Asymptomatic birds can shed the virus for years before exhibiting any clinical signs. Peracute, acute, and chronic forms of PBFD occur in parrots. Generally, the progression of the disease is dictated by the age of the bird when clinical signs first appear. Younger birds have a faster progression of the disease. Chronic PBFD is most common and is characterized by symmetrical, slowly progressive dystrophy of developing feathers that worsens with each successive molt. The feather dystrophy includes retained feather sheaths, hemorrhage within the pulp, curled feathers, and circumferential constrictions of the feather shaft. Usually the down and contour feathers are affected first, and then the primaries. Birds can go on to develop complete alopecia and sometimes beak abnormalities consisting of progressive elongation of the beak and necrosis of the palate rostrally, near the upper beak. These birds are often immunocompromised and die of secondary bacterial or fungal infection. A PBFD variant (PsCV-2) has been described in lories that is not as pathogenic as the originally described PBFD. Lories with PsCV-2 had clinical feather lesions similar to PBFD but had less severe clinical signs, and, most important, they recovered. Bird species other than lories may be infected with PsCV-2.

Top Differentials

Any damage to the developing feather, such as a bacterial or fungal infection of the follicle, or trauma to the follicle, can cause constriction of the feather shafts.

Diagnosis

- PBFD DNA probe tests are performed on whole blood and detect viral DNA; therefore a positive test means there was PBFD viral DNA in the blood at the time of sampling.
- If a bird is positive but has no clinical signs, it is recommended to retest the bird in 90 days to see if the viral DNA is still present. If it is still present, then the bird is infected; if not, then the bird was transiently infected and overcame the infection.
- Any bird displaying feather abnormalities should have a feather follicle biopsy and DNA in situ hybridization performed, in addition to the DNA probe blood test, because some clinical birds are so viremic that they will have a negative blood test. This can also occur if a bird is extremely leukopenic. Intracytoplasmic inclusion bodies are seen in the bone marrow, thymus, and bursa.
- PCR available at the University of Georgia Infectious Disease Laboratory can distinguish between PBFD and PsCV-2.

Treatment and Prognosis

- Because the virus is nonenveloped, it is very stable, can survive years in the environment, and is resistant to destruction by common disinfectants.
- A cell culture–derived circovirus was killed by 1% iodine, sodium hypochlorite, 0.4% B-propiolactone, and 1% glutaraldehyde at 80°C for 1 hour.
- A PCR test can be used to detect viral DNA on a swab of the environment to assist in determining the effectiveness of disinfection efforts.
- Once clinical signs develop, treatment for PBFD-1 consists of supportive care and antimicrobials for secondary infection for the immunosuppresion, but the diagnosis eventually leads to death weeks to years later.
- Once clinical signs develop, the disease is always fatal if infected with PBFD-1.
- Some birds after exposure will mount an immune response and recover and never show clinical signs. These birds do not shed and are considered naturally vaccinated.
- Prevention through testing and isolation is currently the best way to control this disease in the United States.

Psittacine Beak and Feather Disease (PBFD)—bird—*cont'd*

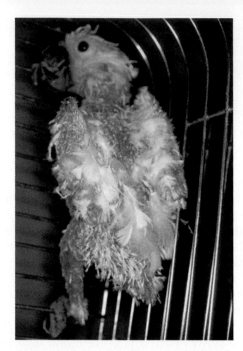

FIGURE 15-41 **Psittacine Beak and Feather Disease.** Adult cockatoo with end-stage psittacine beak and feather disease. Note that the feathers over the entire body, including the head, are affected.

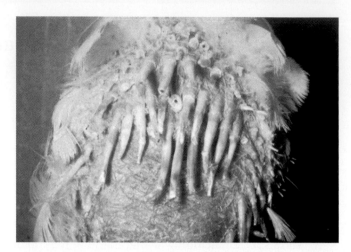

FIGURE 15-42 **Psittacine Beak and Feather Disease.** Adult cockatoo with end-stage psittacine beak and feather disease. The feathers over the top of the head are growing abnormally with retained, constricted sheaths.

Papillomavirus—ferret (toe), rabbit (oral/rectal), rabbit (facial)

Features

In ferrets, papillomas are dry, proliferative lesions on the plantar surfaces of the feet. In rabbits, an oral form of papilloma may be found within the oral cavity and is usually self-limiting. Rabbits also occasionally present with rectal papillomas that are not self-limiting and usually need to be treated. The papillomavirus of rabbits that affects the face causes proliferative, keratinized, hornlike projections on the face that have been shown to predispose the rabbit to squamous cell carcinoma later. Rabbit facial papilloma is spread by mosquitoes feeding on infected cottontail rabbits in the area, so house rabbits indoors.

Top Differentials

The facial papilloma in rabbits initially, with minimal keratinization, may look like rabbit syphilis. No other red, raised, irregular surface masses are found in the oral or rectal area of rabbits.

Diagnosis

Histopathologic examination of biopsy.

Treatment and Prognosis

- Ferret toe papillomas usually do not require treatment unless large or constantly traumatized.
- Rabbit oral papillomas are usually monitored until they resolve several months later. Seldom do they interfere with mastication.
- Rabbit rectal papillomas can be monitored; if associated with tenesmus, they are best treated by weekly silver nitrate applications to the mass while the rabbit is under anesthesia. Immediately after applying the silver nitrate, deactivate the chemical burning by rinsing with water. After three or four treatments, the rectal papilloma is gone, but it can recur. Meloxicam can be given after treatment to decrease minor pain and inflammation.
- Rabbit facial papillomas need to be surgically removed to prevent later squamous cell carcinoma, but this is often difficult because there is little spare tissue for adequate closure after surgical resection of the masses. The prognosis is good, except in rabbits that get squamous cell carcinoma secondary to the facial form.

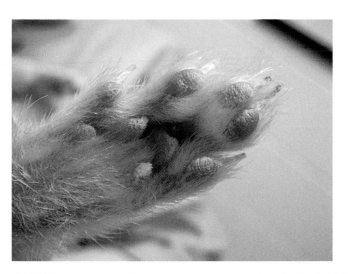

FIGURE 15-43 Papillomavirus. Ferret with hyperkeratotic area on the toe thought to be caused by a papillomavirus.

Papillomavirus—ferret, rabbit, rabbit—*cont'd*

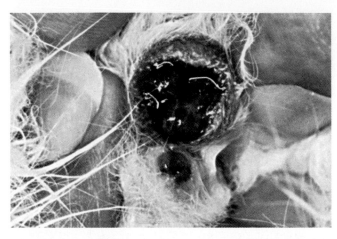

FIGURE 15-44 Papillomavirus. Rabbit with proliferative growth just inside the anus thought to be caused by a papillomavirus. Similar masses can be found within the oral cavity.

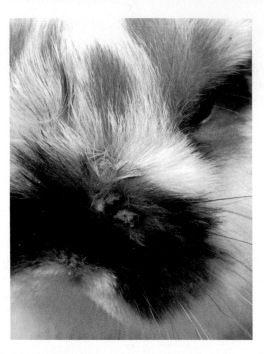

FIGURE 15-45 Papillomavirus. Rabbit with facial papillomavirus that is a different virus from the oral papillomavirus of rabbits. Facial papillomavirus is spread by mosquitoes that have fed on an infected wild cottontail rabbit. The masses continue to grow and can predispose pet rabbits to squamous cell carcinoma. This rabbit was housed in an outdoor hutch.

Papillomatous Cloacal/Oral Masses—bird

Features

Now known to be caused by psittacine herpesvirus-3, papillomatous masses of the cloaca and oral cavity of parrots, mostly Amazon parrots and macaws, look like papillomas, but histopathologically lack the rete pegs seen with true papillomas. Red, proliferative, irregular surface masses are usually seen in the proctodeum part of the cloaca just inside the vent, but can also be found within the oral cavity, or worse, but rarely, anywhere along the GI tract. The disease can be sexually transmitted. Amazon parrots can present with concomitant bile duct carcinoma caused by the same virus.

Top Differentials

None. Typical clinical signs do not resemble other diseases.

Diagnosis

Direct observation of typical clinical signs, or histopathologic examination of fine needle aspiration or biopsy. Amazon parrots should always have serum chemistry evaluation of lever enzymes and bile acids; some veterinarians may aggressively pursue endoscopic evaluation and biopsy of the liver to diagnose concomitant bile duct carcinoma.

Treatment and Prognosis

- Cloacal and even oral papillomatosis is best treated with weekly silver nitrate application to the mass while the bird is under anesthesia. Immediately after applying the silver nitrate, deactivate the chemical burning by rinsing with water. After three or four treatments, rectal papillomatosis is gone, but it does recur, especially after bouts of stress as are typical with herpesviruses, so prognosis is guarded.
- Papillomatosis in the GI tract may require surgical resection.
- Amazon parrots with concomitant bile duct carcinoma carry a grave prognosis. Acyclovir may help, but this has not been proved.

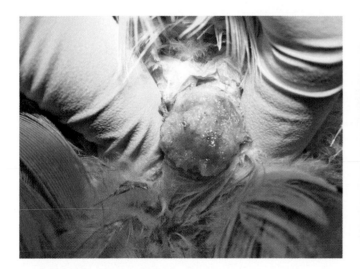

FIGURE 15-46 Papillomatous Mass. Large papillomatous mass in the cloaca of a blue and gold macaw caused by psittacine herpesvirus.

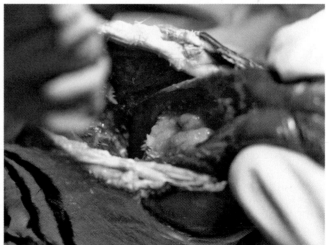

FIGURE 15-47 Papillomatous Mass. Papillomatous mass in the choana (roof of mouth) of the blue and gold macaw in Figure 15-46. The choanal masses are less common than the cloacal masses.

Papillomatous Cloacal/Oral Masses—bird—*cont'd*

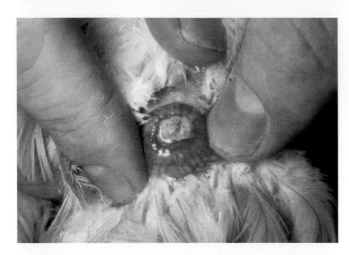

FIGURE 15-48 Papillomatous Mass. Papillomatous mass caused by psittacine herpesvirus after treatment under anesthesia with the chemical cautery agent silver nitrate. Water was flushed over the area to deactivate the burn. Weekly treatments for 5 weeks cleared the infection, but stress, such as that seen whenever the owner moved, would cause the mass to return.

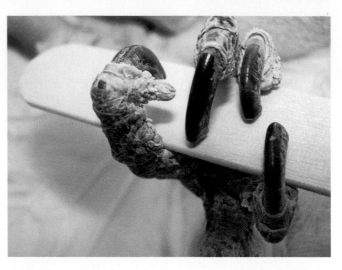

FIGURE 15-49 Papillomatous Mass. A cockatoo with a hyperkeratotic mass on the toes consistent with adenovirus. No treatment is needed.

Inclusion Body Disease (IBD)—snake

Features

Usually boas rather than pythons present with neurologic signs and dysecdysis (abnormal shedding) caused by a retrovirus-like agent. Dysecdysis, dermatitis, and respiratory disease in these snakes is thought to be due to secondary bacterial infections.

Top Differentials

Many factors can contribute to dysecdysis, most notably low environmental humidity. Rule-outs for neurologic signs in snakes are toxins, trauma, neoplasia, and infectious brain disease.

Diagnosis

Demonstration of inclusion bodies in esophageal tonsil, kidney, or liver.

Treatment and Prognosis

There is no treatment for this contagious virus, so prognosis is grave. Treatment consists of prevention of spread to other snakes.

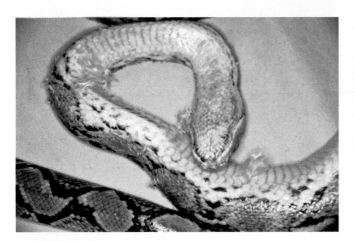

FIGURE 15-50 Inclusion Body Disease. Besides neurologic signs, snakes with inclusion body disease commonly exhibit dysecdysis (abnormal shed in pieces).

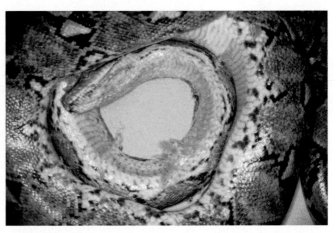

FIGURE 15-51 Inclusion Body Disease. Same snake as in Figure 15-50.

FUNGAL

Fungal Dermatitis (ringworm)—**chinchilla**

Features

Clinical signs or ringworm in small mammals is very similar in appearance to what is seen in a dog or cat. The most common exotic animal species presenting with ringworm is the chinchilla, although any small mammal species can present with ringworm. Generally *Trichophyton* spp. are more common than the *Microsporum* spp.

Top Differentials

Trauma or bacterial dermatitis.

Diagnosis

A dermatophyte test medium (DTM) culture can be performed. Cytology/biopsy can also be performed but is more invasive.

Treatment and Prognosis

Topical miconazole is typically used daily for 3 months or at least 1 month past resolution of clinical signs. Griseofulvin given orally is described in the older literature but generally is avoided now because of hepatic side effects.

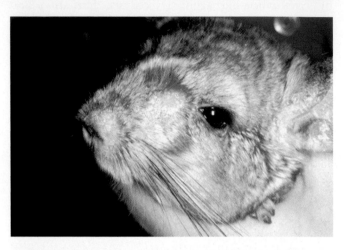

FIGURE 15-52 Fungal Dermatitis. Chinchilla with dermatophytosis on the face that responded to long-term topical miconazole cream.

Fungal Dermatitis (*Chrysosporium* spp.)—reptile

Features

Chrysosporium spp. fungus can cause slow-growing granulomas, as seen in this box turtle, or can cause a dermatitis and yellowing of the skin commonly called "Yellow Skin Disease" in inland bearded dragons (Pogona Vitticeps).

Top Differentials

Trauma or bacterial dermatitis.

Diagnosis

A biopsy of the granuloma will show the fungal organisim, or it can be grown by fungal culture.

Treatment and Prognosis

Surgical removal of granulomas, if possible. Long-term oral and topical antifungal therapy such as fluconazole, itraconazole, or voraconazole. Prognosis is typically poor.

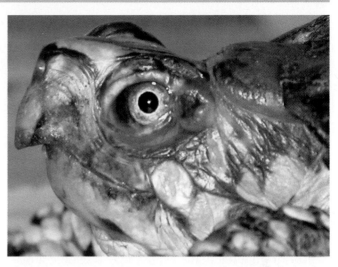

FIGURE 15-53 **Fungal (*Chrysosporium* spp.)** Wild box turtle with multiple fungal granulomas, including one in the dorsal cervical area (shown here) caused by *Chrysosporium*, a pigmented fungus.

NEOPLASIA

Mast Cell Tumor—ferret

Features

In ferrets, mast cell tumors are very common and appear as round, red to pink, erosive skin lesions that may or may not be raised, that may worsen or spontaneously resolve. Unlike dogs, mast cell tumors in ferrets are not known to metastasize.

Top Differentials

A slow-healing traumatic wound may resemble a mast cell tumor in a ferret or, rarely, a skin tumor of another type.

Diagnosis

Because the disease is very common and has a typical presentation of a "scab that comes and goes or does not quite heal," many veterinarians diagnose by clinical signs. A definitive diagnosis is based on histopathologic examination.

Treatment and Prognosis

If the mass causes irritation or excessive bleeding because of its location, then removal is recommended.

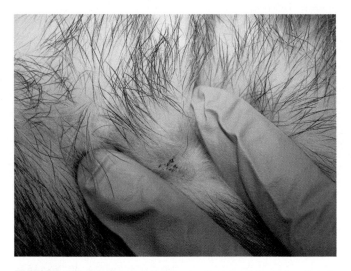

FIGURE 15-54 Mast Cell Tumor. Ferret with pink, slightly raised mast cell tumor—a very common but benign finding in ferrets.

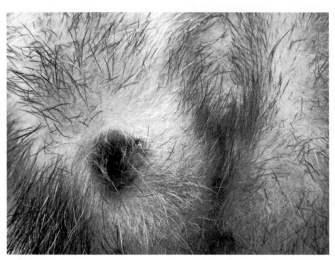

FIGURE 15-55 Mast Cell Tumor. Ferret with red, scabbed, and erosive mast cell tumor. These benign tumors need to be removed only if they are in a high-motion area and are causing pain or discomfort, such as on a toe.

Adrenal Cortical Tumor—ferret

Features

The incidence of adrenal gland disease in pet ferrets in the United States is estimated to be approximately 43% among ferrets over 3 years of age; the disease sometimes involves both glands. The cause of the high incidence of this and other tumors of ferrets is unknown, although theories include inbreeding and spaying/neutering at any age. Adrenal tissue and gonadal tissue arise from the same stem cells, and neutering/spaying in the ferret chronically stimulates the adrenal glands. Generally, the disease is common in ferrets over 3 years of age, but adrenal tumor has been diagnosed as early as 10 months. Clinical signs include bilateral, symmetrical alopecia, a harsh dry hair coat, muscle atrophy, a pendulous abdomen, and splenomegaly (extramedullary hematopoiesis). Clinical signs may also include vulvar enlargement even in spayed females, prostatic hyperplasia and subsequent urethral blockage in males, pruritus, aggressiveness, return to male behavior in neutered males, and bone marrow suppression in males or females.

Top Differentials

Affected adrenal glands have been shown to have hyperplasia (a possible pre-neoplastic condition), adenoma, or adenocarcinoma. Occasionally, other tumors, including leiomyosarcoma and pheochromocytoma, have been diagnosed. Aplastic anemia in an intact female ferret may present with bilaterally symmetrical alopecia.

Diagnosis

Diagnosis is based on clinical signs, a hormone panel, and/or ultrasound. The advantage of ultrasound is that it can identify which of the adrenal glands is affected, as this influences treatment decisions. Cortisol levels, adrenocorticotropic hormone (ACTH) stimulation test, and dexamethasone suppression test are all inconsistent and of little value in the ferret. In one study, 14 of 17 ferrets known to have an adrenal tumor had a normal ACTH stimulation test. In ferrets, a "ferret hormone panel" (available from the University of Tennessee Endocrinology Laboratory) is a sensitive test that can be used to determine if adrenal disease is present (Table 15-2).

Hormone panels may be a more sensitive indicator of adrenal disease, but they do not provide information as to which adrenal gland is affected. If surgery is an option, then ultrasound should be performed before surgery is performed. Identifying which adrenal gland is affected via ultrasound has several advantages, including knowing which adrenal to remove at surgery (sometimes early in the disease, this is difficult to determine grossly), knowing what type of surgery to expect (relatively simple left or difficult right adrenalectomy), and providing the owner with an initial cost estimate and suspected outcome of surgery and/or medical treatment. Normally, the adrenal gland is pinkish-yellow and elliptical in shape, about 3 mm wide and 5 mm long. If the gland takes on a "plump" appearance, or the diameter is ≥3 mm, then disease should be suspected. The right adrenal gland is dorsal and is attached to the vena cava. Sometimes the dorsal vena caval wall is affected and a pedunculated mass of tumor is intraluminal, partially or completely obstructing blood flow.

TABLE 15-2 Ferret Adrenal Hormone Panel (University of Tennessee)

Ferret Adrenal Panel	Reference Interval
Estrogen	30–180.0 pmol/L
17-OH progesterone	0–0.8 pmol/L
Androstenedione	0–15.0 pmol/L

Treatment and Prognosis

Treatment of adrenal gland disease in ferrets involves either to completely remove the affected gland or hormonal therapy to alleviate the clinical signs associated with the disease. If the tumor involves the left adrenal gland, then the treatment of choice is a relatively simple left adrenalectomy. If the tumor involves the right adrenal gland, complete surgical removal carries risk and is often difficult because of its very close association with the dorsal surface of the caudal vena cava. Magnifying loupes and microsurgical instruments such as a pediatric Statinsky clamp and an 8-0 nylon vascular suture are required to clamp off the vena cava during complete removal of the right adrenal gland. Incomplete debulking of the gland will result in regrowth. Therefore, treatment options for a right adrenal tumor include surgery and hormonal therapy. Hormonal therapy does not stop the growth of the tumor, it only improves clinical signs by reducing the production of hormones through a negative-feedback mechanism. Mitotane and other drugs utilized in dogs to decrease adrenal hyperplasia rarely decrease clinical signs in ferrets, and therefore are not recommended. Mitotane affects hyperplastic adrenal tissue, and in most cases, ferrets have adrenal adenoma or adenocarcinoma. Hormonal therapy with leuprolide acetate (Depo-Lupron),

Adrenal Cortical Tumor—ferret—*cont'd*

a gonadotropin-releasing hormone (GnRh) agonist, works well to counteract the clinical signs encountered with adrenal disease in ferrets. The dose for leuprolide acetate is 100 micrograms/kg IM q 1 month with the 1-month form, and 2 mg/kg with the 4-month form. The human injection of leuprolide acetate can be divided into ferret-sized doses and frozen for up to 3 months, or individual doses can be purchased through Professional Arts Pharmacy (410-747-6870). Deslorelin, another GnRh agonist that is available as an implant lasting about 9 months, has just recently become available in Australia and England and can be imported into the United States under "compassionate use" on a case-by-case basis. The dose for deslorelin is a 4.7 mg implant that lasts about 9 months.

Prognosis is good because even adrenal adenocarcinoma in the ferret rarely metastasizes. Prognosis in male ferrets with associated prostatic involvement is guarded, but poor if bacterial prostatitis is present.

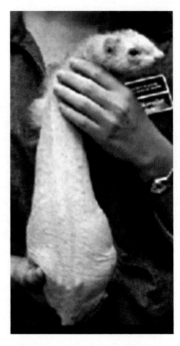

FIGURE 15-56 Adrenal Cortical Tumor. Ferret with adrenal cortical tumor causing bilateral symmetrical alopecia, pendulous abdomen, thin skin, and splenomegaly. The tail of the spleen can be seen wrapping around to the caudal right abdomen.

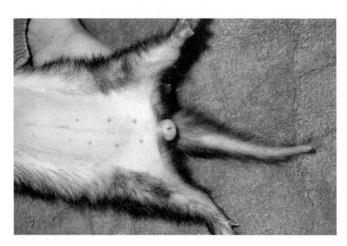

FIGURE 15-57 Adrenal Cortical Tumor. Three-year-old female spayed ferret with adrenal cortical tumor causing tail alopecia and vulvar swelling (usually the vulva is only barely visible).

Mammary Fibroadenoma—rat, mouse

Features

The incidence and types of tumors vary dramatically with the strain of the rat, as well as with age, sex, diet, caloric intake, and environment. Unfortunately, the genetic background of pet rats is unknown. The most common tumor of rats is the mammary gland tumor, described as having an incidence of 30% to 57% in female Sprague-Dawley rats, 50% to 90% in female aged rats, and 16% in male rats. Most rat mammary tumors are fibroadenomas (prolactin sensitive); about 10% are adenocarcinomas (estrogen sensitive). In mice, occurrence is opposite—90% are fibroadenocarcinomas and 10% are fibroadenomas. Unlike rats, mice more commonly are affected by mammary adenocarcinomas than by fibroadenomas. The tumors are located in the neck (even in the dorsum of the neck), flank, and inguinal and axillary regions, and often metastasize to the lung. These mammary adenocarcinomas are usually soft, fleshy, highly vascular, and infiltrative. It generally is not recommended to remove mouse mammary tumors because they are difficult to remove surgically without significant tissue damage and hemorrhage, and they have a high rate of metastasis. In rats, fibroadenoma tumors are well demarcated, are ovoid or discoid in shape, and usually are associated with one large vessel; they can quickly reach 10 cm in diameter. The tumors are well tolerated by the rat until they reach such a size that they interfere with ambulation, or until they become ulcerated, hemorrhagic, and necrotic and contribute to secondary bacterial infection or sepsis.

Top Differentials

The primary differential is abscess, or other SC tumor.

Diagnosis

Histopathologic examination of fine needle aspiration or incisional or preferably excisional biopsy.

Treatment and Prognosis

- Mammary fibroadenomas in rats are easily removed surgically, but often recur in nearby mammary tissue.
- Some inguinal masses are more difficult to remove if associated with the urethra.
- Mammary tissue can occur anywhere along the shoulder, neck, ventrum, flank, or tail base. One study showed that rats ovariectomized at 90 days of age had a significantly lower incidence of mammary tumor than intact female rats—2/47 versus 24/29, respectively—but there is no evidence that spaying an adult rat prevents the occurrence, or recurrence, of fibroadenoma or fibroadenocarcinoma.
- Because 90% of rat mammary tumors are fibroadenomas that are prolactin sensitive, the administration of antiestrogen drugs such as tamoxifen has not been shown to be helpful unless the tumor is a fibroadenocarcinoma, as is found in mice or in 10% of rats.
- Energy consumption restriction has been shown to decrease tumor incidence in mice.

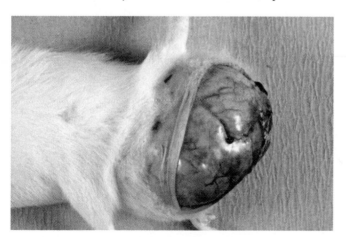

FIGURE 15-58 Mammary Fibroadenoma. Two-year-old rat with large mammary fibroadenoma. This rat was euthanized because of urethral involvement/impingement, but most of these tumors in rats easily shell out with one cord of vessels to ligate. Recurrence is common.

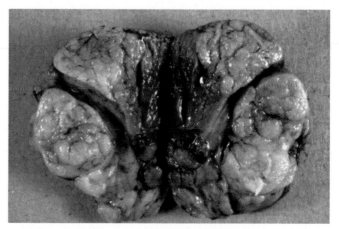

FIGURE 15-59 Mammary Fibroadenoma. Most rat mammary tumors are fibroadenomas, such as this one with a mix of fibrous tissue and adenomatous tissue.

Hamster Cheek Pouch

Features

A cheek pouch, which may extend halfway down the length of the body, is used to temporarily store food, and when full, it should not be mistaken for a tumor. An entire shelled peanut can fit inside a Syrian hamster cheek pouch.

Top Differentials

Tumor of the cheek pouch is rare, but a nearby SC mass could be in the same area as a cheek pouch.

Diagnosis

The cheek pouch can be everted or explored with a cotton applicator to determine if an SC mass or food is present.

Treatment

None, if normal food-storing behavior. Remove food if it is necrotic and adhered.

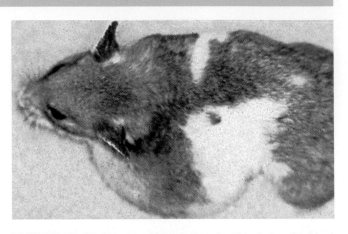

FIGURE 15-60 Hamster Cheek Pouch. This Syrian (Golden) hamster has a peanut in the cheek pouch, which can extend halfway down the length of the body. Do not misinterpret this as a neoplastic mass.

Tumor of Ventral Scent Gland—gerbil

Features

It is important to know the appearance of a normal gerbil ventral abdominal gland compared with a cancerous one. Benign adenomas of the ventral abdominal gland have been reported to be the third most common spontaneously occurring tumor in the gerbil.

Top Differential

Be able to differentiate a normal versus an abnormal ventral abdominal gland. If ulcerated, histopathologic evaluation of fine needle aspiration or incisional or excisional biopsy gives a definitive diagnosis.

Diagnosis

Oftentimes tumors of the ventral abdominal scent gland are inflamed and ulcerated and easily become secondarily infected with bacteria.

Treatment and Prognosis

Surgical removal of the mass if the gland is abnormal. Prognosis after complete surgical removal is good.

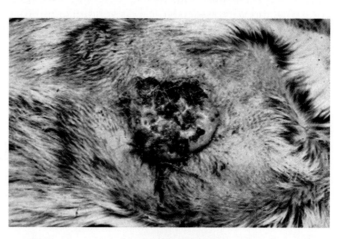

FIGURE 15-61 Tumor of Ventral Scent Gland. Tumor of ventral abdominal scent gland in a gerbil.

Squamous Cell Carcinoma—bird, turtle

Features

Among birds, squamous cell carcinoma (SCC) tends to occur more frequently in Amazon parrots, macaws, and African grey parrots, and can involve the uropygial (preen) gland with associated excess keratinization that almost looks hornlike. Birds with a chronic history of hypovitaminosis A from a lifelong seed-only diet tend to develop SCC in the oral cavity (especially Amazon parrots), presumably secondary to chronic squamous metaplasia. In turtles, an SC or dermal mass is present.

Top Differentials

Other tumors or fungal granuloma.

Diagnosis

Histopathologic examination of fine needle aspiration or incisional or excisional biopsy.

Treatment and Prognosis

If possible, remove with large margins. If this is not possible, then remove most of the tumor and combine with radiation and chemotherapy. Birds and especially reptiles seem to be refractory to even high doses of radiation. Strontium-90 radiation in a box turtle destroyed tumor tissue only within 1 mm of the probe. Intralesional and IV cisplatin has been attempted in birds with variable success.

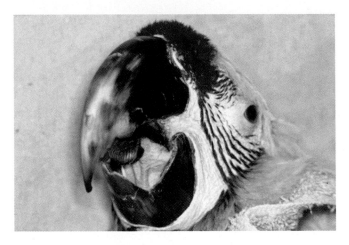

FIGURE 15-62 Squamous Cell Carcinoma. Squamous cell carcinoma of the beak and surrounding tissues in a Buffon's macaw. Radiation and chemotherapy did not slow the growth of the tumor.

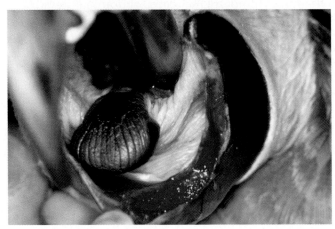

FIGURE 15-63 Squamous Cell Carcinoma. Close up of bird in Figure 15-62.

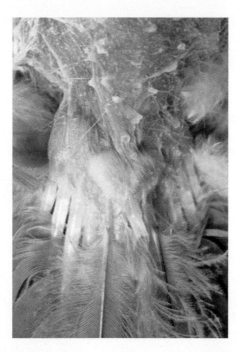

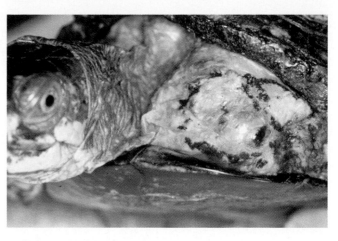

FIGURE 15-65 Squamous Cell Carcinoma. Squamous cell carcinoma in a wild, caught, captive box turtle. Strontium radiation therapy was unsuccessful, and the tumor spread into the cranial coelomic cavity.

FIGURE 15-64 Squamous Cell Carcinoma. Normal uropygial (preen) gland in a conure, demonstrating the bilobed appearance of the gland. It is good to know normal so that an abnormal preen gland, such as one that is infected or neoplastic, can be recognized.

Lipoma—bird

Features

Lipoma is common in budgerigars and rose-breasted cockatoos, but it can be seen in any species of bird. Typically, it presents as a light yellow to tan , soft mass over the cranial end of the keel, or over the coelomic area ventrally.

Top Differentials

Rarely, a liposarcoma can present that has a similar appearance.

Diagnosis

Histopathologic examination of fine needle aspiration or biopsy.

Treatment and Prognosis

Weight loss through diet and exercise is recommended if the bird is overweight and if on a seed-only diet. The use of thyroid supplementation is controversial; it should not be used unless it has been proved that the bird has hypothyroidism. One study evaluated the use of L-carnitine with variable results. Surgery has been tried in severe cases where the mass was interfering with normal activity.

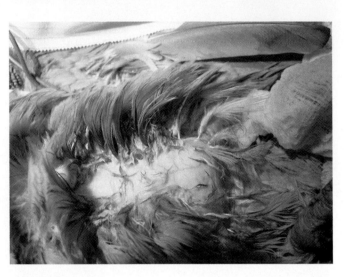

FIGURE 15-66 **Lipoma.** Amazon parrot with an SC lipoma just caudal to the sternum.

Xanthoma—bird

Features

Xanthomas are bright yellow, locally invasive tumors of the skin of birds, usually associated with a past history of trauma to the skin of the affected area.

Top Differentials

No other mass is bright yellow like a xanthoma.

Diagnosis

Histopathologic examination shows characteristic cholesterol clefts.

Treatment and Prognosis

Surgical excision of the mass with margins is needed to prevent further spread.

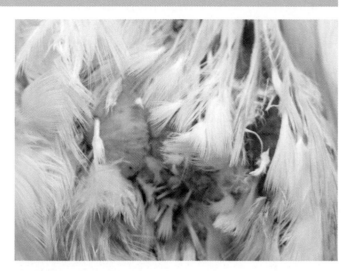

FIGURE 15-67 Xanthoma. A cockatiel with a xanthoma—a bright yellow tumor associated with an area of chronic trauma. No known trauma was found in this case. Xanthomas are aggressively locally invasive, so surgery is highly recommended to completely remove the mass.

Brown Hypertrophy of the Cere—budgerigar (parakeet)

Features

The cere, the area around the nostrils in a bird, is normally blue in male budgerigars and pink to pinkish-brown in female budgerigars. If a male's blue cere turns brown later in life, then suspect a commonly occurring estrogen-secreting testicular tumor. If a female's cere becomes darker brown and proliferative, then suspect an increase in estrogen due to impending egg laying, a cystic ovary, or an estrogen-secreting ovarian tumor.

Top Differentials

A female's cere may darken and become hypertrophied as the result of any cause of increased estrogen.

Diagnosis

Clinical signs: palpation, radiograph ± barium in GI tract, or ultrasound may help diagnose reproductive diseases in birds. Estrogen levels can also be evaluated.

Treatment and Prognosis

Surgery to remove gonads in any psittacine bird is not recommended because of potential complications from the small size and close arterial/aorta involvement. A depot form of leuprolide acetate has been used with some success with cystic ovary, giving a fair prognosis. Tumors carry a grave prognosis.

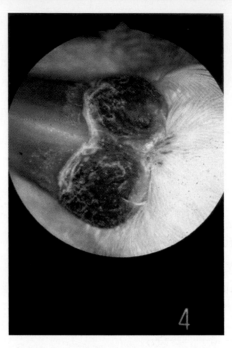

FIGURE 15-68 **Brown Hypertrophy of the Cere.** Adult female budgerigar (parakeet) with brown hypertrophy of the cere secondary to increased estrogen.

TRAUMA

Bruise—bird

Features

Birds bruise green rather than purple. This should not be mistaken for gangrene. After approximately 3 days, a bruise will turn green in birds because they lack biliverdin reductase, an enzyme that converts biliverdin to bilirubin. This phenomenon helps to age a bruise in a bird.

Top Differentials

Gangrene.

Diagnosis

Direct visualization.

Treatment and Prognosis

Treat the trauma appropriately as for other animals.

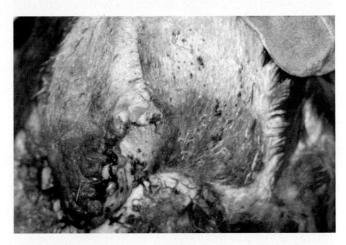

FIGURE 15-69 Bruise. A captive great horned owl that had a wing amputated after severe trauma and bleeding 3 days previously. Birds bruise bright green because they lack biliverdin reductase to convert biliverdin to bilirubin.

Necrosis From Injectable Enrofloxacin

Features

After IM injection of enrofloxacin, an area of necrosis can occur that may be visible, especially in birds. Injectable enrofloxacin is for IM use only; a switch to the oral form as soon as possible is recommended. The IM form of enrofloxacin given subcutaneously to rabbits can cause necrosis.

Top Differentials

Trauma from other causes.

Diagnosis

Visual appearance. Commonly diagnosed via histopathogy on a necropsy report in birds that died of other causes but were given IM enrofloxacin before death.

Treatment and Prognosis

Use the injectable form of enrofloxacin for as short a time as possible, then switch to an oral form.

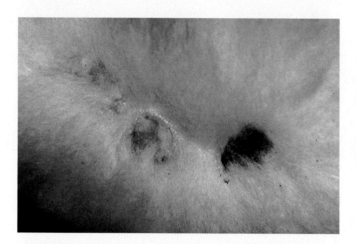

FIGURE 15-70 Necrosis From Injectable Enrofloxacin. Subcutaneous necrosis in a rabbit from SC administration of enrofloxacin. The pH of enrofloxacin is not physiologic, and it can cause necrosis. Enrofloxacin can be given PO, IM, or in a large amount of saline SC.

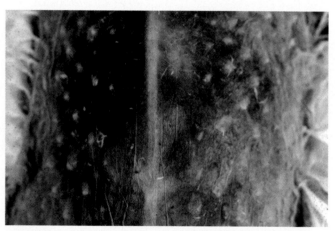

FIGURE 15-71 Necrosis From Injectable Enrofloxacin. Necrosis in a parrot from IM administration of enrofloxacin as prescribed. The pH of enrofloxacin is not physiologic, and it can cause necrosis even if given as directed. Enrofloxacin can also be given PO, or in a large amount of saline SC.

Air Sac Rupture—bird

Features

Rupture of the cervicocephalic air sac in a parrot can occur secondary to blunt trauma to the head or neck area, or secondary to an erosive lesion of the air sac. This disease is characterized by an air-filled swelling on one or both sides of the neck. It is not painful, but may be associated with some dyspnea.

Top Differentials

Air in crop from aerophagia.

Diagnosis

Clinical appearance.

Treatment and Prognosis

If recent trauma, then can deflate with a 25-gauge needle repeatedly until refilling of air does not occur. If refilling of the air sac continues past several days of deflating with a needle, then surgery to place a Teflon stent may be needed to permanently deflate.

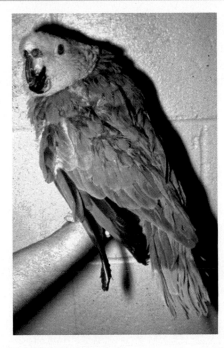

FIGURE 15-73 Air Sac Rupture. The Amazon parrot with air sac rupture in Figure 15-72.

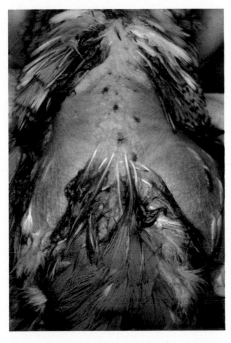

FIGURE 15-72 Air Sac Rupture. Close-up of an Amazon parrot with a cervicocephalic air sac rupture. Note the air trapped in the air sac under the skin. Trauma, such as a bad fall in this case, can rupture an air sac.

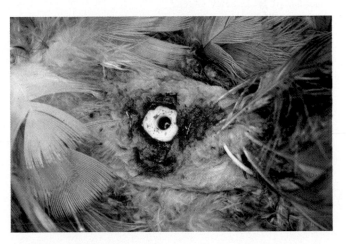

FIGURE 15-74 Air Sac Rupture. A stent was placed in the cervicocephalic air sac to resolve air sac rupture of the Amazon parrot in Figure 15-72.

Constricted Toe Syndrome—bird

Features

A circumferential section of skin around the toe causes constriction, impaired venous return, and swelling of the toe distal to the constriction. Young, hand-raised parrots kept in a dry environment are most often affected. Eclectus parrots tend to present with this disease more often than other species.

Top Differentials

Thread or fiber constriction around the toe. Use a magnifying glass or loupe to determine if dry skin or a thread is causing the constriction.

Diagnosis

Visual inspection.

Treatment and Prognosis

Treatment consists of surgery to break down the dry skin constriction by creating four release cuts. Avoid cutting directly laterally where the digital vessels run. Suture the skin as needed, but still maintain the release cuts and then bandage. Soaking feet in water may prevent this disease, or treat early cases.

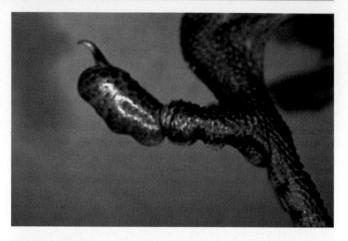

FIGURE 15-75 Constricted Toe Syndrome. A juvenile Eclectus parrot with constricted toe syndrome subsequent to being in a dry environment. Surgery resolved the problem. Increasing humidity in the environment prevented additional problems.

Hernia—bird

Features

Female birds, after excessive egg laying, can develop a coelomic cavity hernia, presenting with a large, sometimes pendulous mass ventrally.

Top Differentials

Tumor.

Diagnosis

A barium GI series helps to determine if the mass is a hernia, and if there is any GI involvement.

Treatment and Prognosis

Surgery to return the coelomic contents to their rightful place and repair the defect. Mersilene mesh or similar can be used if there is not enough muscle to cover the defect.

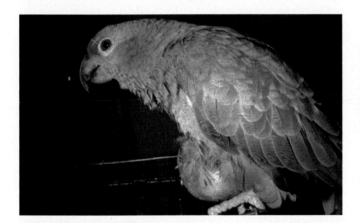

FIGURE 15-76 Hernia. A 20+-year-old Amazon parrot with a chronic hernia. It had been slowly growing for 7 years. The owner had been told that nothing could be done for the mass.

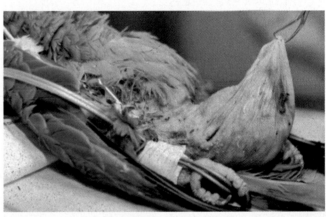

FIGURE 15-77 Hernia. Same bird as in Figure 15-76. Surgery to correct the hernia and Mersilene mesh to repair the defect were successful.

Cloacal Prolapse—bird

Features

The cloaca is the endpoint of three systems—the renal, reproductive, and GI systems. Prolapse, or eversion, of the cloaca can also involve any of these systems. It is normal for a female bird to have a mild, temporary prolapse immediately after laying an egg, but otherwise a cloacal prolapse is abnormal. Causes for prolapse include papillomatous lesions, tenesmus (diarrhea or constipation), genetic predisposition (cockatoos, African grey parrot) leading to a collagen synthesis defect, chronic irritation of the cloaca from masturbation, egg laying, and idiopathic atony (cockatoos).

Top Differentials

Other tissues can be prolapsed, including the uterus, which is very red, has longitudinal striations, and has a lumen, and GI organs, such as the colon, which is smooth and has a lumen. A papillomatous lesion will be pinkish red with an irregular surface.

Diagnosis

Based on clinical examination and history.

Treatment and Prognosis

Many options are available to prevent re-prolapse after the prolapse is reduced, including laterally suturing the vent with a stay suture on either side, and cloacopexy, where the cloaca is surgically attached via suture to the rib (not recommended because of movement of the rib) or lateral coelomic wall, or is incorporated into the closure of the incision after removal of any fat between the cloaca and the coelomic wall. Ventplasty, which is removing a portion of the vent and suturing it into a smaller opening, can be performed.

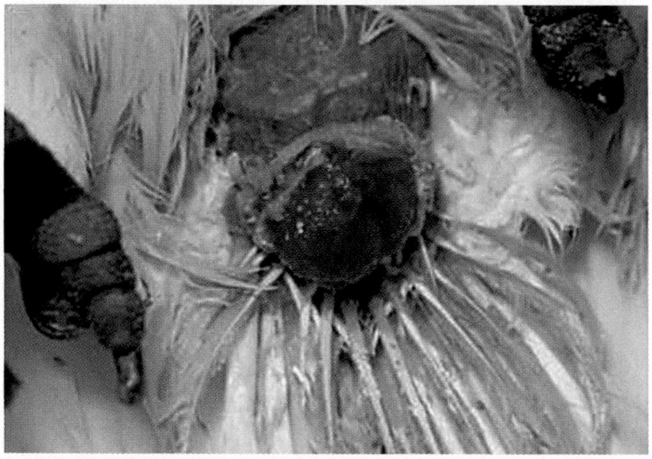

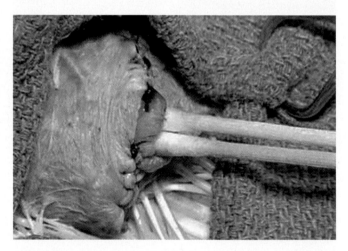

FIGURE 15-78 Cloacal Prolapse. An adult male sulfur-crested cockatoo developed a chronic cloacal prolapse secondary to chronic masturbation. Multiple surgeries, including internal pexies, external vent tacking, and ventplasty to permanently tighten the cloaca, all eventually failed. Leuprolide acetate hormonal injections finally curbed the excessive behavior and resolved the prolapse.

FIGURE 15-79 Cloacal Prolapse. The cockatoo in Figure 15-78 after a ventplasty surgery.

Bite Trauma—snake, iguana

Features

If a cold or otherwise not hungry snake is left alone with its dinner—a live mouse or rat—then the "dinner" can become the "diner" and can get hungry and chew on the snake; therefore it is always recommended to feed dead prey to a snake. Rodents have chisel-shaped incisor teeth that inflict severe damage to the snake, including damage to the bone of the spine. Small exotic pets sometimes present after a cat or dog bite.

Top Differentials

The history and appearance of the wound are typical with no other rule-outs.

Diagnosis

Radiographs may be needed to determine the extent of the lesion.

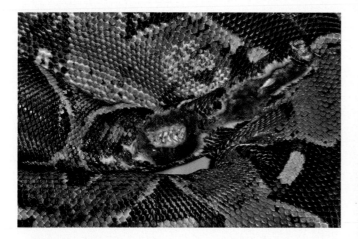

FIGURE 15-80 Bite Trauma. A boa snake with trauma to skin, muscle and bone from a rat bite. This is a case where the "dinner" for the snake (the rat) became the "diner" by chewing on the snake after it was not eaten by the snake and became hungry after hours of being left in the cage. Snakes may not eat because of illness or because they are cold, so always feed dead prey items.

Treatment and Prognosis

In reptiles, clean and débride the wound with the patient under anesthesia. Offer pain relief as needed, and always prescribe long-term (6–10 weeks), broad-spectrum, bactericidal antibiotics.

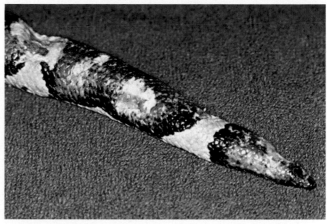

FIGURE 15-81 Bite Trauma. Tail of the snake in Figure 15-80.

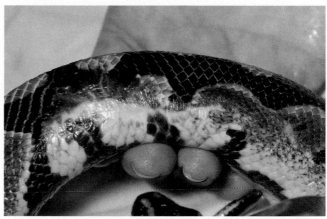

FIGURE 15-82 Bite Trauma. A ball python years after trauma to the skin had occurred. Snakes heal well, but very slowly. Scarring to cover the defect shown took over a year.

Bite Trauma—snake, iguana—*cont'd*

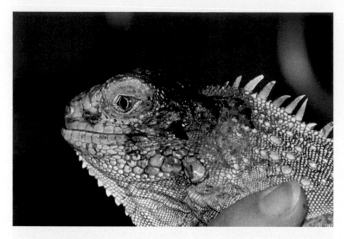

FIGURE 15-83 **Bite Trauma.** Green iguana immediately after a cat attack. There are puncture wounds about the head and neck, including a puncture of the tympanic membrane.

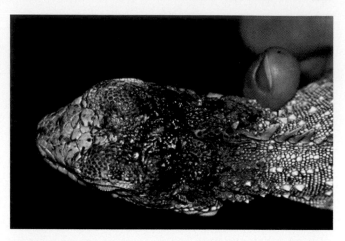

FIGURE 15-84 **Bite Trauma.** Dorsal view of the iguana shown in Figure 15-83.

Shell Repair—turtle, tortoise

Features

Wild and captive turtles may require shell repair after trauma from a car or from being chewed by a dog. The top shell is called the *carapace*, and the bottom shell is called the *plastron*. Both are made of bone covered with a thin layer of keratin. If the pigmented keratin is missing, the white bone underneath will be exposed. Fractures occur through both bone and keratin.

Diagnosis

Sometimes radiographs are needed, but rarely, because the bone of the shell is external.

Treatment and Prognosis

Various treatment options are available, including (1) wiring closed after placement of a hole in the shell or after a pin is placed on which to wrap the wire around, (2) using bone plates with screws, (3) applying the glue/epoxy attachment of braces or an upside-down screw or anything that the cerclage wire can be wrapped around, or (4) using 5-minute epoxy with fiberglass mesh or plumber's epoxy to bridge the fracture gap. A fracture must be sterile if it is to be covered completely by a repair. Systemic antibiotics and pain relievers are given.

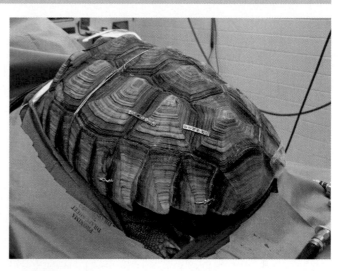

FIGURE 15-86 Shell Repair. Seven-year-old male spur-thighed tortoise hit by a car with multiple carapace and plastron fractures reduced by metal plates, screws with cerclage wires, and cerclage wires alone through holes drilled in the shell.

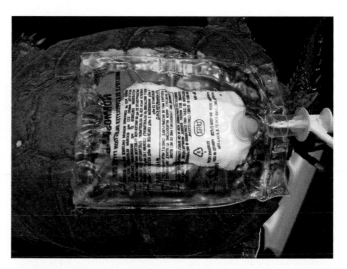

FIGURE 15-87 Shell Repair. A slider turtle with a severe carapace (shell) defect. An empty sterile IV fluid bag was cut to fit over the wound and was sealed to the shell, so that a needle hooked to suction could be attached to a vacuum device to encourage healing of the open, infected, wet wound.

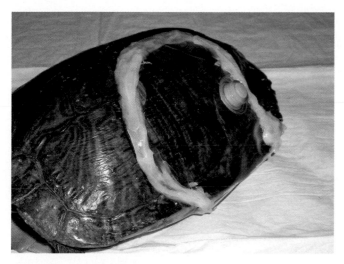

FIGURE 15-85 Shell Repair. A slider turtle with a severe carapace (shell) defect. An empty sterile IV fluid bag was cut to fit over the wound and was sealed to the shell, so that a needle hooked to suction could be attached to a vacuum device to encourage healing of the open, infected, wet wound.

Shell Repair—turtle, tortoise—*cont'd*

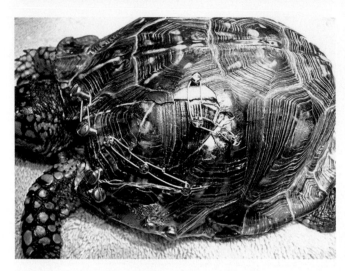

FIGURE 15-88 **Shell Repair.** A wild box turtle with carapace fractures reduced with screws and cerclage wire.

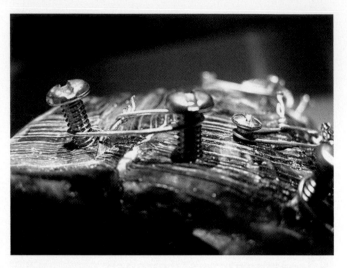

FIGURE 15-89 **Shell Repair.** Close-up of the box turtle shown in Figure 15-88.

METABOLIC/NUTRITIONAL/ENDOCRINE RELATED

Vitamin A Deficiency—bird, turtle

Features

Liver disease in birds is very common and is usually secondary to chronic hypovitaminosis A. First indications are blackening of the feathers from not being formed normally and being unable to refract light normally for us to perceive the color green. The beak and nails may also become elongated. Plantar erosions can develop and predispose the bird to ulcerative pododermatitis. White oral plaques can form secondary to squamous metaplasia of the salivary ducts at the base of the tongue. Squamous metaplasia can occur in any epithelial tissue, including renal tubules. Turtles present with thickened, swollen eyelids.

Top Differentials

Any trauma to the feathers can cause blackening of the feathers, including overpetting by the owner. Head trauma in turtles may cause swollen lids.

Diagnosis

Blood chemistry, including aspartate aminotransferase (AST), lactate dehydrogenase (LDH), and creatine kinase (CK), to determine liver enzyme activity or muscle activity, along with a bile acid. Liver biopsy can be performed via endoscopy. Vitamin A levels can be determined in birds. History is helpful.

Treatment and Prognosis

Slowly change the diet to include vitamin A–containing foods such as pellets made for birds, or add cooked sweet potato to the diet. Giving lactulose treats any concurrent liver disease and helps by converting NH_3 to NH_4 so the liver is spared. Colchicine prevents any further hepatic fibrosis from forming, but it has a very narrow therapeutic margin; milk thistle with its active ingredient silymarin is also helpful. There is controversy regarding the old practice of giving a vitamin A injection rather than slowly increasing the body's vitamin A levels via dietary means. Some small debilitated turtles have died after vitamin A injection. An overgrown beak can be trimmed with a rotary tool to remove excess keratin growth.

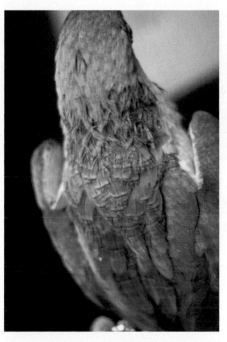

FIGURE 15-91 Vitamin A Deficiency. Blue and gold macaw with evidence of hypovitaminosis A causing weakened feathers that break down and turn black in color.

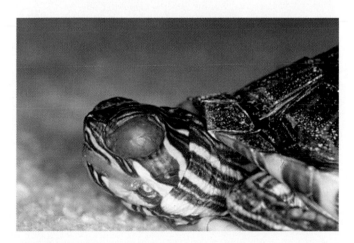

FIGURE 15-90 Vitamin A Deficiency. A pet red-eared slider turtle with swollen eyelids secondary to hypovitaminosis A.

Vitamin A Deficiency—bird, turtle—_cont'd_

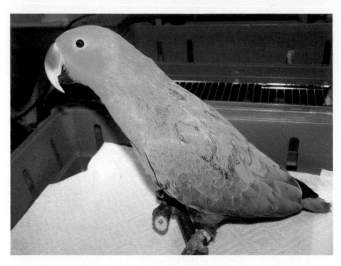

FIGURE 15-92 **Vitamin A Deficiency.** Male Eclectus with evidence of hypovitaminosis A causing weakened feathers that break down and turn black in color.

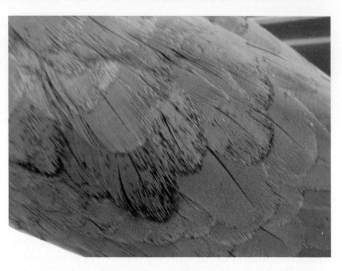

FIGURE 15-93 **Vitamin A Deficiency.** Close-up of the bird shown in Figure 15-92.

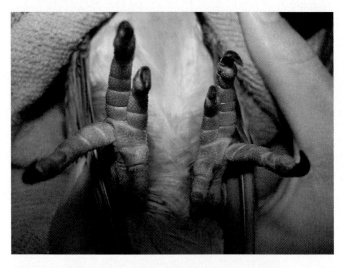

FIGURE 15-94 **Vitamin A Deficiency.** Senegal parrot showing a normal plantar surface to the right foot and, on the bird's left foot, plantar erosions consistent with hypovitaminosis A.

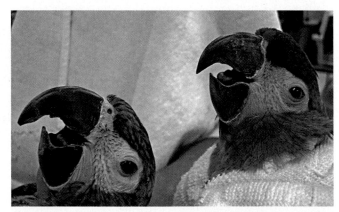

FIGURE 15-95 **Vitamin A Deficiency.** Young macaws from the same clutch. The bird on the right has a normal beak; the bird on the left has an overgrown, thickened beak secondary to suspected liver disease or hypovitaminosis A.

Cystic Ovary—guinea pig

Features

The incidence of cystic ovary in intact female guinea pigs over 5 years of age is approximately 80%. Generally the left ovary is involved, but this condition can affect the right ovary, or both. The ovarian cyst can commonly reach 5 × 5 cm in size. Clinical signs include lethargy, painful abdomen, partial anorexia, enlarged abdomen, enlarged nipples, and bilaterally symmetrical alopecia along the flanks and ventrum.

Top Differentials

This similar pattern of alopecia can occur in female guinea pigs that have had many successive litters.

Diagnosis

Palpation or radiograph or ultrasound demonstrates the large cyst.

Treatment and Prognosis

Some veterinarians give leuprolide acetate or human chorionic gonadotropin (HCG); others recommend a complete spay procedure; others suggest that only an ovariectomy is needed and that it is a quicker surgery.

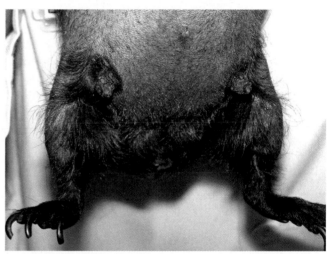

FIGURE 15-97 Cystic Ovary. A 5-year-old, female intact guinea pig with bilateral symmetrical lateral and ventral alopecia secondary to increased hormone levels from a cystic ovary. Note that the nipples are enlarged.

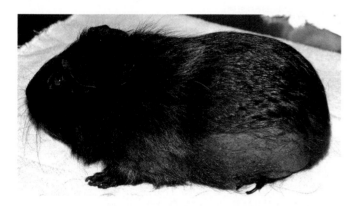

FIGURE 15-96 Cystic Ovary. A 5-year-old, female intact guinea pig with bilateral symmetrical lateral and ventral alopecia secondary to increased hormone levels from a cystic ovary.

OTHER DISEASES

Feather Picking/Chewing/Self-Mutilation—bird

Features

Birds feather pick or chew for many reasons, including medical causes and behavioral causes. They usually chew the breast feathers and areas under the wing and around the legs, but any pattern can present. Usually feathers on the head are intact. Picking of the feathers over the ventral coelomic cavity is sometimes seen with *Giardia* spp. intestinal infection. Zinc toxicosis has been shown to be linked to feather picking. Anecdotal reports suggest that a unilateral pattern of picking may indicate a disease process under the area of picking, such as testicular or renal, viral (PBFD or polyomavirus), bacterial folliculitis, dermal yeast infection, or topical irritant. Rarely do birds feather pick with external parasites. There are many rule-outs for behavioral feather picking, as well as improper socialization when raised by humans resulting in phobic birds or those with obsessive-compulsive disorder. A traumatic event can cause a bird to become "nervous" and pick; anecdotal examples abound, such as witnessing an attack by a hawk outside the window at a bird feeder, the owner leaving for vacation, a change in the color of the cage, a nervous owner, the death of a mate or owner, and so forth. Some birds improve in a new home with a new owner for unknown reasons. Self-mutilation is a serious, life-threatening disease; the help of a board-certified behaviorist familiar with birds is recommended.

Top Differentials

Generally, feather-picking birds cannot reach the feathers on their head, so these feathers are normal, unless another bird is picking their feathers for them, or viral PBFD or bacterial disease or trauma occurs.

Diagnosis

All possible medical causes for a bird's feather picking are evaluated first; then if no medical cause is found, behavioral causes are explored. A complete blood count (CBC) profile, blood lead and serum zinc test (Louisiana Veterinary Medical Diagnostic Laboratory can run this test on 0.1 mL of blood and serum), radiographs, Psittacine Beak and Feather Test, and fecal float and fecal enzyme-linked immunosorbent assay (ELISA) test for *Giardia* spp., if necessary, are performed, along with a feather follicle biopsy and culture. Ask about any history of toxins in the environment.

Treatment and Prognosis

- Many treatment options exist. Treat any underlying medical causes.
- Remove any stressors. Improve the bird's diet, and restore what the bird perceives as a normal environment.
- If a bird is self-mutilating, then some medications may help, including clomipramine (this works well in true obsessive-compulsive disorder), haloperidol, or other tricyclic antidepressants.
- Distracting the bird with toys, a "sweater" over the area, etc., may help, but be sure the bird can also engage in normal and necessary preening behavior.
- A collar is not recommended in birds as it does not allow them to engage in normal preening behavior, normal feeding behavior, and normal ambulation. A collar should be used only if the bird is in imminent danger of hurting itself (self-mutilating).

Consult *Carpenter's Exotic Animal Formulary* for further drug information.

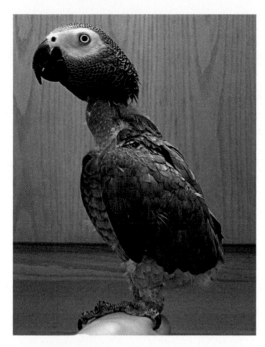

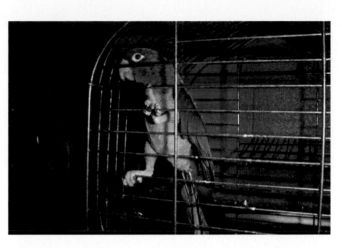

FIGURE 15-99 Feather Picking/Chewing/Self-Mutilation. Mitred conure with alopecia over the ventral breast area and legs due to feather picking by the bird. This is a typical pattern of feather picking in parrots.

FIGURE 15-98 Feather Picking/Chewing/Self-Mutilation. African grey parrot with alopecia over the ventral cervical area and the tail due to feather picking by the bird.

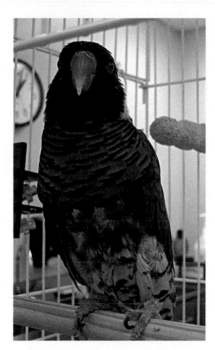

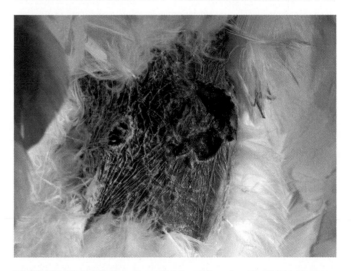

FIGURE 15-101 Feather Picking/Chewing/Self-Mutilation. Cockatoo with alopecia over the ventral breast area and bites of skin and muscle picking by the bird. Self-mutilation is a serious, life-threatening problem that requires multiple modalities to treat, including a collar to prevent further trauma, medications to calm the bird, and behavioral/environmental investigation and modification to determine why the bird is self-destructive. Clomipramine helped in this case, but after a year of attempted treatments, the owners elected euthanasia.

FIGURE 15-100 Feather Picking/Chewing/Self-Mutilation. Rainbow lory with alopecia over the ventral abdominal area and the legs due to feather picking by the bird. It is unknown why the bird picked.

Feather Cyst—bird

Features

A firm mass usually found at the wing tip, consisting of an ingrown feather that has continued to grow and has curled up into a ball under the skin. The follicle is greatly stretched and inflamed over the cyst.

Top Differentials

Neoplasia or abscess.

Diagnosis

Typical appearance and mass do not change over a long time.

Treatment and Prognosis

Surgery to lance the follicle to remove the ingrown feather material. It is important to not use cautery within a follicle, as this can traumatize the follicle and cause further feather cyst formation. Bleeding can be controlled with gelfoam packing. The follicle should be left open to heal by second intention healing. It can be bandaged during this healing time.

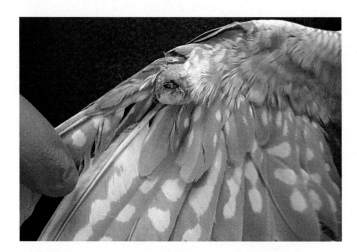

FIGURE 15-102 Feather Cyst. Cockatiel with a feather cyst over the right carpus and main digit.

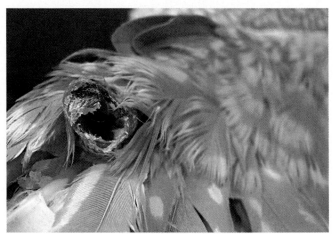

FIGURE 15-103 Feather Cyst. Same cockatiel as in Figure 15-102 after surgical lancing and débridement. The wound is left open for second intention healing.

Excess Keratin—guinea pig foot

Features

Sometimes excess keratin is seen where the fifth toenail would be if guinea pigs had five toes on each of the front feet (they only have four toes on each of the front feet). It is similar to a chestnut in a horse.

Top Differentials

None.

Diagnosis

Typical appearance.

Treatment and Prognosis

It can be trimmed just as a toenail because it is just excess keratin.

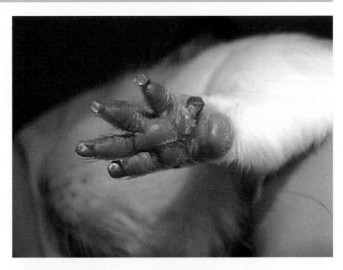

FIGURE 15-104 **Excess Keratin.** Adult guinea pig that presented for a nail trim for elongated nails and a commonly seen keratin growth on the lateral side of the foot, where the fifth digit would be if guinea pigs still had one. This keratin is also trimmed as part of the nail trim.

Porphyrin Tears—rat

Features

Red tears occur in rats as the result of stress causing excess Harderian gland secretions, which contain red porphyrins that look like blood.

Top Differentials

Blood.

Diagnosis

Typical appearance; usually occur with a concurrent disease.

Treatment and Prognosis

Treat underlying disease. Clean the face to determine if any new porphyrin tears are being formed.

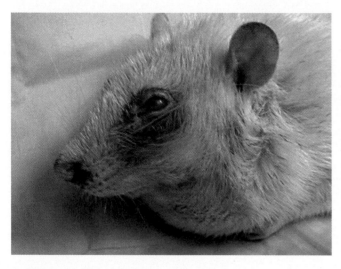

FIGURE 15-105 Porphyrin Tears. Severe case of porphyrin tears in a sick rat. Stress and illness cause increased secretions from the Harderian gland, which are often mistaken for blood.

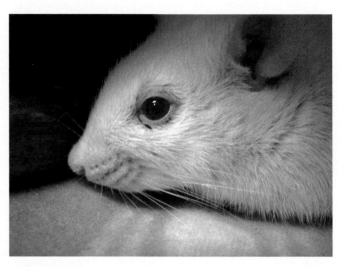

FIGURE 15-106 Porphyrin Tears. Mild case of porphyrin tears in a sick rat. This rat had *Mycoplasma* pneumonia and was mildly dyspneic.

Improper Vaccine Delivery—bird

Features

Small, firm SC masses over the caudal pectoral muscles where one commonly administers an SC vaccine. A granuloma occurs if a vaccine is given to a bird not SC, but rather intradermally or in the muscle, or if the sarcolemma is damaged when the vaccine is given.

Top Differentials

Neoplasia or abscess.

Diagnosis

Typical appearance and mass do not change over a long time.

Treatment and Prognosis

None. The granuloma can be surgically removed if causing a problem, but this would be rare. Care to prevent damage to the underlying muscle is imperative. Using a 22-gauge needle will ensure an SC injection, rather than an intradermal injection. If a 25-gauge needle is used, an intradermal injection may be given inadvertently, leaving a white bleb.

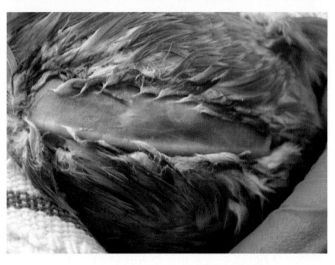

FIGURE 15-107 **Inappropriate Vaccine Delivery.** An Amazon parrot with SC granulomas from a polyoma vaccine that was given inappropriately. The vaccine is to be given SC, but if the sarcolemma is damaged, or if the vaccine is given IM or intradermally, then a granuloma can form.

Hairless Varieties

Features

Realize that there are hairless varieties of guinea pigs, mice, etc.

Top Differentials

None.

Diagnosis

Typical appearance.

Treatment and Prognosis

None. Hairless varieties may be more sensative to cooler temperatures, sunlight, trauma, and dryness than haired varieties.

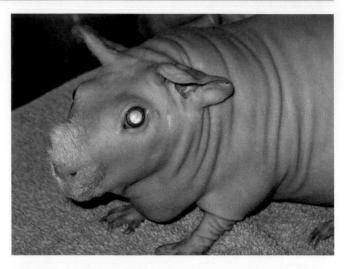

FIGURE 15-108 Hairless Varieties. Several species can be purchased hairless, including mice and, as in this case, guinea pigs. Hairless varieties seem less immunocompetent than their haired relatives.

Tattoo—ferret, rabbit, bird

Features

Two dot tattoos in the right ear of a ferret signify that it has been spayed or neutered and de-scented. Occasionally, show rabbits will present with a tattoo in the ear that is used for identification. Years ago, when birds were sexed via laparoscopy rather than blood sexing, a tattoo was placed in the left wing web to signify a female and in the right wing web to signify a male.

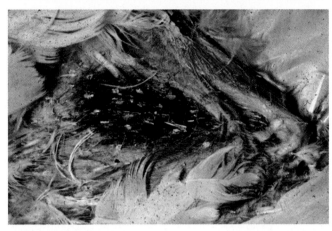

FIGURE 15-110 **Tattoo.** A tattoo in the wing web of a bird signifies that it has been surgically or blood sexed and marked as a female (left wing web) or a male (right wing web).

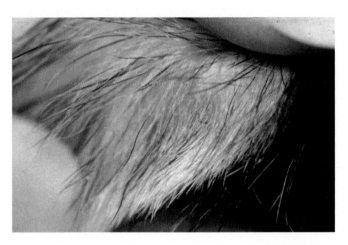

FIGURE 15-109 **Tattoo.** Two dot tattoos in the right ear of a ferret signify that it has been neutered/spayed and de-scented.

Suggested Readings

Adamcak A, Kaufman A, Quesenberry K: What's your diagnosis? Generalized alopecia in a Syrian (golden) hamster, *Lab Anim* 27:19, 1998.

Bauck L, Orr JP, Lawrence KH: Hyperadrenocorticism in three teddy bear hamsters, *Can Vet J* 25:247, 1984.

Collins BR: Common diseases and medical management of rodents and lagomorphs. In Jacobson ER, Kollias GV editor: *Exotic Animals*, New York, 1988, Churchill Livingstone, p 261.

Cooper JE: Dermatology. In Mader DR, editor: *Reptile Medicine and Surgery*, ed 2, St. Louis, 2006, Elsevier, p 196.

Derrell CJ: Biology and diseases of other rodents. In Fox JG, Cohen BJ, Loew FM, editors: *Laboratory Animal Medicine*, Orlando, 1984, Academic Press, p 183.

Diethelm G: Reptiles. In Carpenter JW, editor: *Exotic Animal Formulary*, ed 3, Philadelphia, 2005, Elsevier Saunders, p 58.

Dirx MJ, Zeegers MP, Dagnelie PC, van den Bogaard T, et al: Energy restriction and the risk of spontaneous mammary tumors in mice: a meta-analysis, *Int J Cancer* 106:766, 2003.

Donnelly TM: Disease problems of small rodents. In Hillyer EV, Quesenberry KE, editors: *Ferrets, Rabbits, and Rodents—Clinical Medicine and Surgery*, Philadelphia, 1997, Saunders, p 307.

Donnelly TM, Quimby FW: Biology and diseases of other rodents. In Fox JG, Anderson LC, Loew FM, Quimby FW, editors: *Laboratory Animal Medicine*, ed 2, San Diego, 2002, Academic Press, p 248.

Fitzgerald KT, Vera R: Reported toxicity in reptiles. In Mader DR, editor: *Reptile medicine and surgery*, ed 2, St. Louis, 2006, Mosby, p 1068.

Fox JG: *Parasitic diseases. In Biology and Diseases of the Ferret*, ed 2, Baltimore, 1998, Williams and Wilkins, p 375.

Gamble C, Morrisey JK: Ferrets. In Carpenter JW, editor: *Exotic Animal Formulary*, ed 3, St. Louis, 2005, Elsevier, p 447.

Georgi JR, Georgi ME: *Parasitology for Veterinarians*, Philadelphia, 1990, Saunders.

Gerlach H: Viruses. In Ritchie BW, Harrison LR, editors: *Avian Medicine, Principles and Application*, Lake Worth, 1994, Wingers Publishing, p 862.

Hankenson FC, Van Hoosier GL: Biology and diseases of hamsters. In Fox JG, Anderson LC, Loew FM, Quimby FW, editors: *Laboratory Animal Medicine*, ed 2, San Diego, 2002, Academic Press, p 168.

Harcourt-Brown F: Skin diseases. In *Textbook of Rabbit Medicine*, Oxford, 2002, Alden Press, p 224.

Harkness JE, Murray KA, Wagner JE: Biology and diseases of guinea pigs. In Fox JG, Anderson LC, Loew FM, Quimby FW, editors: *Laboratory Animal Medicine*, ed 2, San Diego, 2002, Academic Press, p 203.

Harkness JE, Wagner JE: Specific diseases and conditions. In Harkness JE, Wagner JE, editors: *The Biology and Medicine of Rabbits and Rodents*, ed 4, Philadelphia, 1995, Williams and Wilkins, p 171.

Hernandez-Divers SJ: Rabbits. In Carpenter JW, editor: *Exotic Animal Formulary*, ed 3, St. Louis, 2005, Elsevier, p 410.

Hotchkiss C: Effect of surgical removal of subcutaneous tumors on survival of rats, *J Am Vet Med Assoc* 206:1575, 1995.

Jacoby RO, Fox JG, Davisson M: Biology and diseases of mice. In Fox JG, Anderson LC, Loew FM, Quimby FW, editors: *Laboratory Animal Medicine*, ed 2, San Diego, 2002, Academic Press, p 35

Kohn DF, Clifford CB: Biology and diseases of rats. In Fox JG, Anderson LC, Loew FM, Quimby FW, editors: *Laboratory Animal Medicine*, ed 2, San Diego, 2002, Academic Press, p 121.

Lipman NS, Foltz C: Hamsters. In Laber-Laird K, Swindle MM, Flecknell P, editors: *Handbook for Rodent and Rabbit Medicine*, New York, 1995, Pergamon, p 65.

Lloyd M: Dermatologic diseases. In *Ferrets—Health, Husbandry and Diseases*, London, 1999, Blackwell Science, p 78.

Marini RP, Otto G, Erdman S, Palley L, Fox JG: Biology and diseases of ferrets. In Fox JG, Anderson LC, Loew FM, Quimby FW, editors: *Laboratory Animal Medicine*, ed 2, San Diego, 2002, Academic Press, p 483.

McTier TL, Hair JA, Walstrom DJ, Thompson L: Efficacy and safety of topical administration of selamectin for treatment of ear mite infestation in rabbits, *J Am Vet Med Assoc* 223:322, 2003.

Morrisey JK: Part II Other diseases. In Quesenberry KE, Carpenter JW, editors: *Ferrets, Rabbits, and Rodents—Clinical Medicine and Surgery*, ed 2, Philadelphia, 2004, Saunders, p 66.

Murray MJ: Aural abscesses. In Mader D, editor: *Reptile Medicine and Surgery*, Philadelphia, 1996, Saunders, p 349.

Ness RD: Rodents. In Carpenter JW, editor: *Exotic Animal Formulary*, ed 3, St. Louis, 2005, Elsevier, p 377.

Orcutt C: Dermatologic diseases. In Hillyer EV, Quesenberry KE, editors: *Ferrets, Rabbits, and Rodents—Clinical Medicine and Surgery*, Philadelphia, 1997, Saunders, p 115.

Pollack C, Carpenter JW, Antinoff N: Birds. In Carpenter JW, editor: *Exotic Animal Formulary*, ed 3, St. Louis, 2005, Elsevier, p 135.

Quesenberry KE, Orcutt C: Basic approach to veterinary care. In Quesenberry KE, Carpenter JW, editors: *Ferrets, Rabbits, and Rodents—Clinical Medicine and Surgery*, ed 2, Philadelphia, 2004, Saunders, p 13.

Ramis A, Latimer KS, Niagro FD, et al: Diagnosis of psittacine beak and feather disease (PBFD) viral infection, avian polyomavirus infection, adenovirus infection and herpesvirus infection in psittacine tissues using DNA in situ hybridization, *Avian Pathol* 23:643, 1994.

Raymond JT, Garner MM: Spontaneous tumours in captive African hedgehogs (Atelerix albiventris): a retrospective study, *Journal Comp Pathol* 124:128, 2001.

Ritchie BW: Circoviridae. In *Avian Viruses, Function and Control*, Lake Worth, 1995, Wingers Publishing, p 223.

Rosenthal KL: Respiratory disease. In Quesenberry KE, Carpenter JW, editors: *Ferrets, Rabbits, and Rodents—Clinical Medicine and Surgery*, ed 2, Philadelphia, 2004, Saunders, p 72.

Schmidt RE (guest editor): In Dermatology. The Veterinary Clinics of North America—Exotic Animal Practice, 4(2), 2001, Philadelphia, WB Saunders.

Shoemaker NJ: Selected dermatologic conditions in exotic pets, *Exotic DVM* 1:5, 1999.

Styles DK, Tomaszewski EK, Jaeger LA, Phalen DN: Psittacid herpesvirus associated with mucosal papillomas in neotropical parrots, *Virology* 325:24, 2004.

Suckow MA, Brammer DW, Rush HG, Chrisp CE: Biology and diseases of rabbits. In Fox JG, Anderson LC, Loew FM, Quimby FW, editors: *Laboratory Animal Medicine*, ed 2, San Diego, 2002, Academic Press, p 329.

Tanaka A, Hisanaga A, Ishinishi N: The frequency of spontaneously-occurring neoplasms in the male Syrian golden hamster, *Vet Hum Toxicol* 33:318, 1991.

CHAPTER 16

Pretreatment and Posttreatment Response Images

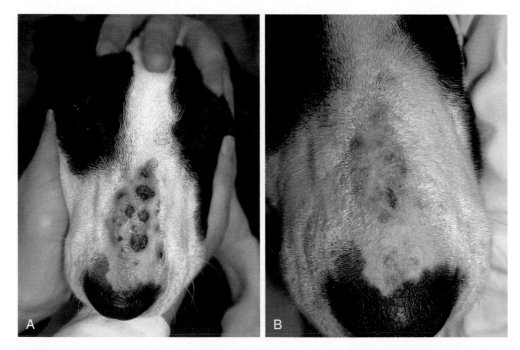

FIGURE 16-1 **Nasal Pyoderma. A,** Alopecic, crusting, papular dermatitis on the nose before treatment is provided. **B,** Following 3 weeks of aggressive antibiotic therapy (high dose, long duration, and optimal frequency), the bacterial folliculitis and furunculosis were resolving.

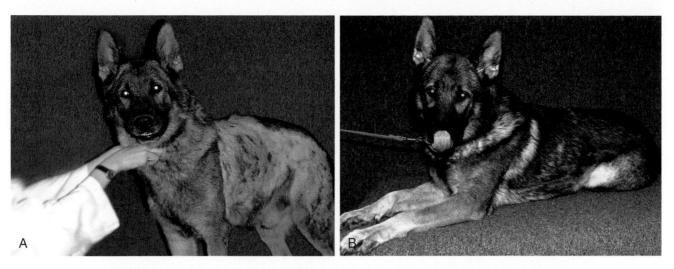

FIGURE 16-2 Pyoderma. A, An adult German shepherd with generalized bacterial folliculitis and furunculosis. The fur has been clipped, revealing numerous crusting, papular lesions with drainage. **B,** After aggressive antibiotic therapy (high dose, long duration, and optimal frequency), the bacterial folliculitis and furunculosis have resolved.

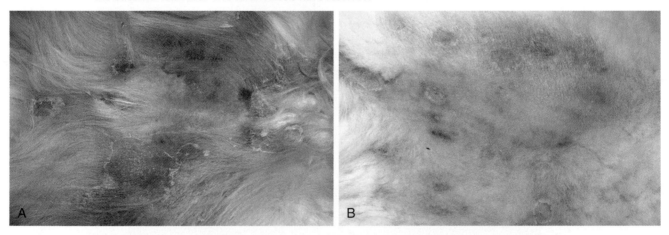

FIGURE 16-3 Pyoderma. A, Severe erythematous dermatitis with numerous epidermal collarettes. **B,** After aggressive antibiotic therapy, the pyoderma has improved, but numerous epidermal collarettes remain apparent. This dog had a multidrug-resistant *Staphylococcus schleiferi* infection.

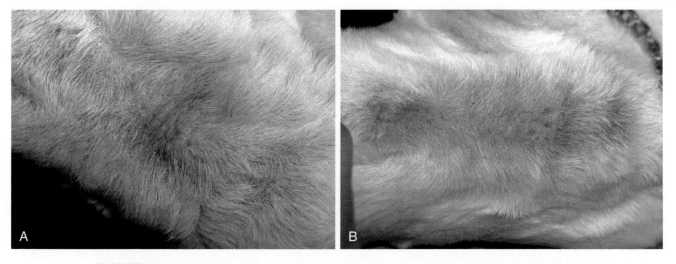

FIGURE 16-4 Pyoderma. A, Alopecia and lichenification on the ventral neck caused by bacterial pyoderma. Note the similarity to *Malassezia* (yeast) dermatitis. **B,** After aggressive antibiotic therapy (high dose, long duration, and optimal frequency), the bacterial folliculitis and furunculosis have resolved.

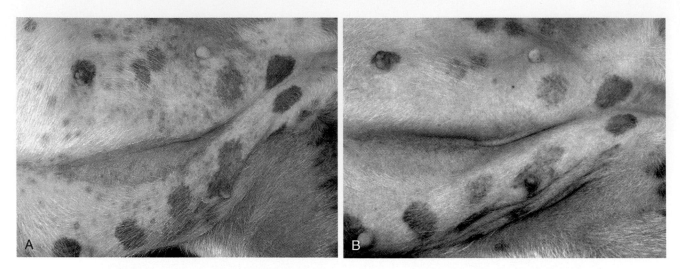

FIGURE 16-5 **Pyoderma. A,** An erythematous papular rash on the abdomen of a dog with bacterial folliculitis is characteristic of pyoderma in dogs. **B,** After aggressive antibiotic therapy (high dose, long duration, and optimal frequency), the bacterial folliculitis and furunculosis have resolved.

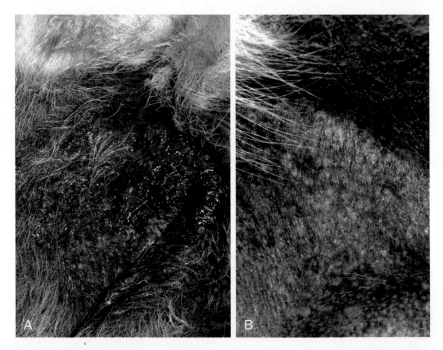

FIGURE 16-6 **Pyoderma. A,** This erosive dermatitis was caused by an aggressive *Staphylococcus* infection in an adult German shepherd. *Staphylococcus* exotoxins are likely responsible for the erosive lesions (similar to *Staphylococcus* scalded skin syndrome). **B,** After aggressive antibiotic therapy (high dose, long duration, and optimal frequency), the bacterial folliculitis and furunculosis have resolved.

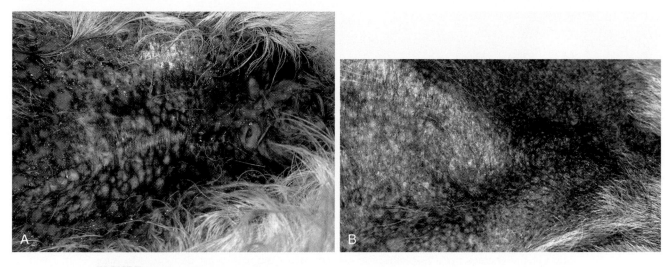

FIGURE 16-7 Pyoderma. Same dog as in Figure 16-6. **A,** Erosive lesions caused by the aggressive *Staphylococcus* infection developed on the abdomen. **B,** After aggressive antibiotic therapy (high dose, long duration, and optimal frequency), the bacterial folliculitis and furunculosis have resolved.

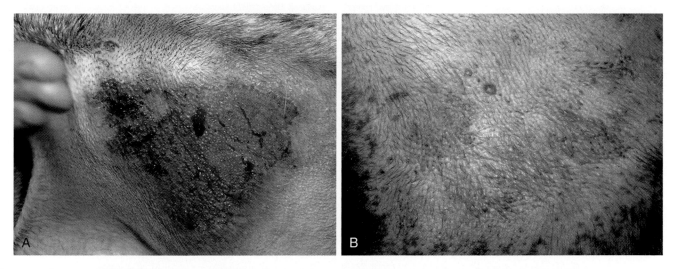

FIGURE 16-8 Nocardiosis. A, An erythematous plaque on the inner thigh with exudate. This plaquelike lesion is unusual for *Nocardia*, which typically causes a more deep cellulitis. **B,** After aggressive therapy with trimethoprim-sulfa, the lesions were resolving.

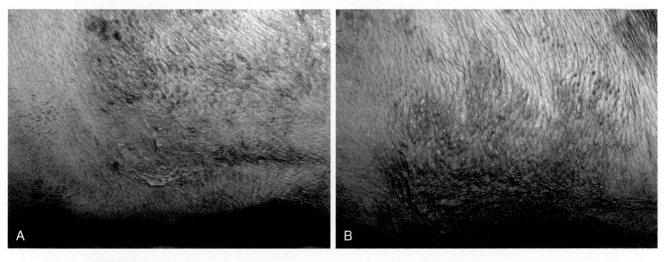

FIGURE 16-9 Nocardiosis. Same dog as in Figure 16-8. **A,** This unusual plaque is not typical of the cellulitis lesions associated with nocardiosis. **B,** After aggressive therapy with trimethoprim-sulfa, the lesions were resolving.

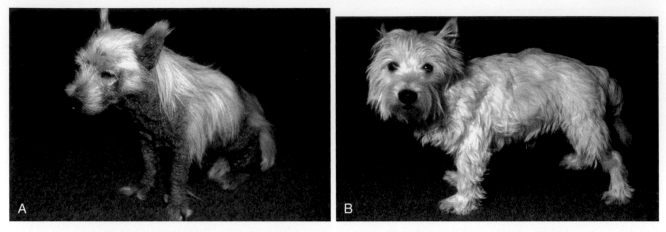

FIGURE 16-10 Malasseziasis. A, Generalized alopecia with hyperpigmentation and lichenification in the characteristic "elephant hide" pattern associated with yeast dermatitis. **B,** After several weeks of systemic ketoconazole and topical antifungal therapy, the yeast dermatitis has resolved. The underlying/primary condition (allergies or endocrine disease) must be controlled to prevent recurrence of the infection.

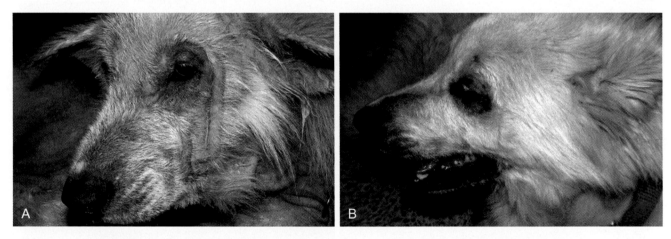

FIGURE 16-11 Malasseziasis. A, Severe erythematous, alopecic, lichenified dermatitis on the face of a dog caused by secondary yeast dermatitis associated with primary allergic dermatitis. **B,** After several weeks of systemic ketoconazole and topical antifungal therapy, the yeast dermatitis has resolved.

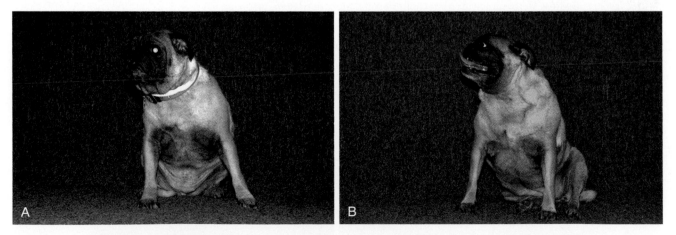

FIGURE 16-12 Malasseziasis. A, Severe alopecia, hyperpigmentation, and lichenification of the face and axilla in the classic "elephant hide" pattern typical of yeast dermatitis. **B,** After several weeks of systemic and topical antifungal and antibacterial therapy, the yeast dermatitis was resolving.

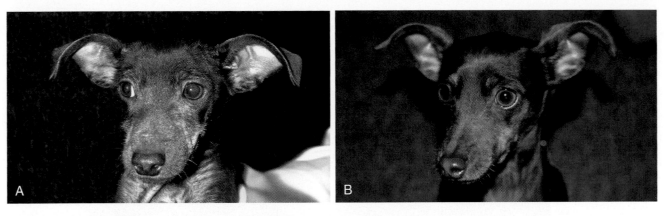

FIGURE 16-13 Malasseziasis. A, Alopecia and lichenification on the face and neck of a young miniature pinscher caused by a secondary yeast infection associated with food allergy. **B,** After several weeks of systemic ketoconazole and topical antifungal therapy, the yeast dermatitis has resolved. The food allergy was treated with a dietary food trial.

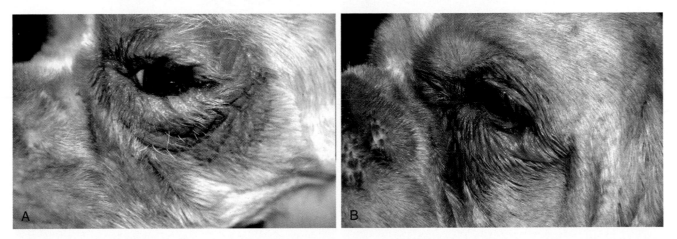

FIGURE 16-14 Malasseziasis. A, Alopecia, hyperpigmentation, and lichenification on the face and periocular skin of an adult Cocker spaniel with allergic dermatitis. **B,** After several weeks of systemic ketoconazole and topical antifungal therapy, the yeast dermatitis has resolved.

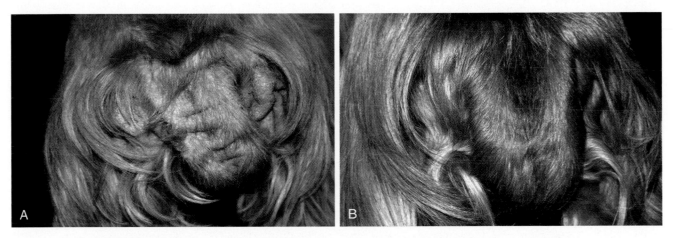

FIGURE 16-15 Malasseziasis. Same dog as in Figure 16-14. **A,** Alopecia and lichenification of the tail base caused by secondary yeast dermatitis. Note the similarity to flea allergy dermatitis. **B,** After several weeks of systemic ketoconazole and topical antifungal therapy, the yeast dermatitis has resolved.

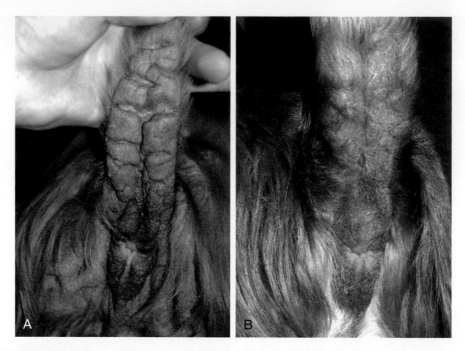

FIGURE 16-16 Malasseziasis. A, Severe alopecia, hyperpigmentation, and lichenification on the ventral tail and perianal region in a dog with severe secondary yeast dermatitis. Based on the perianal distribution, food allergy dermatitis should be considered as a possible primary condition. **B,** After several weeks of systemic ketoconazole and topical antifungal therapy, the yeast dermatitis has resolved.

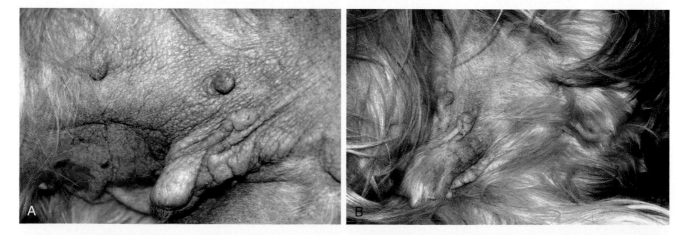

FIGURE 16-17 Malasseziasis. A, Alopecia, hyperpigmentation, and lichenification in the characteristic "elephant skin" pattern associated with secondary yeast infection. **B,** After several weeks of systemic ketoconazole and topical antifungal therapy, the yeast dermatitis has resolved.

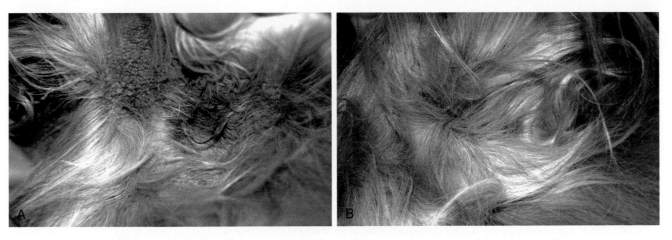

FIGURE 16-18 Malasseziasis. A, Alopecia and lichenification of the axillary region are characteristic of yeast dermatitis. **B,** After several weeks of systemic ketoconazole and topical antifungal therapy, the yeast dermatitis has resolved.

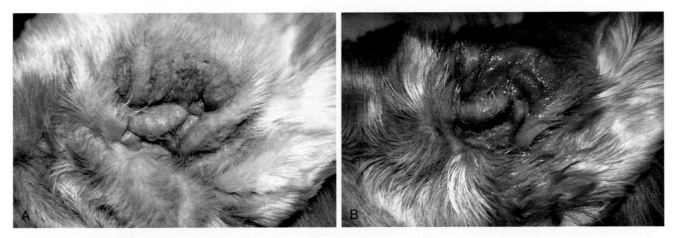

FIGURE 16-19 *Malassezia* **Otitis. A,** Erythema, lichenification, and stenosis of the external ear canal with a moist exudate. Cytologic evaluation demonstrated a predominant secondary yeast infection. **B,** After several weeks of systemic ketoconazole and topical Otomax therapy, the yeast otitis has resolved. The moist material is Otomax. Note that with resolution of the infection and treatment with topical steroids, the ear canal swelling has decreased considerably.

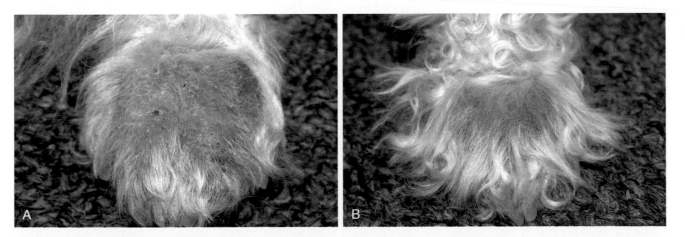

FIGURE 16-20 Malasseziasis. A, Alopecia and lichenification on the foot of an allergic dog with secondary yeast pododermatitis. The interdigital space is usually the predominant site of secondary bacterial and yeast infections; however, in this patient, the dermatitis extended to the dorsal surface of the foot. **B,** After several weeks of systemic ketoconazole and topical antifungal therapy, the yeast dermatitis has resolved.

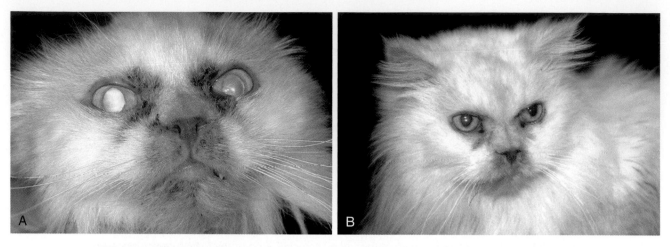

FIGURE 16-21 Malasseziasis. A, A dark exudate has caused clumping of the hairs and crust formation of the periocular skin and muzzle in this cat with secondary yeast dermatitis. Note the similarity to feline pemphigus and idiopathic facial dermatitis of Persians. **B,** After several weeks of systemic itraconazole (ketoconazole produces many adverse effects in cats) and topical antifungal therapy, the yeast dermatitis resolved.

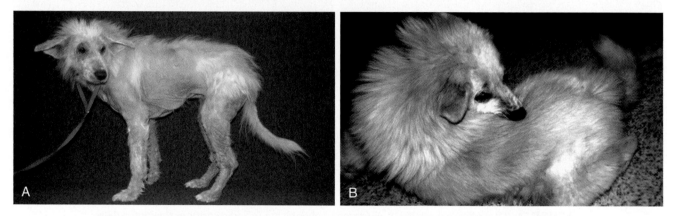

FIGURE 16-22 Malasseziasis. A, Generalized alopecia, erythema, and lichenification in an adult dog with secondary yeast dermatitis associated with an underlying allergy. **B,** After several weeks of systemic ketoconazole and topical antifungal therapy, the yeast dermatitis has resolved. Note that the dog was still pruritic from the underlying allergic disease, which remains uncontrolled.

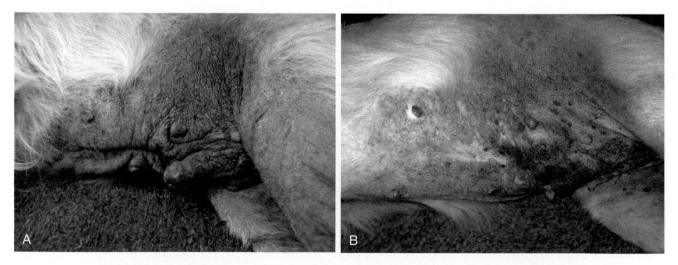

FIGURE 16-23 Malasseziasis. A, Alopecia, hyperpigmentation, and lichenification in the characteristic "elephant hide" pattern associated with yeast dermatitis. **B,** After several weeks of systemic ketoconazole and topical antifungal therapy, the yeast dermatitis has resolved.

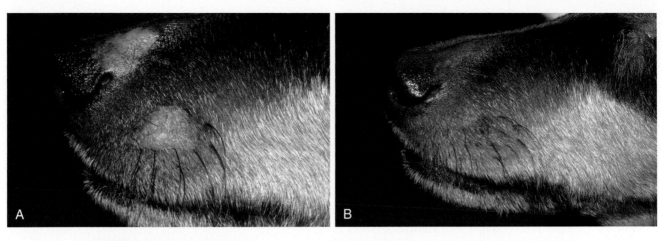

FIGURE 16-24 **Dermatophytosis. A,** Focal alopecia and erythema on the muzzle of an adult Dachshund. **B,** After several weeks of systemic ketoconazole and topical antifungal therapy, the dermatophytosis has resolved.

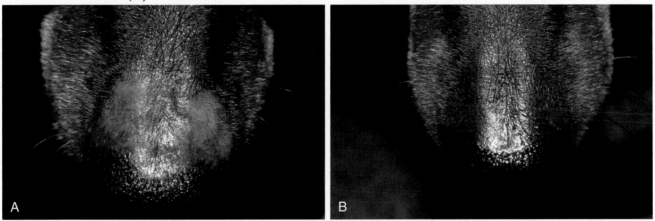

FIGURE 16-25 **Dermatophytosis.** Same dog as in Figure 16-24. **A,** The alopecia and erythema caused by folliculitis affect only the haired portion of the nose, unlike autoimmune skin disease, which would affect nonhaired nasal planum. **B,** After several weeks of systemic ketoconazole and topical antifungal therapy, the dermatophytosis has resolved.

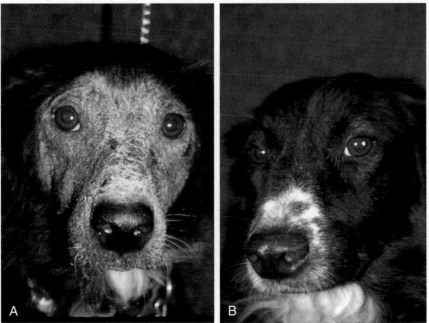

FIGURE 16-26 **Demodicosis. A,** Generalized alopecia and crusting papular rash on the face caused by demodicosis. **B,** After several months of systemic miticidal therapy, the *Demodex* infection resolved (based on two consecutive negative skin scrapes 3 weeks apart).

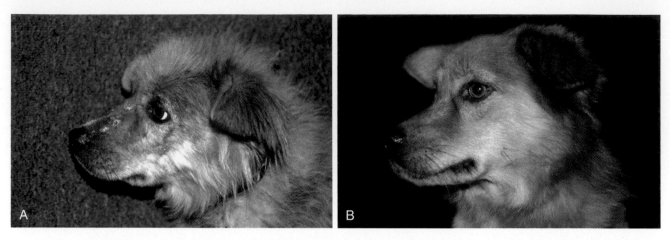

FIGURE 16-27 Demodicosis. A, Generalized alopecia, crusting, and papular dermatitis affecting an adult dog. **B,** After several months of systemic miticidal therapy, the *Demodex* infection resolved (based on two consecutive negative skin scrapes 3 weeks apart).

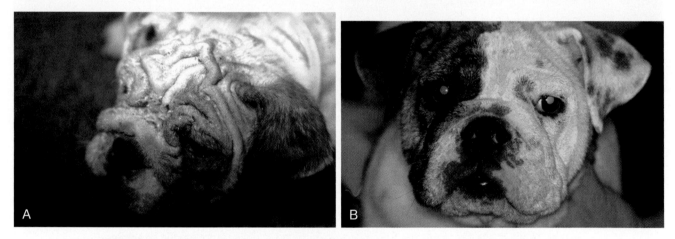

FIGURE 16-28 Demodicosis. A, Generalized alopecia, crusting, and papular dermatitis on the head of an English bulldog puppy. **B,** After several months of systemic miticidal therapy (ivermectin), the *Demodex* infection resolved (based on two consecutive negative skin scrapes 3 weeks apart).

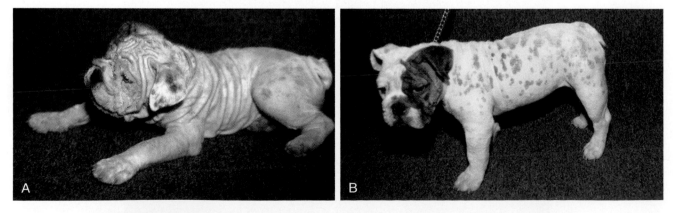

FIGURE 16-29 Demodicosis. A, Generalized alopecia and papular dermatitis covering the entire body. **B,** After several months of systemic miticidal therapy (ivermectin), the *Demodex* infection resolved (based on two consecutive negative skin scrapes 3 weeks apart).

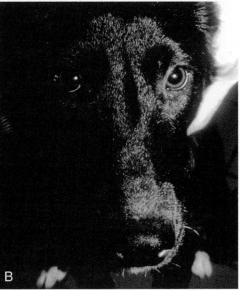
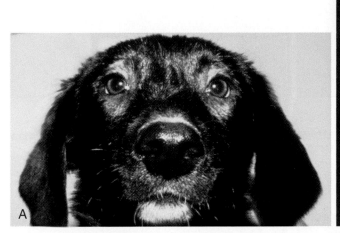

FIGURE 16-30 Demodicosis. A, Periocular alopecia in a young mixed-breed dog. **B,** After several months of systemic miticidal therapy (ivermectin), the *Demodex* infection resolved (based on two consecutive negative skin scrapes 3 weeks apart).

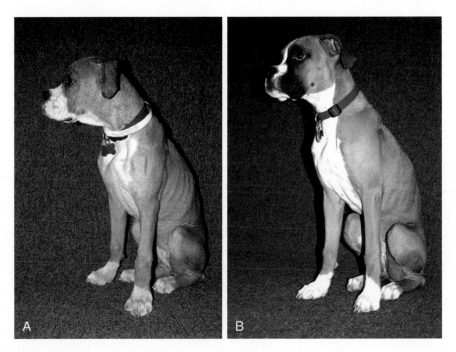

FIGURE 16-31 Demodicosis. A, Generalized alopecia and papular rash in a Boxer puppy. **B,** After several months of systemic miticidal therapy (ivermectin), the *Demodex* infection resolved (based on two consecutive negative skin scrapes 3 weeks apart).

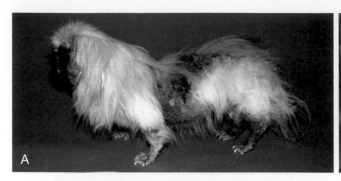
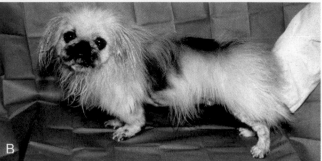

FIGURE 16-32 Demodicosis. A, Generalized alopecia, hyperpigmentation, and crusting papular dermatitis in a dog with iatrogenic Cushing's (caused by numerous long-acting injectable steroid treatments). **B,** After several months of systemic miticidal therapy (ivermectin), the *Demodex* infection is improving. The alopecia and hyperpigmentation will take longer to resolve because of iatrogenic Cushing's.

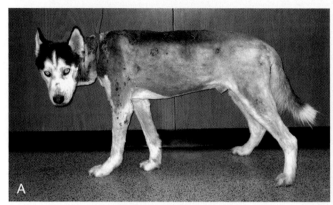
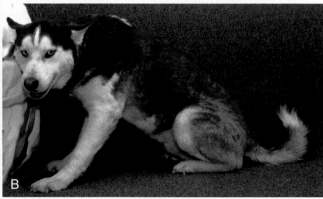

FIGURE 16-33 Demodicosis. A, Generalized crusting papular dermatitis with draining tracts caused by severe folliculitis and furunculosis. **B,** After several months of systemic miticidal therapy, the *Demodex* infection resolved (based on two consecutive negative skin scrapes 3 weeks apart).

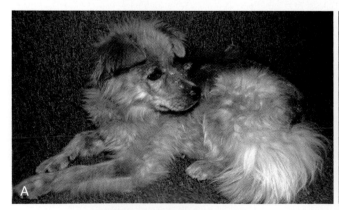
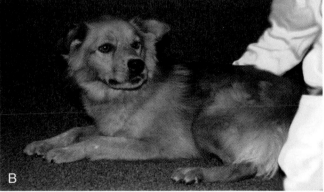

FIGURE 16-34 Demodicosis. A, Generalized alopecia with a crusting papular rash. **B,** After several months of systemic miticidal therapy, the *Demodex* infection resolved (based on two consecutive negative skin scrapes 3 weeks apart).

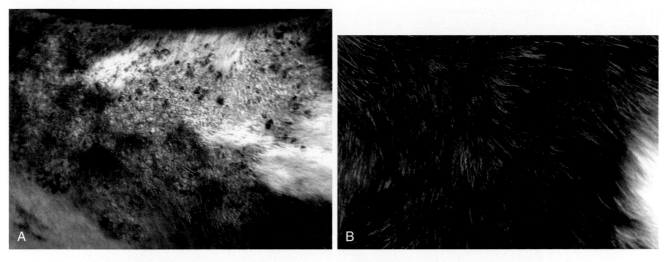

FIGURE 16-35 Demodicosis. A, Alopecia with a severe, crusting papular dermatitis on the trunk of an adult dog. **B,** After several months of systemic miticidal therapy, the *Demodex* infection resolved (based on two consecutive negative skin scrapes 3 weeks apart).

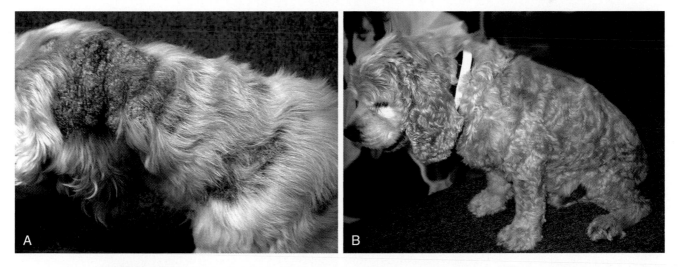

FIGURE 16-36 Demodicosis. A, Alopecia with hyperpigmentation and lichenification on the head, neck, and shoulder of an adult Cocker spaniel. Note the similar lesion type to *Malassezia* (yeast) dermatitis, which would typically occur on the ventrum. **B,** After several months of systemic miticidal therapy, the *Demodex* infection resolved (based on two consecutive negative skin scrapes 3 weeks apart).

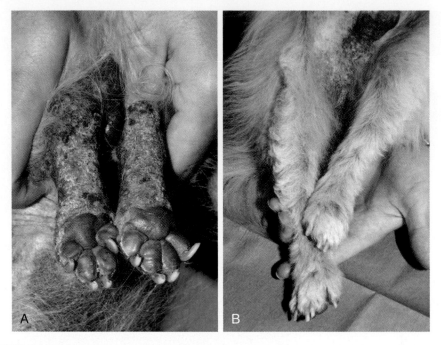

FIGURE 16-37 **Demodicosis.** Same dog as in Figure 16-32. **A,** Generalized alopecia, hyperpigmentation, and crusting papular dermatitis cover most of the cutaneous surface area. **B,** After several months of systemic miticidal therapy (ivermectin), the *Demodex* infection resolved (based on two consecutive negative skin scrapes 3 weeks apart).

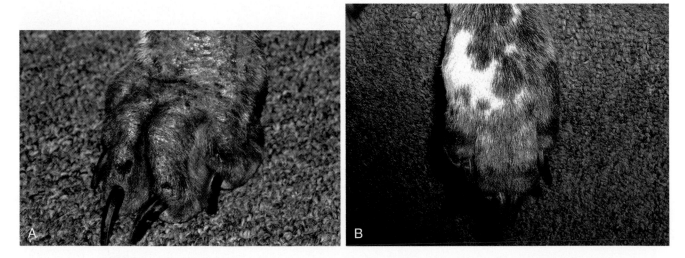

FIGURE 16-38 **Demodicosis. A,** Alopecia, erythema, hyperpigmentation, and lichenification on the foot of a dog with iatrogenic Cushing's disease. **B,** After several months of systemic miticidal therapy (ivermectin) and discontinuation of the steroids, the *Demodex* infection resolved (based on two consecutive negative skin scrapes 3 weeks apart).

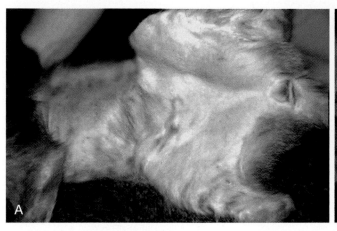
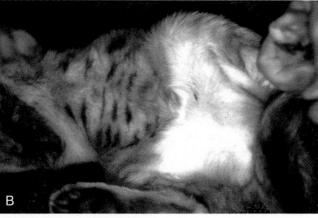

FIGURE 16-39 Feline Demodicosis. A, Alopecia of the abdominal region in a cat with feline demodicosis (*Demodex gatoi*). Note the similarity in lesion pattern (allergic alopecia) to other causes (e.g., ectoparasitism, flea allergy, food allergy, atopy). **B,** The alopecia responded to weekly lime sulfur dips. It is interesting to note that *Demodex gatoi* seems to be less sensitive to systemic miticides (e.g., ivermectin, milbemycin, selamectin) than other mites.

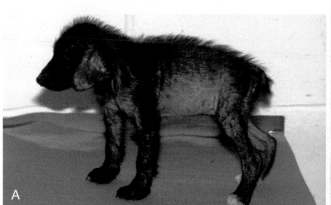
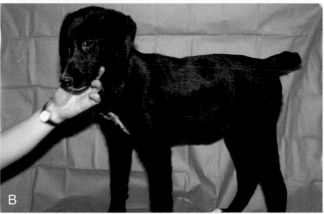

FIGURE 16-40 Canine Scabies. A, Generalized alopecia of a papular crusting rash in a stray puppy. **B,** After several weeks of systemic miticidal therapy (ivermectin), the infection resolved.

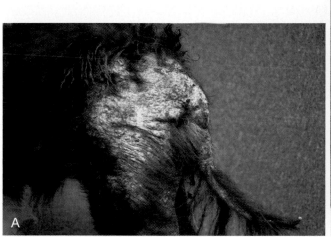
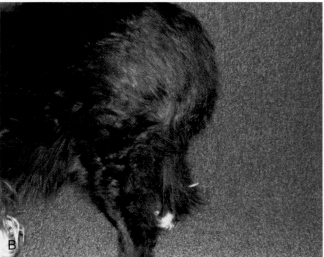

FIGURE 16-41 Flea Allergy Dermatitis. A, Severe alopecia, lichenification, and crusting papular dermatitis on the lumbar area. The lumbar distribution (lesions caudal to the rib cage) is characteristic of flea allergy dermatitis in dogs. **B,** After several weeks of aggressive treatment with topical spot-on flea control, the flea allergy dermatitis was resolving.

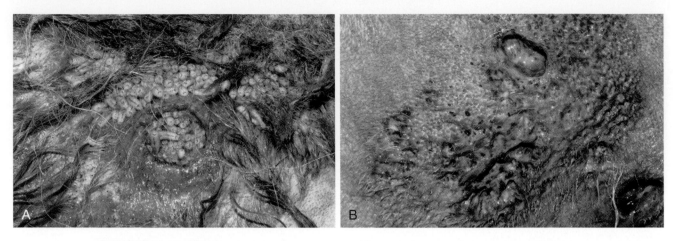

FIGURE 16-42 Myiasis. **A,** Numerous maggots filling a cutaneous lesion in an adult dog. **B,** The patient has been bathed and the maggots removed, leaving open cutaneous lesions.

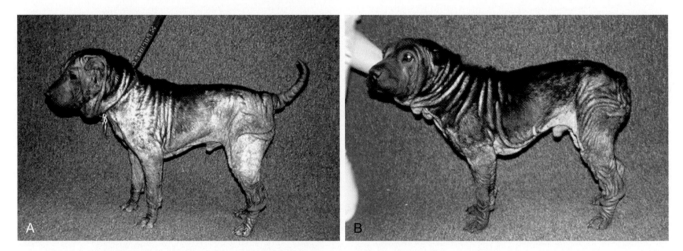

FIGURE 16-43 Allergic Dermatitis. **A,** An adult Shar pei with atopy and food allergy, demonstrating generalized alopecia and papular dermatitis. **B,** The cutaneous lesions were resolving with cyclosporine therapy. This patient had failed to improve with numerous allergy tests and hyposensitization attempts, food trials, and symptomatic therapy.

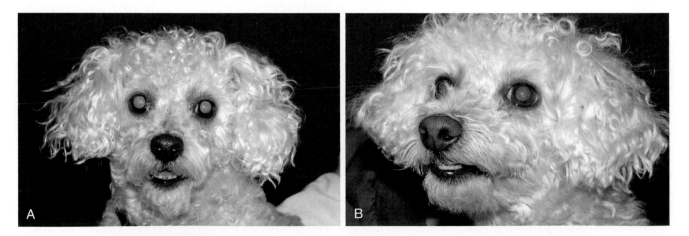

FIGURE 16-44 Canine Atopy. **A,** Periocular alopecia and erythema typical of allergic dermatitis (atopy or food allergy). Note the similarity to other causes of blepharitis (e.g., demodicosis, contact dermatitis). **B,** The periocular alopecia and erythema improved when the underlying allergic disease was controlled.

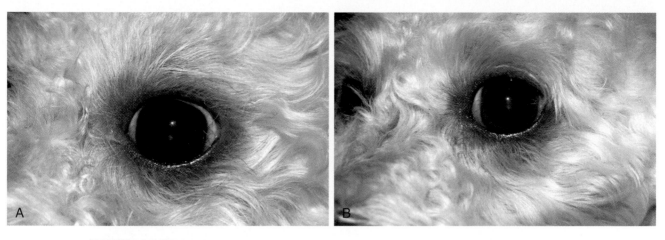

FIGURE 16-45 Canine Atopy. Same dog as in Figure 16-44. **A,** Periocular alopecia and erythema caused by the underlying allergy are apparent. **B,** The periocular alopecia and erythema improved when the underlying allergic disease was controlled.

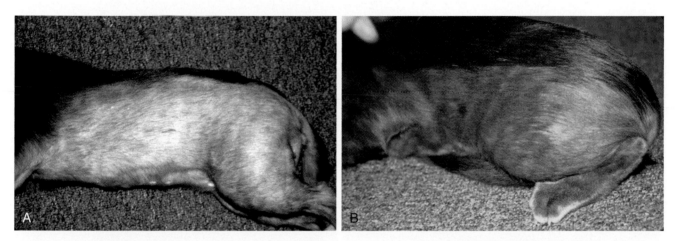

FIGURE 16-46 Feline Allergic Dermatitis. A, Alopecia with or without apparent inflammatory dermatitis can have many causes in cats (e.g., ectoparasitism, flea allergy, food allergy, atopy). **B,** When the primary cause was identified and controlled, the overgrooming (pruritus) was diminished and the hair regrew.

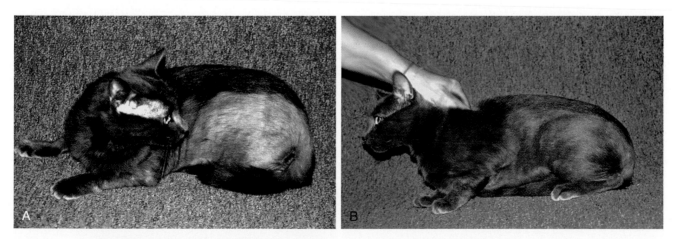

FIGURE 16-47 Feline Allergic Dermatitis. Same cat as in Figure 16-46. **A,** Allergic alopecia with or without apparent inflammatory dermatitis can have many causes in a cat (e.g., ectoparasitism, flea allergy, food allergy, atopy). **B,** When the primary cause is identified and controlled, the overgrooming (pruritus) is diminished and the hair regrows.

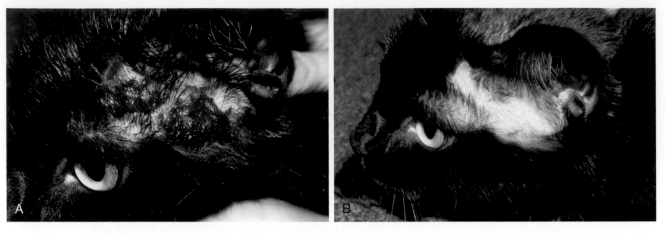

FIGURE 16-48 **Feline Allergic Dermatitis. A,** Eosinophilic plaques are common lesions caused by allergic dermatitis in cats, regardless of the underlying cause (e.g., ectoparasitism, flea allergy, food allergy, atopy). This eosinophilic plaque was likely caused by acute exposure to fleas or other ectoparasites. **B,** These eosinophilic plaques resolved with aggressive flea control and injectable steroid therapy.

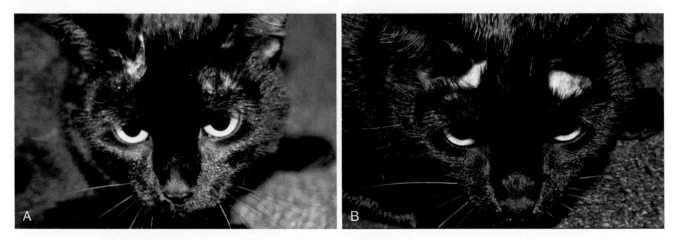

FIGURE 16-49 **Feline Allergic Dermatitis.** Same cat as in Figure 16-48. **A,** These symmetrical eosinophilic plaques developed acutely. **B,** These eosinophilic plaques resolved with aggressive flea control and injectable steroid therapy.

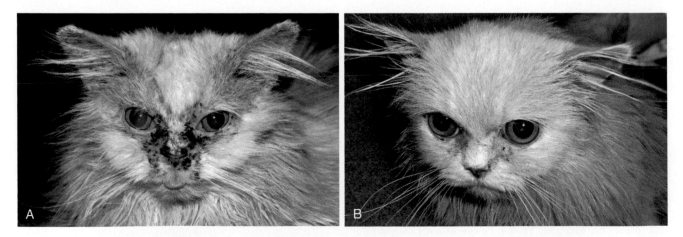

FIGURE 16-50 **Pemphigus Foliaceus. A,** Crusting papular dermatitis on the face and ear pinnae of a cat with pemphigus foliaceus. **B,** The crusting papular dermatitis was resolving after several weeks of traditional immunosuppressive therapy.

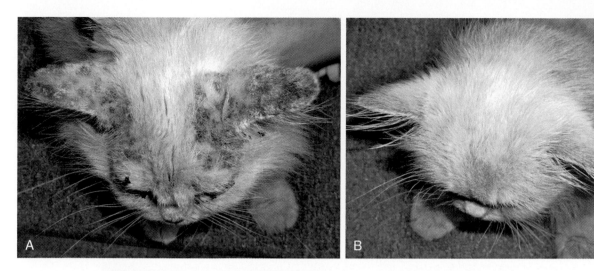

FIGURE 16-51 Pemphigus Foliaceus. Same cat as in Figure 16-50. **A,** Alopecic, crusting, papular dermatitis covering the ear pinnae is characteristic of autoimmune skin disease. Note (in cats) the similarity to other causes of head and neck crusting dermatitis (e.g., ectoparasitism, flea allergy, food allergy, atopy). **B,** The crusting papular dermatitis was resolving after several weeks of traditional immunosuppressive therapy.

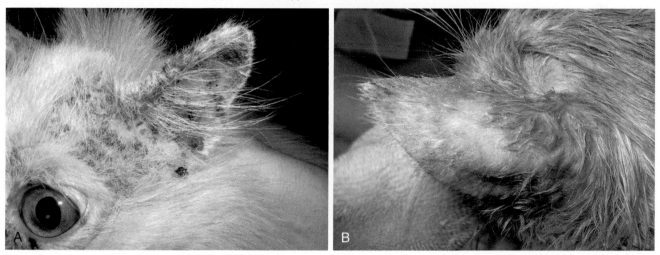

FIGURE 16-52 Pemphigus Foliaceus. Same cat as in Figure 16-50. **A,** Crusting papular dermatitis on the ear pinna and preauricular skin is apparent. **B,** The crusting papular dermatitis was resolving after several weeks of traditional immunosuppressive therapy.

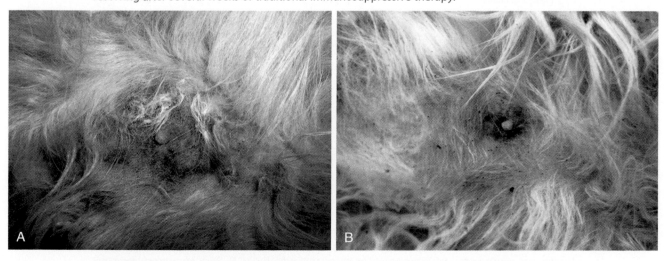

FIGURE 16-53 Pemphigus Foliaceus. A, Alopecic, erythematous, moist dermatitis around the nipples is a unique and common characteristic feature of pemphigus foliaceus in cats. **B,** The dermatitis was resolving after several weeks of traditional immunosuppressive therapy.

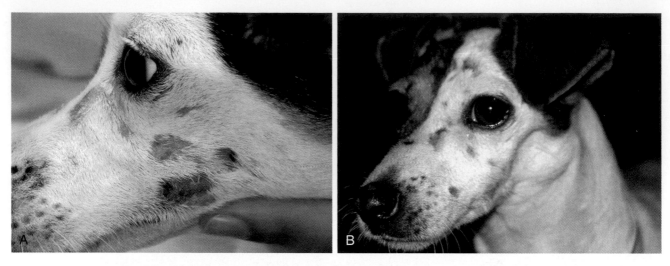

FIGURE 16-54 Systemic Lupus Erythematosus. A, Multiple alopecic, erythematous areas of erosive dermatitis on the face of a Jack Russell terrier. Note the similarity to lesions typical of vasculitis, which can be familial in Jack Russell terriers. **B,** Multiple alopecic scars persisted despite resolution of the active autoimmune skin disease with traditional immunosuppressive therapy.

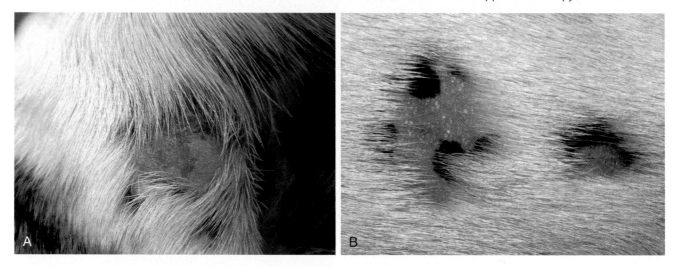

FIGURE 16-55 Systemic Lupus Erythematosus. Same dog as in Figure 16-54. **A,** A focal area of alopecia and erythema. Note that the presence of erythema suggests an inflammatory response and active disease. **B,** With immunosuppressive therapy, the active inflammation and associated erythema should resolve. Depending on the severity of the lesion, alopecic scars may persist.

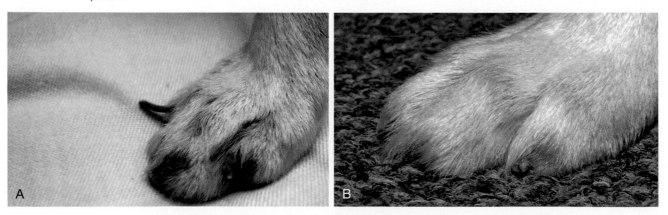

FIGURE 16-56 Systemic Lupus Erythematosus. Same dog as in Figure 16-54. **A,** Onychodystrophy was caused by concurrent vasculitis associated with lupus. **B,** With immunosuppressive therapy, the onychodystrophy improved and the claws became more normal.

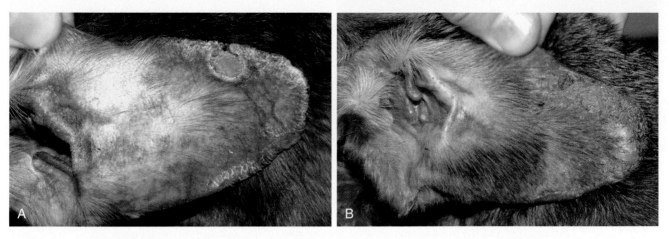

FIGURE 16-57 Systemic Lupus Erythematosus. A, Alopecic, crusting ear margin dermatitis with a circular area of necrosis caused by vascular thrombosis. **B,** With immunosuppressive therapy, the vasculitis associated with lupus resolved, allowing the skin to heal.

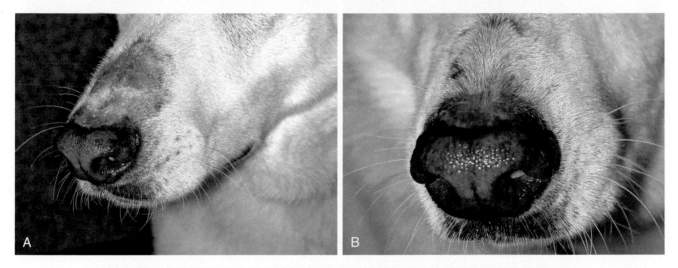

FIGURE 16-58 Discoid Lupus Erythematosus. A, Depigmentation of the nasal planum is unique and characteristic of autoimmune skin diseases. The alopecic, erythematous dermatitis on the haired portion of the nose could be caused by folliculitis (pyoderma, *Demodex*, and dermatophyte) but was associated with the autoimmune skin disease in this patient. **B,** The nasal depigmentation and alopecic dermatitis were resolving after several weeks of therapy with topical tacrolimus.

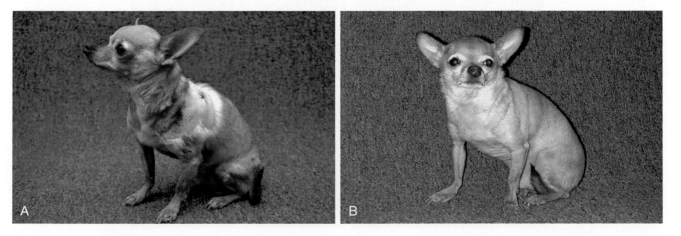

FIGURE 16-59 Sterile Nodular Panniculitis. A, Multiple draining nodules on the shoulders of an adult Chihuahua. **B,** The nodular lesions have resolved and the hair has regrown after several weeks of immunosuppressive therapy.

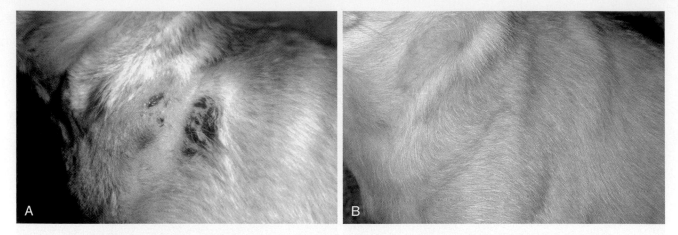

FIGURE 16-60 Sterile Nodular Panniculitis. Same dog as in Figure 16-59. **A,** Numerous draining nodules with crust formation on the shoulders of an adult Chihuahua. **B,** The nodular lesions have resolved and the hair has regrown after several weeks of immunosuppressive therapy.

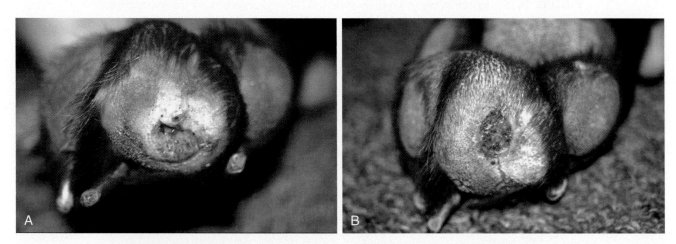

FIGURE 16-61 Cutaneous Vasculitis. A, This ulcerative lesion close to the center of the digital footpad is characteristic of vasculitis. **B,** The ulcerative lesion in the center of the digital footpad improved after several weeks of therapy with pentoxifylline.

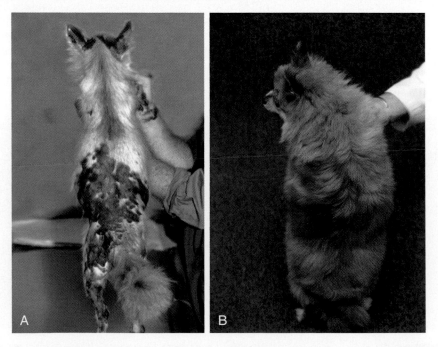

FIGURE 16-62 Erythema Multiforme. A, Generalized alopecia with erosive, hyperpigmenting lesions in an adult Pomeranian. Note that the well-demarcated serpentine borders of the lesions are characteristic of cutaneous drug reaction, vasculitis, and autoimmune skin disease. **B,** Complete resolution of the lesions after several months of immunosuppressive therapy with cyclosporine (Atopica).

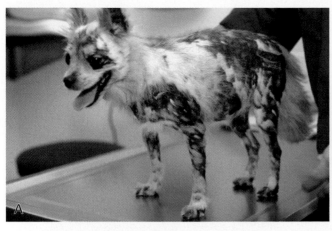
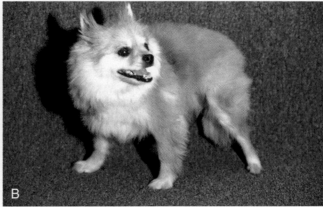

FIGURE 16-63 Erythema Multiforme. Same dog as in Figure 16-62. **A,** The generalized alopecic, hyperpigmenting lesions with well-demarcated borders are characteristic of this disease. **B,** Complete resolution of the lesions after several months of immunosuppressive therapy with cyclosporine (Atopica).

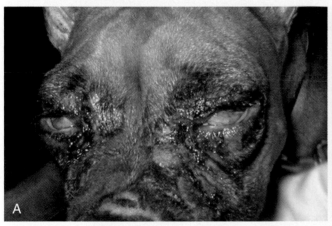
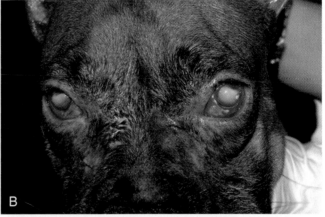

FIGURE 16-64 Erythema Multiforme. A, Severe erosive dermatitis on the periocular skin and face of an adult Boxer. The dog also had a methicillin-resistant *Staphylococcus aureus* infection, likely contracted from the owner, who worked in the human health care industry. **B,** Moderate improvement in erosive dermatitis after several weeks of aggressive antibiotic therapy (based on culture, high dose, long duration, and optimal frequency) and immunosuppressive treatment.

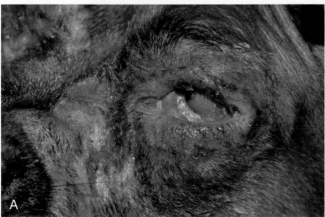
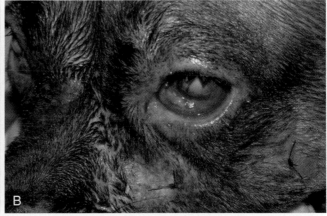

FIGURE 16-65 Erythema Multiforme. Same dog as in Figure 16-64. **A,** Severe erosive dermatitis on the periocular skin with concurrent corneal edema and uveitis. The dog also had a methicillin-resistant *Staphylococcus aureus* infection, likely contracted from the owner, who worked in the human health care industry. **B,** Moderate improvement in erosive dermatitis after several weeks of aggressive antibiotic therapy (based on culture, high dose, long duration, and optimal frequency) and immunosuppressive treatment.

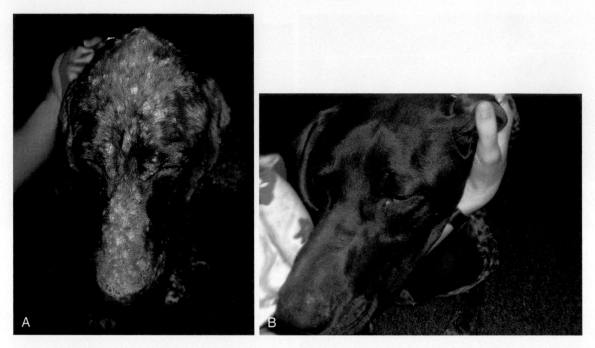

FIGURE 16-66 Cutaneous Drug Reaction. A, A crusting nodular dermatitis covering the entire head and body, likely caused by an idiosyncratic drug reaction. **B,** Complete resolution of crusting nodular dermatitis after discontinuation of the suspected drug and several weeks of immunosuppressive therapy.

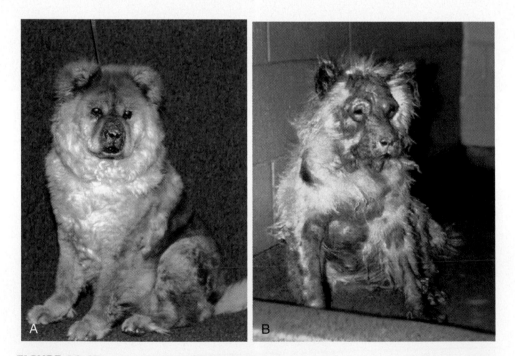

FIGURE 16-67 Canine Hyperadrenocorticism. A, An adult Chow with pemphigus foliaceus demonstrating the characteristic depigmentation and erosive dermatitis on the nasal planum and ear pinnae. **B,** Generalized alopecia and hyperpigmentation after overly aggressive (too long duration) immunosuppressive therapy with steroids. Iatrogenic Cushing's disease caused a secondary bacterial pyoderma and adult-onset demodicosis.

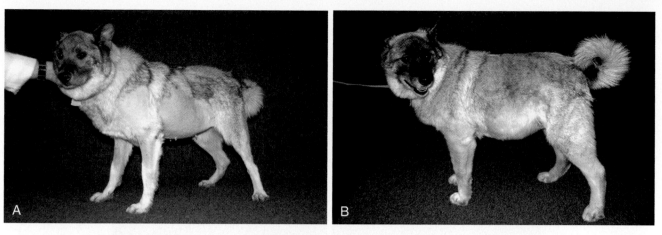

FIGURE 16-68 **Canine Hyperadrenocorticism. A,** Symptoms of Cushing's disease can often be subtle. This dog demonstrates a relatively normal fur coat but has poor body confirmation. **B,** After treatment with mitotane, the subtle symptoms of Cushing's disease resolved. The dog's muscle tone and body posture were greatly improved.

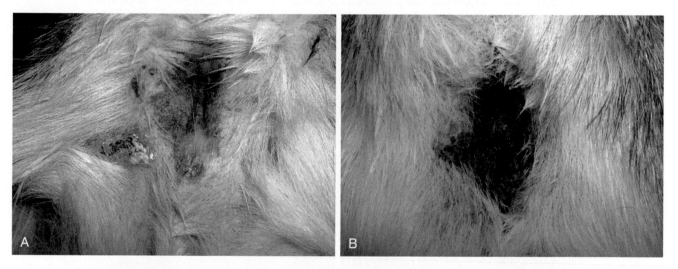

FIGURE 16-69 **Canine Hyperadrenocorticism. A,** Secondary bacterial pyoderma with alopecia and a crusting papular dermatitis on the perianal skin. **B,** When Cushing's disease was treated and antibiotics administered, the secondary bacterial pyoderma resolved.

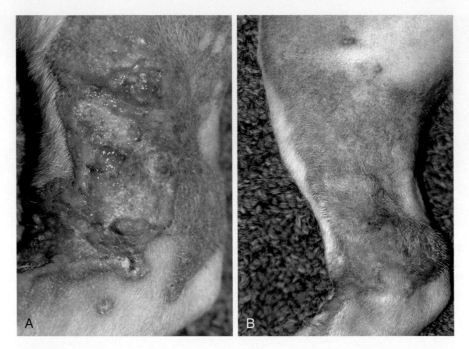

FIGURE 16-70 Calcinosis Cutis. A, Severe alopecic, hyperpigmented, erosive dermatitis caused by calcium deposition and secondary bacterial infection associated with iatrogenic Cushing's disease due to injectable long-acting steroid treatments. **B,** After discontinuation of the steroids and several weeks of aggressive antibiotic therapy, the infection resolved and the calcium was reabsorbed, allowing the skin to heal.

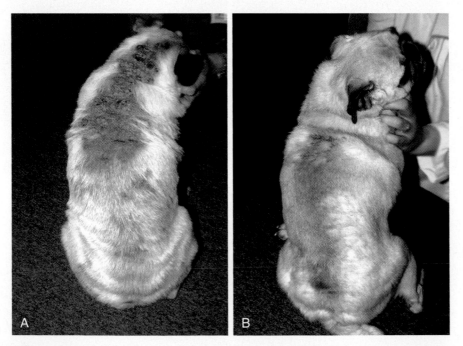

FIGURE 16-71 Calcinosis Cutis. A, Severe alopecic, erythematous, papular dermatitis with calcium deposition on the dorsum of a dog with iatrogenic Cushing's disease. **B,** After discontinuation of the steroids and several weeks of aggressive antibiotic therapy, the active inflammatory process was diminished and the skin was healing.

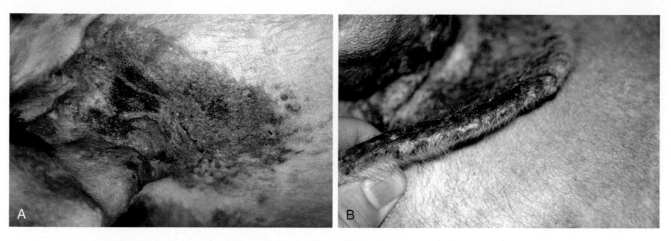

FIGURE 16-72 Calcinosis Cutis. A, Severe erythematous papular dermatitis caused by a secondary bacterial infection associated with iatrogenic Cushing's disease (caused by numerous injectable long-acting steroid treatments) and calcium deposition. **B,** After discontinuation of the steroids and several weeks of aggressive antibiotic therapy, the active inflammatory process was diminished and the skin has become hyperpigmented. The calcium deposits organized, forming a solid plate that could be lifted as a single sheet.

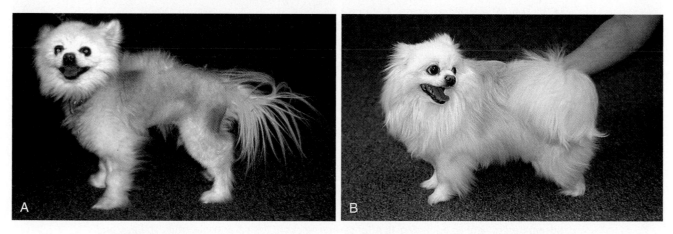

FIGURE 16-73 Sex Hormone Alopecia. A, Generalized alopecia and hyperpigmentation without apparent inflammatory dermatitis are typical of endocrine disease. **B,** Following castration, the fur coat regrew normally.

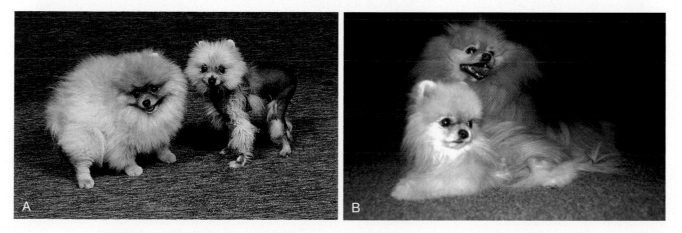

FIGURE 16-74 Alopecia X. A, Two related male Pomeranians with alopecia X. The Pomeranian on the left was recently treated, causing temporary regrowth of hair. **B,** The Pomeranian in front has the noninflammatory alopecia with cutaneous hyperpigmentation characteristic of this disorder.

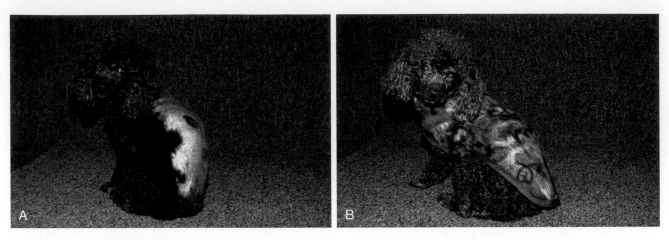

FIGURE 16-75 **Alopecia X. A,** An adult Poodle with persistent dorsal alopecia despite several treatment attempts. Note the biopsy-induced areas of hair regrowth typical of this syndrome. **B,** The Poodle after sweater therapy.

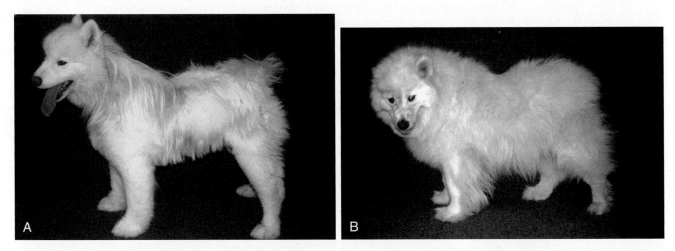

FIGURE 16-76 **Sebaceous Adenitis. A,** Generalized alopecia with erythematous, crusting dermatitis on the trunk of an adult dog. **B,** After several weeks of topical antiseborrheic therapy and systemic vitamin A supplementation, the dermatitis resolved.

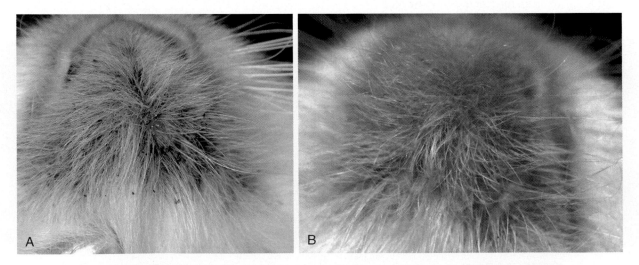

FIGURE 16-77 **Feline Acne. A,** Numerous comedones and papular dermatitis typical of feline acne complicated by a secondary bacterial infection. **B,** After frequent comedolytic cleansing and topical mupirocin ointment, the acne improved.

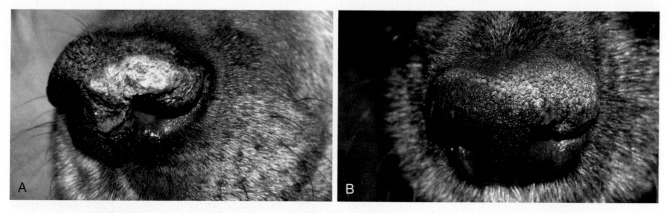

FIGURE 16-78 **Parasympathetic Nasal Hyperkeratosis. A,** Severe focal hyperkeratosis affecting predominantly one side of the nasal planum seems to be a common lesion pattern of this syndrome. **B,** After several weeks of topical mupirocin ointment therapy, the focal hyperkeratosis was markedly improved.

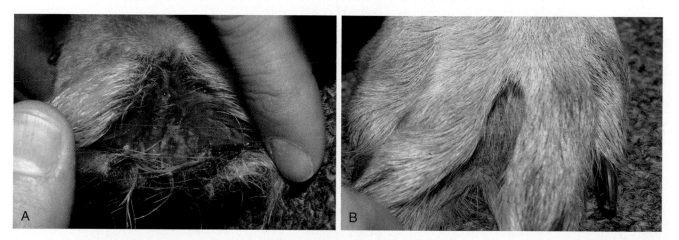

FIGURE 16-79 **Canine Interdigital Pyogranuloma. A,** Severe erosive interdigital dermatitis with a secondary bacterial pyoderma in an adult German shepherd. **B,** The interdigital lesions completely resolved after several weeks of aggressive topical and systemic antibacterial therapy, suggesting that the secondary infection was the main cause of the severe dermatitis.

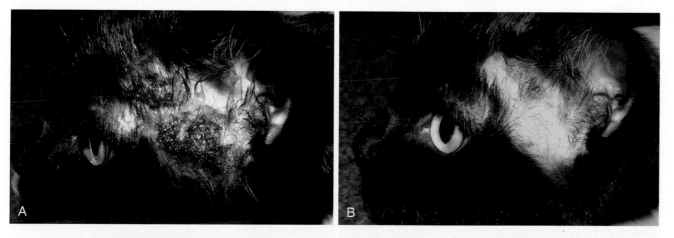

FIGURE 16-80 **Eosinophilic Plaque. A,** This eosinophilic plaque (erosive dermatitis with crust formation) on the preauricular skin developed acutely and was likely caused by exposure to fleas or other ectoparasites. **B,** After aggressive flea control and treatment with injectable steroids, the eosinophilic plaque completely resolved.

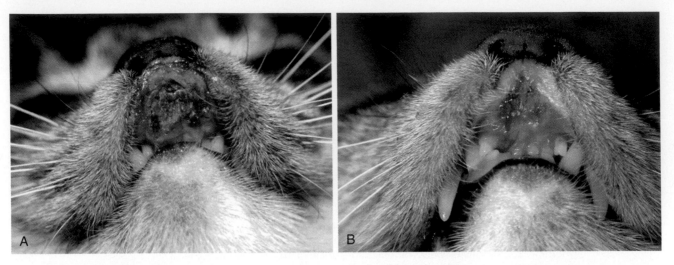

FIGURE 16-81 Indolent Ulcer. A, Severe tissue destruction of the upper lip is characteristic of this disease. **B,** After several weeks of treatment with trimethoprim-sulfa (used as an antibiotic and immune-modulating agent), the indolent ulcer was improving.

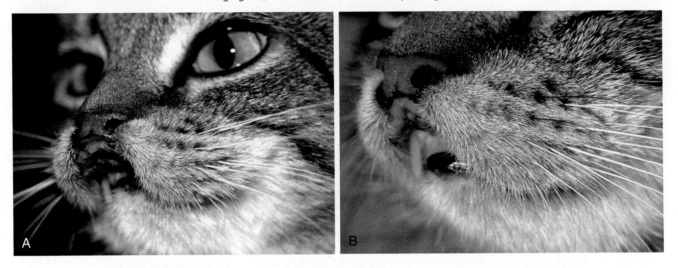

FIGURE 16-82 Indolent Ulcer. Same cat as in Figure 16-81. **A,** Swelling and severe tissue destruction of the upper lip are apparent. This cat had failed to respond to numerous treatment attempts with traditional therapies for indolent ulcers. **B,** After several weeks of treatment with trimethoprim-sulfa (used as an antibiotic and immune-modulating agent), the indolent ulcer was improving.

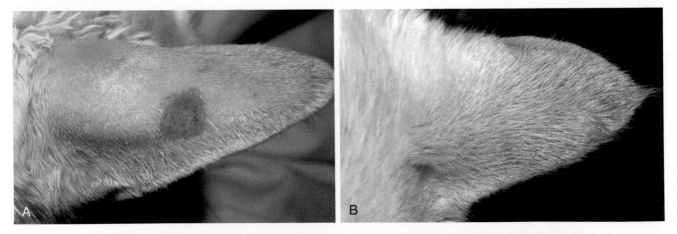

FIGURE 16-83 Feline Solar Dermatosis. A, A focal area of carcinoma in situ on the pinna of an adult cat. **B,** Several weeks after laser ablation, the skin was completely healed and hair was regrowing. Early detection and therapeutic intervention produced excellent cosmetic outcomes.

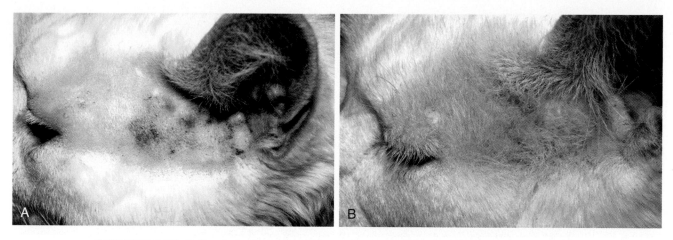

FIGURE 16-84 **Feline Solar Dermatosis.** Same cat as in Figure 16-83. **A,** A papular rash on the preauricular skin was caused by multiple solar lesions and foci of carcinoma in situ. **B,** Several weeks after laser ablation, the skin was completely healed and the hair was regrowing. Early detection and therapeutic intervention produced excellent cosmetic outcomes.

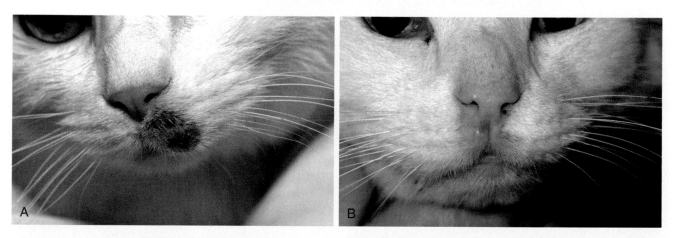

FIGURE 16-85 **Feline Solar Dermatosis. A,** A focal area of carcinoma in situ on the upper lip of an adult cat. *(Courtesy R. Seamen.)* **B,** Several weeks after laser ablation, the skin was completely healed and hair was regrowing. Early detection and therapeutic intervention produced excellent cosmetic outcomes. *(Courtesy R. Seamen.)*

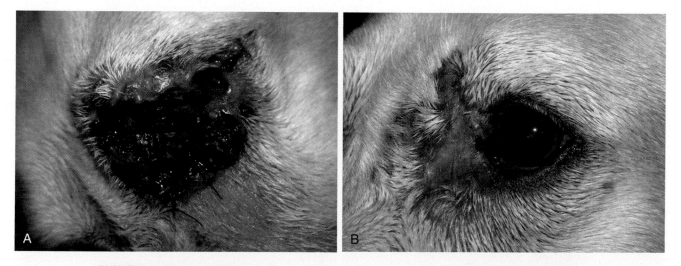

FIGURE 16-86 **Blepharitis. A,** Severe proliferative, erosive dermatitis on the eyelids and periocular skin of an adult Labrador. *(Courtesy K. Tobias.)* **B,** After several weeks of immunosuppressive therapy (doxycycline), the severe erosive dermatitis resolved, leaving alopecic, scarred skin. Note that the absence of erythema indicates resolution of the active inflammatory process.

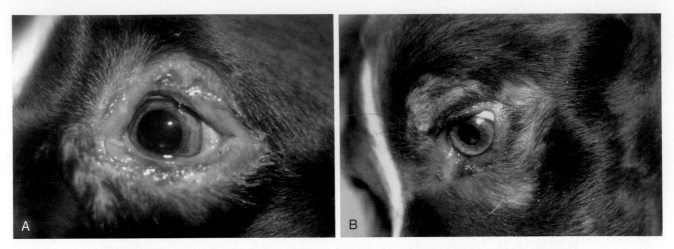

FIGURE 16-87 Blepharitis. A, Alopecic, erythematous, erosive dermatitis on the eyelids and periocular skin caused by marginal blepharitis. This immune-mediated skin disease is an unusual manifestation of an aberrant immune response. **B,** After several weeks of immunosuppressive therapy, the severe erosive dermatitis resolved, leaving alopecic, scarred skin.

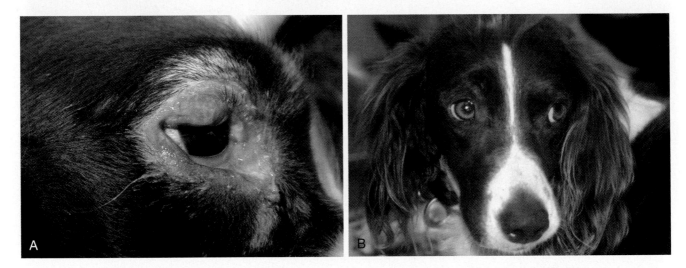

FIGURE 16-88 Blepharitis. Same dog as in Figure 16-87. **A,** Alopecic, erythematous dermatitis affecting the eyelid margins is apparent. **B,** After several weeks of immunosuppressive therapy, the severe erosive dermatitis resolved, leaving alopecic, scarred skin.

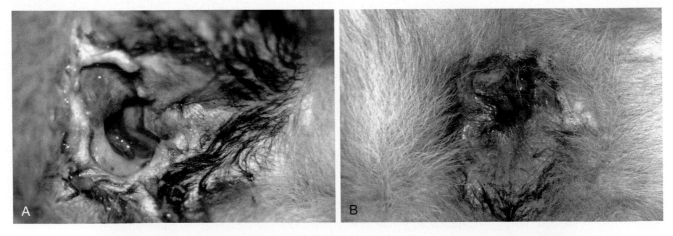

FIGURE 16-89 Perianal Fistulae. A, Deep fistulous track with tissue proliferation completely destroying the normal anal architecture. **B,** After several weeks of immunosuppressive therapy, the perianal fistula was greatly improved.

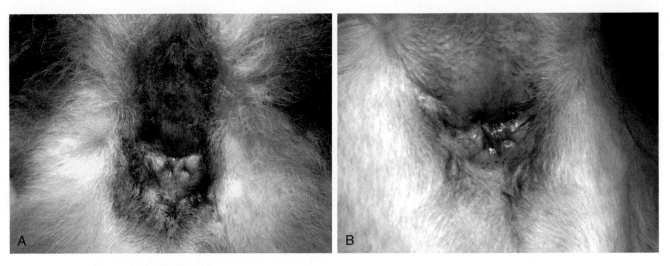

FIGURE 16-90 **Perianal Fistulae. A,** Tissue proliferation surrounding a persistent fistula in an adult German shepherd. **B,** After several weeks of immunosuppressive therapy, the perianal fistula was greatly improved.

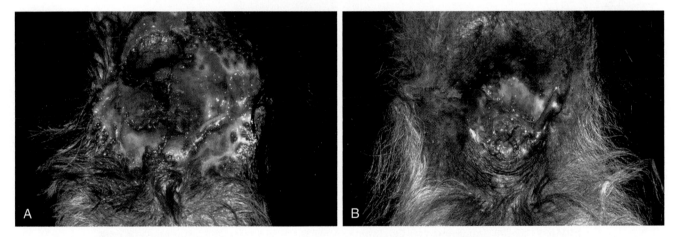

FIGURE 16-91 **Perianal Fistulae. A,** Severe destruction of the perianal tissue. **B,** After several weeks of immunosuppressive therapy, the perianal fistulae were greatly improved.

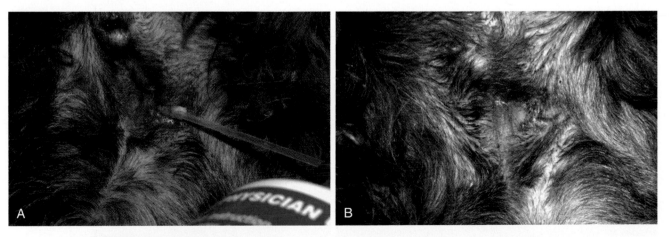

FIGURE 16-92 **Perianal Fistulae. A,** Cryosurgery (using a canned cryogen, Verruca-Freeze) is being performed to re-stimulate wound healing and resolve persistent perianal fistulae (which had persisted despite several months of topical and systemic immunosuppressive treatment). **B,** Several weeks after the cryosurgical procedure, the perianal fistulae have almost resolved.

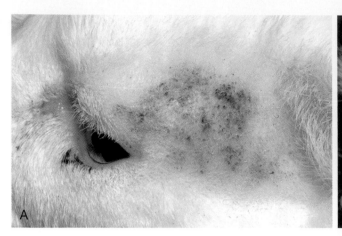
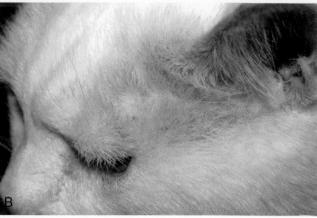

FIGURE 16-93 Squamous Cell Carcinoma. A, Multiple crusting papular lesions caused by solar dermatitis and squamous cell carcinoma. **B,** Several weeks after laser ablation, the skin was completely healed and hair was regrowing. Early detection and therapeutic intervention produced excellent cosmetic outcomes.

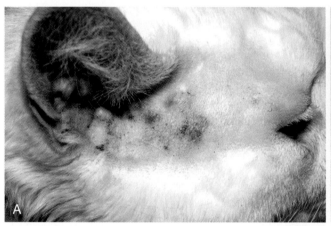
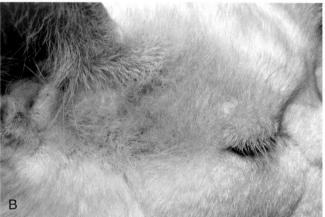

FIGURE 16-94 Squamous Cell Carcinoma. Same cat as in Figure 16-93. **A,** Papular lesions caused by solar dermatitis and carcinoma are apparent on the preauricular skin. **B,** Several weeks after laser ablation, the skin was completely healed and hair was regrowing. Early detection and therapeutic intervention produced excellent cosmetic outcomes.

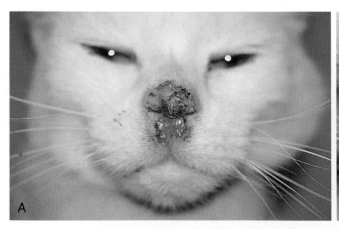
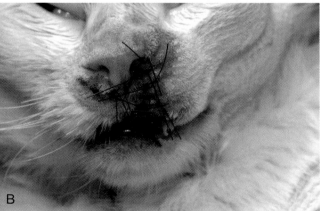

FIGURE 16-95 Squamous Cell Carcinoma. A, Severe crusting, ulcerative dermatitis associated with invasive squamous cell carcinoma on the nasal planum and upper lip of an adult cat. **B,** Radical surgical excision was necessary to remove the entire tumor. Surgical correction would have been much easier if performed earlier. *(Courtesy R. Seamen.)*

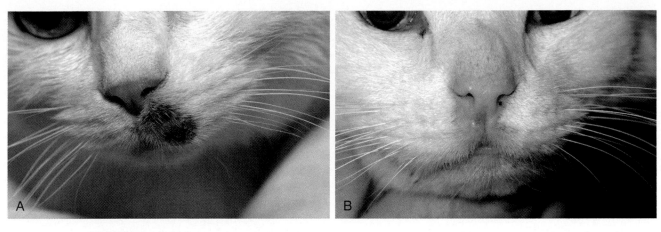

FIGURE 16-96 **Squamous Cell Carcinoma. A,** Focal area of carcinoma in situ on the upper lip of an adult cat. *(Courtesy R. Seamen.)* **B,** Several weeks after laser ablation, the skin was completely healed and hair was regrowing. Early detection and therapeutic intervention produced excellent cosmetic outcomes. *(Courtesy R. Seamen.)*

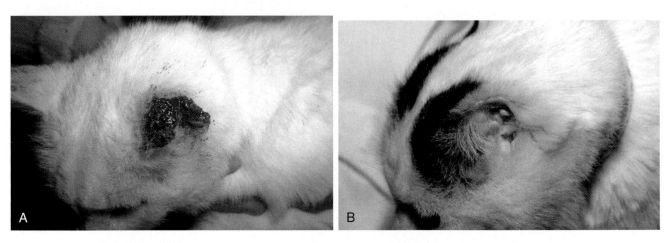

FIGURE 16-97 **Squamous Cell Carcinoma. A,** Severe tissue destruction of the entire distal ear pinna caused by progression of the squamous cell carcinoma. **B,** Amputation of this cat's ear pinna was performed to remove the tumor. Early detection and therapeutic intervention provide better cosmetic outcomes.

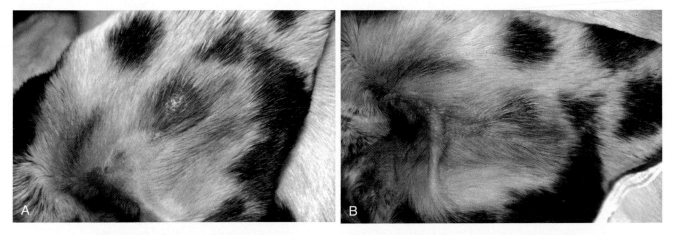

FIGURE 16-98 **Mast Cell Tumor. A,** Alopecic, erythematous tumor on the ear pinna of a Dalmatian. **B,** After several weeks of steroid therapy, the mast cell tumor was reduced in size.

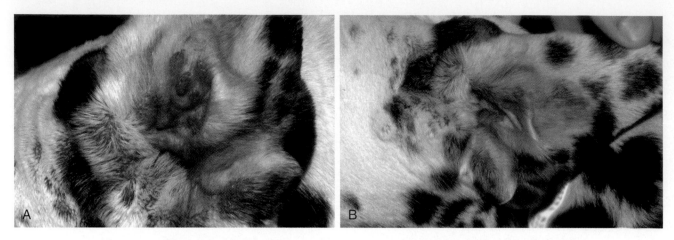

FIGURE 16-99 **Mast Cell Tumor. A,** Multiple alopecic, erythematous tumors on the head and ear pinna of a Dalmatian. **B,** After several weeks of steroid therapy, the mast cell tumors were reduced in size.

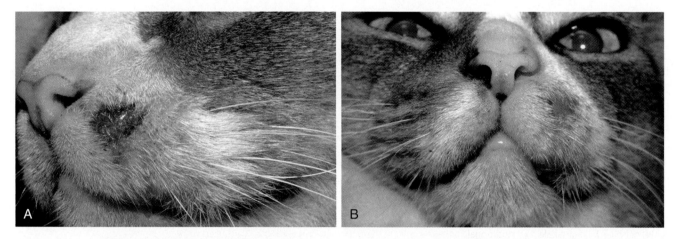

FIGURE 16-100 **Epitheliotropic Lymphoma. A,** Focal, alopecic, ulcerated lesions on a cat's lip. Note that the entire lip is swollen—a condition that is caused by infiltrating neoplastic cells. **B,** After several weeks of topical steroid therapy, the inflammation associated with the tumor was improved.

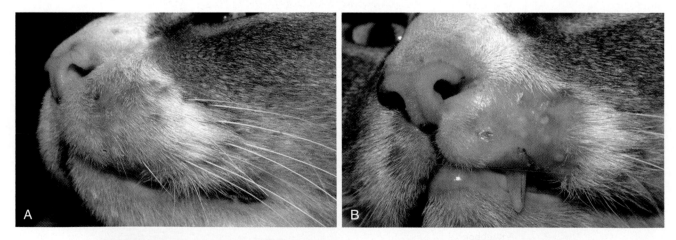

FIGURE 16-101 **Epitheliotropic Lymphoma.** Same cat as in Figure 16-100. **A,** Despite transient improvement associated with topical steroids, the lymphoma continued to spread. This image was taken several weeks after chemotherapy was used to slow the tumor. **B,** Despite the transient improvement associated with topical steroids and chemotherapy, the lymphoma continued to spread. This image was taken several weeks after aggressive radiation therapy was provided. The tumor had improved, but the skin was left alopecic and scarred from the radiation damage.

Antimicrobial, Antiseborrheic, and Antipruritic Shampoo Therapy

Antimicrobial, Antiseborrheic, and Antipruritic Shampoo Therapy

Ingredient	Therapeutic Effects	Usage	Disadvantages
Chlorhexidine	Antibacterial Antifungal Antiviral	Mild shampoo with excellent antimicrobial activity	
Benzoyl peroxide	Antibacterial Follicular flushing Degreasing Keratolytic	Potent degreasing, follicular flushing shampoo with excellent antibacterial effects Mildly antiseborrheic Good for crusting and oily seborrheic disorders	Drying May irritate skin May bleach fabrics
Chlorhexidine/miconazole combinations	Antifungal Antibacterial	Superior antifungal efficacy compared with single-ingredient products	
Chlorhexidine/ketoconazole combinations	Antifungal Antibacterial	Superior antifungal efficacy compared with single-ingredient products	
Triclosan	Antibacterial	Moderately effective antibacterial ingredient added to shampoos	
Ethyl lactate	Antibacterial Decreases skin pH Degreasing Comedolytic	Mild degreasing, antiseborrheic shampoo with good antibacterial activity Good for dry, scaling seborrhea	
Povidone-iodine	Antibacterial Antifungal Antiviral	Mild shampoo with excellent antimicrobial activity but limited duration of effect	Short duration of effect Staining May irritate skin Thyroid dysfunction Metabolic acidosis
Acetic acid Boric acid	Antimicrobial	Good therapy for *Malassezia* dermatitis	May be irritating
Ketoconazole	Antifungal	Mild shampoo with good antifungal activity	
Miconazole	Antifungal	Mild shampoo with good antifungal activity	
Phytosphingosine	Antimicrobial Antisebborrheic	Mild shampoo	
Lactoferrin Lactoperoxidase Zinc gluconate Lysozymes Potassium iodide	Antimicrobial	Mild shampoo with antimicrobial effects	May be irritating

Continued

Antimicrobial, Antiseborrheic, and Antipruritic Shampoo Therapy—cont'd

Ingredient	Therapeutic Effects	Usage	Disadvantages
Sulfur/salicylic acid	Keratolytic Keratoplastic	Moderately well-tolerated shampoo with good antiseborrheic activity Good for crusting or dry seborrheic disorders	
Sodium salicylate Zinc gluconate Pyridoxine	Antiseborrheic Antimicrobial	Good antiseborrheic shampoo without the adverse effects of tar	
Tar	Keratolytic Keratoplastic Degreasing Antipruritic Vasoactive	Potent degreasing and antiseborrheic shampoo Good for severe oily seborrheic disorders	Toxic to cats Drying May irritate skin Staining Photosensitization Carcinogenic
Selenium sulfide	Keratolytic Keratoplastic Degreasing	Potent degreasing shampoo with good antiseborrheic activity Good for oily seborrheic disorders Moderate activity against yeast	Drying May irritate skin
Oatmeal	Decreases prostaglandins Antipruritic Soothing	Mild shampoo with moderate antipruritic activity	
Diphenhydramine	Antipruritic	Mild shampoo with moderate antipruritic activity	Contact sensitivity
Pramoxine	Antipruritic	Mild shampoo with good antipruritic activity	
Hydrocortisone	Anti-inflammatory Antipruritic	Mild shampoo with good antipruritic activity	Immunosuppression Cutaneous atrophy
L-rhamnose	Antiallergic	Mild shampoo that helps prevent allergen penetration	
Menthol	Antipruritic	Added to products to decrease pruritus	May be irritating
Aloe vera	Anti-inflammatory Antibacterial	Added to many products for mild anti-inflammatory effects	
Melaleuca oil Tea tree oil	Anti-inflammatory Antimicrobial	Moderately effective anti-inflammatory with good antimicrobial properties	May be irritating Excessive application may cause toxicity (salivation, neurologic symptoms, hepatotoxicity)

Humectants
  Propylene glycol
  Urea
  Lactic acid
  Glycerin
	Moisturizers	Hygroscopic agents that actively pull water into the skin	

Emollients
  Oils
  Lanolin
  Paraffin
  Waxes
	Moisturizers	Occlusive agents that decrease transepidermal water loss.	

Topical Brands With Active Ingredients

Brand Name	How Supplied
Antimicrobials/Antifungals	
Malaseb Shampoo (DVM)	2% miconazole nitrate, 2% chlorhexidine gluconate in a surfactant base
Malaseb Spray & Pledgets (DVM)	2% miconazole nitrate, 2% chlorhexidine gluconate
Oxydex Shampoo (DVM)	2.5% benzoyl peroxide
Sulfoxydex Shampoo (DVM)	2.5% benzoyl peroxide, 2% sulfur
Oxydex Gel (DVM)	5% benzoyl peroxide
Micropearls Benzoyl Plus (Vetoquinol)	2.5% benzoyl peroxide in a Novasome base
Pyoben Shampoo (Virbac)	3% benzoyl peroxide, nonlathering
Pyoben Gel (Virbac)	5% benzoyl peroxide in a water-based gel
BPO 3 Shampoo (Vet's Solution)	3% benzoyl peroxide
Benzoyl Peroxide Shampoo (Animal Pharm)	2.5% benzoyl peroxide, sulfur, drying
Chlorhexiderm Shampoo (DVM)	2% chlorhexidine gluconate
Chlorhexiderm Max Shampoo (DVM)	4% chlorhexidine gluconate
Chlorhexidine Shampoo (Animal Pharm)	4% chlorhexidine
Sebozole (Vet's Solution)	2% miconazole nitrate, 1% chloroxylenol, 2% solubilized sulfur, 2% salicylic acid
Ketochlor Shampoo (Virbac)	2.3% chlorhexidine gluconate, 1% ketoconazole
Pharmaseb Shampoo (Animal Pharm)	2% chloroxylenol, 1% ketoconazole
Micropearls Sebahex (Vetoquinol)	2% chlorhexidine, 2% sulfur (elemental), 2% salicylic acid
Hexadine Shampoo (Virbac)	3% chlorhexidine gluconate
Resichlor Leave-on Lotion (Virbac)	2% chlorhexidine gluconate in a leave-on base
Micropearls Miconazole Shampoo (Vetoquinol)	1% miconazole nitrate in a Novasome base
Micropearls Miconazole Spray (Vetoquinol)	1% miconazole nitrate spray
Dermazole Shampoo (Virbac)	2% miconazole, 2% salicylic acid
Resizole Leave-on Lotion (Virbac)	2% miconazole in a leave-on lotion base
Etiderm Shampoo (Virbac)	10% ethyl lactate
Douxo Chlorhexidine PS Shampoo (Sogeval)	Phytosphingosine salicyloyl 0.05%, chlorhexidine 3%
Antiseborrheics	
Sebalyt Shampoo (DVM)	2% sulfur (elemental), 2% salicylic acid, 0.5% triclosan
Nu-Sal T Shampoo (DVM)	2% coal tar, 3% salicylic acid, 1% menthol
Micropearls Sebahex Shampoo (Vetoquinol)	2% sulfur (elemental), 2% salicylic acid, 2% Chlohexidine in a Novasome base
Sebolux Shampoo (Virbac)	2% sulfur (solubilized), 2% salicylic acid
Keratolux Shampoo (Virbac)	1% salicylic acid, 0.5% zinc gluconate, 0.5% pyridoxine
DermaSebS Shampoo (DermaPet)	Sulfur (solubilized), salicylic acid
Universal Medicated Shampoo (Vet's Solution)	2% chloroxylenol, 3.1% sodium thiosulfate (equivalent to 2% solubilized sulfur), 2% salicylic acid
Douxo Seborrhea Shampoo (Sogeval)	Phytosphingosine 0.1%
Douxo Seborrhea Micro-emulsion Spray (Sogeval)	Phytosphingosine 0.2%
Souxo Seborrhea Spot-on (Sogeval)	Phytosphingosine 1%
Antipruritics	
Relief Shampoo & Cream Rinse (DVM)	1% pramoxine HCL in a colloidal oatmeal base
Relief Spray (DVM)	1% pramoxine HCL with colloidal oatmeal
Relief HCSpray (DVM)	1% pramoxine HCL, 1% hydrocortisone HCL, colloidal oatmeal
Micropearls Dermal Soothe Shampoo (Vetoquinol)	1% pramoxine HCL, 2% colloidal oatmeal in a Novasome base
Micropearls Dermal Soothe Cream Rinse (Vetoquinol)	1% pramoxine HCL, 2% colloidal oatmeal in a Novasome base
Micropearls Dermal Soothe Spray (Vetoquinol)	1% pramoxine HCL, lactic acid, in a Novasome base
Epi-Soothe Shampoo & Cream Rinse (Virbac)	20% colloidal oatmeal
DermAllay Oatmeal Shampoo And Conditioner (DermaPet)	Soluble oatmeal
Aloe and Oatmeal Shampoo (Vet's Solution)	Aloe, 2% colloidal oatmeal
Aloe & Oatmeal Shampoo (Animal Pharm)	Aloe, colloidal oatmeal
CortiSpray (DVM)	1% hydrocortisone acetate, lactic acid
Resisoothe Leave-on Lotion (Virbac)	Colloidal oatmeal, omega-6 fatty acids
Resiprox Leave-on Lotion (Virbac)	1.5% pramoxine HCL, colloidal oatmeal
Resihist Leave-on Lotion (Virbac)	2% diphenhydramine HCL
Resicort Leave-on Lotion (Virbac)	1% hydrocortisone
Dermacool Spray (Virbac)	1.5% lidocaine HCL in an astringent base
Dermacool HC Spray (Virbac)	1% hydrocortisone in an astringent base
Histacalm Shampoo (Virbac)	2% diphenhydramine HCL, colloidal oatmeal base
Allerspray w/Bittran (Vetoquinol)	2.4% lidocaine, Bittran, aloe, lanolin

Continued

Topical Brands With Active Ingredients—*cont'd*

Brand Name	How Supplied
Hypoallergenic/Moisturizing/Normal Skin	
Hylyt EFA Shampoo & Rinse (DVM)	EFA, sodium lactate, lanolin, glycerin, coconut oil, Hypoallergenic
Hylyt EFA Bath Oil Spray (DVM)	Emollients, sodium lactate, EFAs
Hylyt Crème Rinse (DVM)	Emollients in a moisturizing base
Pearlyte Shampoo (DVM)	Pearlized whitening shampoo with colloidal oatmeal
DVM Tearless Shampoo (DVM)	Hypoallergenic, tearless shampoo
Micropearls Hydrapearls Shampoo (Vetoquinol)	Mild shampoo in a Novasome base
Micropearls Hydrapearls Cream Rinse (Vetoquinol)	Mild cream rinse in a Novasome base
Micropearls Hydrapearls Spray (Vetoquinol)	Lactic acid moisturizing spray in a Novasome base
Allergroom Shampoo (Virbac)	Moisturizing, hypoallergenic
Humilac Spray (Virbac)	Lactic acid
Ultragroom Shampoo (Virbac)	Peach fragrance
Essential Fatty Acid Shampoo (Animal Pharm)	Soap-free, "hypoallergenic"
Groom-Aid 35X Shampoo (Vetoquinol)	Dilutable, affordable kennel baths
D-Basic Shampoo (DVM)	Affordable kennel baths, premedicated bath
DermaLyte Shampoo (DermaPet)	Hypoallergenic, vitamin E, EFAs
Douxo Maintenance Shampoo (Sogeval)	Mild shampoo

Courtesy Debbie Corral, DVM Pharmaceuticals, TEVA, Inc.

Topical Therapeutic Drugs

Topical Therapeutic Drugs

Drug Name	Brand Name	How Supplied
Aluminum Acetate 5% Solution	Otic Domeboro Solution: Bayer; West Haven, Connecticut	2% Acetic Acid in Aqueous Aluminum, 2 fl oz dropper bottles
Amitraz Collars	Preventic Collar: Allerderm/Virbac; Fort Worth, Texas	9% Amitraz 25 inch plastic collar
Amitraz Solution	Mitaban: Pfizer Animal Health; Exton, Pennsylvania	19.9% Amitraz in 10.6 mL bottles
	Ectodex: Hoechst Roussel Vet (not available in United States)	5% Amitraz in 50 mL bottles
	Taktic EC: Hoechst Roussel Vet; Warren, New Jersey	12.5% Amitraz in 760 mL containers
Amphotericin B 3% Lotion, Cream, and Ointment	Fungizone: Apothecon; Princeton, New Jersey	Lotion: 30 mL bottles Cream: 20 g tubes Ointment: 20 g tubes
Benzoyl Peroxide 5% Gel	Cytoxyl-AQ Gel: VetGenix; Coral Gables, Florida	Benzoyl Peroxide in 170 g bottle with dispensing tip
	Pyoben Gel: Allerderm/Virbac; Fort Worth, Texas	Benzoyl Peroxide in 30 g plastic tubes
	Oxydex Gel: DVM; Miami, Florida	Benzoyl Peroxide in 30 g tubes
Burow's Solution/ Hydrocortisone	Bur-O-Cort 2:1: QA Labs; Kansas City, Missouri	10 oz and 16 oz bottles
	Burow's H Solution: Vetus; Farmer's Branch, Texas	1 oz squeeze bottles, 2 oz spray bottles, and 16 oz bottles
	Cort/Astrin Solution: Vedco; St. Joseph, Missouri	1 oz dropper bottles and 16 oz bottles
	Corti-Derm Solution: First Priority; Elgin, Illinois	16 oz bottles
	Hydro-Plus: Phoenix; St. Joseph, Missouri (many other generics)	1 oz and 1 pint bottles
Chlorhexidine Ointment	Chlorhexidine Ointment: Davis Veterinary Products; Scottsdale, Georgia	2% ointment in 4 oz containers
	Nolvasan Antiseptic Ointment: Wyeth; Fort Dodge, Iowa (many other generics)	1% ointment in 1 oz, 7 oz, and 16 oz tubes
Chlorhexidine 2% Solution	Nolvasan Solution: Wyeth; Fort Dodge, Iowa	1 gal containers
	Hexasol: Vetus; Farmer's Branch, Texas (many other generics)	1 gal containers
Clindamycin 1% Gel, Lotion, and Solution	Clindamycin Phosphate: Geneva; Broomfield, Colorado	Gel: 30 g tubes Lotion: 60 mL bottles Solution: 30 mL and 60 mL bottles
	Cleocin T: Pfizer	Gel: 7.5 g and 30 g tubes Lotion: 60 mL bottles Solution: 30 mL and 60 mL bottles
	Clindaderm: Paddock; Minneapolis, Minnesota	Solution: 60 mL bottles
	C/T/S: Hoechst Marion Roussel; Kansas City, Missouri	Solution: 30 mL and 60 mL containers

Continued

Topical Therapeutic Drugs—*cont'd*

Drug Name	Brand Name	How Supplied
Clotrimazole 1% Cream, Lotion, and Solution	Clotrimazole: Taro; Hawthorne, New York	Cream: 15 g, 30 g, and 45 g tubes Solution: 30 mL bottles
	Fungoid: Pedinol; Farmingdale, New York	Cream: 30 g tubes Solution: 30 mL bottles
	Lotrimin: Schering-Plough; Kenilworth, New Jersey	Lotion: 30 mL containers Solution: 10 mL, 30 mL containers
	Lotrimin AF: Schering-Plough; Kenilworth, New Jersey (OTC)	Lotion: 20 mL bottles Solution: 10 mL bottles
Dimethyl Sulfoxide 20% Gel	Domoso: Wyeth; Fort Dodge, Iowa	2.1 oz and 4.2 oz tubes and 15 oz containers
Econazole 1% Cream	Spectazole: Ortho Pharmaceutical Corporation; Raritan, New Jersey	15 g, 30 g, and 85 g tubes
Enilconazole 1% Solution	Imaverol: Janssen Pharmaceutica (not available in United States)	100 mL and 1 L containers
Erythromycin Solution	Staticin: Westwood Squibb; Buffalo, New York	1.5% Erythromycin in 60 mL bottles with applicators
	Erythromycin Topical: Bausch & Lomb; Claremont, California (many other generics)	2% Erythromycin in 60 mL bottles
Fipronil Spray and Solution	Frontline Spray and TopSpot: Merial; Iselin, New Jersey	29% Spray: 3.4 oz and 8.5 oz containers 9.7% Solution: 0.5 mL, 0.67 mL, 1.3 mL, and 0.68 mL pipettes
Fipronil/ (S)-Methoprene Solution	Frontline-Plus: Merial: Iselin, New Jersey	9.8% Fipronil and 9.8% (S)-Methoprene (dogs) or 11.8% Methoprene (cats): 0.5 mL, 0.67 mL, 1.34 mL, 2.68 mL, and 4.02 mL pipettes
Gentamicin-Betamethasone Valerate Spray	Genta-Spray: Vetus; Farmer's Branch, Texas	60 mL, 120 mL, and 240 mL bottles
	GentaVed Topical Spray: Vedco; St. Joseph, Missouri	
	Gentocin Topical Spray: Schering- Plough; Union, New Jersey	
Icthamol 20% Ointment	Icthamol: Butler; Dublin, Ohio, and Phoenix; St. Joseph, Missouri	1 lb jars
	Icthamol Ointment: First Priority; Elgin, Ohio	4 oz and 1 lb jars
	Icthamol Ointment: Aspen; Kansas City, Missouri (many other generics)	1 lb jars
Imidacloprid Solution	Advantage: Bayer; Shawnee Mission, Kansas	9.1% Solution Cats: 0.4 mL and 0.8 mL pipettes Dogs: 0.4 mL, 0.8 mL, 1.0 mL, 2.5 mL, and 4.0 mL pipettes
Imidacloprid/ Permethrin Solution	K9 Advantix: Bayer; Shawnee Mission, Kansas	Imidacloprid/Permethrin Combination (no concentration given) in 0.4 mL, 1.0 mL, 2.0 mL, and 4.0 mL pipettes
Imiquimod Cream	Aldara Cream: 3M Pharmaceuticals; St. Paul, Minnesota	5% Cream in 250 mg single-use packets (box of 12)
Ketoconazole 2% Cream	Nizoral 2% Cream: Janssen Pharmaceutica; Titusville, New Jersey	15 g, 30 g, and 60 g tubes
Lidocaine Spray and Gel	Allerspray: Evsco; Buena, New Jersey	2.5% Lidocaine HCl in 4 oz and 12 oz containers
	Dermacool With Lidocaine HCl: Allerderm/Virbac; Fort Worth, Texas	Hamamelis Extract and Lidocaine HCl (no concentration given) in 4 oz bottles
	VetMark Anti-itch Gel and Spray: Bioderm; Longview, Texas	Gel: 2.46% Lidocaine HCl in 2 oz bottles Spray: 2.46% Lidocaine HCl in 4 oz containers
Lime-Sulfur Solution	Lymdyp: DVM, Miami, Florida	16 oz and 1 gal containers
Metronidazole 0.75% Gel	Metro Gel: Galderma; Fort Worth, Texas	28.4 g tubes

Topical Therapeutic Drugs—*cont'd*

Drug Name	Brand Name	How Supplied
Miconazole 1% Spray, Lotion, and Cream	Micaved: Vedco; St. Joseph, Missouri	Spray: 120 mL and 240 mL containers
	Micazole: Vetus; Carrollton, Texas	Lotion: 60 mL bottles
	Miconosol: Med-Pharmex; Pomona, California	Cream: 15 g tubes
	Conofite: Schering-Plough; Union, New Jersey	Spray: 60 mL bottles Lotion: 30 mL containers
Mupirocin 2% Ointment	Bactoderm: Pfizer Animal Health; Exton, Pennsylvania	15 g tubes
Neomycin Ointment and Powder	Forte-Topical: Pfizer Animal Health; Exton, Pennsylvania	Neomycin Sulfate/Procaine Penicillin G/Polymyxin B Sulfate/Hydrocortisone Acetate/Hydrocortisone Sodium Succinate in 10 mL tubes
	Neo-Predef: Pfizer Animal Health; Exton, Pennsylvania	Neomycin Sulfate/Isoflupredone Acetate/Tetracaine HCl Topical Powder in 15 g bottles
	Triple Antibiotic Ointment: Legere; Scottsdale, Arizona	Neomycin Sulfate/Polymyxin B Sulfate/Bacitracin in ½ oz tubes
	Tritop: Pfizer Animal Health; Exton, Pennsylvania (many other generics)	Neomycin Sulfate/Isoflupredone Acetate/Tetracaine HCl in 10 g tubes
Nystatin-Neomycin-Thiostrepton-Triamcinolone Acetonide	Animax: Pharmaderm; Melville, New York	Ointment: 7.5 mL, 15 mL, 30 mL tubes and 240 mL bottles
	Panalog: Solvay; Mendota Heights, Minnesota (many other generics)	Ointment: 75 mL, 15 mL, 30 mL, and 240 mL Cream: 7.5 g and 15 g tubes
Povidine-Iodine 10% Solution	Betadine: Perdue-Frederick; Norwalk, Connecticut	15 mL, 120 mL, 237 mL, 1 pint, 1 quart, and 1 gal containers
	Poviderm Solution: Vetus; Farmer's Branch, Texas (many other generics)	1 gal containers
Pramoxine HCl 1% Solution	Heska Pramoxine Spray: Heska; Fort Collins, Texas	12 oz bottles
	Relief Spray: DVM; Miami, Florida	8 oz containers
	Corium-Tx: VRx; Harbor City, California	2 oz bottles
Selamectin Solution	Revolution: Pfizer; Exton, Pennsylvania	6%–12% Solution in 0.25 mL, 0.75 mL, 0.5 mL, and 2 mL tubes
	Stronghold: Pfizer Ltd, Kent, United Kingdom	
Salicylic Acid-Sodium Lactate-Urea Gel	KeraSolv: DVM; Miami, Florida	1 oz tubes
Silver Sulfadiazine 1% Cream	SSD Cream: Boots (Knoll); Mount Olive, New Jersey	25 g, 50 g, 85 g, 400 g, and 1000 g tubes
	Silvadene: Hoechst Marion Roussel; Kansas City, Missouri	20 g, 50 g, 85 g, 400 g, and 1000 g tubes
	Thermazene: Sherwood (Kendall): Mansfield, Massachusetts	50 g, 400 g, and 1000 g tubes
Tetracycline Solution and Ointment	Topicycline: Roberts; Eatontown, New Jersey	2.2 mg/mL Solution when reconstituted; supplied as Powder with Diluent for 70 mL
	Achromycin: Lederle; Pearl River, New York	3% Ointment in 14.2 g and 30 g tubes
Tretinoin Gel and Cream	Retin-A: Ortho; Raritan, New Jersey	Gel: 0.01% in 15 g and 45 g tubes; 0.025% in 15 g and 45 g tubes; 0.1% in 20 g and 45 g tubes Cream: 0.025% in 20 g and 45 g tubes; 0.1% in 20 g and 45 g tubes
Triamcinolone Cream	Vetalog Cream: Wyeth; Fort Dodge, Iowa	15 g tubes

Otic Therapeutic Drugs

Otic Therapeutic Drugs

Drug Name	Brand Name	How Supplied
Acetic Acid-Hydrocortisone	Clear X Ear Drying Solution: DVM; Miami, Florida	25% Acetic Acid; 2% Colloidal Sulfur; 1% Hydrocortisone in 30 mL containers
	Bur-Otic Ear Treatment: Allerderm/Virbac; Fort Worth, Texas (many other generics)	1% Hydrocortisone; also contains Burow's Solution, Acetic Acid, and Benzalkonium Chloride in 30 mL containers
Chloramphenicol/ Prednisolone (otic)	Chlora-Otic: Vetus; Farmer's Branch, Texas	10 mL tubes and 12 oz bottles
	Liquichlor: Evsco; Buena, New Jersey	
Clotrimazole 1% (otic)	Otobiotic Ointment: Vetus; Farmer's Branch, Texas	Gentamicin Sulfate/Betamethasone Valerate/Clotrimazole Ointment in 7.5 mL, 15 mL, 30 mL, and 240 mL
	Tri-Otic: Med-Pharmex; Pomona, California	
	Otomax: Schering-Plough; Union, New Jersey	
Enrofloxacin/Silver Sulfadiazine	Baytril Otic: Bayer; Shawnee Mission, Kansas	0.5% Enrofloxacin and 1.0% Silver Sulfadiazine in 15 and 30 mL bottles
Fluocinolone-Dimethyl Sulfoxide (otic)	Synotic Solution: Wyeth; Fort Dodge, Iowa	0.01% Fluocinolone Acetonide, 0.01 Dimethyl Sulfoxide in 8 mL and 60 mL dropper vials
Gentamicin	Genta-Otic: Vetus; Farmer's Branch, Texas	Gentamicin Sulfate/Betamethasone Valerate in 7.5 mL, 15 mL, and 240 mL squeeze bottles
	Gentaved Otic: Vedco; St. Joseph, Missouri	Gentamicin Sulfate/Betamethasone Valerate/Clotrimazole in 7.5 mL, 15 mL, and 240 mL squeeze bottles
	Gentocin Otic: Schering-Plough; Union, New Jersey	
	Otibiotic: Vetus; Farmer's Branch, Texas	
	Otomax: Schering-Plough; Union, New Jersey	
	Tri-Otic: Med-Pharmex; Pomona, California	
Gentamicin-Betamethasone Valerate	Genta-Spray: Vetus; Farmer's Branch, Texas	60 mL, 120 mL, and 240 mL bottles
	GentaVed Topical Spray: Vedco; St. Joseph, Missouri	
	Gentocin Topical Spray: Schering-Plough; Union, New Jersey	
Nystatin-Neomycin-Thiostrepton-Triamcinolone Acetonide Cream and Ointment	Animax: Pharmaderm; Melville, New York	Ointment: 7.5 mL, 15 mL, and 30 mL tubes and 240 mL bottles
	Panalog: Fort Dodge; Mendota Heights, Minnesota (many other generics)	Ointment: 7.5 mL, 15 mL, 30 mL, and 240 mL Cream: 7.5 g and 15 g tubes

Otic Therapeutic Drugs—*cont'd*

Drug Name	Brand Name	How Supplied
Otic miticides	Acarexx: IDEXX; Blue Ridge Pharmaceuticals; Greensboro, North Carolina	0.01% Ivermectin in 0.5 mL ampules
	Aurimite: Schering-Plough; Union, New Jersey	Pyrethrin/Piperonyl Butoxide in 1 fl oz and 16 oz bottles
	Cerumite: Evsco; Buena, New Jersey	Pyrethrin/Piperonyl Butoxide in 0.5 fl oz bottles
	Ear Miticide: Phoenix Pharmaceutical; St. Joseph, Missouri	Rotenone/Cube Resins in 2 oz
	Ear Mite Lotion: Duravet; Blue Springs, Missouri	Same as above in 4 oz containers
	Mita-Clear; Pfizer Animal Health; Exton, Pennsylvania	N-Octyl Bicycloheptene Dicarboximide/Di-n-Propyl Isocinchomeronate in 22 mL bottles
	Mitaplex-R: Tomlyn; Buena, New Jersey	Rotenone in 2 oz and 4 oz bottles
	Otomite Plus Ear Mite Treatment: Allerderm/Virbac; Fort Worth, Texas (many others)	Pyrethrin/Piperonyl Butoxide/N-Octyl Bicycloheptene Dicarboxide/Di-n-Propyl Isocinchomeronate in $\frac{1}{2}$ oz bottles
Silver Sulfadiazine	Silvadene: Hoechst Marion Roussel; Kansas City, Missouri	1.0% Cream in 20 g, 50 g, 85 g, 400 g, and 1000 g tubes
	Silver Sulfadiazine, Micronized: Spectrum Laboratory Products; Gardena, California	Powder in 10 g, 25 g, 100 g, and 1 kg containers
Thiabendazole-Dexamethasone-Neomycin Solution	Tresaderm: Merial; Rahway, New Jersey	7.5 mL and 15 mL dropper bottles
Tobramycin 0.3% Solution	Tobramycin: Bausch & Lomb; Tampa, Florida	5 mL bottles
	AKTob: Akorn; Buffalo Grove, Illinois	
	Tobradex: Alcon Laboratories; Fort Worth, Texas (many other generics)	
Tricide	Molecular Therapeutics, Inc.; Ann Arbor, Michigan	Powder 5.4 g (dissolved in 1 L yields 8 mM EDTA with 20 mM Tris)

Systemic Therapeutic Drugs

Systemic Therapeutic Drugs

Drug Name	Brand Name	How Supplied
Acitretin	Soriatane: Roche; Nutley, New Jersey	Capsules: 10 mg and 25 mg
Allopurinol	Allopurinol: Boots (Knoll); Mount Olive, New Jersey	Tablets: 100 mg and 200 mg
	Geneva; Broomfield, Colorado. Major; Livonia, Michigan	
	Mylan; Morgantown, West Virginia Parmed; Niagara Falls, New York Vangard; Glasgow, Kentucky	
	Zyloprim: GlaxoWellcome; Research Triangle Park, North Carolina	Tablets (scored): 100 mg and 200 mg
Amikacin Sulfate	Amiglyde-V Injection: Wyeth; Fort Dodge, Iowa	Injectable Solution: 50 mg/mL in 50 mL vials
	Amiject D: Vetus; Farmer's Branch, Texas	
	Amikacin C: Phoenix; St. Joseph, Missouri	
	Amikacin Sulfate Injection: Vet-Tek; Blue Springs, Missouri	
Amino Acid 10% Infusion (crystalline)	Aminosyn 10%: Abbott; Abbott Park, Illinois	Injectable Solution: 500 mL and 1000 mL containers
Amitriptyline HCl	Elavil: AstraZeneca; Westboro, Massachusetts	Tablets: 10 mg, 25 mg, 50 mg, 75 mg, 100 mg, and 150 mg
	Amitriptyline HCl: Geneva; Broomfield, Colorado (many other generics)	
Amoxicillin (clavulanated)	Clavamox: Pfizer Animal Health—Manufactured by SmithKline Beecham; Exton, Pennsylvania	Oral Suspension: 62.5 mg/mL (12.5 mg clav acid, 50 mg amox) 15 mL bottles Tablets: 62.5 mg (50 mg amox/12.5 mg clav acid) 125 mg (100 mg amox/25 mg clav acid) 250 mg (200 mg amox/50 mg clav acid) 375 mg (300 mg amox/75 mg clav acid)
Amphotericin B Injection	Amphotericin B: Pharm-Tek; Huntington, New York	Powder for Injection: 50 mg vials
	Fungizone IV: Bristol-Myers Squibb; Princeton, New Jersey	Powder for Injection: 50 mg vials
	Amphotec: Sequus Pharmaceuticals; Menlo Park, California	Powder for Injection: 50 mg and 100 mg vials
	AmBisome: Fujisawa; Deerfield, Illinois	Powder for Injection: 50 mg in 20 mL vials and 100 mg in 50 mL vials
	Abelcet: Liposome; Princeton, New Jersey	Powder for Injection (liposomal complex): 50 mg vials Suspension for Injection (lipid complex): 100 mg vials

Systemic Therapeutic Drugs—*cont'd*

Drug Name	Brand Name	How Supplied
Asparaginase	Elspar: Merck; West Point, Pennsylvania	Powder for Injection: 10,000 U in 10 mL vials
Auranofin	Ridaura: Connetics; Palo Alto, California	Capsules: 3 mg
Azathioprine	Imuran: GlaxoWellcome; Research Triangle Park, North Carolina	Tablets (scored): 50 mg
Betamethasone	Betasone: Schering-Plough; Union, New Jersey	Injection Suspension: Betamethasone Dipropionate (2 mg/mL) and Betamethasone Sodium Phosphate (2 mg/mL) in 5 mL vials
Brompheniramine Maleate	Dimetane-DX: AH Robins; Richmond, Virginia	Oral Syrup: 0.4 mg/mL in 1 pint bottles
Buspirone	BuSpar: Bristol-Myers Squibb; Princeton, New Jersey	Tablets (scored): 5 mg, 10 mg, 15 mg, and 30 mg
Calcitriol	Rocaltrol: Roche; Nutley, New Jersey	Capsules: 0.25 mcg and 0.5 mcg Oral Solution: 1 mcg/mL in 15 mL bottles
Cefadroxil	Cefa-Tabs, Cefa-Drops: Wyeth; Fort Dodge, Iowa	Tablets: 50 mg, 100 mg, and 200 mg Tablets (scored): 1 g Oral Suspension: 50 mg/mL in 15 mL and 50 mL dropper bottles
Ceftazidime Sodium	Fortaz: GlaxoSmithKline; Research Triangle Park, North Carolina	Injection Suspension: 1 g and 2 g Powder for Injection: 500 mg, 1 g, 2 g, and 6 g
Cephalexin	Keflex: Dista; Indianapolis, Indiana	Oral Suspension: 25 mg/mL and 50 mg/mL in 100 mL and 200 mL bottles
	Cephalexin: Novopharm; Schaumberg, Illinois	Capsules: 250 mg and 500 mg
Cephradine	Velosef: Bristol-Myers Squibb; Princeton, New Jersey	Powder for Injection: 250 mg, 500 mg, 1 g, and 2 g vials
	Cephradine: Geneva; Broomfield, Colorado (many other generics)	Oral Suspension: 25 mg/mL in 100 mL and 200 mL bottles Capsules: 250 mg and 500 mg
Cetirizine HCl	Zyrtec: Pfizer; New York, New York	Oral Syrup: 1 g/mL in 120 mL, 473 mL (1 pint) bottles Tablets: 5 mg and 10 mg
Chlorambucil	Leukeran: GlaxoWellcome; Research Triangle Park, North Carolina	Tablets: 2 mg
Chloramphenicol	Chloramphenicol Capsules: V.P.C.; Pomona, New York	Capsules: 100 mg, 250 mg, 500 mg, and 1 g
	Duricol Chloramphenicol Capsules USP: Nylos; Pomona, New York	Capsules: 50 mg, 100 mg, 250 mg, and 500 mg
Chlorpheniramine Maleate	Chlor-Trimeton Allergy: Schering-Plough; Union, New Jersey	Tablets: 4 mg, 8 mg, and 12 mg Chewable Tablets: 2 mg Oral Syrup: 0.4 mg/mL in 118 mL bottles
	Chlorpheniramine Maleate: Geneva; Broomfield, Colorado	Tablets: 4 mg
Cimetidine	Tagamet: SmithKline Beecham; Philadelphia, Pennsylvania (many other generics)	Tablets: 100 mg, 200 mg, 300 mg, 400 mg, and 800 mg Oral Liquid: 60 mg/mL
Ciprofloxacin	Cipro: Bayer; Shawnee Mission, Kansas	Tablets: 100 mg, 250 mg, 500 mg, and 750 mg Injectable Solution: 2 mg/mL in 100 mL and 200 mL bottles and 10 mg/mL in 20 mL and 40 mL vials
Clarithromycin	Biaxin: Abbott Laboratories; North Chicago, Illinois	Tablets: 250 mg and 500 mg Oral Suspension: 25 mg/mL and 50 mg/mL in 50 mL and 100 mL bottles

Continued

Systemic Therapeutic Drugs—*cont'd*

Drug Name	Brand Name	How Supplied
Clemastine	Tavist: Novartis; East Hanover, New Jersey	Tablets (scored): 2.68 mg Oral Syrup: 0.134 mg/mL syrup in 118 mL bottles
	Clemastine Fumarate, various manufacturers	Tablets: 1.34 mg
	Antihist-1: Rugby (Watson); Corona, California	Tablets: 1.34 mg
	Clemastine Fumarate, various manufacturers	Tablets: 2.68 mg
Clindamycin HCl	Antirobe: Pfizer Animal Health; Exton, Pennsylvania	Capsules: 25 mg, 75 mg, and 150 mg Oral Solution: 25 mg/mL in 30 mL bottles
	Clindrops: Vetus; Farmer's Branch, Texas (many other generics)	Oral Solution: 25 mg/mL in 30 mL bottles
Clofazimine	Lamprene: Geigy (Novartis); East Hanover, New Jersey	Capsules: 50 mg
Clomipramine HCl	Clomicalm: Novartis; East Hanover, New Jersey	Tablets: 20 mg, 40 mg, and 80 mg
	Clomipramine HCl: Teva; Montgomeryville, Pennsylvania	Capsules: 25 mg, 50 mg, and 75 mg
	Anafranil: Novartis; East Hanover, New Jersey	Capsules: 25 mg, 50 mg, and 75 mg
Cyclophosphamide	Cytoxan: Mead Johnson Oncology (Bristol-Myers Oncology), Princeton, New Jersey	Tablets: 25 mg and 50 mg Powder for Injection: 100 mg, 200 mg, and 500 mg vials and 1 g and 2 g vials
	Neosar: Pfizer Animal Health; Exton, Pennsylvania	Powder for Injection: 100 mg, 200 mg, 500 mg, and 1 g and 2 g vials
Cyclosporine	Atopica: Novartis; East Hanover, New Jersey	Gelatin Capsules: 10 mg, 25 mg, 50 mg, and 100 mg
	Neoral: Novartis; East Hanover, New Jersey (other generics may not be interchangeable)	Gelatin Capsules: 25 mg and 100 mg Oral Solution: 100 mg/mL in 50 mL vials
Cyproheptadine HCL	Periactin: Merck; West Point, Pennsylvania	Tablets (scored): 4 mg Oral Solution: 0.4 mg/mL
	Cyproheptadine HCl: Moore Medical Corp; New Britain, Connecticut	Tablets: 4 mg
	Cyproheptadine HCl: Geneva; Broomfield, Colorado (many other generics)	Syrup: 0.4 mg/mL in 118 mL, 1 pint, and 1 gal containers
Dapsone	Dapsone: Jacobus; Princeton, New Jersey	Tablets (scored): 25 mg and 100 mg
Dexamethasone	Pet-Derm III Chewable Tablets: King Pharmaceutical; Bristol, Tennessee	Tablets (scored): 0.25 mg, 0.5 mg, 0.75 mg, and 1 mg
	Dexamethasone: Rugby; Livonia, Michigan	Tablets: 0.25 mg and 0.50 mg
	Azium Solution: Schering-Plough; Union, New Jersey	Injectable Solution: 2 mg/mL IV/IM in 100 mL vials
	Aspen: Kansas City, Missouri. Butler; Dublin, Ohio	Injectable Solution: 2 mg/mL in 100 mL vials
	Phoenix; St. Joseph, Missouri	
	Dexaject: Vetus; Farmer's Branch, Texas	
Diazepam	Valium: Roche Products; Manati, Puerto Rico (many other generics)	Tablets (scored): 2 mg, 5 mg, and 10 mg Injectable Solution: 5 mg/mL in 10 mL vials
Diphenhydramine HCl	Benadryl: Warner-Lambert; Morris Plains, New Jersey	Capsules (OTC): 25 mg Tablets (OTC): 12.5 mg and 25 mg Oral Solution (OTC): 2.5 mg/mL Injectable Solution: 50 mg/mL in 1 mL and 10 mL vials
	Diphenhydramine HCl: Geneva; Broomfield, Colorado	Capsules: 25 mg and 50 mg
	Diphenhydramine HCl: Rugby; Corona, California (many other generics)	Syrup: 2.5 mg/mL
Doramectin	Dectomax Injectable Solution; Pfizer Animal Health; Exton, Pennsylvania	Injectable Solution: 10 mg/mL in 100 mL, 250 mL, and 500 mL vials

Systemic Therapeutic Drugs—*cont'd*

Drug Name	Brand Name	How Supplied
Doxepin HCl	Sinequan: Roering-Pfizer; New York, New York	Capsules: 10 mg, 25 mg, 50 mg, 75 mg, 100 mg, and 150 mg
	Doxepin HCl: UDL Laboratories; Loves Park, Illinois	Capsules: 10 mg, 25 mg, 50 mg, 75 mg, 100 mg, and 150 mg Oral Concentrate: 10 mg/mL in 120 mL bottle
Doxycycline	Vibramycin: Pfizer; New York, New York	Tablets: 100 mg Oral Suspension: 5 mg/mL in 60 mL bottles Oral Syrup: 10 mg/mL in 60 mL bottles
	Doxycycline: Lederle; Pearl River, New York	Capsules: 50 mg
	Periostat: CollaGenex; Newtown, Pennsylvania	Capsules: 20 mg
Enrofloxacin	Baytril: Bayer; Shawnee Mission, Kansas	Tablets (double scored): 22.7 mg, 68 mg, and 136 mg Injectable Solution: 22.7 mg/mL in 20 mL vials
Epinephrine	Many manufacturers	Injectable Solution: 1 mg/mL
Erythromycin	Erythromycin: Abbott; North Chicago, Illinois (many other generics)	Tablets: 250 mg, 500 mg
Estrogen	Premarin: Wyeth-Ayerst; Philadelphia, Pennsylvania	Tablets: 0.3 mg, 0.625 mg, 0.9 mg, 1.25 mg, and 2.5 mg
Ethambutol HCl	Myambutol: Lederle; Pearl River, New York	Tablets: 100 mg Tablets (scored): 400 mg
Fenbendazole	Panacur: Hoechst Roussel Vet (Global); Warren, New Jersey	Granules: 22 mg/g in 1 g, 2 g, and 4 g packages and 454 g jars
Fluconazole	Diflucan: Roering-Pfizer; New York, New York	Tablets: 50 mg, 100 mg, 150 mg, and 200 mg Oral Suspension: 10 mg/mL in 30 mL bottles and 40 mg/mL in 35 mL bottles Injectable Solution: 2 mg/mL in 100 mL and 200 mL bottles
Flucytosine	Ancoban: Roche; Nutley, New Jersey	Capsules: 250 mg and 500 mg
Fluoxetine HCl	Prozac: Dista; Indianapolis, Indiana	Tablets (scored): 10 mg Capsules: 10 mg, 20 mg, and 40 mg Oral Solution: 4 mg/mL in 120 mL bottles
Gentamicin	Gentaject: Vetus; Farmer's Branch, Texas	Injectable Solution: 50 mg/mL in 50 mL vials and 100 mg/mL in 250 mL vials
	Gentocin Injection: Schering-Plough; Union, New Jersey	
	Gentaved 50: Vedco; St. Joseph, Missouri	
Gold Sodium Thiomalate	Myochrysine: Merck and King Pharmaceuticals; West Point, Pennsylvania	Injectable Solution: 50 mg/mL in 10 mL vials
Goserelin Acetate	Zoladex: AstraZeneca; Wayne, Pennsylvania	Implants: 3.6 mg and 10.8 mg
Griseofulvin, Microsize	Fulvicin U/F: Schering-Plough; Liberty Corner, New Jersey	Tablets (scored): 250 mg and 500 mg
	Grifulvin V: Ortho-Derm; Raritan, New Jersey	Tablets (scored): 250 mg and 500 mg Oral Suspension: 125 mg/mL in 120 mL bottles
	Grisactin: Wyeth-Ayerst; Philadelphia, Pennsylvania	Capsules: 250 mg and 500 mg
Griseofulvin, Ultramicrosize	Fulvicin P/G: Schering-Plough; Liberty Corner, New Jersey	Tablets (scored): 125 mg, 165 mg, and 250 mg
	Grisactin Ultra: Wyeth-Ayerst; Philadelphia, Pennsylvania	Tablets (scored): 125 mg, 250 mg, and 330 mg
Hydrocodone	Hycodan: DuPont; Wilmington, Delaware	Tablets (scored): 5 mg
	Hydrocodone Compound Syrup, various manufacturers	Oral Syrup: 1 mg/mL in 473 mL bottles

Continued

Systemic Therapeutic Drugs—*cont'd*

Drug Name	Brand Name	How Supplied
Hydroxyzine	Atarax: Pfizer; New York, New York	Tablets: 10 mg, 25 mg, 50 mg, and 100 mg Oral Syrup: 2 mg/mL in 1 pint bottles
	Vistaril: Pfizer; New York, New York (many other generics)	Capsules: 25 mg, 50 mg, and 100 mg Oral Suspension: 5 mg/mL in 120 mL and 473 mL bottles
Ibafloxacin	Ibaflin Tablets: Intervet International; Boxmeer, Netherlands	Tablets: 150 mg and 300 mg Gel: 3% Oral Gel—15 mL prefilled syringes
Imipramine HCl	Tofranil: Novartis; Summit, New Jersey Imipramine HCl, various manufacturers	Tablets: 10 mg, 25 mg, and 50 mg
Interferon-alpha 2B	Intron A: Schering-Plough; Liberty Corner, New Jersey	Powder for Injection: 3 million U, 5 million U, 10 million U, 18 million U, 25 million U, and 50 million U in vials Injectable Solution: 3 million U, 5 million U, 10 million U, 18 million U, and 25 million U in vials
Isoniazid (isonicotinic acid hydrazide)	Isoniazid: Schein; Florham Park, New Jersey	Tablets: 50 mg
	Laniazid: Lannett; Philadelphia, Pennsylvania	Tablets (scored): 50 mg Oral Syrup: 10 mg/mL in 480 mL bottles
	Isoniazid: Carolina Medical; Farmville, North Carolina (many other generics)	Tablets: 100 mg Tablets: 300 mg
Isotretinoin	Accutane: Roche; Nutley, New Jersey	Capsules: 10 mg, 20 mg, and 40 mg
Itraconazole	Sporanox: Janssen Pharmaceutica; Titusville, New Jersey	Capsules: 100 mg Oral Solution: 10 mg/mL in 150 mL containers
Ivermectin	Ivomec: Merial; Iselin, New Jersey	Injectable Solution: 2.7 mg/mL in 200 mL collapsible soft packs; 10 mg/mL in 50 mL bottles; and 200 mL, 500 mL, and 1000 mL collapsible soft packs
	Double Impact: Agrilabs; St Joseph, Missouri	Injectable Solution: 10 mg/mL in 50 mL bottles; and 200 mL and 500 mL collapsible soft packs
	Eqvalen: Merial; Iselin, New Jersey	Oral Suspension: 10 mg/mL in 100 mL bottles
Ketoconazole	Nizoral: Janssen Pharmaceutica; Titusville, New Jersey	Tablets (scored): 200 mg
	Ketoconazole: Novopharm; Schaumburg, Illinois	Tablets: 200 mg
Ketotifen Fumarate	Zaditor: Ciba Vision; Duluth, Georgia	0.025% Solution in 5 mL, 7.5 mL for ophthalmic use
Leuprolide Acetate	Lupron: TAP Pharma; Deerfield, Illinois	Injectable Solution: 5 mg/mL in 2.8 mL vials Injection Depot: 3.75 mg, 7.5 mg, 11.25 mg, 22.5 mg, and 30 mg
Levamisole	Levasole Sheep Wormer: Schering-Plough; Union, New Jersey	Boluses: 184 mg
Levothyroxine	Soloxine: Daniels; St. Louis, Missouri	Tablets: 0.1 mg, 0.2 mg, 0.3 mg, 0.4 mg, 0.5 mg, 0.6 mg, 0.7 mg, and 0.8 mg
Lincomycin HCl	Licocin: Pfizer Animal Health; Exton, Pennsylvania	Tablets (scored): 100 mg, 200 mg, and 500 mg Oral Solution: 50 mg/mL in 20 mL bottles Injectable Solution: 100 mg/mL in 20 mL vials
Loratadine	Claritin: Schering-Plough; Liberty Corner, New Jersey	Tablets: 10 mg Oral Syrup: 1 mg/mL in 480 mL bottles
Lufenuron	Program: Ciba; Greensboro, North Carolina	Oral Suspension: 135 mg and 270 mg packets Tablets: 45 mg, 90 mg, 204.9 mg, and 409.8 mg Injectable Suspension: 40 mg (0.4 mL) and 80 mg (0.8 mL) in syringes
Lufenuron-Milbemycin Oxime	Sentinel: Novartis; Greensboro, North Carolina	Tablets: 46 mg Lufenuron/2.3 mg Milbemycin Oxime 115 mg Lufenuron/5.75 mg Milbemycin Oxime 230 mg Lufenuron/115 mg Milbemycin Oxime 460 mg Lufenuron/230 mg Milbemycin Oxime

Systemic Therapeutic Drugs—*cont'd*

Drug Name	Brand Name	How Supplied
Marbofloxacin	Zeniquin: Pfizer Animal Health; Exton, Pennsylvania	Tablets (scored): 25 mg, 50 mg, 100 mg, and 200 mg
Mebendazole	Vermox: Janssen Pharmaceutica; Titusville, New Jersey	Tablets: 100 mg
	Mebendazole: Copley; Canton, Massachusetts (many other generics)	
Medroxyprogesterone Acetate	Depo-Provera: Pharmacia Corp, Kalamazoo, Michigan	Injectable Suspension: 150 mg/mL-1 mL prefilled syringe
	Medroxyprogesterone Acetate, several manufacturers	Injectable Suspension: 150 mg/mL-1 mL vial
Meropenem	Merrem: AstraZeneca Pharmaceuticals LP; Wilmington, Delaware	Powder for Infusion: 500 mg/1 g vial
Methylprednisolone	Medrol: Pfizer Animal Health; Exton, Pennsylvania	Tablets (double scored): 4 mg
	Methylprednisolone Tablets: Boehringer Ingelheim; Sioux City, Iowa	Tablets: 2 mg
	Methylprednisolone Tablets, Vedco; St. Joseph, Missouri	Tablets: 2 mg
	Depo-Medrol: Pfizer Animal Health; Exton, Pennsylvania	Injectable Suspension: 20 mg/mL in 10 mL and 20 mL vials
	Methylprednisolone Acetate Injection: Boehringer Ingelheim; Sioux City, Iowa	Injectable Suspension: 40 mg/mL in 5 mL and 30 mL vials
Methyltestosterone	Android: ICN Pharma; Costa Mesa, California	Tablets: 10 mg and 25 mg
	Oreton Methyl: Schering-Plough; Liberty Corner, New Jersey	Tablets: 10 mg
	Testred: ICN Pharma; Costa Mesa, California	Capsules: 10 mg
	Methyltestosterone, various: Goldline; Miami, Florida (many other generics)	Tablets: 10 mg and 25 mg
Metronidazole	Flagyl: Searle; Chicago, Illinois	Tablets: 250 mg and 500 mg Capsules: 375 mg
	Metronidazone: Geneva; Broomfield, Colorado	Tablets (scored): 250 mg and 500 mg
Metyrapone	Metopirone: Novartis; East Hanover, New Jersey	Gelatin Capsules: 250 mg
Milbemycin Oxime	Interceptor: Novartis; Greensboro, North Carolina	Tablets: 2.3 mg, 5.75 mg, 11.5 mg, and 23.0 mg Sentinel: Same color coding as above plus Lufenuron at 10 mg/kg (46 mg, 115 mg, 230 mg, 460 mg of lufenuron, respectively)
Minocycline	Minocin: Lederle; Pearl River, New York	Capsules: 50 mg and 100 mg Oral Suspension: 10 mg/mL in 60 mL bottles
	Dynacin: Medicis Dermatologics; Phoenix, Arizona	Capsules: 50 mg and 100 mg
	Minocycline HCl: Warner Chilcott; Rockaway, New Jersey (many other generics)	Capsules: 50 mg and 100 mg
Misoprostol	Cytotec: Searle; Chicago, Illinois	Tablets: 100 mg Tablets (scored): 200 mg
Mitotane	Lysodren: Bristol-Myers Squibb; Princeton, New Jersey	Tablets (scored): 500 mg
Naltrexone	ReVia: DuPont; Wilmington, Delaware	Tablets (scored): 50 mg
	Depade: Mallinckrodt: St Louis, Missouri	
Niacinamide	OTC, many manufacturers	Tablets: 100 mg and 500 mg
Nitenpyram	Capstar: Novartis Animal Health; Basel, Switzerland	Tablets: 11.4 mg and 57 mg
Orbifloxacin	Orbax: Schering-Plough; Union, New Jersey	Tablets: 5.7 mg Tablets (scored): 22.7 mg and 68 mg
Ormetoprim/ Sulfadimethoxine	Primor: Pfizer Animal Health; Exton, Pennsylvania	Tablets (scored): 120 mg, 240 mg, 600 mg, and 1200 mg
Oxacillin	Oxacillin Sodium: Teva Pharmaceuticals; Montgomeryville, Pennsylvania	Capsules: 250 mg and 500 mg

Continued

Systemic Therapeutic Drugs—*cont'd*

Drug Name	Brand Name	How Supplied
Pentoxifylline	Trental: Hoechst Marion Roussel; Kansas City, Missouri Pentoxifylline: Copley; Canton, Massachusetts Many other generics	Tablets: 400 mg
Phenobarbital	Many manufacturers	Tablets: 15 mg, 30 mg, 60 mg, and 100 mg Oral Elixir: 3–4 mg/mL Injectable Solution: 130 mg/mL
Potassium Iodide	Potassium Iodide: Roxane; Columbus, Ohio	Oral Solution: 1 g/mL in 30 mL and 240 mL bottles
	PIMA: Fleming; Fenton, Missouri (many other generics)	Oral Solution: 65 mg/mL
Prednisolone	Prednistabs: Vedco; St. Joseph, Missouri	Tablets: 5 mg
	Prednistabs: Vet-A-Mix; Shenandoah, Iowa	Tablets: 5 mg and 20 mg
	Predate-50: Legere; Scottsdale, Arizona	Oral Suspension (prednisolone acetate): 50 mg/mL in 10 mL vials
	Sterisol-20: Anthony; Arcadia, California	Injectable Solution (prednisolone sodium phosphate): 20 mg/mL in 50 mL vials
	Solu-Delta-Cortef: Pfizer Animal Health; Exton, Pennsylvania (many other generics)	Powder for Injection (prednisolone sodium succinate): 100 mg/mL and 500 mg/mL in 10 mL vials
Prednisone	Prednisone: Geneva; Broomfield, Colorado	Tablets: 5 mg, 10 mg, 20 mg, and 50 mg
	Prednisone: Roxane; Columbus, Ohio (many other generics)	Tablets: 1 mg Oral Solution: 1 mg/mL in 5 mL and 500 mL bottles
Proligestone	Delvosteron: Intervet; United Kingdom	Injectable Solution: 100 mg/mL in 20 mL vials
Pyrantel Pamoate	Nemex: Pfizer; Exton, Pennsylvania (many other generics)	Tablets: 22.7 mg and 113.5 mg Oral Suspension: 4.54 mg/mL in 2 fl oz bottles
Pyrazinamide	Pyrazinamide: Lederle; Pearl River, New York	Tablets (scored): 500 mg
Selegiline HCl (L-deprenyl)	Anipryl: Pfizer; Exton, Pennsylvania	Tablets: 2 mg, 5 mg, 10 mg, 15 mg, and 30 mg
	Carbex: DuPont Pharma; Wilmington, Delaware	Tablets: 5 mg
	Eldepryl: Somerset; Tampa, Florida	Capsules: 5 mg
	Selegiline HCl: Apothecon; Princeton, New Jersey	Tablets: 5 mg
Sulfadiazine	Sulfadiazine: Eon; Laurelton, New York	Tablets: 500 mg
	Sulfadiazine: Major; Livonia, Michigan (many other generics)	
Sulfamethizole	Thiosulfil Forte: Wyeth-Ayerst; Philadelphia, Pennsylvania	Tablets (scored): 500 mg
Sulfisoxazole	Sulfisoxazole: Moore; New Britain, Connecticut	Tablets: 500 mg
	Sulfisoxazole: Geneva; Broomfield, Colorado (many other generics)	
Terbafine HCl	Lamisil: Sandoz/Novartis; East Hanover, New Jersey	Tablets: 250 mg
Tetracycline HCl	Achromycin: Lederle Laboratories; Pearl River, New York	Capsules: 250 mg and 500 mg Oral Suspension: 25 mg/mL Injectable Solution: 100 mg, 250 mg, and 500 mg vials
	Panmycin Aquadrops: Pfizer Animal Health; Exton, Pennsylvania	Oral Suspension: 100 mg/mL in 15 mL and 30 mL bottles
	Tetracycline HCl: Global; Philadelphia, Pennsylvania	Capsules: 250 mg
Thiabendazole	Mintezol: Merck; West Point, Pennsylvania	Tablets (scored): 500 mg Oral Solution: 50 mg/mL in 120 mL bottles
Ticarcillin	Ticar: SmithKline Beecham; Philadelphia, Pennsylvania	Powder for Injection: 1 g, 3 g, 6 g, 20 g, and 30 g vials
Ticarcillin-Clavulanate Potassium	Timentin: SmithKline Beecham; Philadelphia, Pennsylvania	Powder for Injection: 3 g ticarcillin, 0.1 g clavulanic acid in 3.1 g vials; 3 g ticarcillin, 0.1 g clav acid per 100 mL in 100 mL premixed vials

Systemic Therapeutic Drugs—*cont'd*

Drug Name	Brand Name	How Supplied
Triamcinolone Acetonide	Vetalog: Wyeth; Fort Dodge, Iowa	Tablets: 0.5 mg and 1.5 mg Injectable Suspension: 2 mg and 6 mg in 5 mL and 25 mL vials
	Cortalone Tablets: Vedco; St. Joseph, Missouri	Tablets: 0.5 mg and 1.5 mg
	Triamcinolone Acetonide Tablets: Boehringer-Ingelheim; Sioux City, Iowa	Tablets: 0.5 mg and 1.5 mg
	Triamtabs: Vetus; Farmer's Branch, Texas	Tablets: 0.5 mg and 1.5 mg
Trilostane	Modrenal: Stegrum Pharmaceuticals; Billinghurst, United Kingdom	Capsules: 10 mg, 60 mg, and 120 mg
	Vetoryl: Arnolds Veterinary Products (Dechra Pharmaceuticals), United Kingdom	
Trimeprazine-Prednisolone	Temeril-P: Pfizer; Exton, Pennsylvania	Tablets: 5 mg trimeprazine/2 mg prednisolone
Trimethoprim-Sulfadiazine	Tribrissen: Schering-Plough; Union, New Jersey	Tablets: 30 mg and 120 mg Tablets (scored): 480 mg and 960 mg
Trimethoprim-Sulfamethoxazole	Bactrim: Roche; Nutley, New Jersey	Tablets (scored): 480 mg and 960 mg Oral Suspension: 48 mg/mL in 16 oz bottles Injectable Solution: 96 mg/mL in 10 mL and 30 mL vials
	Septra: Monarch Pharmaceuticals; Bristol, Tennessee (many other generics)	Tablets (scored): 480 mg and 960 mg Oral Suspension: 48 mg/mL in 16 oz bottles Injectable Solution: 96 mg/mL in 5 mL, 10 mL, and 20 mL vials
Vincristine Sulfate	Oncovin: Lily; Indianapolis, Indiana	Injectable Solution: 1 mg/mL in 1 mL, 2 mL, and 5 mL vials
	Vincristine Sulfate, various: Akorn; Buffalo Grove, Illinois	
	Vincasar: Pfizer Animal Health; Exton, Pennsylvania	

Index